POISONS:
THEIR EFFECTS AND DETECTION

A Manual for the Use of Analytical Chemists and Experts.

With an Introductory Essay on the Growth of Modern Toxicology.

by

Alexander Wynter Blyth,
M.R.C.S., F.I.C., F.C.S., &c.,

Barrister-At-Law; Public Analyst for the County of Devon; and Medical Officer of Health and Public Analyst for St. Marylebone.

Third Edition, Revised and Enlarged.
With Tables and Illustrations.

NATAL PUBLISHING LLC
ARS LONGA, VITA BREVIS

PREFACE TO THE THIRD EDITION.

The present edition, which appears on the same general plan as before, will yet be found to have been in great part re-written, enlarged, and corrected.

Analytical methods which experience has shown to be faulty have been omitted, and replaced by newer and more accurate processes.

The intimate connection which recent research has shown to exist between the arrangement of the constituent parts of an organic molecule and physiological action, has been considered at some length in a separate chapter.

The cadaveric alkaloids or ptomaines, bodies playing so great a part in food-poisoning and in the manifestations of disease, are in this edition treated of as fully as the limits of the book will allow.

The author, therefore, trusts that these various improvements, modifications, and corrections will enable "Poisons" to maintain the position which it has for so many years held in the esteem of toxicologists and of the medical profession generally.

The Court House, St. Marylebone, W.
June, 1895.

CONTENTS.

PART I.—INTRODUCTORY.

I. THE OLD POISON-LORE.

VII. CHLORAL.

VIII. BISULPHIDE OF CARBON.

IX. THE TAR ACIDS—PHENOL—CRESOL.

Tests for Carbolic Acid.

LIST OF ILLUSTRATIONS.

PART I.—INTRODUCTORY.

I.—The Old Poison-Lore.

§ 1. It is significant that the root "*tox*" of the modern word *toxicology* can be traced back to a very ancient word meaning "bow" or "arrow," or, in its broadest sense, some "tool" used for slaying: hence it is no far-fetched supposition that the first poison-knowledge was that of the septic poisons. Perchance the savage found that weapons soiled with the blood of former victims made wounds fatal; from this observation the next step naturally would be that of experiment—the arrow or spear would be steeped in all manner of offensive pastes, and smeared with the vegetable juices of those plants which were deemed noxious; and as the effects were mysterious, they would be ascribed to the supernatural powers, and covered with a veil of superstition.

The history of the *poison-lehre*, like all history, begins in the region of the myths: there was a dark saga prevailing in Greece, that in the far north existed a land ruled by sorcerers—all children of the sun—and named Aeëtes, Perses, Hecate, Medea, and Circe. Later on, the enchanted land was localised at Colchis, and Aeëtes and Perses were said to be brothers. Hecate was the daughter of Perses; she was married to Aeëtes, and their daughters were Medea and Circe. Hecate was the discoverer of poisonous herbs, and learned in remedies both evil and good. Her knowledge passed to Medea, who narcotised the dragon, the guardian of the golden fleece, and incited Jason to great undertakings.

In the expedition of the Argonauts, the poets loved to describe Hecate's garden, with its lofty walls. Thrice-folding doors of ebony barred the entrance, which was guarded by terrible forms: only the initiated few, only they who bore the leavened rod of expiation, and the concealed conciliatory offering of the Medea, could enter into the sanctuary. Towering above all was the temple of the dread Hecate, whose priestesses offered to the gods ghastly sacrifices.

§ 2. The oldest Egyptian king, Menes, and Attalus Phylometer, the last king of Pergamus, were both famous for their knowledge of plants. Attalus Phylometer was acquainted with hyoscyamus, aconite, conium, veratrum, and others; he experimented on the preparation of poisons, and occupied himself in compounding medicines. Mithradetes Eupator stood yet higher: the receipt for the famous *theriaca*, prepared in later years at an enormous price, and composed of fifty-four different ingredients, is ascribed to him. The wonderful skill shown by the Egyptians in embalming and technical works is sufficient to render it fairly certain that their chemical knowledge was considerable; and the frequent operations of one caste upon the dead must have laid the foundations of a pathological and anatomical culture, of which only traces remain.

The Egyptians knew prussic acid as extracted in a dilute state from certain plants, among the chief of which was certainly the peach; on a papyrus preserved at the Louvre, M. Duteil read, "Pronounce not the name of I. A. O. under the penalty of the peach!" in which dark threat, without doubt, lurks the meaning that those who revealed the religious mysteries of the priests were put to death by waters distilled from the peach. That the priests actually distilled the peach-leaves has been doubted by those who consider the art of distillation a modern invention; but this process was well known to adepts of the third and fourth centuries, and there is no inherent improbability in the supposition that the Egyptians practised it.

§ 3. From the Egyptians the knowledge of the deadly drink appears to have passed to the Romans. At the trial of Antipater,[1] Verus brought a potion derived from Egypt, which had been intended to destroy Herod; this was essayed on a criminal, he died at once. In the reign of Tiberius, a Roman knight, accused of high treason, swallowed a poison, and fell dead at the feet of the senators: in both cases the rapidity of action appears to point to prussic acid.

The use of poison by the Greeks, as a means of capital punishment, without doubt favoured suicide by the same means; the easy, painless death of the state prisoner would be often preferred to the sword by one tired of life. The ancients looked indeed upon suicide, in certain instances, as something noble, and it was occasionally formally

---

[1] Jos. Ant., B. xvii. c. 5.

sanctioned. Thus, Valerius Maximus tells us that he saw a woman of quality, in the island of Ceos, who, having lived happily for ninety years, obtained leave to take a poisonous draught, lest, by living longer, she should happen to have a change in her good fortune; and, curiously enough, this sanctioning of self-destruction seems to have been copied in Europe. Mead relates that the people of Marseilles of old had a poison, kept by the public authorities, in which cicuta was an ingredient: a dose was allowed to any one who could show why he should desire death. Whatever use or abuse might be made of a few violent poisons, Greek and Roman knowledge of poisons, their effects and methods of detection, was stationary, primitive, and incomplete.

Nicander of Colophon (204-138 B.C.) wrote two treatises, the most ancient works on this subject extant, the one describing the effects of snake venom; the other, the properties of opium, henbane, certain fungi, colchicum, aconite, and conium. He divided poisons into those which kill quickly, and those which act slowly. As antidotes, those medicines are recommended which excite vomiting—*e.g.*, lukewarm oil, warm water, mallow, linseed tea, &c.

Apollodorus lived at the commencement of the third century B.C.: he wrote a work on poisonous animals, and one on deleterious medicines; these works of Apollodorus were the sources from which Pliny, Heraclitus, and several of the later writers derived most of their knowledge of poisons.

Dioscorides (40-90 A.D.) well detailed the effects of cantharides, sulphate of copper, mercury, lead, and arsenic. By arsenic he would appear sometimes to mean the sulphides, sometimes the white oxide. Dioscorides divided poisons, according to their origin, into three classes, viz.:—

1. **Animal Poisons.**—Under this head were classed cantharides and allied beetles, toads, salamanders, poisonous snakes, a particular variety of honey, and the blood of the ox, probably the latter in a putrid state. He also speaks of the "*sea-hare*." The sea-hare was considered by the ancients very poisonous, and Domitian is said to have murdered Titus with it. It is supposed by naturalists to have been one of the genus *Aplysia*, among the *gasteropods*. Both Pliny and Dioscorides depict the animal as something very formidable: it was not to be looked at, far less touched. The aplysiæ exhale a very nauseous and fœtid odour when they are approached: the best known of the species resembles, when in a state of repose, a mass of unformed flesh; when in motion, it is like a common slug; its colour is reddish-brown; it has four horns on its head; and the eyes, which are very small, are situated between the two hinder ones. This aplysia has an ink reservoir, like the sepia, and ejects it in order to escape from its enemies; it inhabits the muddy bottom of the water, and lives on small crabs, mollusca, &c.

2. **Poisons from Plants.**—Dioscorides enumerates opium, black and white hyoscyamus (especially recognising the activity of the seeds), mandragora, which was probably a mixture of various solanaceæ, conium (used to poison the condemned by the people of Athens and the dwellers of ancient Massilia), elaterin, and the juices of a species of euphorbia and apocyneæ. He also makes a special mention of aconite, the name of which is derived from *Akon*, a small city in Heraclea. The Greeks were well aware of the deadly nature of aconite, and gave to it a mythical origin, from the foam of the dog Cerberus. Colchicum was also known to Dioscorides: its first use was ascribed to Medea. Veratrum album and nigrum were famous medicines of the Romans, and a constituent of their "*rat and mice powders*;" they were also used as insecticides. According to Pliny, the Gauls dipped their arrows in a preparation of veratrum.[2] Daphne mezereon, called by the Romans also smilax and taxus, appears to have been used by Cativolcus, the king of the Eburones, for the purpose of suicide, or possibly by "taxus" the yew-tree is meant.[3]

The poisonous properties of certain fungi were also known. Nicander calls the venomous mushrooms the "evil fermentation of the earth," and prescribes the identical antidotes which we would perhaps give at the present time—viz., vinegar and alkaline carbonates.

3. **Mineral Poisons.**—Arsenic has been already alluded to. The ancients used it as a caustic and depilatory. Copper was known as sulphate and oxide; mercury only as cinnabar: lead oxides were used, and milk and olive-oil prescribed as an antidote for their poisonous properties. The *poison-lehre* for many ages was considered as something forbidden. Galen, in his treatise "On Antidotes," remarks that the only authors who dared to treat of poisons were Orpheus, Theologus, Morus, Mendesius the younger, Heliodorus of Athens, Aratus, and a few others; but none of these treatises have come down to us. From the close similarity of the amount of information in the treatises of Nicander, Dioscorides, Pliny, Galen, and Paulus Ægineta, it is probable that all were derived from a common source.

§ 4. If we turn our attention to early Asiatic history, a very cursory glance at the sacred writings of the East will

[2] Pliny, xxv. 5.

[3] *De Bello Gallico*, vi. 31.

prove how soon the art of poisoning, especially in India, was used for the purpose of suicide, revenge, or robbery.

The ancient practice of the Hindoo widow—self-immolation on the burning pile of her husband—is ascribed to the necessity which the Brahmins were under of putting a stop to the crime of domestic poisoning. Every little conjugal quarrel was liable to be settled by this form of secret assassination, but such a law, as might be expected, checked the practice.

Poison was not used to remove human beings alone, for there has been from time immemorial in India much cattle-poisoning. In the Institutes of Menu, it is ordained that when cattle die the herdsman shall carry to his master their ears, their hides, their tails, the skin below their navels, their tendons, and the liquor oozing from their foreheads. Without doubt these regulations were directed against cattle-poisoners.

The poisons known to the Asiatics were arsenic, aconite, opium, and various solanaceous plants. There has been a myth floating through the ages that a poison exists which will slay a long time after its introduction. All modern authors have treated the matter as an exaggerated legend, but, for my own part, I see no reason why it should not, in reality, be founded on fact. There is little doubt that the Asiatic poisoners were well acquainted with the infectious qualities of certain fevers and malignant diseases. Now, these very malignant diseases answer precisely to the description of a poison which has no immediate effects. Plant small-pox in the body of a man, and for a whole fortnight he walks about, well and hearty. Clothe a person with a garment soaked in typhus, and the same thing occurs—for many days there will be no sign of failure. Again, the gipsies, speaking a tongue which is essentially a deformed *prakrit*, and therefore Indian in origin, have long possessed a knowledge of the properties of the curious "*mucor phycomyces*." This was considered an alga by Agaron, but Berkeley referred it to the fungi. The gipsies are said to have administered the spores of this fungi in warm water. In this way they rapidly attach themselves to the mucous membrane of the throat, all the symptoms of a phthisis follow, and death takes place in from two to three weeks. Mr Berkeley informed me that he has seen specimens growing on broth which had been rejected from the stomach, and that it develops in enormous quantities on oil-casks and walls impregnated with grease. The filaments are long, from 12 to 18 inches, and it is capable of very rapid development.

There is also a modern poison, which, in certain doses, dooms the unfortunate individual to a terrible malady, simulating, to a considerable extent, natural disease,—that is phosphorus. This poison was, however, unknown until some time in the eleventh century, when Alchid Becher, blindly experimenting on the distillation of urine and carbon, obtained his "*escarboucle*," and passed away without knowing the importance of his discovery, which, like so many others, had to be rediscovered at a later period.

§ 5. The Hebrews were acquainted with certain poisons, the exact nature of which is not quite clear. The words "*rosch*" and "*chema*" seem to be used occasionally as a generic term for poison, and sometimes to mean a specific thing; "*rosch*," especially, is used to signify some poisonous parasitic plant. They knew yellow arsenic under the name of "*sam*," aconite under the name of "*boschka*," and possibly "*son*" means *ergot*.[4] In the later period of their history, when they were dispersed through various nations, they would naturally acquire the knowledge of those nations, without losing their own.

§ 6. The part that poison has played in history is considerable. The pharmaceutical knowledge of the ancients is more graphically and terribly shown in the deaths of Socrates, Demosthenes, Hannibal, and Cleopatra, than in the pages of the older writers on poisons.

In the reign of Artaxerxes II. (Memnon), (B.C. 405-359), Phrysa poisoned the queen Statira by cutting food with a knife poisoned on one side only. Although this has been treated as an idle tale, yet two poisons, aconite and arsenic, were at least well known; either of these could have been in the way mentioned introduced in sufficient quantity into food to destroy life.

In the early part of the Christian era professional poisoners arose, and for a long time exercised their trade with impunity. Poisoning was so much in use as a political engine that Agrippina (A.D. 26) refused to eat of some apples offered to her at table by her father-in-law, Tiberius.

It was at this time that the infamous Locusta flourished. She is said to have supplied, with suitable directions, the poison by which Agrippina got rid of Claudius; and the same woman was the principal agent in the preparation of the poison that was administered to Britannicus, by order of his brother Nero. The details of this interesting case have been recorded with some minuteness.

It was the custom of the Romans to drink hot water, a draught nauseous enough to us, but, from fashion or habit, considered by them a luxury; and, as no two men's tastes are alike, great skill was shown by the slaves in

[4] R. J. Wunderbar, *Biblisch-talmudische Medicin*. Leipzig, 1850-60.

bringing the water to exactly that degree of heat which their respective masters found agreeable.[5]

The children of the Imperial house, with others of the great Roman families, sat at the banquets at a smaller side table, while their parents reclined at the larger. A slave brings hot water to Britannicus; it is too hot; Britannicus refuses it. The slave adds cold water; and it is this cold water that is supposed to have been poisoned; in any case, Britannicus had no sooner drunk of it than he lost voice and respiration. Agrippina, his mother, was struck with terror, as well as Octavia, his sister. Nero, the author of the crime, looks coldly on, saying that such fits often happened to him in infancy without evil result; and after a few moments' silence the banquet goes on as before. If this were not sudden death from heart or brain disease, the poison must have been either a cyanide or prussic acid.

In those times no autopsy was possible: although the Alexandrian school, some 300 years before Christ, had dissected both the living and the dead, the work of Herophilus and Erasistratus had not been pursued, and the great Roman and Greek writers knew only the rudiments of human anatomy, while, as to pathological changes and their true interpretation, their knowledge may be said to have been absolutely *nil*. It was not, indeed, until the fifteenth century that the Popes, silencing ancient scruples, authorised dissections; and it was not until the sixteenth century that Vesalius, the first worthy of being considered a great anatomist, arose. In default of pathological knowledge, the ancients attached great importance to mere outward marks and discolorations. They noted with special attention spots and lividity, and supposed that poisons singled out the heart for some quite peculiar action, altering its substance in such a manner that it resisted the action of the funeral pyre, and remained unconsumed. It may, then, fairly be presumed that many people must have died from poison without suspicion, and still more from the sudden effects of latent disease, ascribed wrongfully to poison. For example, the death of Alexander was generally at that time ascribed to poison; but Littré has fairly proved that the great emperor, debilitated by his drinking habits, caught a malarious fever in the marshes around Babylon, and died after eleven days' illness. If, added to sudden death, the body, from any cause, entered into rapid putrefaction, such signs were considered by the people absolutely conclusive of poisoning: this belief, indeed, prevailed up to the middle of the seventeenth century, and lingers still among the uneducated at the present day. Thus, when Britannicus died, an extraordinary lividity spread over the face of the corpse, which they attempted to conceal by painting the face. When Pope Alexander VI. died, probably enough from poison, his body (according to Guicciardini) became a frightful spectacle—it was livid, bloated, and deformed; the gorged tongue entirely filled the mouth; from the nose flowed putrid pus, and the stench was horrible in the extreme.

All these effects of decomposition, we know, are apt to arise in coarse, obese bodies, and accompany both natural and unnatural deaths; indeed, if we look strictly at the matter, putting on one side the preservative effects of certain metallic poisons, it may be laid down that generally the corpses of those dying from poison are *less* apt to decompose rapidly than those dying from disease—this for the simple reason that a majority of diseases cause changes in the fluids and tissues, which render putrefactive changes more active, while, as a rule, those who take poison are suddenly killed, with their fluids and tissues fairly healthy.

When the Duke of Burgundy desired to raise a report that John, Dauphin of France, was poisoned (1457), he described the imaginary event as follows:—

"One evening our most redoubtable lord and nephew fell so grievously sick that he died forthwith. His lips, tongue, and face were swollen; his eyes started out of his head. It was a horrible sight to see—for so look people that are poisoned."

The favourite powder of the professional poisoner, arsenic, was known to crowned heads in the fourteenth century; and there has come down to us a curious document, drawn out by Charles le Mauvais, King of Navarre. It is a commission of murder, given to a certain Woudreton, to poison Charles VI., the Duke of Valois, brother of the king, and his uncles, the Dukes of Berry, Burgundy, and Bourbon:—

"Go thou to Paris; thou canst do great service if thou wilt: do what I tell thee; I will reward thee well. Thou shalt do thus: There is a thing which is called sublimed arsenic; if a man eat a bit the size of a pea he will never survive. Thou wilt find it in Pampeluna, Bordeaux, Bayonne, and in all the good towns through which thou wilt pass, at the apothecaries' shops. Take it and powder it; and when thou shalt be in the house of the king, of the Count de Valois, his brother, the Dukes of Berry, Burgundy, and Bourbon, draw near, and betake thyself to the kitchen, to the larder, to the cellar, or any other place where thy point can be best gained, and put the powder in the soups, meats, or wines, provided that thou canst do it secretly. Otherwise, do it not." Woudreton was detected, and executed

[5] Tacitus, lib. xii., xiii. Mentioned also by Juvenal and Suetonius.

in 1384.[6]

A chapter might be written entitled "royal poisoners." King Charles IX. even figures as an experimentalist.[7] An unfortunate cook has stolen two silver spoons, and, since there was a question whether "*Bezoar*" was an antidote or not, the king administers to the cook a lethal dose of corrosive sublimate, and follows it up with the antidote; but the man dies in seven hours, although Paré also gives him oil. Truly a grim business!

The subtle method of removing troublesome subjects has been more often practised on the Continent than in England, yet the English throne in olden time is not quite free from this stain.[8] The use of poison is wholly opposed to the Anglo-Saxon method of thought. To what anger the people were wrought on detecting poisoners, is seen in the fact that, in 1542, a young woman was boiled alive in Smithfield for poisoning three households.[9]

§ 7. Two great criminal schools arose from the fifteenth to the seventeenth centuries in Venice and Italy. The Venetian poisoners are of earlier date than the Italian, and flourished chiefly in the fifteenth century. Here we have the strange spectacle, not of the depravity of individuals, but of the government of the State formally recognising secret assassination by poison, and proposals to remove this or that prince, duke, or emperor, as a routine part of their deliberations. Still more curious and unique, the dark communings of "*the council of ten*" were recorded in writing, and the number of those who voted for and who voted against the proposed crime, the reason for the assassination, and the sum to be paid, still exist in shameless black and white. Those who desire to study this branch of secret history may be referred to a small work by Carl Hoff, which gives a brief account of what is known of the proceedings of the council. One example will here suffice. On the 15th of December 1513 a Franciscan brother, John of Ragubo, offered a selection of poisons, and declared himself ready to remove any objectionable person out of the way. For the first successful case he required a pension of 1500 ducats yearly, which was to be increased on the execution of future services. The presidents, Girolando Duoda and Pietro Guiarina, placed the matter before the "ten" on the 4th of January 1514, and on a division (10 against 5) it was resolved to accept so patriotic an offer, and to experiment first on the Emperor Maximilian. The bond laid before the "ten" contained a regular tariff—for the great Sultan 500 ducats, for the King of Spain 150 ducats, but the journey and other expenses were in each case to be defrayed; the Duke of Milan was rated at 60, the Marquis of Mantua at 50, the Pope could be removed at 100 ducats. The curious offer thus concludes:—"The farther the journey, the more eminent the man, the more it is necessary to reward the toil and hardships undertaken, and the heavier must be the payment." The council appear to have quietly arranged thus to take away the lives of many public men, but their efforts were only in a few cases successful. When the deed was done, it was registered by a single marginal note, "*factum*."

What drugs the Venetian poisoners used is uncertain. The Italians became notorious in the sixteenth and seventeenth centuries for their knowledge of poisons, partly from the deeds of Toffana and others, and partly from the works of J. Baptista Porta, who wrote a very comprehensive treatise, under the title of *Natural Magic*,[10] and managed to slide into the text, in the sections on cooking (*De Re Coquinaria*, lib. xiv.), a mass of knowledge as to

[6] *Trésor de Chartes*. Charles de Navarre. P. Mortonval, vol. ii. p. 384.

[7] *Œuvres de Paré*, 2nd ed., liv. xx. *Des Vennes*, chap. xliv. p. 507.

[8] For example, King John is believed to have poisoned Maud Fitzwalter by "a poisoned egg."

"In the reign of King John, the White Tower received one of the first and fairest of a long line of female victims in that Maud Fitzwalter who was known to the singers of her time as Maud the Fair. The father of this beautiful girl was Robert, Lord Fitzwalter, of Castle Baynard, on the Thames, one of John's greatest barons. Yet the king, during a fit of violence with the queen, fell madly in love with this young girl. As neither the lady herself nor her powerful sire would listen to his disgraceful suit, the king is said to have seized her by force at Dunmow, and brought her to the Tower. Fitzwalter raised an outcry, on which the king sent troops into Castle Baynard and his other houses; and when the baron protested against these wrongs, his master banished him from the realm. Fitzwalter fled to France with his wife and his other children, leaving his daughter Maud in the Tower, where she suffered a daily insult in the king's unlawful suit. On her proud and scornful answer to his passion being heard, John carried her up to the roof, and locked her in the round turret, standing on the north-east angle of the keep. Maud's cage was the highest, chilliest den in the Tower; but neither cold, nor solitude, nor hunger could break her strength. In the rage of his disappointed love, the king sent one of his minions to her room with a poisoned egg, of which the brave girl ate and died."—*Her Majesty's Tower*, by Hepworth Dixon. Lond., 1869; i. p. 46.

[9] "This yeare, the 17th of March, was boyled in Smithfield one Margaret Davie, a mayden, which had pouysoned 3 householdes that she dwelled in. One being her mistress, which dyed of the same, and one Darington and his wyfe, which she also dwelled with in Coleman Street, which dyed of the same, and also one Tinleys, which dyed also of the same."—Wriotherley's *Chronicle*, A.D. 1542.

[10] J. Bapt. Porta, born 1537, died 1615. *Neapolitani Magiæ Naturalis*. Neapoli, 1589.

the preparation of poisons. There are prescriptions that little accord with the title, unless indeed the trades of cook and poisoner were the same. He gives a method of drugging wine with belladonna root, for the purpose of making the loaded guest loathe drink; he also gives a list of solanaceous plants, and makes special mention of nux vomica, aconite, veratrum, and mezereon. Again, in the section (*De Ancupio*, lib. xv.) he gives a recipe for a very strong poison which he calls "*venenum lupinum*;" it is to be made of the powdered leaves of *Aconitum lycoctonum*, *Taxus baccata*, powdered glass, caustic lime, sulphide of arsenic, and bitter almonds, the whole to be mixed with honey, and made into pills the size of a hazel-nut.

In the section *De Medicis Experimentis* he gives a process to poison a sleeping person: the recipe is curious, and would certainly not have the intended effect. A mixture of hemlock juice, bruised datura, stramonium, belladonna, and opium is placed in a leaden box with a perfectly fitting cover, and fermented for several days; it is then opened under the nose of the sleeper. Possibly Porta had experimented on small animals, and had found that such matters, when fermented, exhaled enough carbonic acid gas to kill them, and imagined, therefore, that the same thing would happen if applied to the human subject. However this may be, the account which Porta gives of the effects of the solanaceous plants, and the general tone of the work, amply prove that he was no theorist, but had studied practically the actions of poisons.

The iniquitous Toffana (or Tophana) made solutions of arsenious acid of varying strength, and sold these solutions in phials under the name of "*Acquetta di Napoli*" for many years. She is supposed to have poisoned more than 600 persons, among whom were two Popes—viz., Pius III. and Clement XIV. The composition of the Naples water was long a profound secret, but is said to have been known by the reigning Pope and by the Emperor Charles VI. The latter told the secret to Dr Garelli, his physician, who, again, imparted the knowledge to the famous Friedrich Hoffman in a letter still extant. Toffana was brought to justice in 1709, but, availing herself of the immunity afforded by convents, escaped punishment, and continued to sell her wares for twenty years afterwards. When Kepfer[11] was in Italy he found her in a prison at Naples, and many people visited her, as a sort of lion (1730). With the *Acqua Toffana*, the "*Acquetta di Perugia*" played at the same time its part. It is said to have been prepared by killing a hog, disjointing the same, strewing the pieces with white arsenic, which was well rubbed in, and then collecting the juice which dropped from the meat; this juice was considered far more poisonous than an ordinary solution of arsenic. The researches of Selmi on compounds containing arsenic, produced when animal bodies decompose in arsenical fluids, lend reason and support to this view; and probably the juice would not only be very poisonous, but act in a different manner, and exhibit symptoms different from those of ordinary arsenical poisoning. Toffana had disciples; she taught the art to Hieronyma Spara, who formed an association of young married women during the popedom of Alexander VII.; these were detected on their own confession.[12]

Contemporaneously with Toffana, another Italian, Keli, devoted himself to similar crimes. This man had expended much as an adept searching for the philosopher's stone, and sought to indemnify himself by entering upon what must have been a profitable business. He it was who instructed M. de St. Croix in the properties of arsenic; and St. Croix, in his turn, imparted the secret to his paramour, Madame de Brinvilliers. This woman appears to have been as cold-blooded as Toffana; she is said to have experimented on the patients at the Hôtel Dieu, in order to ascertain the strength of her powders, and to have invented "les poudres de succession." She poisoned her father, brothers, sister, and others of her family; but a terrible fate overtook both her and St. Croix. The latter was suffocated by some poisonous matters he was preparing, and Madame de Brinvilliers' practices having become known, she was obliged to take refuge in a convent. Here she was courted by a police officer disguised as an abbé, lured out of the convent, and, in this way brought to justice, was beheaded[13] and burnt near Nôtre Dame, in the middle of the

---

[11] Kepfer's *Travels*. Lond., 1758.

[12] Le Bret's *Magazin zu Gebrauche der Staat u. Kirchen-Geschichte*, Theil 4. Frankfort and Leipzig, 1774.

[13] The Marchioness was imprisoned in the Conciergerie and tortured. Victor Hugo, describing the rack in that prison, says, "The Marchioness de Brinvilliers was stretched upon it stark naked, fastened down, so to speak, quartered by four chains attached to the four limbs, and there suffered the frightful extraordinary torture by water," which caused her to ask "How are you going to contrive to put that great barrel of water in this little body?"—*Things seen by Victor Hugo*, vol. i.

The water torture was this:—a huge funnel-like vessel was fitted on to the neck, the edge of the funnel coming up to the eyes; on now pouring water into the funnel so that the fluid rises above the nose and mouth, the poor wretch is bound to swallow the fluid or die of suffocation; if indeed the sufferer resolve to be choked, in the first few moments of unconsciousness the fluid is swallowed automatically, and air again admitted to the lungs; it is therefore obvious that in this way prodigious quantities of fluid might be taken.

reign of Louis XIV.[14]

The numerous attempts of the Italian and Venetian poisoners on the lives of monarchs and eminent persons cast for a long time a cloud over regal domestic peace. Bullets and daggers were not feared, but in their place the dish of meat, the savoury pasty, and the red wine were regarded as possible carriers of death. No better example of this dread can be found than, at so late a period as the reign of Henry VII.,[15] the extraordinary precautions thought necessary for preserving the infant Prince of Wales.

"No person, of whatsoever rank, except the regular attendants in the nursery, should approach the cradle, except with an order from the king's hand. The food supplied to the child was to be largely '*assayed*,' and his clothes were to be washed by his own servants, and no other hand might touch them. The material was to be submitted to all tests. The chamberlain and vice-chamberlain must be present, morning and evening, when the prince was washed and dressed, and nothing of any kind bought for the use of the nursery might be introduced until it was washed and perfumed. No person, not even the domestics of the palace, might have access to the prince's rooms except those who were specially appointed to them, nor might any member of the household approach London, for fear of their catching and conveying infection."[16]

However brief and imperfect the foregoing historical sketch of the part that poison has played may be, it is useful in showing the absolute necessity of a toxicological science—a science embracing many branches of knowledge. If it is impossible now for Toffanas, Locustas, and other specimens of a depraved humanity to carry on their crimes without detection; if poison is the very last form of death feared by eminent political persons; it is not so much owing to a different state of society, as to the more exact scientific knowledge which is applied during life to the discrimination of symptoms, distinguishing between those resulting from disease and those due to injurious substances, and after death to a highly developed pathology, which has learned, by multiplied observations, all the normal and abnormal signs in tissues and organs; and, finally, to an ever-advancing chemistry, which is able in many instances to separate and detect the hurtful and noxious thing, although hid for months deep in the ground.

II.—Growth and Development of the Modern Methods of Chemically Detecting Poisons.

§ 8. The history of the detection of poisons has gone through several phases. The first phase has already been incidentally touched upon—*i.e.*, detection by antecedent and surrounding circumstances, aided sometimes by experiments on animals. If the death was sudden, if the post-mortem decomposition was rapid, poison was indicated: sometimes a portion of the food last eaten, or the suspected thing, would be given to an animal; if the animal also died, such accumulation of proof would render the matter beyond doubt. The modern toxicologists are more sceptical, for even the last test is not of itself satisfactory. It is now known that meat may become filled with bacilli and produce rapid death, and yet no poison, as such, has been added.

In the next phase, the doctors were permitted to dissect, and to familiarise themselves with pathological appearances. This was a great step gained: the apoplexies, heart diseases, perforations of the stomach, and fatal internal hæmorrhages could no longer be ascribed to poison. If popular clamour made a false accusation, there was more chance of a correct judgment. It was not until the end of the eighteenth and the beginning of the present century, however, that chemistry was far enough advanced to test for the more common mineral poisons; the modern phase was then entered on, and toxicology took a new departure.

§ 9. From the treatise of Barthélémy d'Anglais[17] in the thirteenth century (in which he noticed the poisonous properties of quicksilver vapour), up to the end of the fifteenth century, there are numerous treatises upon poison, most of which are mere learned compilations, and scarcely repay perusal. In the sixteenth century, there are a few

[14] For the court of poisoners (*chambre ardente*) and the histories of St. Croix, De Brinvilliers, the priest Le Sage, the women La Voisin, and La Vigoureux, the reader may be referred to Voltaire's *Siècle de Louis XIV.*, Madame de Sévigné's *Lettres*, Martinière's *Hist. de la Règne de Louis XIV.*, Strutzel, *De Venenis*, &c.

[15] Henry VIII., at one time of his life, was (or pretended to be) apprehensive of being poisoned; it was, indeed, a common belief of his court that Anne Boleyn attempted to dose him. "The king, in an interview with young Prince Henry, burst into tears, saying that he and his sister (meaning the Princess Mary) might thank God for having escaped from the hands of that accursed and venomous harlot, who had intended to poison them."—*A Chronicle of England during the Reign of the Tudors*, by W. J. Hamilton. Introduction, p. xxi.

[16] Froude's *History of England*, vol. iii. p. 262.

[17] *De Rerum Proprietaribus.*

works, such, for example, as Porta, which partook of the general advancement of science, and left behind the stereotyped doctrine of the old classical schools.[18]

In the seventeenth century the Honourable Robert Boyle made some shrewd observations, bearing on toxicology, in his work on "The usefulness of Natural Philosophy," &c.: Oxford, 1664. Nicolas L'Emery also wrote a *Cours de Chimie*,—quite an epitome of the chemical science of the time.[19]

In the eighteenth century still further advances were made. Richard Mead published his ingenious *Mechanical Theory of Poisons*. Great chemists arose—Stahl, Marggraf, Brandt, Bergmann, Scheele, Berthollet, Priestley, and lastly, Lavoisier—and chemistry, as a science, was born. Of the chemists quoted, Scheele, in relation to toxicology, stands chief. It was Scheele who discovered prussic acid,[20] without, however, noting its poisonous properties; the same chemist separated oxalic acid from sorrel,[21] and made the important discovery that arsenic united with hydrogen, forming a fœtid gas, and, moreover, that this gas could be decomposed by heat.[22] From this observation, a delicate test for arsenic was afterwards elaborated, which for the first time rendered the most tasteless and easily administered poison in the whole world at once the easiest of detection. The further history of what is now called "Marsh's Test" is as follows:—

Bergmann first described oxalic acid as obtained by the oxidation of saccharine bodies; but Scheele recognised its identity with the acid contained in sorrel.

§ 10. Proust[23] observed that a very fœtid hydrogen gas was disengaged when arsenical tin was dissolved in hydrochloric acid, and that arsenic was deposited from the inflamed gas on cold surfaces which the flame touched. Trommsdorff next announced, in 1803, that when arsenical zinc was introduced into an ordinary flask with water and sulphuric acid, an arsenical hydrogen was disengaged; and if the tube was sufficiently long, arsenic was deposited on its walls.[24] Stromeyer, Gay-Lussac, Thénard, Gehlen, and Davy later studied this gas, and Serullas in 1821 proposed this reaction as a toxicological test. Lastly, in 1836, Marsh published his Memoir.[25] He elaborated a special apparatus of great simplicity, developed hydrogen by means of zinc and sulphuric acid, inflamed the issuing gas, and obtained any arsenic present as a metal, which could be afterwards converted into arsenious acid, &c.

This brief history of the so-called "Marsh's Test" amply shows that Marsh was not the discoverer of the test. Like many other useful processes, it seems to have been evolved by a combination of many minds. It may, however, be truly said that Marsh was the first who perfected the test and brought it prominently forward.

§ 11. Matthieu Joseph Bonaventura Orfila must be considered the father of modern toxicology. His great work, *Traité de Toxicologie*, was first published in 1814, and went through many editions. Orfila's chief merit was the discovery that poisons were absorbed and accumulated in certain tissues—a discovery which bore immediate fruit, and greatly extended the means of seeking poisons. Before the time of Orfila, a chemist not finding anything in the stomach would not have troubled to examine the liver, the kidney, the brain, or the blood. The immense number of experiments which Orfila undertook is simply marvellous. Some are of little value, and teach nothing accurately as to the action of poisons—as, for example, many of those in which he tied the gullet in order to prevent vomiting, for such are experiments under entirely unnatural conditions; but there are still a large number which form the very basis of our pathological knowledge.

Orfila's method of experiment was usually to take weighed or measured quantities of poison, to administer them to animals, and then after death—first carefully noting the changes in the tissues and organs—to attempt to recover by chemical means the poison administered. In this way he detected and recovered nearly all the organic and inorganic poisons then known; and most of his processes are, with modifications and improvements, in use at

[18] In the sixteenth century it was not considered proper to write upon poisons. Jerôme Cardan declared a poisoner worse than a brigand, "and that is why I have refused not only to teach or experiment on such things, but even to know them."—*J. Cardan: De Subtilitate*. Basel, 1558.

[19] *Cours de Chimie, contenant la manière de faire les opérations qui sont en usage dans la Médecine.* Paris, 1675.

[20] *Opuscula Chemica*, vol. ii. pp. 148-174.

[21] *De Terra Rhubarbi et Acido Acetosellæ. Nova Acta Acad. Veg. Sued. Anni*, 1784. *Opuscula Chemica*, vol. ii. pp. 187-195.

[22] *Mémoires de Scheele*, t. i., 1775.

[23] Proust, *Annales de Chimie*, t. xxviii., 1798.

[24] *Nicholson's Journal*, vol. vi.

[25] "Description of a New Process of Separating Small Quantities of Arsenic from Substances with which it is mixed." *Ed. New. Phil. Journal*, 1836.

the present time.[26]

§ 12. The discovery of the alkaloids at the commencement of this century certainly gave the poisoner new weapons; yet the same processes (slightly modified) which separated the alkaloids from plants also served to separate them from the human body. In 1803 Derosne discovered narcotine and morphine, but he neither recognised the difference between these two substances, nor their basic properties. Sertürner from 1805 devoted himself to the study of opium, and made a series of discoveries. Robiquet, in 1807, recognised the basic characters of narcotine. In 1818 Pelletier and Caventou separated strychnine; in 1819 brucine; and in the same year delphinine was discovered simultaneously by Brande, Lassaigne, and Feneuille. Coniine was recognised by Giesecke in 1827, and in the following year, 1828, nicotine was separated by Reimann and Posselt. In 1832 Robiquet discovered codeine; and in 1833 atropine, aconitine, and hyoscyamine were distinguished by Geiger and Hesse. Since then, every year has been marked by the separation of some new alkaloid, from either animal or vegetable substances. So many workers in different countries now began to study and improve toxicology, that it would exceed the limits and be foreign to the scope of this treatise to give even a brief *résumé* of their labours. It may, notwithstanding, be useful to append a short bibliography of the chief works on toxicology of the present century.

§ 13.—BIBLIOGRAPHY OF THE CHIEF WORKS ON TOXICOLOGY (NINETEENTH CENTURY).

Anglada, Jos.—"Traité de Toxicologie Générale, &c." Montpellier et Paris, 1835.

Autenrieth.—"Kurze Anleitung zur Auffindung der Gifte." Freiburg, 1892.

Bandlin, O.—"Die Gifte." Basel, 1869-1873.

Baumert, G.—"Lehrbuch der gerichtl. Chemie." Braunschweig, 1889-92.

Bayard, Henri.—"Manuel Pratique de Médecine Légale." Paris, 1843.

Bellini, Ranieri.—"Manuel de Tossicologia." Pisa, 1878.

Berlin, N. J.—"Nachricht, die gewöhnlichen Gifte chemisch zu entdecken." Stockholm, 1845.

Bernard, C.—"Leçons sur les Effets des Substances Toxiques et Médicamenteuses." Paris, 1857.

Bertrand, C. A. R. A.—"Manuel Médico-Légale des Poisons introduits dans l'Estomac, et les Moyens Thérapeutiques qui leur conviennent: suivi d'un Plan d'Organisation Médico-Judiciaire, et d'un Tableau de la Classification Générale des Empoisonnemens." Paris, 1818.

Binz, C.—"Intoxicationen" in Gerhardt's "Handbuch der Kinderkrankheiten." iii. Heft. Tübingen, 1878.

Blyth, A. Wynter.—"A Manual of Practical Chemistry: The Analysis of Foods and the Detection of Poisons." London, 1879.

Bocker, Frieder. Wilhelm.—"Die Vergiftungen in forensischer u. klinischer Beziehung." Iserlohn, 1857.

Böhm, R., Naunyn, B., und Von Boeck, H.—"Handbuch der Intoxicationen." (Bd. 15 of the German edition of Ziemssen's Cyclopædia.)

Brandt, Phöbus, und Ratzeburg.—"Deutschlands Giftgewächse." Berlin, 1834-38 (2 vols. with 56 coloured plates).

Briand, J., et Chaude, Ern.—"Manuel Complet de Médecine Légale." (The latest edition, 1879.) The chemical portion is by J. Bouis.

Buchner, E.—"Lehrbuch der gerichtlichen Medicin für Aerzte u. Juristen." 3rd ed. München, 1872.

Casper, J. L.—"Handbuch der gerichtlichen Medicin." 7th ed. Berlin, 1881.

Chevallier, A.—"Traité de Toxicologie et de Chimie Judiciaire." Paris, 1868.

Chiaje, Stef.—"Enchiridis di Tossicologia teorico-pratica." 3rd ed. Napoli, 1858.

Christison, Robert.—"A Treatise on Poisons." Edinburgh, 1830. (A third edition appeared in 1836.)

Cornevin, C.—"Des Plantes Vénéneuses." Paris, 1887.

Devergie, Alphonse.—"Médecine Légale, Théorique, et Pratique." 3rd ed. Paris, 1852.

Dragendorff, Jean Georges.—"Die gerichtlich-chemische Ermittelung von Giften in Nahrungsmitteln, Luftgemischen, Speiseresten, Körpertheilen." &c. St. Petersburg, 1868. 3rd ed. Göttingen, 1888.

[26] Orfila's chief works are as follows:—

Traité de Toxicologie. 2 vols. 8vo. Paris, 1814.

Leçons de Chimie, appliquées à la Méd. Pratique. 16mo. Brussels, 1836.

Mémoire sur la Nicotine et la Conicine. Paris, 1851.

Leçons de la Méd. Légale. 8vo. Paris, 1821.

Traité des Exhumations Juridiques, et Considérations sur les Changemens Physiques que les Cadavres éprouvent en se pourrissant. 2 tom. Paris, 1831.

—— "Untersuchungen aus dem Pharmaceutischen Institute in Dorpat. Beiträge zur gerichtlichen Chemie einzelner organischer Gifte." Erstes Heft. St. Petersburg, 1871.
—— "Jahresbericht über die Fortschritte der Pharmacognosie, Pharmacie, und Toxicologie." Herausgegeben von Dr. Dragendorff. 1876.
Duflos, A.—"Handbuch der angewandten gerichtlich-chemischen Analyse der chemischen Gifte, ihre Erkennung in reinem Zustande u. in Gemengen betreffend." Breslau u. Leipzig, 1873.
Eulenberg, Dr. Hermann.—"Handbuch der Gewerbe-Hygiene." Berlin, 1876.
Falck, C. Ph.—"Die Klinischwichtigen Intoxicationen." (Handbuch der spec. Pathologie u. Therapie red. von R. Virchow, Bd. 2.) Erlangen, 1854.
Falck, Ferd. Aug.—"Lehrbuch der praktischen Toxicologie." Stuttgart, 1880.
Flandin, C.—"Traité des Poisons, ou Toxicologie appliquée à la Médecine Légale, à la Physiologie, et à la Thérapeutique." Paris, 1847, 1853.
Fröhner, Eug.—"Lehrbuch der Toxicologie für Thierärzte." Stuttgart, 1890.
Galtier, C. P.—"Traité de Toxicologie Médico-Légale et de la Falsification des Aliments," &c. Paris, 1845.
—— "Traité de Toxicologie Médicale, Chimique et Légale," &c. Paris, 1855. A later edition of the same work.
Greene, Will. H.—"A Practical Handbook of Medical Chemistry, applied to Clinical Research and the Detection of Poisons." Philadelphia, 1880.
Guérin, G.—"Traité Pratique d'Analyse Chimique et de Recherches Toxicologiques." Paris, 1893.
Guy, W. A., and Ferrier, David.—"Principles of Forensic Medicine." London, 1874.
Harnack, Erich.—"Lehrbuch der Arzneimittellehre," &c. Hamburg, 1883.
Hasselt, van, A. W. M.—"Handbuch der Giftlehre für Chemiker, Aerzte, Apotheker, u. Richtspersonen." (A German translation of the original Dutch edition, edited by J. B. Henkel. Braunschweig, 1862. Supplemental vol. by N. Husemann, Berlin, 1867.)
Helwig, A.—"Das Mikroskop in der Toxicologie." 64 photographs, roy. 8vo, Mainz, 1865.
Hemming, W. D.—"Aids to Forensic Medicine and Toxicology." London, 1877.
Hermann, L.—"Lehrbuch der experimentellen Toxicologie." 8vo. Berlin, 1874.
Hoffmann, E. R.—"Lehrbuch der gerichtlichen Medicin." 5th ed. Wien, 1890-91.
Husemann and A. Hilger.—"Die Pflanzenstoffe in chemischer, pharmakologischer, u. toxicologischer Hinsicht." 2nd ed. Berlin, 1882.
Husemann, Th., and Husemann, A.—"Handbuch der Toxicologie." Berlin, 1862. (Suppl. Berlin, 1867.)
Kobert, Rud.—"Lehrbuch der Intoxicationen." Stuttgart, 1893.
Koehler, R.—"Handbuch der speciellen Therapie, einschliesslich der Behandlung der Vergiftungen." 3rd ed. 2 vols. roy. 8vo. Tübingen, 1869.
Lesser, Adolf.—"Atlas der gerichtlichen Medicin." Berlin, 1883.
Loew, Oscar.—"Ein natürliches System der Gift-Wirkungen." München, 1893.
Ludwig, E.—"Medicinische Chemie in Anwendung auf gerichtliche Untersuchungen."
Mahon, A.—"Médecine Légale et Police Médicale." Paris, 1807.
Marx, K. F. H.—"Die Lehre von den Giften." Göttingen, 1827-29.
Maschka, J.—"Handbuch der gerichtlichen Medicin." Tübingen, 1881-82. This work is under the editorship of Dr. Maschka, and contains separate articles on medico-legal and toxicological questions by various eminent toxicologists, somewhat after the manner of Ziemssen's Cyclopædia.
Mende, Lud. Jul. Casp.—"Ausführliches Handbuch der gerichtlichen Medicin." 1819-32.
Mohr, Fried.—"Chemische Toxicologie." Braunschweig, 1874.
Montgarny, H. de.—"Essai de Toxicologie, et spécialement avec la Jurisprudence Médicale." Paris, 1878.
Montmahon, E. S. de.—"Manuel Médico-Légale des Poisons," &c. Paris, 1824.
Mutel, D. Ph.—"Des Poisons, considérés sous le rapport de la Médecine Pratique," &c. Montpellier et Paris, 1835.
Nacquet, A.—"Legal Chemistry: A guide to the detection of Poisons, Examination of Stains, &c., as applied to Chemical Jurisprudence." New York, 1876.
A translation from the French; see "Foods, their Composition and Analysis," page 43.
Nicolai, Joh. Ant. Heinr.—"Handbuch der gerichtlichen Medicin." Berlin, 1841.
The chemical portion is by F. R. Simon.
Ogston, F.—"Lectures on Medical Jurisprudence." London, 1878.
Orfila, Matthieu Jos. Bonaventura.—"Traité des Poisons, ou Toxicologie Générale." Paris, 1st ed., 1814; 5th ed.,

1852.
Orfila et Lesueur.—"Traité de Médecine légale." Paris, 1821; 4th ed., Paris, 1848.
Otto, F. G.—"Anleitung zur Ausmittelung der Gifte." Braunschweig, 1856; 5th ed., 1875. 6th ed. by Robert Otto, Braunschweig, 1884.
Praag van, Leonides, u. Opwyrda, R. J.—"Leerboek voor practische giftleer." In Zwei Theilen. Utrecht, 1871.
Rabuteau, A.—"Élémens de Toxicologie et de Médecine Légale, appliquées à l'Empoisonnement." Paris, 1873. 2nd ed. by Ed. Bourgoing. Paris, 1888.
Reese, John J.—"Manual of Toxicology, including the consideration of the Nature, Properties, Effects, and Means of Detection of Poisons, more especially in their Medico-legal relations." Philadelphia, 1874.
Remer, W. H. G.—"Lehrbuch der polizeilich-gerichtlichen Chemie." Bd. 1 u. 2. 3. Auflage, Helmstadt, 1824.
Schneider, F. C.—"Die gerichtliche Chemie für Gerichtsärzte u. Juristen." Wien, 1852.
Schneider, P. J.—"Ueber die Gifte in medicinisch-gerichtlicher u. gerichtlich-polizeilicher Rücksicht." 2nd ed., 1821.
Selmi, F.—"Studi di Tossicologia Chimica." Bologna, 1871.
Sobernheim, Jos. Fr. u. Simon, J. F.—"Handbuch der praktischen Toxicologie," &c. Berlin, 1838.
Sonnenschein, L.—"Handbuch der gerichtlichen Medicin." Berlin, 1860. A new edition by Dr. A. Classen. Berlin, 1881.
Tardieu, A.—"Étude Médico-Légale et Clinique sur l'Empoisonnement, avec la Collaboration de M. T. Roussin pour la partie de l'expertise relative à la Recherche Chimique des Poisons." Paris, 1867.
Taylor, Alfred Swaine.—"On Poisons in relation to Medical Jurisprudence and Medicine." 3rd ed. 1875. Manual, 1879.
—— "Principles and Practice of Medical Jurisprudence." 3 vols. London, 1873.
Werber, Ant.—"Lehrbuch der praktischen Toxicologie." Erlangen, 1869.
Wood, Horatio C.—"Therapeutics, Materia Medica, and Toxicology." Philadelphia, 1874.
Woodmann, W. Bathurst, and Tidy, Ch.—"A Handy-Book of Forensic Medicine and Toxicology." London, 1877.
Wormley, Theodore G.—"Micro-Chemistry of Poisons, including their Physiological, Pathological, and Legal Relations." New York, 1857.
Wurtz, A.—"Traité Elémentaire de Chimie Médicale, comprenant quelques notions de Toxicologie," &c. 2nd ed. Paris, 1875.

Part II.

I.—Definition of Poison.

§ 14. The term "*Poison*" may be considered first in its legal, as distinct from its scientific, aspect.

The legal definition of "poison" is to be gathered from the various statute-books of civilised nations.

The English law enacts that: "Whoever shall administer, or cause to be administered to, or taken by any person, any poison or other destructive thing, with intent to commit murder, shall be guilty of felony."

Further, by the Criminal Consolidation Act, 1861: "Whosoever shall, by any other means other than those specified in any of the preceding sections of this Act, attempt to commit murder, shall be guilty of felony."

It is therefore evident that, by implication, the English law defines a poison to be a destructive thing administered to, or taken by, a person, and it must necessarily include, not only poisons which act on account of their inherent chemical and other properties after absorption into the blood, but mechanical irritants, and also specifically-tainted fluids. Should, for example, a person give to another milk, or other fluid, knowing, at the same time, that such fluid is contaminated by the specific poison of scarlet fever, typhoid, or any serious malady capable of being thus conveyed, I believe that such an offence could be brought under the first of the sections quoted. In fine, the words "*destructive thing*" are widely applicable, and may be extended to any substance, gaseous, liquid, or solid, living or dead, which, if capable at all of being taken within the body, may injure or destroy life. According to this view, the legal idea of "poison" would include such matters as boiling water, molten lead, specifically-infected fluids, the flesh of animals dying of diseases which may be communicable to man, powdered glass, diamond dust, &c. Evidence must, however, be given of guilty intent.

The words, "administered to or taken by," imply obviously that the framers of the older statute considered the mouth as the only portal of entrance for criminal poisoning, but the present law effectually guards against any attempt to commit murder, no matter by what means. There is thus ample provision for all the strange ways by which poison has been introduced into the system, whether it be by the ear, nose, brain, rectum, vagina, or any other conceivable way, so that, to borrow the words of Mr. Greaves (*Notes on Criminal Law Consolidation*), "the malicious may rest satisfied that every attempt to murder which their perverted ingenuity may devise, or their fiendish malignity suggest, will fall within some clause of this Act, and may be visited with penal servitude for life."

Since poison is often exhibited, not for the purpose of taking life, but from various motives, and to accomplish various ends—as, for example, to narcotise the robber's victim (this especially in the East), to quiet children, to create love in the opposite sex (love philters), to detect the secret sipper by suitably preparing the wine, to expel the inconvenient fruit of illicit affection, to cure inebriety by polluting the drunkard's drink with antimony, and, finally, to satisfy an aimless spirit of mere wantonness and wickedness, the English law enacts "that whosoever shall unlawfully or maliciously administer to, or cause to be taken by, any other person, any poison or other destructive or noxious thing, so as thereby to endanger the life of such person, or so as thereby to inflict upon such person any grievous bodily harm, shall be guilty of felony."

There is also a special provision, framed, evidently, with reference to volatile and stupefying poisons, such as chloroform, tetrachloride of carbon, &c.:—

"Whoever shall unlawfully apply, or administer to, or cause to be taken by any person, any chloroform, laudanum, or other stupefying or overpowering drug, matter, or thing, with intent, in any such case, thereby to enable himself or any other person to commit, or with intent, &c., to assist any other person in committing, any indictable offence, shall be guilty of felony."

§ 15. The German statute, as with successive amendments it now stands, enacts as follows:[27]—

---

[27] "Wer vorsätzlich einem Andern, um dessen Gesundheit zu beschädigen, Gift oder andere Stoffe beibringt, welche die Gesundheit zu zerstören geeignet sind, wird mit Zuchthaus von zwei bis zu zehn Jahren bestraft.

"Ist durch die Handlung eine schwere Körperverletzung verursacht worden, so ist auf Zuchthaus nicht unter fünf Jahren, und wenn durch die Handlung der Tod verursacht worden, auf Zuchthaus nicht unter zehn Jahren oder auf lebenslängliches

"Whoever wilfully administers (*beibringt*) to a person, for the purpose of injuring health, poison, or any other substance having the property of injuring health, will be punished by from two to ten years' imprisonment.

"If by such act a serious bodily injury is caused, the imprisonment is not to be less than five years; if death is the result, the imprisonment is to be not under ten years or for life.

"If the death is wilfully caused by poison, it comes under the general law: 'Whoever wilfully kills a man, and if the killing is premeditated, is on account of murder punishable with death.'"

The French law runs thus (Art. 301, *Penal Code*): — "Every attempt on the life of a person, by the effect of substances which may cause death, more or less suddenly, in whatever manner these substances may have been employed or administered, and whatever may have been the results, is called poisoning."[28]

There is also a penalty provided against any one who "shall have occasioned the illness or incapacity for personal work of another, by the voluntary administration, in any manner whatever, of substances which, without being of a nature to cause death, are injurious to health."[29]

§ 16. **Scientific Definition of a Poison.**—A true scientific definition of a poison must exclude all those substances which act mechanically,—the physical influences of heat, light, and electricity; and parasitic diseases, whether caused by the growth of fungus, or the invasion of an organism by animal parasites, as, for example, "trichinosis," which are not, so far as we know, associated with any poisonous product excreted by the parasite;—on the other hand, it is now recognised that pathogenic micro-organisms develop poisons, and the symptoms of all true infections are but the effects of "toxines." The definition of poison, in a scientific sense, should be broad enough to comprehend not only the human race, but the dual world of life, both animal and vegetable.

Husemann and Kobert are almost the only writers on poisons who have attempted, with more or less success, to define poison by a generalisation, keeping in view the exclusion of the matters enumerated. Husemann says—"We define poisons as such inorganic, or organic substances as are in part capable of artificial preparation, in part existing, ready-formed, in the animal or vegetable kingdom, which, without being able to reproduce themselves, through the chemical nature of their molecules under certain conditions, change in the healthy organism the form and general relationship of the organic parts, and, through annihilation of organs, or destruction of their functions, injure health, or, under certain conditions, destroy life." Kobert says:—"Poisons are organic or inorganic unorganised substances originating in the organism itself, or introduced into the organism, either artificially prepared, or ready formed in nature, which through their chemical properties, under certain conditions, so influence the organs of living beings, that the health of these beings is seriously influenced temporarily or permanently."

In the first edition of this work I made an attempt to define a poison thus:—*A substance of definite chemical composition, whether mineral or organic, may be called a poison, if it is capable of being taken into any living organism, and causes, by its own inherent chemical nature, impairment or destruction of function.* I prefer this definition to Kobert's, and believe that it fairly agrees with what we know of poisons.

II.—Classification of Poisons.

§ 17. At some future time, with a more intimate knowledge of the way in which each poison acts upon the various forms of animal and vegetable life, it may be possible to give a truly scientific and philosophical classification of poisons—one based neither upon symptoms, upon local effects, nor upon chemical structure, but upon a collation and comparison of all the properties of a poison, whether chemical, physical, or physiological. No

Zuchthaus zu erkennen.

"Ist die vorsätzliche rechtswidrige Handlung des Gift—&c.,—Beibringens auf das 'Tödten' gerichtet, soll also durch dieselbe gewollter Weise der Tod eines Anderen herbeigeführt werden, so kommt in betracht: Wer vorsätzlich einen Menschen tödtet, wird, wenn er die Tödtung mit Ueberlegung ausgeführt hat, wegen Mordes mit dem Tode bestraft."

[28] "Est qualifié *empoisonnement*—tout attentat à la vie d'une personne par l'effet de substances qui peuvent donner la mort plus ou moins promptement, de quelque manière que ces substances aient été employées ou administrées, et quelles qu'en aient été les suites."—Art. 301, *Penal Code*.

[29] "Celui qui aura occasionné à autrui une maladie ou incapacité de travail personnel en lui administrant volontairement, de quelque manière que ce soit, des substances qui, sans être de nature à donner la mort, sont nuisibles à la santé."—Art. 317, *Penal Code*.

perfect systematic arrangement is at present attainable: we are either compelled to omit all classification, or else to arrange poisons with a view to practical utility merely.

From the latter point of view, an arrangement simply according to the most prominent symptoms is a good one, and, without doubt, an assistance to the medical man summoned in haste to a case of real or suspected poisoning. Indeed, under such circumstances, a scheme somewhat similar to the following, probably occurs to every one versed in toxicology:—

A. Poisons causing Death immediately, or in a few minutes.

There are but few poisons which destroy life in a few minutes. Omitting the strong mineral acids, carbon monoxide, carbon dioxide, with the irrespirable gases,—*Prussic acid, the cyanides, oxalic acid*, and occasionally *strychnine*, are the chief poisons coming under this head.

B. Irritant Poisons (symptoms mainly pain, vomiting, and purging).

Arsenic, antimony, phosphorus, cantharides, savin, ergot, digitalis, colchicum, zinc, mercury, lead, copper, silver, iron, baryta, chrome, yew, laburnum, and putrid animal substances.

C. Irritant and Narcotic Poisons (symptoms those of an irritant nature, with the addition of more or less pronounced cerebral indications).

To this class more especially belong *oxalic acid* and *the oxalates*, with several poisons belonging to the purely narcotic class, but which produce occasionally irritant effects.

D. Poisons more especially affecting the Nervous System.

1. Narcotics (chief symptom insensibility, which may be preceded by more or less cerebral excitement): *Opium, Chloral, Chloroform.*

2. Deliriants (delirium for the most part a prominent symptom): *Belladonna, hyoscyamus, stramonium, with others of the Solanaceæ*, to which may be added—*poisonous fungi, Indian hemp, lolium temulentum, œnanthe crocata*, and *camphor.*

3. Convulsives.—Almost every poison has been known to produce convulsive effects, but the only true convulsive poisons are the *alkaloids of the strychnos class.*

4. Complex Nervous Phenomena: *Aconite, digitalis, hemlock, calabar bean, tobacco, lobelia inflata*, and *curara.*

§ 18. Kobert's Classification.—The latest authority on poisons—Kobert—has classified poisons according to the following scheme:—

I. POISONS WHICH CAUSE COARSE ANATOMICAL CHANGES OF THE ORGANS.

A. Those which specially irritate the part to which they are applied.

1. *Acids.*

2. *Caustic alkalies.*

3. *Caustic salts*, especially those of the heavy metals.

4. Locally irritating organic substances which neither can be classified as corrosive acids nor alkalies, nor as corrosive salts; such are:—*cantharidine, phrynine*, and others in the animal kingdom, *croton oil* and *savin* in the vegetable kingdom. Locally irritating colours, such as the *aniline dyes.*

5. Gases and vapours which cause local irritation when breathed, such as *ammonia, chlorine, iodine, bromine*, and *sulphur dioxide.*

B. Those which have but little effect locally, but change anatomically other parts of the body; such as *lead, phosphorus*, and others.

II. BLOOD POISONS.

1. Blood poisons interfering with the circulation in a purely physical manner, such as *peroxide of hydrogen, ricine, abrine.*

2. Poisons which have the property of dissolving the red blood corpuscle, such as the *saponins.*

3. Poisons which, with or without primary solution of the red blood corpuscles, produce in the blood methæmoglobin; such as *potassic chlorate, hydrazine, nitrobenzene, aniline, picric acid, carbon disulphide.*

4. Poisons having a peculiar action on the colouring matter of the blood, or on its decomposition products, such as *hydric sulphide, hydric cyanide*, and the *cyanides* and *carbon monoxide.*

III. POISONS WHICH KILL WITHOUT THE PRODUCTION OF COARSE ANATOMICAL CHANGE.

1. Poisons affecting the cerebro-spinal system; such as *chloroform, ether, nitrous oxide, alcohol, chloral, cocaine, atropine, morphine, nicotine, coniine, aconitine, strychnine, curarine*, and others.

2. Heart Poisons; such as, *digitalis*, *helleborin*, *muscarine*.

IV. POISONOUS PRODUCTS OF TISSUE CHANGE.

1. Poisonous albumin.
2. Poisons developed in food.
3. Auto-poisoning, *e.g.* uræmia, glycosuria, oxaluria.
4. The more important products of tissue change; such as, *fatty acids*, *oxyacids*, *amido-fatty acids*, *amines*, *diamines*, and *ptomaines*.

§ 19. I have preferred an arrangement which, as far as possible, follows the order in which a chemical expert would search for an unknown poison—hence an arrangement partly chemical and partly symptomatic. First the chief gases which figure in the mortality statistics are treated, and then follow in order other poisons.

A chemist, given a liquid to examine, would naturally test first its reaction, and, if strongly alkaline or strongly acid, would at once direct his attention to the mineral acids or to the alkalies. In other cases, he would proceed to separate volatile matters from those that were fixed, lest substances such as prussic acid, chloroform, alcohol, and phosphorus be dissipated or destroyed by his subsequent operations.

Distillation over, the alkaloids, glucosides, and their allies would next be naturally sought, since they can be extracted by alcoholic and ethereal solvents in such a manner as in no way to interfere with an *after*-search for metals.

The metals are last in the list, because by suitable treatment, after all organic substances are destroyed, either by actual fire or powerful chemical agencies, even the volatile metals may be recovered. The metals are arranged very nearly in the same order as that in which they would be separated from a solution—viz., according to their behaviour to hydric and ammoniac sulphides.

There are a few poisons, of course, such as the oxalates of the alkalies, which might be overlooked, unless sought for specially; but it is hoped that this is no valid objection to the arrangement suggested, which, in greater detail, is as follows:—

A.—POISONOUS GASES.

1. Carbon monoxide.
2. Chlorine.
3. Hydric sulphide.

B.—ACIDS AND ALKALIES.

1. Sulphuric acid.
2. Hydrochloric acid.
3. Nitric acid.
4. Potash.
5. Soda.
6. Ammonia.
7. Neutral sodium, potassium, and ammonium salts.

In nearly all cases of death from any of the above, the analyst, from the symptoms observed during life, from the surrounding circumstances, and from the pathological appearances and evident chemical reactions of the fluids submitted, is put at once on the right track, and has no difficulty in obtaining decided results.

C.—POISONOUS SUBSTANCES CAPABLE OF BEING SEPARATED BY DISTILLATION FROM EITHER NEUTRAL OR ACID LIQUIDS.

1. Hydrocarbons.
2. Camphor.
3. Alcohols.
4. Amyl-nitrite.
5. Chloroform and other anæsthetics.
6. Carbon disulphide.
7. Carbolic acid.
8. Nitro-benzene.
9. Prussic acid.
10. Phosphorus.

The volatile alkaloids, which may also be readily distilled by strongly alkalising the fluid, because they admit of a rather different mode of treatment, are not included in this class.

D.—ALKALOIDS AND POISONOUS VEGETABLE PRINCIPLES SEPARATED FOR THE MOST PART BY ALCOHOLIC SOLVENTS.

DIVISION I.—Vegetable Alkaloids.

1. Liquid volatile alkaloids, alkaloids of hemlock, nicotine, piturie, sparteine, aniline.
2. The opium group of alkaloids.
3. The strychnine or tetanic group of alkaloids—strychnine, brucine, igasurine.
4. The aconite group of alkaloids.
5. The mydriatic group of alkaloids—atropine, hyoscyamine, solanin, cytisine.
6. The alkaloids of the veratrines.
7. Physostigmine.
8. Pilocarpine.
9. Taxine.
10. Curarine.
11. Colchicin.
12. Muscarine and the active principles of certain fungi.

There would, perhaps, have been an advantage in arranging several of the individual members somewhat differently—*e.g.*, a group might be made of poisons which, like pilocarpine and muscarine, are antagonistic to atropine; and another group suggests itself, the physiological action of which is the opposite of the strychnos class; solanin (although classed as a mydriatic, and put near to atropine) has much of the nature of a glucoside, and the same may be said of colchicin; so that, if the classification were made solely on chemical grounds, solanin would have followed colchicin, and thus have marked the transition from the alkaloids to the glucosides.

DIVISION II.—Glucosides.

1. The digitalis group.
2. Other poisonous glucosides acting on the heart.
3. Saponin.

The glucosides, when fairly pure, are easily recognised; they are destitute of nitrogen, neutral in reaction, and split up into sugar and other compounds when submitted to the action of saponifying agents, such as boiling with dilute mineral acids.

DIVISION III.—Certain Poisonous Anhydrides of the Organic Acids.

1. Santonin.
2. Mezereon.

It is probable that this class will in a few years be extended, for several other organic anitrogenous poisons exist, which, when better known, will most likely prove to be anhydrides.

DIVISION IV.—Various Vegetable Poisonous Principles not admitting of Classification under the previous Three Divisions.

Ergot, picrotoxin, the poison of *Illicium religiosum*, cicutoxin, *Æthusa cynapium*, *Œnanthe crocata*, croton oil, savin oil, the toxalbumins of castor oil and *Abrus*.

The above division groups together various miscellaneous toxic principles, none of which can at present be satisfactorily classified.

E.—POISONS DERIVED FROM LIVING OR DEAD ANIMAL SUBSTANCES.

DIVISION I.—Poisons Secreted by the Living.

1. Poisonous amphibia.
2. Poison of the scorpion.
3. Poisonous fish.
4. Poisonous insects—spiders, wasps, bees, beetles, &c.
5. Snake poison.

DIVISION II.—Poisons formed in Dead Animal Matters.

1. Ptomaines.
2. Poisoning by putrid or changed foods—sausage poisoning.

F.—THE OXALIC ACID GROUP.

G.—INORGANIC POISONS.

DIVISION I.—Precipitated from a Hydrochloric Acid Solution by Hydric Sulphide—Precipitate, Yellow or

Orange.

- Arsenic, antimony, cadmium.

DIVISION II.—Precipitated by Hydric Sulphide in Hydrochloric acid Solution—Black.

- Lead, copper, bismuth, silver, mercury.

DIVISION III.—Precipitated from a Neutral Solution by Hydric Sulphide.

- Zinc, nickel, cobalt.

DIVISION IV.—Precipitated by Ammonia Sulphide.

- Iron, chromium, thallium, aluminium.

DIVISION V.—Alkaline Earths.

- Barium.

III.—Statistics.

§ 20. The number of deaths from poison (whether accidental, suicidal, or homicidal), as compared with other forms of violent, as well as natural deaths, possesses no small interest; and this is more especially true when the statistics are studied in a comparative manner, and town be compared with town, country with country.

The greater the development of commercial industries (especially those necessitating the use or manufacture of powerful chemical agencies), the more likely are accidents from poisons to occur. It may also be stated, further, that the higher the mental development of a nation, the more likely are its homicides to be caused by subtle poison—its suicides by the euthanasia of chloral, morphine, or hemlock.

Other influences causing local diversity in the kind and frequency of poisoning, are those of race, of religion, of age and sex, and the mental stress concomitant with sudden political and social changes.

In the ten years from 1883-1892, there appear to have died from poison, in England and Wales, 6616 persons, as shown in the following tables:—

DEATHS FROM POISON IN ENGLAND AND WALES DURING THE TEN YEARS 1883-92.

	Accident or Negligence.		Suicide.		Murder.		Total.	
	M.	F.	M.	F.	M.	F.	M.	F.
Metals.								
Arsenic,	37	14	37	20	1	1	75	35
Antimony,	3	...	1	2	...	...	4	2
Copper,	4	1	2	1	...	...	6	2
Lead,	831	209	1	2	...	...	832	211
Silver Nitrate,	1	...	...	...	...	...	1	...
Zinc Chloride (or Sulphate),	7	...	4	...	...	...	11	...
Mercury,	22	11	16	8	2	1	40	20
Chromic Acid,	1	...	...	...	...	...	1	...
Iron Perchloride,	...	...	...	1	...	...	...	1
Alkaline Earths.								
Lime,	2	...	...	1	...	...	2	1
Barium Chloride,	1	...	...	...	...	...	1	...
The Alkalies and their Salts.								
Ammonia,	39	25	18	16	...	...	57	41

Caustic Soda,	3	4	...	1	...	...	3	5
„ Potash,	8	10	1	...	...	...	9	10
Potassic Chlorate,	1	...	...	...	...	...	1	...
„ Bichromate,	2	2	7	3	...	...	9	5
„ Bromide,	1	...	...	...	...	...	1	...
„ Binoxalate (Sorrel),	1	3	1	4	...	...	2	7
Acids.								
Sulphuric Acid,	30	9	29	24	1	...	60	33
Nitric „	18	7	18	9	...	...	36	16
Hydrochloric„	48	18	83	55	...	...	131	73
Oxalic„	17	6	114	86	...	...	131	92
Tartaric „	...	1	...	...	...	...	...	1
Acetic„	4	3	...	2	...	...	4	5
Carbolic „	169	101	219	271	...	1	388	373
Hydrofluoric„	...	...	...	1	...	...	...	1
Phosphorus (including Lucifer matches),	24	47	28	56	...	...	52	103
Iodine,	6	7	1	1	...	...	7	8
Volatile Liquids.								
Paraffin (Petroleum),	9	2	1	...	...	...	10	2
Benzoline,	3	2	...	1	...	...	3	3
Naphtha,	1	...	...	...	...	...	1	...
Carbon Bisulphide,	...	...	1	...	...	...	1	...
Turpentine,	5	1	...	3	...	...	5	4
Methylated Spirit,	...	2	1	2	...	...	1	4
Alcohol,	81	24	1	2	...	...	82	26
Chloroform,	57	41	9	5	1	...	67	46
Ether,	5	2	...	...	...	...	5	2
Spt. Etheris Nitrosi,	1	...	...	...	...	...	1	...
Anæsthetic (kind not stated),	4	3	...	...	...	...	4	3
Oil of Juniper,	1	...	...	...	...	...	1	...
Opiates and Narcotics.								
Opium, Laudanum—Morphia,	503	373	330	167	4	2	837	542
Soothing Syrup, Paregoric, &c.	18	22	2	3	...	...	20	25
Chlorodyne,	56	30	8	8	...	...	64	38
Chloral,	89	22	14	1	1	...	104	23
Cyanides.								
Prussic Acid, and Oil of Almonds,	17	11	203	19	2	8	222	38
Potassium Cyanide,	19	21	100	22	3	1	122	44

Alkaloids.								
Strychnine and Nux Vomica,	22	21	65	85	4	4	91	110
Vermin-Killer,	2	6	49	69	1	...	52	75
Atropine,	2	...	1	...	...	...	3	...
Belladonna,	36	20	11	9	...	...	47	29
Aconite,	19	21	9	10	...	...	28	31
Ipecacuanha,	1	1	...	...	...	...	1	1
Cocaine,	3	...	...	...	...	...	3	...
Miscellaneous.								
Antipyrine,	1	...	...	...	...	...	1	...
Cantharides,	1	...	...	1	...	...	1	1
Camphorated Oil,	1	...	...	...	...	...	1	...
Croton Oil,	1	...	...	...	...	...	1	...
Cayenne Pepper,	1	...	...	...	...	...	1	...
Syrup of Rhubarb,	1	...	...	...	...	...	1	...
Colchicum,	2	...	...	...	...	...	2	...
Hemlock,	3	1	...	...	...	...	3	1
Water Hemlock,	5	6	...	...	...	...	5	6
Colocynth,	...	2	...	...	...	...	...	2
Castor Oil Seeds,	1	1	...	...	...	...	1	1
Laburnum Seeds,	2	1	...	...	...	...	2	1
Thorn Apple,	1	...	...	...	...	...	1	...
Yew Leaves or Berries,	3	2	...	...	...	...	3	2
Crow-foot,	...	1	...	...	...	...	...	1
Whin-flower,	1	...	...	...	...	...	1	...
Pennyroyal,	...	1	...	...	...	...	...	1
Meadow Crow-foot,	...	1	...	...	...	...	...	1
Arum Seeds,	...	1	...	...	...	...	...	1
Bitter Aloes,	...	1	...	1	...	...	...	2
Cocculus Indicus,	...	...	1	...	...	...	1	...
Horse Chestnut,	...	1	...	...	...	...	...	1
Creosote,	1	...	...	...	...	...	1	...
Spirits of Tar (Oil of Tar),	2	1	...	...	...	...	2	1
Nitro-Glycerine,	1	...	...	...	...	...	1	...
Camphor,	...	1	...	...	...	...	...	1
Tobacco,	4	...	1	...	...	...	5	...
Lobelia,	1	...	...	...	...	...	1	...
Fungi,	13	10	...	...	...	...	13	10
Poisonous Weeds,	2	...	...	...	...	...	2	...
Hellebores,	...	...	1	1	...	...	1	1
Kind not stated,	216	158	256	167	3	1	475	326
	2498	1292	1644	1140	23	19	4165	2551
	3790		2784		42		6616	

Although so large a number of substances destroy life by accident or design, yet there are in the list only about 21 which kill about 2 persons or above each year: the 21 substances arranged in the order of their fatality are as follows:—

	Actual deaths in ten years ending 1892.
Caustic potash	19
Poisonous fungi	23
Aconite	59
Mercury	60
Belladonna	76
Sulphuric acid	93
Ammonia	98
Chlorodyne	102
Alcohol	108
Arsenic	110
Chloroform	113
Vermin-killer	127
Chloral	127
Phosphorus	155
Cyanide of potassium	166
Strychnine	201
Nitric acid	204
Prussic acid	260
Carbolic acid	762
Lead	1043
Opiates	1324

In each decade there are changes in the position on the list. The most significant difference between the statistics now given and the statistics for the ten years ending 1880, published in the last edition of this work, is that in the former decade carbolic acid occupied a comparatively insignificant place; whereas in the ten years ending 1892, deaths from carbolic acid poisoning are the most frequent form of fatal poisoning save lead and opiates.

§ 21. The following table gives some German statistics of poisoning:

TABLE SHOWING THE ADMISSIONS INTO VARIOUS MEDICAL INSTITUTIONS[30] IN BERLIN OF PERSONS SUFFERING FROM THE EFFECTS OF POISON DURING THE THREE YEARS 1876, 1877, 1878.

	Males.	Females.	Total.
Charcoal Vapour,	77	78	155
Sulphuric Acid,	24	54	93
Hydrochloric Acid,	4	4	
Nitric Acid, and Aqua Regia,	7	...	
Phosphorus,	13	28	41
Cyanide of Potassium,	29	3	38

[30] Viz., the Königl. Charité, Allg. Städtisches Krankenhaus, Städtisches Baracken-Lazareth, Bethanien, St. Helwög's-Lazarus, Elisabethen-Krankenhaus, Augusta Hospital, and the Institut für Staatsarzneikunde.

Prussic Acid,	5	1	19
Oxalic Acid, and Oxalate of Potash,	11	8	
Alcohol,	12	2	14
Arsenic,	7	5	12
Morphine,	8	1	12
Opium,	2	1	
Potash or Soda Lye,	2	6	8
Chloral,	3	4	7
Chloroform,	4	2	6
Sewer Gas,	5	...	5
Strychnine,	...	4	4
Atropine,	1	2	3
Copper Sulphate,	1	2	3
Nitrobenzol,	2	...	2
Carbolic Acid,	...	2	2
Chromic Acid,	1	1	2
Burnt Alum,	...	1	1
Ammonium Sulphide,	1	...	1
Datura Stramonium,	...	1	1
Petroleum,	...	1	1
Benzine,	1	...	1
Ether,	1	...	1
Prussic Acid and Morphine,	1	...	1
Prussic Acid and Chloral,	1	...	1
Turpentine and Sal Ammoniac,	...	1	1
	223	212	435

Suicidal Poisoning.—Poisons which kill more than one person suicidally each year are only 19 in number, as follows:—

	Deaths from suicide during the ten years ending 1892.
Potassic bichromate	10
Chloroform	14
Chloral	15
Chlorodyne	16
Aconite	19
Belladonna	20
Mercury	24
Nitric acid	27
Ammonia	34
Sulphuric acid	53
Arsenic	77
Phosphorus	84
Vermin-killer	118
Prussic acid	122

Hydrochloric acid	138
Strychnine	150
Oxalic acid	200
Prussic acid	222
Opiates	281
Phenol	290

In the ten years ending 1880, suicidal deaths from vermin-killers, from prussic acid, from cyanide of potassium, and from opiates were all more numerous than deaths from phenol, whereas at present phenol appears to be the poison most likely to be chosen by a suicidal person.

Criminal Poisoning.

§ 22. Some useful statistics of criminal poisoning have been given by Tardieu[31] for the 21 years 1851-1871, which may be summarised as follows:—

Total accusations of Poisoning in the 21 years,			793
Results of the Poisoning:—			
Death,		280	
Illness,		346	- 872
Negative,		246	
Accused:—			
Men,		304	- 703
Women,		399	
Nature of Poison Employed:—			
Arsenic,			287
Phosphorus,			267
Copper -	Sulphate,	120	- 159
	Acetate (Verdigris),	39	
Acids -	Sulphuric Acid,	36	- 47
	Hydrochloric Acid,	8	
	Nitric Acid,	3	
Cantharides,			30
Nux Vomica,		5	- 12
Strychnine,		7	
Opiates -	Opium,	6	- 10
	Laudanum,	3	

[31] *Étude Médico-Légale sur l'Empoisonnement*, Paris, 1875.

	Sedative Water,	1	
Salts of Mercury,			8
Sulphate of Iron,			6
Preparations of Antimony,			5
Ammonia,			4
Cyanides -	Prussic Acid,	2	4
	Cyanide of Potassium,	2	
Hellebore,			3
Datura Stramonium,			3
Powdered Glass,			3
Digitalin,			2
Potash,			2
Sulphate of Zinc,			2
Eau de Javelle (a solution of Hypochlorite of Potash),			1
Tincture of Iodine,			1
Croton Oil,			1
Nicotine,			1
Belladonna,			1
"Baume Fiovarenti,"			1
Euphorbia,			1
Acetate of Lead,			1
Carbonic Acid Gas,			1
Laburnum Seeds,			1
Colchicum,			1
Mushrooms,			1
Sulphuric Ether,			1
Total,			867

It hence may be concluded, according to these statistics of criminal poisoning, that of 1000 attempts in France, either to injure or to destroy human life by poison, the following is the most probable selective order:—

Arsenic,	331
Phosphorus,	301
Preparations of Copper,	183
The Mineral Acids,	54
Cantharides,	35
Strychnine,	14
Opiates,	12
Mercurial preparations,	9
Antimonial preparations,	6
Cyanides (that is, Prussic Acid and Potassic Cyanide),	5
Preparations of Iron,	5

This list accounts for 955 poisonings, and the remaining 45 will be distributed among the less used drugs and chemicals.

IV.—The Connection between Toxic Action and Chemical Composition.

§ 23. Considerable advance has been made of late years in the study of the connection which exists between the chemical structure of the molecule of organic substances and physiological effect. The results obtained, though important, are as yet too fragmentary to justify any great generalisation; the problem is a complicated one, and as Lauder Brunton justly observes:—

"The physiological action of a drug does not depend entirely on its chemical composition nor yet on its chemical structure, so far as that can be indicated even by graphic formula, but upon conditions of solubility, instability, and molecular relations, which we may hope to discover in the future, but with which we are as yet imperfectly acquainted."[32]

The occurrence of hydroxyl, whether the substance belong to the simpler chain carbon series or to the aromatic carbon compounds, appears to usually endow the substance with more or less active and frequently poisonous properties, as, for example, in the alcohols, and as in hydroxylamine. It is also found that among the aromatic bodies the toxic action is likely to increase with the number of hydroxyls: thus phenol has one hydroxyl, resorcin two, and phloroglucin three; and the toxic power is strictly in the same order, for, of the three, phenol is least and phloroglucin most poisonous.

Replacing hydrogen by a halogen, especially by chlorine, in the fatty acids mostly produces substances of narcotic properties, as, for instance, monochloracetic acid. In the sulphur compounds, the entrance of chlorine modifies the physiological action and intensifies toxicity: thus ethyl sulphide $(C_2H_5)_2S$ is a weak poison, monochlorethyl sulphide $C_2H_5C_2H_4ClS$ a strong poison, and dichlorethyl sulphide $C_4H_8Cl_2S$ a very strong poison: the vapour kills rabbits within a short time, and a trace of the oil applied to the ear produces intense inflammation of both the eyes and the ear.[33]

The weight of the molecule has an influence in the alcohols and acids of the fatty series; for instance, ethyl, propyl, butyl, and amyl alcohols show as they increase in carbon a regular increase in toxic power; the narcotic actions of sodium propionate, butyrate, and valerianate also increase with the rising carbon. Nitrogen in the triad condition in the amines is far less poisonous than in the pentad condition.

Bamberger[34] distinguishes two classes of hydrogenised bases derived from α and β naphthylamine, by the terms "acylic" and "aromatic." The acylic contains the four added hydrogens in the amidogen nucleus, the aromatic in the other nucleus, thus

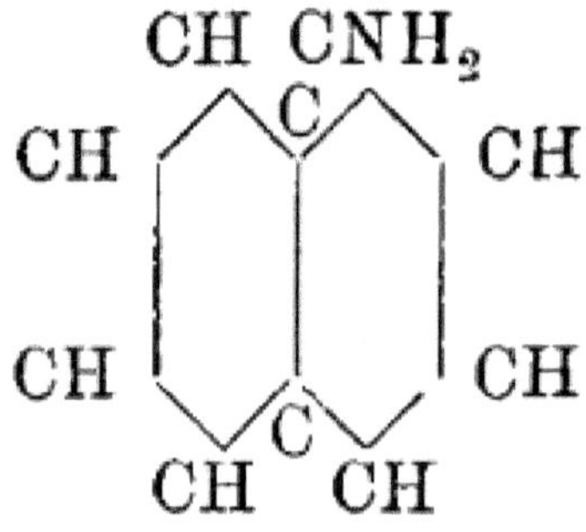

α Naphthylamine.

[32] *Introduction to Modern Therapeutics*, Lond., 1892. 136.
[33] V. Meyer, *Ber. d. Chem. Ges.*, XX., 1725.
[34] *Ber.*, xxii. 777-778.

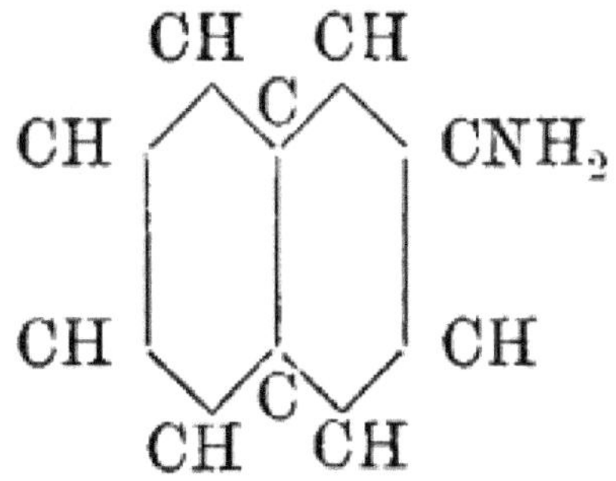

β Naphthylamine.

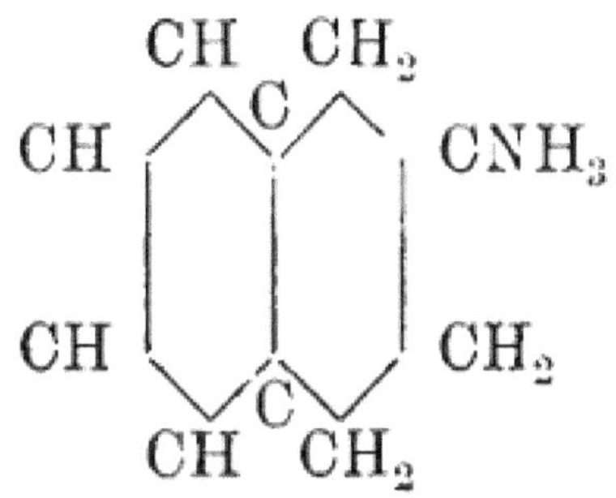

Acylic tetrahydro-α Naphthylamine.

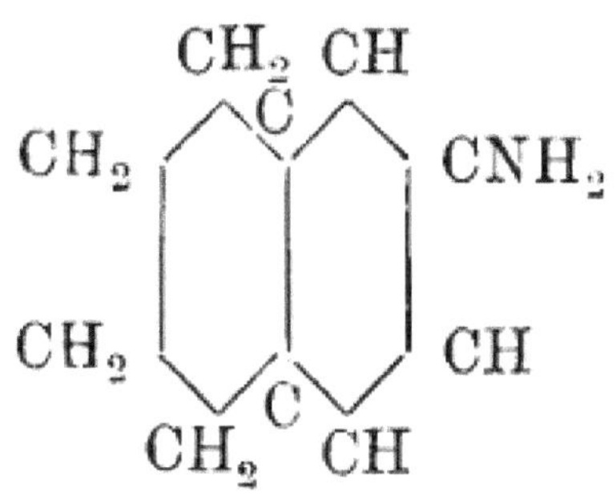

Aromatic tetrahydro-β Naphthylamine.

The acylic β tetrahydro-naphthylamine, the β tetrahydroethylnaphthylamine, and the β tetrahydromethylnaphthylamine all cause dilatation of the pupil and produce symptoms of excitation of the cervical sympathetic nerve; the other members of the group are inactive.

§ 24. The result of replacing hydrogen by alkyls in aromatic bodies has been studied by Schmiedeberg and others; replacing the hydrogen of the amidogen by ethyl or methyl, usually results in a body having a more or less pronounced narcotic action. The rule is that methyl is stronger than ethyl, but it does not always hold good; ortho-amido-phenol is not in itself poisonous, but when two hydrogens of the amidogen group are replaced by two methyls thus—

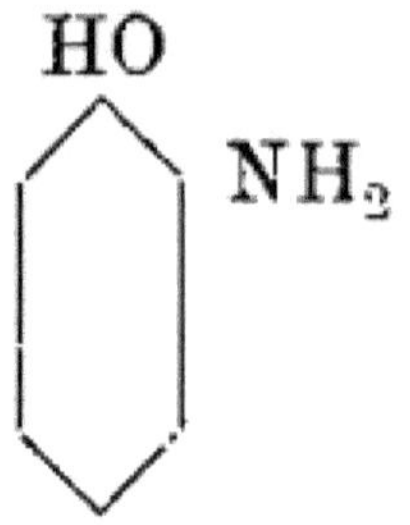

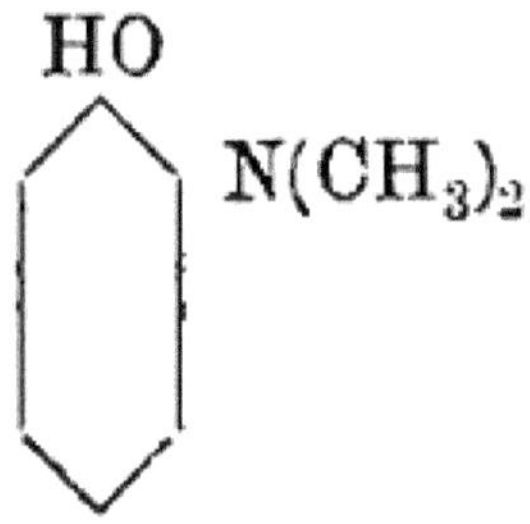

the resulting body has a weak narcotic action.

It would naturally be inferred that the replacement of the H in the hydroxyl by a third methyl would increase this narcotic action, but this is not so: on the other hand, if there are three ethyl groups in the same situation a decidedly narcotic body is produced.

The influence of position of an alkyl in the aromatic bodies is well shown in ortho-, para- and meta-derivatives. Thus the author proved some years ago that with regard to disinfecting properties, ortho-cresol was more powerful than meta-; meta-cresol more powerful than para-; so again ortho-aceto-toluid is poisonous, causing acute nephritis; meta-aceto-toluid has but feeble toxic actions but is useful as an antipyretic; and para-aceto-toluid is inactive.

In the trioxybenzenes, in which there are three hydroxyls, the toxic action is greater when the hydroxyls are consecutive, as in pyrogallol, than when they are symmetrical, as in phloroglucin.

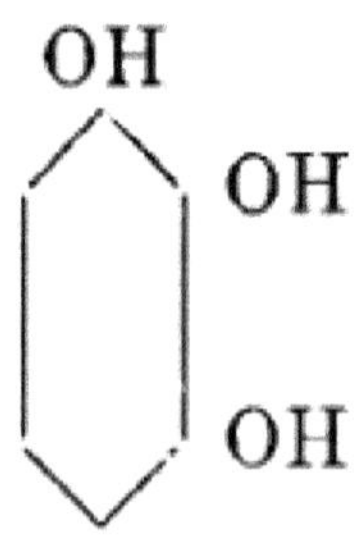

Pyrogallol.

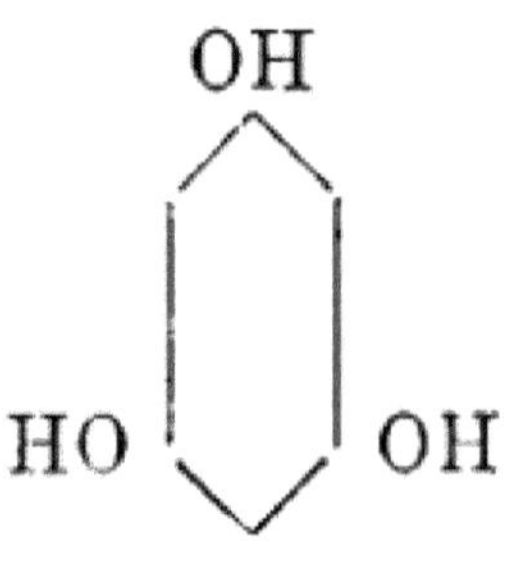

Phloroglucin.

The introduction of methyl into the complicated molecule of an alkaloid often gives curious results: thus methyl strychnine and methyl brucine instead of producing tetanus have an action on voluntary muscle like curare.

Benzoyl-ecgonine has no local anæsthetic action, but the introduction of methyl into the molecule endows it with a power of deadening the sensation of the skin locally; on the other hand, cocethyl produces no effect of this kind.

Drs. Crum Brown and Fraser[35] have suggested that there is some relation between toxicity and the saturated or non-saturated condition of the molecule.

Hinsberg and Treupel have studied the physiological effect of substituting various alkyls for the hydrogen of the hydroxyl group in para-acetamido-phenol.

Para-aceto-amido-phenol when given to dogs in doses of 0.5 grm. for every kilogr. of body weight causes slight narcotic symptoms, with slight paralysis; there is cyanosis and in the blood much methæmoglobin.

In men doses of half a gramme (7.7 grains) act as an antipyretic, relieve neuralgia and have weak narcotic effects.

The following is the result of substituting certain alkyls for H in the HO group.

(1) **Methyl.**—The narcotic action is strengthened and the antipyretic action unaffected. The methæmoglobin in the blood is somewhat less.

(2) **Ethyl.**—Action very similar, but much less methæmoglobin is produced.

(3) **Propyl.**—Antipyretic action a little weaker. Methæmoglobin in the blood smaller than in para-acetamido-phenol, but more than when the methyl or ethyl compound is administered.

(4) **Amyl.**—Antipyretic action decreased.

The smallest amount of toxicity is in the ethyl substitution; while the maximum antipyretic and antineuralgic action belongs to the methyl substitution.

Next substitution was tried in the Imid group. It was found that substituting ethyl for H in the imid group annihilated the narcotic and antipyretic properties. No methæmoglobin could be recognised in the blood.

Lastly, simultaneous substitution of the H of the HO group by ethyl and the substitution of an alkyl for the H in the NH group gave the following results:—

Methyl.—In dogs the narcotic action was strengthened, the methæmoglobin in the blood diminished. In men the narcotic action was also more marked as well as the anti-neural action. The stomach and kidneys were also stimulated.

Ethyl.—In dogs the narcotic action was much strengthened, while the methæmoglobin was diminished. In men the antipyretic and anti-neural actions were unaffected.

Propyl.—In dogs the narcotic action was feebler than with methyl or ethyl, and in men there was diminished antipyretic action.

Amyl.—In dogs the narcotic action was much smaller.

From this latter series the conclusion is drawn that the maximum of narcotic action is obtained by the introduction of methyl and the maximum antipyretic action by the introduction of methyl or ethyl. The ethyl substitution is, as before, the less toxic.[36]

The effect of the entrance of an alkyl into the molecule of a substance is not constant; sometimes the action of the poison is weakened, sometimes strengthened. Thus, according to Stolnikow, dimethyl resorcin, $C_6H_4(OCH_3)_2$, is more poisonous than resorcin $C_6H_4(OH)_2$. Anisol $C_6H_5OCH_3$, according to Loew, is more poisonous to algæ, bacteria, and infusoria than phenol C_6H_5OH. On the other hand, the replacement by methyl of an atom of hydrogen in the aromatic oxyacids weakens their action; methyl salicylic acid $C_6H_4<^{O.CH_3}_{COOH}$ is weaker than salicylic acid $C_6H_4<^{OH}_{COOH}$.

Arsen-methyl chloride, $As(CH_3)Cl_2$, is strongly poisonous, but the introduction of a second methyl $As(CH_3)_2Cl$

[35] *Journ. Anat. and Phys.*, vol. ii. 224.

[36] *Ueber die physiologische Wirkung des p-amido-phenol u. einiger Derivate desselben.* O. Hinsberg u. G. Treupel, *Archiv f. Exp. Pathol. u. Pharm.*, B. 33, S. 216.

makes a comparatively weak poison.

§ 25. In some cases the increase of CO groups weakens the action of a poison; thus, in allantoin there are three carbonyl (CO) groups; this substance does not produce excitation of the spinal cord, but it heightens muscular irritability and causes, like xanthin, muscular rigidity; alloxantin, with a similar structure but containing six carbonyl groups, does not possess this action.

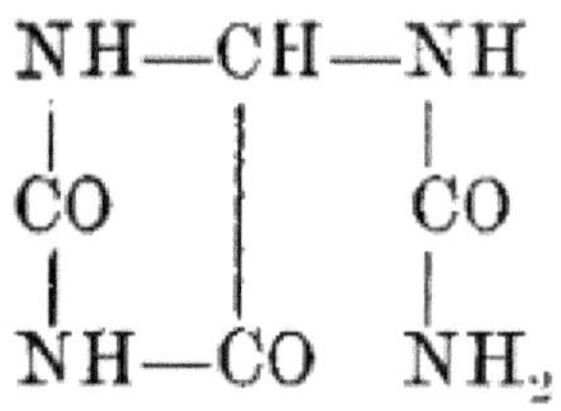

Allantoin.

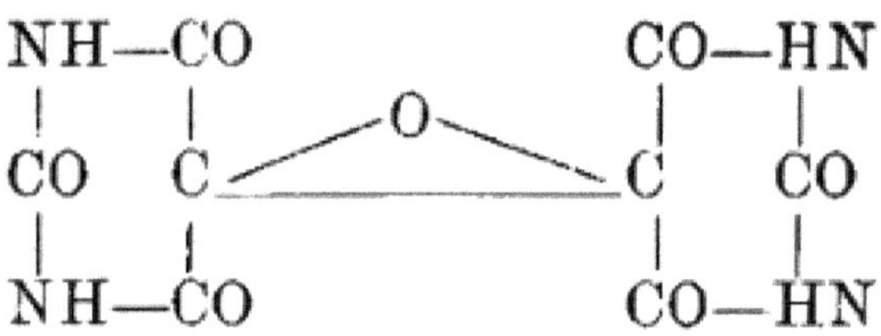

Alloxantin.

§ 26. A theory of general application has been put forward and supported with great ability by Oscar Loew[37] which explains the action of poisons by presuming that living has a different composition to dead albumin; the albumin of the chemist is a dead body of a definite composition and has a stable character; living albumin, such as circulates in the blood or forms the protoplasm of the tissues, is not "stable" but "labile"; Loew says:—"If the old idea is accepted that living albumin is chemically the same substance as that which is dead, numerous toxic phenomena are inexplicable. It is impossible, for instance, to explain how it is that diamide N_2H_4 and hydroxylamine NH_2OH are toxic, even with great dilution, on all living animals; whilst neither of those substances have the smallest action on dead plasma or the ordinary dissolved passive albumin, there must therefore be present in the albumin of the living plasma a grouping of atoms in a "*labile*" condition (*Atomgruppirungen labiler Art*) which are capable of entering into reactions; such, according to our present knowledge, can only be the aldehyde and the ketone groups. The first mentioned groups are more labile and react in far greater dilution than the latter groups."

Loew considers that all substances which enter into combination with aldehyde or ketone groups must be poisonous to life generally. For instance, hydroxylamine, diamide and its derivatives, phenylhydrazine, free ammonia, phenol, prussic acid, hydric sulphide, sulphur dioxide and the acid sulphites all enter into combination with aldehyde.

So again the formation of imide groups in the aromatic ring increases any poisonous properties the original substance possesses, because the imide group easily enters into combination with aldehyde; thus piperidine $(CH_2)_5NH$ is more poisonous than pyridine $(CH)_5N$; coniine $NH(CH_2)_4CH\text{-}CH_2\text{-}CH_2CH_3$, is more poisonous than collidine $N(CH)_4C\text{-}CH\text{-}(CH_3)_2$; pyrrol $(CH)_4NH$ than pyridine $(CH)_5N$; and amarin,[38]

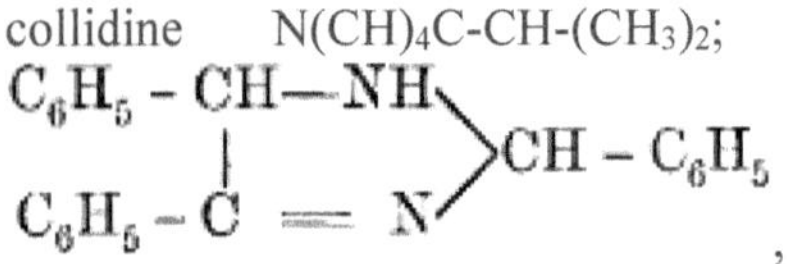

, than hydrobenzamide

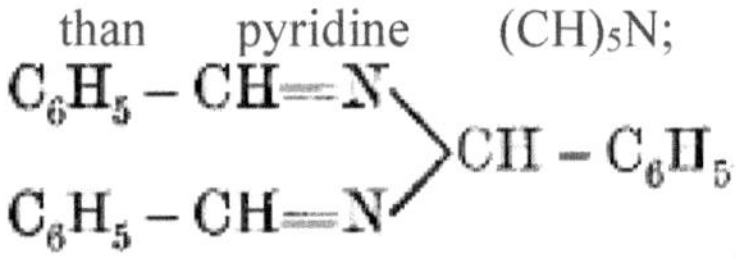

.

[37] *Ein natürliches System der Gift-Wirkungen*, München, 1893.

[38] Th. Weyl (*Lehrbuch der organischen Chemie*) states (p. 385) that amarin is not poisonous, but Baccheti (*Jahr. d. Chemie*, 1855) has shown that 250 mgrms. of the acetate will kill a dog, 80 mgrms. a guinea-pig; and that it is poisonous to fishes, birds, and frogs: hydrobenzamide in the same doses has no effect.

If the theory is true, then substances with "labile" amido groups, on the one hand, must increase in toxic activity if a second amido group is introduced; and, on the other, their toxic qualities must be diminished if the amido group is changed into an imido group by the substitution of an atom of hydrogen for an alkyl.

Observation has shown that both of these requirements are satisfied; phenylenediamine is more poisonous than aniline; toluylenediamine more poisonous than toluidine. Again, if an atom of hydrogen in the amido (NH_2) group in aniline be replaced by an alkyl, *e.g.* methyl or ethyl, the resulting substance does not produce muscular spasm; but if the same alkyl is substituted for an atom of hydrogen in the benzene nucleus the convulsive action remains unaffected.

If an acidyl, as for example the radical of acetic acid, enter into the amido group, then the toxic action is notably weakened; thus, acetanilide is weaker than aniline, and acetylphenylhydrazine is weaker than phenylhydrazine. If the hydrogen of the imido group be replaced by an alkyl or an acid radical, and therefore tertiary bound nitrogen restored, the poisonous action is also weakened.

In xanthin there are three imido groups; the hydrogen of two of these groups is replaced by methyl in theobromin; and in caffein the three hydrogens of the three imido groups are replaced by three methyls, thus:—

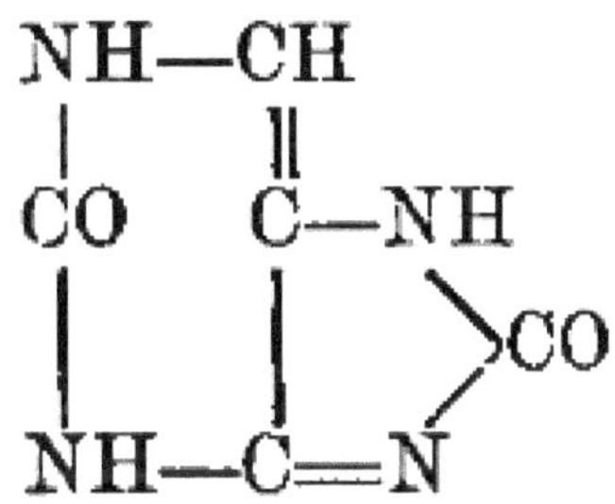

Xanthin.

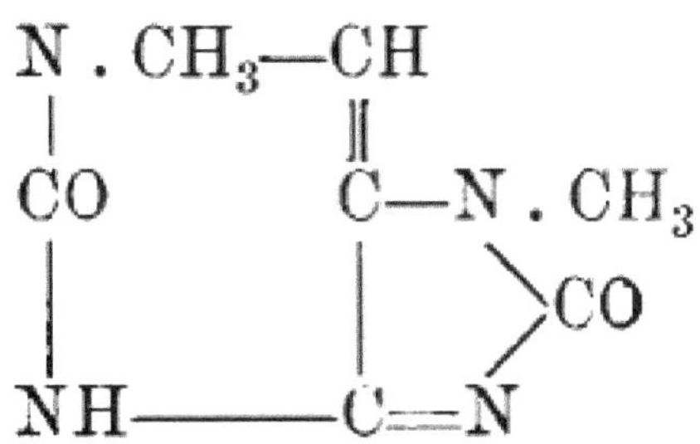

Theobromin.

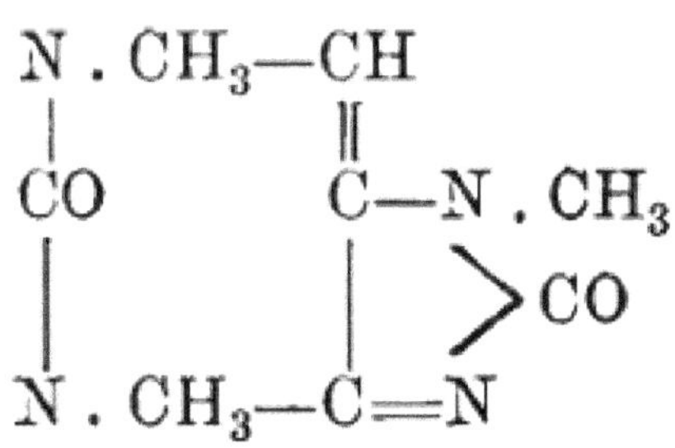

Caffein.

and experiment has shown that theobromin is weaker than xanthin, and caffein still weaker than theobromin.

Loew[39] makes the following generalisations:—

1. Entrance of the carboxyl or sulpho groups weakens toxic action.

2. Entrance of a chlorine atom exalts the toxic character of the catalytic poisons (Loew's catalytic poisons are alcohols, ether, chloroform, chloral, carbon tetrachloride, methylal, carbon disulphide and volatile hydrocarbons).

3. Entrance of hydroxyl groups in the catalytic poisons of the fatty series weakens toxic character; on the other hand, it exalts the toxicity of the substituting poisons. (Examples of Loew's class of "substituting" poisons are hydroxylamine, phenylhydrazine, hydric cyanide, hydric sulphide, aldehyde, and the phenols.)

4. A substance increases in poisonous character through every influence which increases its power of reaction with aldehyde or amido groups. If, for example, an amido or imido group in the poison molecule be made more "labile," or if thrice linked nitrogen is converted into nitrogen connected by two bands, whether through addition of water or transposition (*umlagerung*) or if a second amido group enters, the poisonous quality is increased. Presence of a negative group may modify the action.

5. Entrance of a nitro group strengthens the poisonous character. If a carboxyl or a sulpho group is present in the molecule, or if, in passing through the animal body, negative groups combine with the poison molecule, or carboxyl groups are formed in the said molecule; in such cases the poisonous character of the nitro group may not be apparent.

6. Substances with double carbon linkings are more poisonous than the corresponding saturated substances. Thus neurine with the double linking of the carbon of CH_2 is more poisonous than choline; vinylamine than ethylamine.

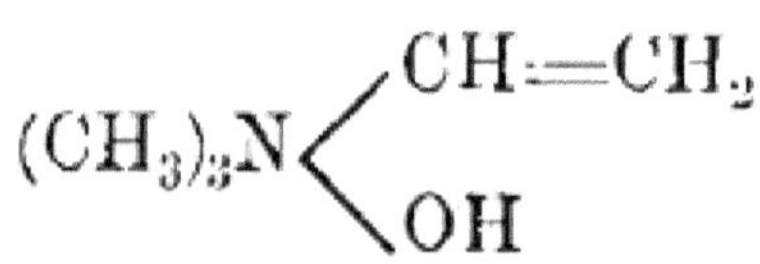

Neurine.

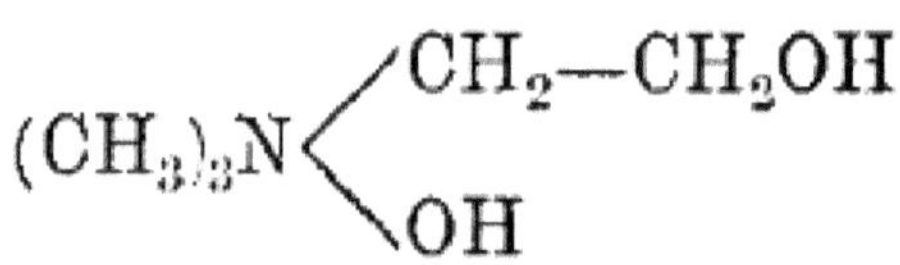

Choline.

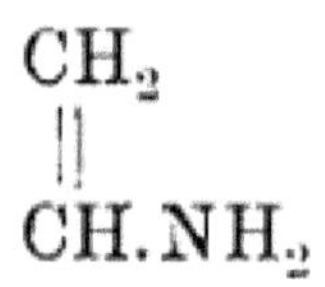

Vinylamine.

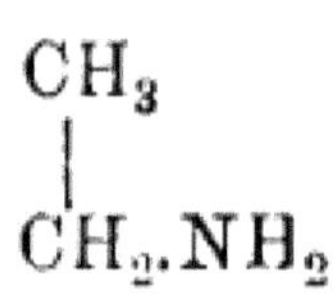

Ethylamine.

§ 27. M. Ch. Michet[40] has investigated the comparative toxicity of the metals by experiments on fish, using

[39] *Ein natürliches System der Gift-Wirkungen*, München, 1893.

[40] "*De la Toxicité comparée des différents Métaux.*" *Note de M. Ch. Michet. Compt. Rend.*, t. xciii., 1881, p. 649.

species of *Serranus*, *Crenolabrus*, and *Julius*. The chloride of the metal was dissolved in water and diluted until just that strength was attained in which the fish would live 48 hours; this, when expressed in grammes per litre, he called "*the limit of toxicity*."

The following is the main result of the inquiry, by which it will be seen that there was found no relation between "the limit of toxicity" and the atomic weight.

TABLE SHOWING THE RESULTS OF EXPERIMENTS ON FISH.

No. of Experiments.	Metal.	Limit of Toxicity.
20.	Mercury,	.00029
7.	Copper,	.0033
20.	Zinc,	.0084
10.	Iron,	.014
7.	Cadmium,	.017
6.	Ammonium,	.064
7.	Potassium,	.10
10.	Nickel,	.126
9.	Cobalt,	.126
11.	Lithium,	.3
20.	Manganese	.30
6.	Barium,	.78
4.	Magnesium,	1 .5
20.	Strontium,	2 .2
5.	Calcium,	2 .4
6.	Sodium,	24 .17

V.—Life-Tests; or the Identification of Poison by Experiments on Animals.

§ 28. A philosophical investigation of poisons demands a complete methodical examination into their action on every life form, from the lowest to the highest. Our knowledge is more definite with regard to the action of poisons on man, dogs, cats, rabbits, and frogs than on any other species. It may be convenient here to make a few general remarks as to the action of poisons on infusoria, the cephalopoda, and insects.

Infusoria.—The infusoria are extremely sensitive to the poisonous alkaloids and other chemical agents. Strong doses of the alkaloids cause a contraction of the cell contents, and somewhat rapid disintegration of the whole body; moderate doses at first quicken the movements, then the body gets perceptibly larger, and finally, as in the first case, there is disintegration of the animal substance.

Rossbach[41] gives the following intimations of the proportion of the toxic principle necessary to cause death:—Strychnine 1 part dissolved in 1500 of water; veratrine 1 in 8000; quinine 1 in 5000; atropine 1 in 1000; the mineral acids 1 in 400-600; salts 1 in 200-300.

The extraordinary sensitiveness of the infusoria, and the small amount of material used in such experiments, would be practically useful if there were any decided difference in the symptoms produced by different poisons. But no one could be at all certain of even the class to which the poison belongs were he to watch, without a previous knowledge of what had been added to the water, the motions of poisoned infusoria. Hence the fact is more curious than useful.

Cephalopoda.—The action of a few poisons on the cephalopoda has been investigated by M. E. Yung.[42] Curara placed on the skin had no effect, but on the branchiæ led to general paralysis. If given in even fifteen times a greater dose than necessary to kill a rabbit, it was not always fatal. Strychnine, dissolved in sea-water, in the proportion of

[41] N. J. Rossbach, *Pharm. Zeitschr. für Russland*, xix. 628.

[42] *Compt. Rend.*, t. xci. p. 306.

1 to 30,000, causes most marked symptoms. The first sign is relaxation of the chromataphore muscle and the closing of the chromataphores; the animal pales, the respiratory movements become more powerful, and at the end of a notable augmentation in their number, they fall rapidly from the normal number of 25 to 5 a minute. Then tetanus commences after a time, varying with the dose of the poison; the arm stiffens and extends in fan-like form, the entire body is convulsed, the respiration is in jerks, the animal empties his pouch, and at the end of a few minutes is dead, in a state of great muscular rigidity. If at this moment it is opened, the venous heart is found still beating. Nicotine and other poisons were experimented with, and the cephalopoda were found to be generally sensitive to the active alkaloids, and to exhibit more or less marked symptoms.

Insects.—The author devoted considerable time, in the autumn of 1882, to observations on the effect of certain alkaloids on the common blow-fly, thinking it possible that the insect would exhibit a sufficient series of symptoms of physiological phenomena to enable it to be used by the toxicologist as a living reagent. If so, the cheapness and ubiquity of the tiny life during a considerable portion of the year would recommend it for the purpose. Provided two blow-flies are caught and placed beneath glass shades—the one poisoned, the other not—it is surprising what a variety of symptoms can, with a little practice, be distinguished. Nevertheless, the absence of pupils, and the want of respiratory and cardiac movements, are, in an experimental point of view, defects for which no amount or variety of merely muscular symptoms can compensate.

From the nature of the case, we can only distinguish in the poisoned fly dulness or vivacity of movement, loss of power in walking on smooth surfaces, irritation of the integument, disorderly movements of the limbs, protrusion of the fleshy proboscis, and paralysis, whether of legs or wings. My experiments were chiefly made by smearing the extracts or neutral solutions of poisons on the head of the fly. In this way some of it is invariably taken into the system, partly by direct absorption, and partly by the insect's efforts to free itself from the foreign substance, in which it uses its legs and proboscis. For the symptoms witnessed after the application of saponin, digitalin, and aconitine, the reader is referred to the articles on those substances.

In poisoning by sausages, bad meat, curarine, and in obscure cases generally, in the present state of science, experiments on living animals are absolutely necessary. In this, and in this way only, in very many instances, can the expert prove the presence of zymotic, or show the absence of chemical poison.

The Vivisection Act, however, effectually precludes the use of life-tests in England save in licensed institutions. Hence the "methods" of applying life-tests described in former editions will be omitted.

§ 29. **Effect of poisons on the heart of Cold-blooded Animals.**—The Vivisection Act does not, however, interfere with the use of certain living tests, such, for instance, as the testing of the action of poisons upon the recently extirpated hearts of cold-blooded animals.

The heart of the frog, of the turtle, of the tortoise, and of the shark will beat regularly for a long time after removal from the body, if supplied with a regular stream of nutrient fluid. The fluids used for this purpose are the blood of the herbivora diluted with common salt solution, or a serum albumin solution, or a 2 per cent. solution of gum arabic in which red blood corpuscles are suspended. The simplest apparatus to use is that known as "Williams'." Williams' apparatus consists of two glass bulbs (see diagram), the one, P, containing nutrient fluid to which a known quantity of the poison has been added; the other, N, containing the same fluid but to which no poison has been added; these bulbs are connected by caoutchouc tubing to a three-way tube, T, and each piece of caoutchouc tubing has a pressure screw clip, V^1 and V; the three-way tube is connected with a wider tube containing a valve float, F, which gives free passage of fluid in one direction only, that is, in the direction of the arrow; this last wide tube is connected with a Y piece of tubing, which again is connected with the aorta of the heart under examination, the other leg of the Y tube is connected with another wide tube, X, having a float valve, F^2: the float containing a drop of mercury and permitting (like the float valve F) passage in one direction only of fluid, it is obvious that if the clip communicating with N is opened and the clip communicating with P is closed, the normal fluid will circulate alone through the heart; if, on the other hand, the P clip is open and the N clip closed, the poisoned blood will alone feed the heart. It is also clear that by raising or depressing the bulbs, the circulating fluid can be delivered at any pressure, high or low. Should a bubble of air get into the tubes, it can be got rid of by removing the cork at S and bringing the fluid up to the level of the top of the aperture. The observation is made by first ascertaining the number and character of the beats when the normal fluid is circulating, and then afterwards when the normal is replaced by the poisoned fluid. A simpler but less accurate process is to pith two frogs, excise their respective hearts, and place the hearts in watch-glasses containing either serum or a solution of common salt (strength 0.75 per cent.); to the one heart is now added a solution of the poison under examination, and the difference in the behaviour and character of the beats noted.

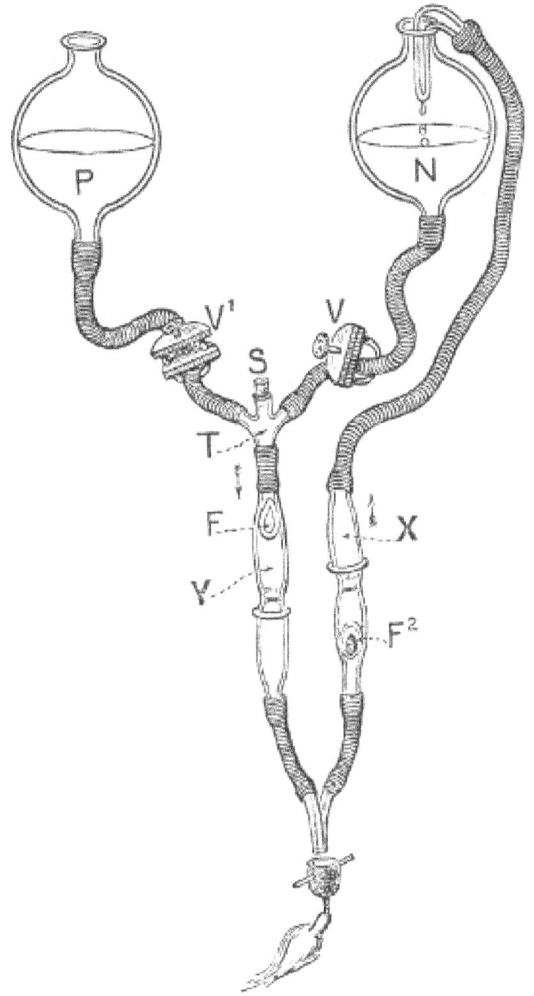

Williams' Apparatus.

The phenomena to be specially looked for are the following:—

1. The heart at the height of the poisoning is arrested in diastole.
2. The heart at the height of the poisoning is arrested in systole.

Arrest in diastole.—The arrest may be preceded by the contractions becoming weaker and weaker, or after the so-called heart peristalsis; or it may be preceded by a condition in which the auricle shows a different frequency to the ventricle.

The final diastole may be the diastole of paralysis or the diastole of irritation.

The diastole of irritation is produced by a stimulus of the inhibitory ganglia, and only occurs after poisoning by the muscarine group of poisons. This condition may be recognised by the fact that contraction may be excited by mechanical and electrical stimuli or by the application of atropine solution; the latter paralyses the inhibitory nervous centres, and therefore sets the mechanism going again. The diastole of paralysis is the most frequent form of death. It may readily be distinguished from the muscarine diastole; for, in muscarine diastole, the heart is full of blood and larger than normal; but in the paralytic form the heart is not fully extended, besides which, although, if normal blood replace that which is poisoned, the beats may be restored for a short time, the response is incomplete, and the end is the same; besides which, atropine does not restore the beats. The diastole of paralysis may depend on paralysis of the so-called excito-motor ganglia (as with iodal), or from paralysis of the muscular structure (as with copper).

§ 30. **The effect of poisons on the iris.**—Several poisons affect the pupil, causing either contraction or dilatation. The most suitable animal is the cat; the pupil of the cat readily showing either state.

Toxic myosis, or toxic contraction of the pupil.—There are two forms of toxic myosis, one of which is central in its origin. In this form, should the poison be applied to the eye itself, no marked contraction follows; the poison must be swallowed or injected subcutaneously to produce an effect. The contraction remains until death.

The contraction in such a case is considered to be due to a paralysis of the dilatation centre; it is a "*myosis paralytica centralis*;" the best example of this is the contraction of the pupil caused by morphine.

In the second case the poison, whether applied direct to the eye or entering the circulation by subcutaneous injection, contracts the pupil; the contraction persists if the eye is extirpated, but in all cases the contraction may be changed into dilatation by the use of atropine. An example of this kind of myosis is the action of muscarine. It is dependent on the stimulation of the ends of the nerves which contract the pupil, especially the ends of the *nervus oculomotorius* supplying the sphincter iridis; this form of myosis is called *myosis spastica periphera*. A variety of this form is the *myosis spastica muscularis*, depending on stimulation of the musc. sphincter iridis, seen in poisoning by physostigmine. This causes strong contraction of the pupil when locally applied; the contraction is not influenced by small local applications of atropine, but it may be changed to dilatation by high doses. Subcutaneous injection of small doses of physostigmine does not alter the pupil, but large poisonous doses contracts the pupil in a marked manner.

Toxic mydriasis, or toxic dilatation of the pupil.—The following varieties are to be noticed:—

1. Toxic doses taken by the mouth or given by subcutaneous injection give rise to strong dilatation; this vanishes before death, giving place to moderate contraction. This form is due to stimulation of the dilatation centre, later passing into paralysis. An example is found in the action of aconite.

2. After subcutaneous or local application, a dilatation neutralised by physostigmine in moderate doses. This is characteristic of β-tetrahydronaphthylamine.

3. After subcutaneous injection, or if applied locally in very small doses, dilatation occurs persisting to death. Large doses of physostigmine neutralise the dilatation, but it is not influenced by muscarine or pilocarpine: this form is characteristic of atropine, and it has been called *mydriasis paralytica periphera*.

The heart at the height of the poisoning stops in systole.

2. Arrest in systole.—The systole preceding the arrest is far stronger than normal, the ventricle often contracting up into a little lump. Contraction of this kind is specially to be seen in poisoning by digitalis. In poisoning by digitalis the ventricle is arrested before the auricle; in muscarine poisoning the auricle stops before the ventricle. If the reservoir of Williams' apparatus is raised so as to increase the pressure within the ventricle the beat may be restored for a time, to again cease.

A frog's heart under the influence of any poison may be finally divided into pieces so as to ascertain if any parts still contract; the significance of this is, that the particular ganglion supplying that portion of the heart has not been affected: the chief ganglia to be looked for are Remak's, on the boundary of the sinus and auricle; Ludwig's, on the auricle and the septum of the auricle; Bidder's, on the atrioventricular border, especially in the valves; and Dogiel's ganglion, between the muscular fibres. According to Dogiel, poisons acting like muscarine affect every portion of the heart, and atropine restores the contractile power of every portion.

VI.—General Method of Procedure in Searching for Poison.

§ 31. Mineral substances, or liquids containing only inorganic matters, can cause no possible difficulty to any one who is practised in analytical investigation; but the substances which exercise the skill of the expert are organic fluids or solids.

The first thing to be done is to note accurately the manner in which the samples have been packed, whether the seals have been tampered with, whether the vessels or wrappers themselves are likely to have contaminated the articles sent; and then to make a very careful observation of the appearance, smell, colour, and reaction of the matters, not forgetting to take the weight, if solid—the volume, if liquid. All these are obvious precautions, requiring no particular directions.

If the object of research is the stomach and its contents, the contents should be carefully transferred to a tall conical glass; the organ cut open, spread out on a sheet of glass, and examined minutely by a lens, picking out any suspicious-looking substance for closer observation. The mucous membrane should now be well cleansed by the aid of a wash-bottle, and if there is any necessity for destroying the stomach, it may be essential in important cases to have it photographed. The washings having been added to the contents of the stomach, the sediment is separated and submitted to inspection, for it must be remembered that, irrespective of the discovery of poison, a knowledge of the nature of the food last eaten by the deceased may be of extreme value.

If the death has really taken place from disease, and not from poison, or if it has been caused by poison, and yet no definite hint of the particular poison can be obtained either by the symptoms or by the attendant circumstances, the analyst has the difficult task of endeavouring to initiate a process of analysis which will be likely to discover any poison in the animal, vegetable, or mineral kingdom. For this purpose I have devised the following process, which differs from those that have hitherto been published mainly in the prominence given to operations in a high vacuum, and the utilisation of biological experiment as a matter of routine. Taking one of the most difficult cases that can occur—viz., one in which a small quantity only of an organic solid or fluid is available—the best method of procedure is the following:—

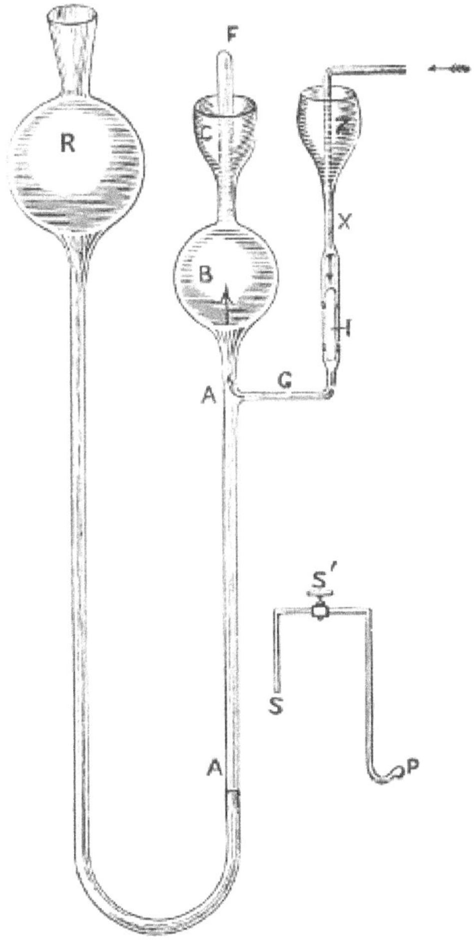

A small portion is reserved and examined microscopically, and, if thought desirable, submitted to various "cultivation" experiments. The greater portion is at once examined for volatile matters, and having been placed in a strong flask, and, if neutral or alkaline, feebly acidulated with tartaric acid, connected with a second or receiving flask by glass tubing and caoutchouc corks. The caoutchouc cork of the receiving flask has a double perforation, so as to be able, by a second bit of angle tubing, to be connected with the mercury-pump described in the author's work on "Foods," the figure of which is here repeated (see the accompanying figure). With a good water-pump having a sufficient length of fall-tube, a vacuum may be also obtained that for practical purposes is as efficient as one caused by mercury; if the fall-tube delivers outside the laboratory over a drain, no offensive odour is experienced when dealing with putrid, stinking liquids. A vacuum having been obtained, and the receiving-flask surrounded with ice, a distillate for preliminary testing may be generally got without the action of any external heat; but if this is too slow, the flask containing the substances or liquid under examination may be gently heated by a water-bath—water, volatile oils, a variety of volatile substances, such as prussic acid, hydrochloric acid, phosphorus, &c., if present, will distil over. It will be well to free in this way the substance, as much as possible, from volatile matters and water. When no more will come over, the distillate may be carefully examined by redistillation and the various appropriate tests.

The next step is to dry the sample thoroughly. This is best effected also in a vacuum by the use of the same apparatus, only this time the receiving-flask is to be half filled with strong sulphuric acid. By now applying very gentle heat to the first flask, and cooling the sulphuric acid receiver, even such substances as the liver in twenty-four hours may be obtained dry enough to powder.

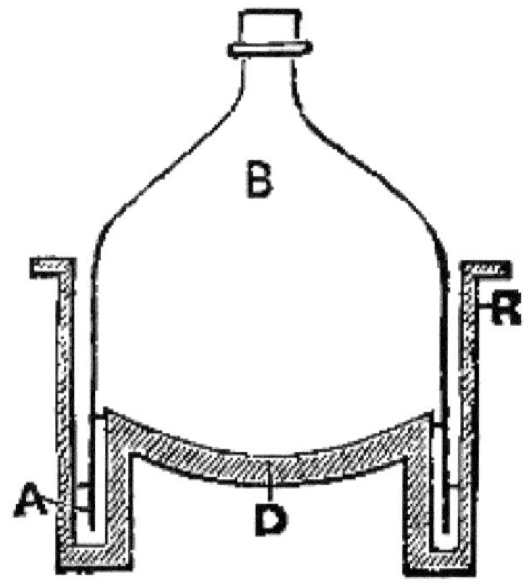

This figure is from "Foods." B is a bell-jar, which can be adapted by a cork to a condenser; R is made of iron; the rim of the bell-jar is immersed in mercury, which the deep groove receives.

Having by these means obtained a nearly dry friable mass, it is reduced to a coarse powder, and extracted with petroleum ether; the extraction may be effected either in a special apparatus (as, for example, in a large "Soxhlet"), or in a beaker placed in the "Ether recovery apparatus" (see fig.), which is adapted to an upright condenser. The petroleum extract is evaporated and leaves the fatty matter, possibly contaminated by traces of any alkaloid which the substance may have contained; for, although most alkaloids are insoluble in petroleum ether, yet they are taken up in small quantities by oils and fats, and are extracted with the fat by petroleum ether. It is hence necessary always to examine the petroleum extract by shaking it up with water, slightly acidulated with sulphuric acid, which will extract from the fat any trace of alkaloid, and will permit the discovery of such alkaloids by the ordinary "group reagents."

The substance now being freed for the most part from water and from fat, is digested in the cold with absolute alcohol for some hours; the alcohol is filtered off, and allowed to evaporate spontaneously, or, if speed is an object, it may be distilled *in vacuo*. The treatment is next with hot alcohol of 90 per cent., and, after filtering, the dry residue is exhausted with ether. The ether and alcohol, having been driven off, leave extracts which may be dissolved in water and tested, both chemically and biologically, for alkaloids, glucosides, and organic acids. It must also be remembered that there are a few metallic compounds (as, for example, corrosive sublimate) which are soluble in alcohol and ethereal solvents, and must not be overlooked.

The residue, after being thus acted upon successively by petroleum, by alcohol, and by ether, is both water-free and fat-free, and also devoid of all organic poisonous bases and principles, and it only remains to treat it for metals. For this purpose, it is placed in a retort, and distilled once or twice to dryness with a known quantity of strong, pure hydrochloric acid.

If arsenic, in the form of arsenious acid, were present, it would distil over as a trichloride, and be detected in the distillate; by raising the heat, the organic matter is carbonised, and most of it destroyed. The distillate is saturated with hydric sulphide, and any precipitate separated and examined. The residue in the retort will contain the fixed metals, such as zinc, copper, lead, &c. It is treated with dilute hydrochloric acid, filtered, the filtrate saturated with SH_2 and any precipitate collected. The filtrate is now treated with sufficient sodic acetate to replace the hydric chloride, again saturated with SH_2 and any precipitate collected and tested for *zinc*, *nickel*, and *cobalt*. By this treatment, viz.:—

1. Distillation in a vacuum at a low temperature,
2. Collecting the volatile products,
3. Dehydrating the organic substances,
4. Dissolving out from the dry mass fatty matters and alkaloids, glucosides, &c., by ethereal and alcoholic solvents,
5. Destroying organic matter and searching for metals,

—a very fair and complete analysis may be made from a small amount of material. The process is, however, somewhat faulty in reference to phosphorus, and also to oxalic acid and the oxalates; these poisons, if suspected, should be specially searched for in the manner to be more particularly described in the sections treating of them. In most cases, there is sufficient material to allow of division into three parts—one for organic poisons generally, one for inorganic, and a third for reserve in case of accident. When such is the case, although, for organic principles, the process of vacuum distillation just described still holds good, it will be very much the most convenient way not to use that portion for metals, but to operate on the portion reserved for the inorganic poisons as follows by destruction of the organic matter.

The destruction of organic matter through simple distillation by means of pure hydrochloric acid is at least equal to that by sulphuric acid, chlorate of potash, and the carbonisation methods. The object of the chemist not being to dissolve every fragment of cellular tissue, muscle, and tendon, but simply all mineral ingredients, the less organic matter which goes into solution the better. That hydrochloric acid would fail to dissolve sulphate of baryta and sulphate of lead, and that sulphide of arsenic is also almost insoluble in the acid, is no objection to the process recommended, for it is always open to the analyst to treat the residue specially for these substances. The sulphides precipitated by hydric sulphide from an acid solution are—arsenic, antimony, tin, cadmium, lead, bismuth, mercury, copper, and silver. Those not precipitated are—iron, manganese, zinc, nickel, and cobalt.

As a rule, one poison alone is present; so that if there should be a sulphide, it will belong only exceptionally to more than one metal.

The colour of the precipitate from hydric sulphide is either yellowish or black. The yellow and orange precipitates are sulphur, sulphides of arsenic, antimony, tin, and cadmium. In pure solutions they may be almost distinguished by their different hues, but in solutions contaminated by a little organic matter the colours may not be distinctive. The sulphide of arsenic is of a pale yellow colour; and if the very improbable circumstance should happen that arsenic, antimony, and cadmium occur in the same solution, the sulphide of arsenic may be first separated by ammonia, and the sulphide of antimony by sulphide of sodium, leaving cadmic sulphide insoluble in both processes.

The black precipitates are—lead, bismuth, mercury, copper, and silver. The black sulphide is freed from arsenic, if present, by ammonia, and digested with dilute nitric acid, which will dissolve all the sulphides, save those of mercury and tin, so that if a complete solution is obtained (sulphur flocks excepted), it is evident that both these substances are absent. The presence of copper is betrayed by the blue colour of the nitric acid solution, and through its special reactions; lead, by the deep yellow precipitate which falls by the addition of chromate of potash and acetate of soda to the solution; bismuth, through a white precipitate on dilution with water. If the nitric acid leaves a black insoluble residue, this is probably sulphide of mercury, and should be treated with concentrated hydrochloric acid to separate flocks of sulphur, evaporated to dryness, again dissolved, and tested for mercury by iodide of potassium, copper foil, &c., as described in the article on *Mercury*. Zinc, nickel, and cobalt are likewise tested for in the filtrate as described in the respective articles on these metals.

AUTENRIETH'S GENERAL PROCESS.

§ 32. A general method of procedure has been published by W. Autenrieth.[43]

He divides poisonous substances, for the purposes of separation and detection, into three classes:—

I. Poisons capable of distillation from an acid aqueous solution.
II. Organic substances which are not capable of distillation from acid solutions.
III. Metallic poisons.

[43] *Kurze Anleitung zur Auffindung der Gifte*, Freiburg, 1892.

Where possible, the fluid or solids submitted to the research are divided into four equal parts, one of the parts to be kept in reserve in case of accident or as a control; one of the remaining three parts to be distilled; a second to be investigated for organic substances; and a third for metals. After the extraction of organic substances from part No. II. the residue may be added to No. III. for the purpose of search after metals; and, if the total quantity is small, the whole of the process may be conducted without division.

I. SUBSTANCES SEPARATED BY DISTILLATION.

The substances are placed in a capacious flask, diluted if necessary with water to the consistence of a thin soup, and tartaric acid added to distinct acid reaction, and distilled.

In this way phosphorus, prussic acid, carbolic acid, chloroform, chloral hydrate, nitrobenzol, aniline,[44] and alcohol may be separated and identified by the reactions given in the sections of this work describing those substances.

II. ORGANIC POISONS NOT VOLATILE IN ACID SOLUTION.

Part No. II. is mixed with double its volume of absolute alcohol, tartaric acid added to distinct acid reaction and placed in a flask connected with an inverted Liebig's condenser; it is then warmed for 15 to 20 minutes on the water-bath. After cooling, the mixture is filtered, the residue well washed with alcohol and evaporated to a thin syrup in a porcelain dish over the water-bath. The dish is then allowed to cool and digested with 100 c.c. of water; fat and resinous matters separate, the watery solution is filtered through Swedish paper previously moistened: if the fluid filtrate is clear it may be at once shaken up with ether, but if not clear, and especially if it is more or less slimy, it is evaporated again on the water-bath to the consistence of an extract: the extract treated with 60 to 80 c.c. of absolute alcohol (which precipitates mucus and dextrin-like substances), the alcohol evaporated off and the residue taken up with from 60 to 80 c.c. of distilled water; it is then shaken up with ether, as in Dragendorff's process, and such substances as digitalin, picric acid, salicylic acid, antipyrin and others separated in this way and identified.

After this treatment with ether, and the separation of the ether extract, the watery solution is strongly alkalised with caustic soda and shaken up again with ether, which dissolves almost every alkaloid save morphine and apomorphine; the ethereal extract is separated and any alkaloid left identified by suitable tests.

The aqueous solution, now deprived of substances soluble in ether both from acid and from solutions made alkaline by soda, is now investigated for morphine and apomorphine; the apomorphine being separated by first acidifying a portion of the alkaline solution with hydrochloric acid, then alkalising with ammonia and shaking out with ether. The morphine is separated from the same solution by shaking out with warm chloroform.[45]

III. METALS.

The substances are placed in a porcelain dish and diluted with a sufficient quantity of water to form a thin soup and 20 to 30 c.c. of pure hydrochloric acid added; the dish is placed on the water-bath and 2 grms. of potassic chlorate added. The contents are stirred from time to time, and successive quantities of potassic chlorate are again added, until the contents are coloured yellow. The heating is continued, with, if necessary, the addition of more acid, until all smell of chlorine has ceased. If there is considerable excess of acid, this is to be evaporated away by diluting with a little water and continuing to heat on the water-bath. The dish with its contents is cooled, a little water added, and the fluid is then filtered.

The metals remaining on the filter are:—

- Silver chloride,
- Lead sulphate,
- Barium sulphate;

in the filtrate will be all the other metals.

The filtrate is put in a flask and heated to from 60 to 80 degrees and submitted to a slow stream of hydric sulphide gas; when the fluid is saturated with the gas, the flask is securely corked and allowed to rest for twelve hours; at the end of that time the fluid is filtered and the filter washed with water saturated with hydric sulphide.

[44] Aniline is a weak base, so that, although a solution be acid, some of the aniline distils over on heating.

[45] Hot amyl alcohol would be better (see "Morphine").

The still moist sulphides remaining on the filter are treated with yellow ammonium sulphide containing some free ammonia and washed with sulphide of ammonium water. Now remaining on the filter, if present at all, will be:—

- Mercury sulphide,
- Lead sulphide,
- Copper sulphide,
- Cadmium sulphide;

in the filtrate may be:—

- Arsenic sulphide,
- Antimony sulphide,
- Tin sulphide,

and there may also be a small portion of copper sulphide, because the latter is somewhat soluble in a considerable quantity of ammonium sulphide.

The filtrate from the original hydric sulphide precipitate will contain, if present, the sulphides of zinc and chromium in solution.

INVESTIGATION OF THE SULPHIDES SOLUBLE IN AMMONIUM SULPHIDE, VIZ., ARSENIC, ANTIMONY, TIN.

The ammonium sulphide solution is evaporated to dryness in a porcelain dish, strong nitric acid added and again dried. To this residue a little strong caustic soda solution is added, and then it is intimately mixed with three times its weight of a mixture composed of 2 of potassic nitrate to 1 of dry sodium hydrate. This is now cast, bit by bit, into a red-hot porcelain crucible. The whole is heated until it has melted into a colourless fluid.

Presuming the original mass contained arsenic, antimony, and tin, the melt contains sodic arseniate, sodic pyro-antimonate, sodic stannate, and tin oxide; it may also contain a trace of copper oxide.

The melt is cooled, dissolved in a little water, and sodium bicarbonate added so as to change any caustic soda remaining into carbonate, and to decompose the small amount of sodic stannate; the liquid is then filtered.

The filtrate will contain the arsenic as sodic arseniate; while on the filter there will be pyro-antimonate of soda, tin oxide, and, possibly, a little copper oxide.

The recognition of these substances now is not difficult (see the separate articles on *Antimony*, *Tin*, *Zinc*, *Arsenic*, *Copper*).

INVESTIGATION OF THE SULPHIDES INSOLUBLE IN SULPHIDE OF AMMONIUM, VIZ., MERCURY, LEAD, COPPER, CADMIUM.

If the precipitate is contaminated with organic matter, it is treated with hydrochloric acid and potassic chlorate in the manner already described.

Afterwards it is once more saturated with hydric sulphide, the precipitate is collected on a filter, well washed, and the sulphides treated with moderately concentrated nitric acid (1 vol. nitric acid, 2 vols. water). The sulphides are best treated with this solvent on the filter; all the sulphides mentioned, save mercury sulphide, dissolve and pass into the filtrate. This mercury sulphide may be dissolved by nitro-muriatic acid, the solution evaporated to dryness, the residue dissolved in water acidified with hydrochloric acid and tested for mercury (see "Mercury").

The filtrate containing, it may be, nitrates of lead, copper and cadmium is evaporated nearly to dryness and taken up in a very little water. The lead is separated as sulphate by the addition of dilute sulphuric acid.

The filtered solution, freed from lead, is treated with ammonia to alkaline reaction; if copper be present, a blue colour is produced, and this may be confirmed by other tests (see "Copper"). To detect cadmium in the presence of copper, potassic cyanide is added to the blue liquid until complete decolorisation, and the liquid treated with SH_2; if cadmium be present, it is thrown down as a yellow sulphide, while potassic cupro-cyanide remains in solution.

SEARCH FOR ZINC AND CHROMIUM.

The filtrate from the hydric sulphide precipitate is divided into two parts; the one half is used in the search for zinc, the other half is used for chromium.

Search for Zinc.—The liquid is alkalised with ammonia and then ammonium sulphide is added. There will always be a precipitate of a dark colour; the precipitate will contain earthy phosphates, iron and, in some cases, manganese. The liquid with the precipitate is treated with acetic acid to strong acid reaction and allowed to stand for several hours. The portion of the precipitate remaining undissolved is collected on a filter, washed, dried and heated to redness in a porcelain crucible. The residue thus heated is cooled and dissolved in a little dilute sulphuric acid. To the acid solution ammonia is added, and any precipitate formed is treated with acetic acid; should the precipitate not completely dissolve, phosphate of iron is present; this is filtered off, and if SH_2 be added to the filtrate, white zinc sulphide will come down (see "Zinc").

Search for Chromium.—The second part of the SH_2 filtrate is evaporated to a thin extract, mixed with double its weight of sodic nitrate, dried and cast, little by little, into a red-hot porcelain crucible. When the whole is fully melted, the crucible is removed from the flame, cooled, and the mass dissolved in water and filtered. Any chromium present will now be in solution in the easily recognised form of potassic chromate (see "Chromium").

INVESTIGATION OF THE RESIDUE AFTER THE TREATMENT OF THE ORIGINAL SUBSTANCE WITH HYDROCHLORIC ACID AND POTASSIC CHLORATE FOR PRESENCE OF SILVER CHLORIDE, LEAD AND BARIUM SULPHATES.

The residue is dried and intimately mixed with three times its weight of a mixture containing 2 parts of sodic nitrate and 1 part of sodium hydrate, This is added, little by little, into a red-hot porcelain crucible. The melted mass is cooled, dissolved in a little water, a current of CO_2 passed through the solution to convert any caustic soda into carbonate, and the solution boiled. The result will be an insoluble portion consisting of carbonates of lead and baryta, and of metallic silver. The mixture is filtered; the insoluble residue on the filter is warmed for some time with dilute nitric acid; the solution of nitrates of silver, lead and barium are concentrated on the water-bath nearly to dryness so as to get rid of any excess of acid, and the nitrates dissolved in water; then the silver is precipitated by hydrochloric acid, the lead by SH_2, and the barium by sulphuric acid.

VII.—The Spectroscope as an aid to the Identification of certain Poisons.

§ 33. The spectra of many of the metals, of phosphine, of arsine and of several other inorganic substances are characteristic and easily obtained.

It is, however, from the employment of the *micro-spectroscope* that the toxicologist is likely to get most assistance.

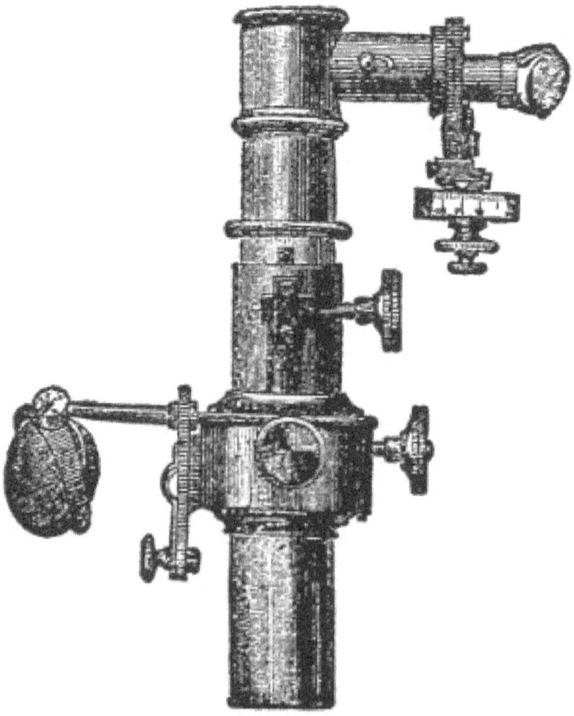

Oscar Brasch[46] has within the last few years studied spectroscopy in relation to the alkaloids and organic poisons. Some of these, when mixed with Froehde's reagent, or with sulphuric acid, or with sulphuric acid and potassic dichromate, or with nitric acid, give characteristic colours, and the resulting solutions, when examined by a spectroscope, for the most part show absorption bands; these bands may, occasionally, assist materially in the identification of a poison. By far the best apparatus is a micro-spectroscope of the Sorby and Browning type, to which is added an apparatus for measuring the position on a scale of the lines and bands. Seibert and Kraft of Wetzlar make an excellent instrument, in which a small bright triangle is projected on the spectrum; this can be moved by a screw, so that the apex may be brought exactly in the centre of any line or band, and its position read on an outside scale. The first thing to be done with such an instrument is to determine the position on the scale of the chief Fraunhofer lines or of the more characteristic lines of the alkalies and alkaline earths,[47] the wave lengths of which are accurately known. If, now, the scale divisions are set out as abscissæ, and the wave lengths in millionths of a millimetre are made the ordinates of a diagram, and an equable curve plotted out, as fully explained in the author's work on "Foods," it is easy to convert the numbers on the scale into wave lengths, and so make the readings applicable to any spectroscope. For the purpose of graphical illustration the curve method is convenient, and is adopted in the preceding diagrams, all taken from Oscar Brasch's monograph. Where the curve is highest there the absorption band is thickest; where the curve is lowest there the band is weak. The fluid to be examined is simply placed in a watch-glass, the watch-glass resting on the microscope stand.

NOTES TO CURVES INDICATING ABSORPTION BANDS.

1. Strychnine, treated with sulphuric acid and potassic dichromate (violet).
2. Brucine, treated with potassic nitrate and sulphuric acid (clear red).
3. Quebrachine, treated with vanadium sulphate (dark blue).
4. Quinine, Vogel's reaction (red).
5. Caffein, Murexid reaction (violet-red).
6. Dephinoidin, Froehde's reagent (cherry-red).
7. Veratrine, treated with sulphuric acid (straw-yellow).
8. ,,,,,, (cherry-red).
9. ,,,,,, (carmine-red).
10. Veratrine, Furfurol reaction (blue-violet).
11. Sabadillin, treated with sulphuric acid (red).
12. Veratroidine,,,,, (brown-red).
13. Jervine, Furfurol reaction (blue).
14. Sabadine, ,,,,(blue).
15. Sabadine, treated with sulphuric acid (cherry-red).
16. Physostigmine,,,,, (grass-green).
17. Morphine, treated with Froehde's reagent and sugar (dark-green).
18. Narcotine, treated with a mixture of sulphuric acid and nitric acid (30 drops of sulphuric to 1 drop of nitric), (red).
19. Codeine, treated with Froehde's reagent and sugar (dark violet).
20. Papaverine, treated with Froehde's reagent (green-blue).
21. Sanguinarin, ,,,, (violet-red).
22. Chelidonin,,, sulphate of vanadium (dark green).
23. Solanin,,, sulphuric acid and allowed to stand 4 hours (brown-red).
24. Digitalin,,, Erdmann's reagent (red).
25. Aniline, ,, sulphuric acid and potassic dichromate (blue).

The wave lengths corresponding to the numbers on the scale in the diagram are as follows:—

[46] *Ueber Verwendbarkeit der Spectroscopie zur Unterscheidung der Farbenreactionen der Gifte im Interesse der forensischen Chemie*, Dorpat, 1890.

[47] The alkalies and earths used for this purpose, with their wave lengths, are as follows: KCl, a line in the red λ 770, in the violet λ 404. Lithium chloride, red line, 670·5; sodium chloride, yellow, 589; strontium chloride, line in the blue, 461. It is also useful to measure the green line of thallium chloride = 535.

	W.L.
0	732
1	656
2	589.2
3	549.8
4	510.2
5	480.0
6	458
7	438

CURVES INDICATING THE POSITION OF ABSORPTION BANDS ON TREATING CERTAIN ALKALOIDS WITH REAGENTS.

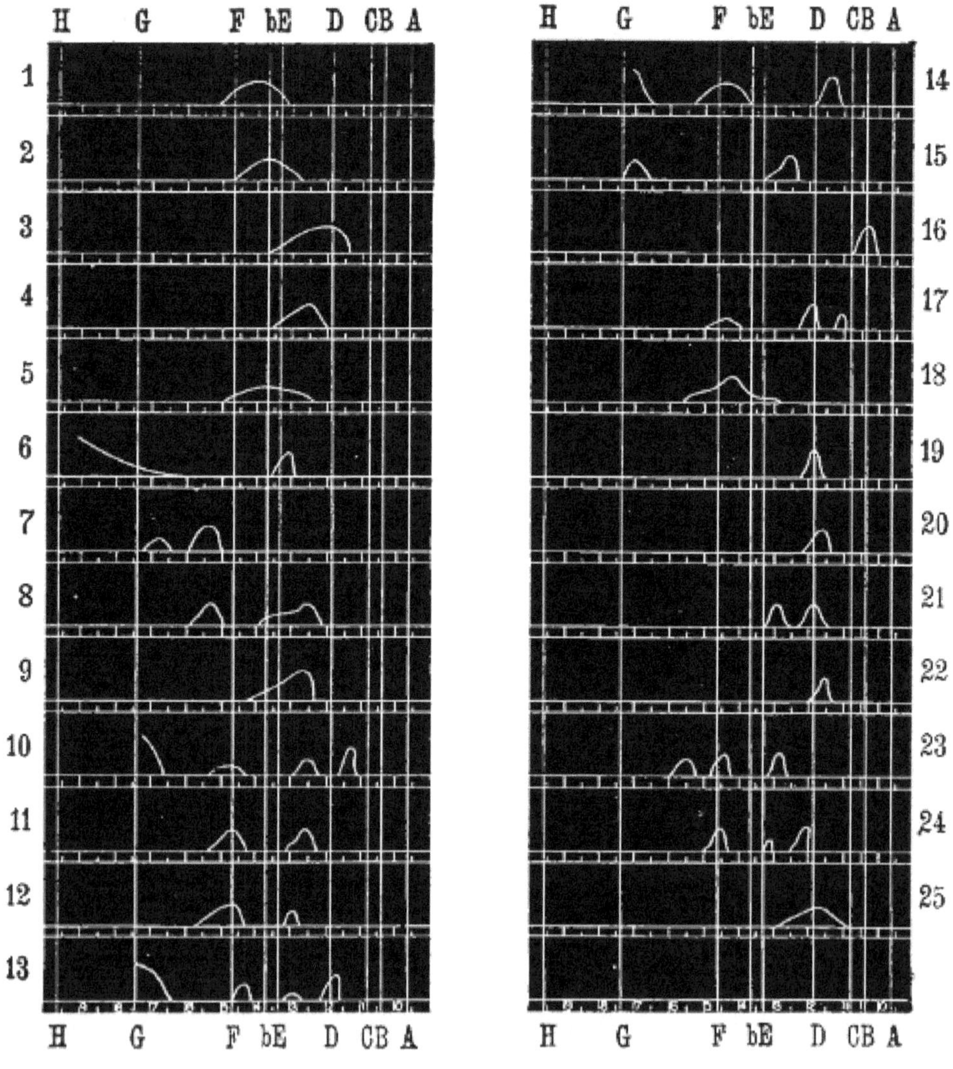

Examination of Blood, or of Blood-Stains.

§ 34. Spots, supposed to be blood—whether on linen, walls, or weapons—should, in any important case, be photographed before any chemical or microscopical examination is undertaken. Blood-spots, according to the nature of the material to which they are adherent, have certain naked eye peculiarities—*e.g.*, blood on fabrics, if dry, has at first a clear carmine-red colour, and part of it soaks into the tissue. If, however, the tissue has been worn some time, or was originally soiled, either from perspiration, grease, or filth, the colour may not be obvious or very distinguishable from other stains; nevertheless, the stains always impart a certain stiffness, as from starch, to the tissue. If the blood has fallen on such substances as wood or metal, the spot is black, has a bright glistening surface, and, if observed by a lens, exhibits radiating fissures and a sort of pattern, which, according to some, is peculiar to each species; so that a skilled observer might identify occasionally, from the pattern alone, the animal whence the blood was derived. The blood is dry and brittle, and can often be detached, or a splinter of it, as it were, obtained. The edges of the splinter, if submitted to transmitted light, are observed to be red. Blood upon iron is frequently very intimately adherent; this is specially the case if the stain is upon rusty iron, for hæmatin forms a compound with iron oxide. Blood may also have to be recovered from water in which soiled articles have been washed, or from walls, or from the soil, &c. In such cases the spot is scraped off from walls, plaster, or masonry, with as little of the foreign matters as may be. It is also possible to obtain the colouring-matter of blood from its solution in water, and present it for farther examination in a concentrated form, by the use of certain precipitating agents.

In the following scheme for the examination of blood-stains, it is presumed that only a few spots of blood, or, in any case, a small quantity, is at the analyst's disposal.

(1) The dried spot is submitted to the action of a cold saturated solution of borax. This medium (recommended by Dragendorff)[48] does certainly dissolve out of linen and cloth blood-colouring matter with great facility. The best way to steep the spots in the solution is to scrape the spot off the fabric, and to digest it in about a cubic centimetre of the borax solution, which must not exceed 40°; the coloured solution may be placed in a little glass cell, with parallel walls, .5 centimetre broad, and .1 deep, and submitted to spectroscopic examination, either by the ordinary spectroscope or by the micro-spectroscope; if the latter is used, a very minute quantity can be examined, even a single drop. In order to interpret the results of this examination properly, it will be necessary to be intimately acquainted with the spectroscopic appearances of both ancient and fresh blood.

§ 35. **Spectroscopic Appearances of Blood.**—If defibrinated blood[49] be diluted with water until it contains about .01 per cent. of oxyhæmoglobin, and be examined by a spectroscope, the layer of liquid being 1 centimetre thick, a single absorption band between the wave lengths 583 and 575 is observed, and, under favourable circumstances, there is also to be seen a very weak band from 550 to 532. With solutions so dilute as this, there is no absorption at either the violet or the red end of the spectrum. A solution containing .09 per cent. of oxyhæmoglobin shows very little absorption in the red end, but the violet end is dark up to about the wave length 428. Two absorption bands may now be distinctly seen. A solution containing .37 per cent. of oxyhæmoglobin shows absorption of the red end to about W.L. 720; the violet is entirely, the blue partly, absorbed to about 453. The bands are considerably broader, but the centre of the bands occupies the same relative position. A solution containing as much as .8 per cent. of oxyhæmoglobin is very dark; the two bands have amalgamated, the red end of the spectrum is absorbed nearly up to Fraunhofer's line a; the green is just visible between W.L. 498 and 518. Venous blood, or arterial blood, which has been treated with reducing agents, such, for example, as an alkaline sulphide, gives the spectrum of reduced hæmoglobin. If the solution is equivalent to about .2 per cent., a single broad band, with the edges very little defined, is seen to occupy the space between W.L. 595 and 538, the band being darkest about 550; both ends of the spectrum are more absorbed than by a solution of oxyhæmoglobin of the same strength. In the blood of persons or animals poisoned with hydric sulphide—to the spectrum of reduced hæmoglobin, there is added a weak absorption band in the red, with its centre nearly corresponding with the Fraunhofer line C. Blood which has been exposed to carbon oxide has a distinct spectrum, due, it would seem, to a special combination of this gas with hæmoglobin; in other words, instead of oxygen, the oxygen of oxyhæmoglobin has been displaced by carbon oxide, and crystals of carbon oxide-hæmoglobin, isomorphous with those of oxyhæmoglobin, may be obtained by suitable treatment. The spectrum of carbon oxide-hæmoglobin, however, differs so little from that of normal blood,

48 *Untersuchungen von Blutspuren* in Maschka's *Handbuch*, Bd. i. Halfband 2.

49 In this brief notice of the spectroscopic appearances of the blood, the measurements in wave lengths are, for the most part, after Gamgee.—*Text-Book of Physiological Chemistry*, London, 1880.

that it is only comparison with the ordinary spectrum, or careful measurements, which will enable any person, not very familiar with the different spectra of blood, to detect it; with careful and painstaking observation the two spectra are seen to be distinct. The difference between the carbon oxide and the normal spectrum essentially consists in a slight moving of the bands nearer to E. According to the measurements of Gamgee, the band α of CO-hæmoglobin has its centre approximately at W.L. 572, and the band β has for its centre W.L. from 534 to 538, according to concentration. If a small quantity of an ammoniacal solution of ferrous tartrate or citrate be added to blood containing carbon oxide, the bands do not wholly fade, but persist more or less distinctly; whereas, if the same solution is added to bright red normal blood, the two bands vanish instantly and coalesce to form the spectrum of reduced hæmoglobin. When either a solution of hæmoglobin or blood is exposed to the air for some time, it loses its bright red colour, becomes brownish-red, and presents an acid reaction. On examining the spectrum, the two bands have become faint, or quite extinct; but there is a new band, the centre of which (according to Gamgee) occupies W.L. 632, but (according to Preyer) 634. In solutions of a certain strength, four bands may be seen, but in a strong solution only one. This change in the spectrum is due to the passing of the hæmoglobin into *methæmoglobin*, which may be considered as an intermediate stage of decomposition, prior to the breaking up of the hæmoglobin into hæmatin and proteids.

A spectrum very similar to that of methæmoglobin is obtained by treating ancient blood-stains with acetic acid—viz., the spectrum of *acid hæmatin*, but the band is nearer to its centre, according to Gamgee, corresponding to W.L. 640 (according to Preyer, 656.6). The portion of the band is a little different in alkaline solution, the centre being about 592. Hæmatin is one of the bodies into which hæmoglobin splits up by the addition of such agents as strong acetic acid, or by the decomposing influence of exposure; the view most generally accepted being that the colouring-matter of the blood is hæmatin in combination with one or more albuminoid bodies. The hæmatin obtained by treating blood with acetic acid may be dissolved out by ether, and the ethereal solution then exhibits a remarkable distinctive spectrum. Hence, in the spectroscopic examination of blood, or solutions of blood, for medico-legal purposes, if the blood is fresh, the spectrum likely to be seen is either that of oxyhæmoglobin or hæmoglobin; but, if the blood-stain is not recent, then the spectrum of either hæmatin or methæmoglobin.

The colouring-matter of cochineal, to which alum, potassic carbonate, and tartrate have been added, gives a spectrum very similar to that of blood (see "Foods," p. 82); but this is only the case when the solution is fresh. The colour is at once discharged by chlorine, while the colour of blood, although changed in hue, remains. The colouring-matter of certain red feathers, purpurin-sulphuric acid, and a few other reds, have some similarity to either the hæmatin or the hæmoglobin spectrum, but the bands do not strictly coincide; besides, no one would trust to a single test, and none of the colouring-matters other than blood yield hæmatin.

The blood in CO poisoning has also other characteristics. It is of a peculiar florid vermilion colour, a colour that is very persistent, lasting for days and even weeks.

Normal blood mixed with 30 per cent. potash solution forms *greenish* streaky clots, while blood charged with CO forms red streaky clots.

Normal blood diluted to 50 times its volume of water, and then treated successively with yellow ammonium sulphide in the proportion of 2 to 25 c.c. of blood, followed by three drops of acetic acid, gives a grey colour, while CO blood remains bright red. CO blood shaken with 4 times its volume of lead acetate remains red, but normal blood becomes brown.[50]

Solutions of platinum chloride or zinc chloride give a bright red colour with CO blood; normal blood is coloured brown or very dark brown.

Phospho-molybdic acid or 5 per cent. phenol gives a carmine-coloured precipitate with CO blood, but a reddish-brown precipitate with normal blood (sensitive to 16 per cent.).

A mixture of 2 c.c. of dilute acetic acid and 15 c.c. of 20 per cent. potassic ferrocyanide solution added to 10 c.c. of CO blood produces an intense bright red; normal blood becomes dark brown.

Four parts of CO blood, diluted with 4 parts of water and shaken with 3 vols. of 1 per cent. tannin solution, become at first bright red with a bluish tinge, and remain so persistently. Normal blood, on the other hand, also strikes bright red at first, but with a yellowish tinge; at the end of 1 hour it becomes brownish, and finally in 24 hours grey. This is stated to be delicate enough to detect 0.0023 per cent. in air.

If blood be diluted with 40 times its volume of water, and 5 drops of phenylhydrazin solution be added, CO

[50] M. Rubner, *Arch. Hyg.*, x. 397.

blood strikes rose-red; normal blood grey-violet.[51]

Gustave Piotrowski[52] has experimented on the length of time blood retains CO. The blood of dogs poisoned by this agent was kept in flasks, and then the gas pumped out by means of a mercury pump on the following dates:—

Date.			Content of gas in CO.	
Jan.	12,	1892,	24.7	per cent.
„	20,	„	23.5	„
„	28,	„	22.2	„
Feb.	8,	„	20.3	„
„	16,	„	15.5	„
„	26,	„	10.2	„
March	3,	„	6.3	„
„	14,	„	4.6	„
„	22,	„	1.2	„

The same dog was buried on the 12th of January, and exhumed on March 28th, and the gas pumped out from some of the blood; this gas gave 11.7 per cent. of CO; hence it is clear that burial preserves CO blood from change to a certain extent.

N. Gréhant[53] treated the poisoned blood of a dog with acetic acid, and found it evolved 14.4 c.c. CO from 100 c.c. of blood.

Stevenson, in one of the cases detailed earlier, found the blood in the right auricle to contain 0.03 per cent. by weight of CO.

(2) **Preparation of Hæmatin Crystals**—(Teichmann's crystals).—A portion of the borax solution is diluted with 5 or 6 parts of water, and one or more drops of a 5 or 6 per cent. solution of zinc acetate added, so long as a brownish-coloured precipitate is thrown down. The precipitate is filtered off by means of a miniature filter, and then removed on to a watch-glass. The precipitate may now be dissolved in 1 or 2 c.c. of acetic acid, and examined by the spectroscope it will show the spectrum of hæmatin. A minute crystal of sodic chloride being then added to the acetic acid solution, it is allowed to evaporate to dryness at the ordinary temperature, and crystals of hæmatin hydrochlorate result. There are other methods of obtaining the crystals. When a drop of fresh blood is simply boiled with glacial acetic acid, on evaporation, prismatic crystals are obtained.

Hæmatin is insoluble in water, alcohol, chloroform, and in cold dilute acetic and hydrochloric acids. It may, however, be dissolved in an alcoholic solution of potassic carbonate, in solutions of the caustic alkalies, and in boiling acetic and hydrochloric acids. Hoppe-Seyler ascribes to the crystals the formula $C_{68}H_{70}N_8Fe_2O_{10}2HCl$. Thudichum considers that the pure crystals contain no chlorine, and are therefore those of hæmatin. It is the resistance of the hæmatin to decomposition and to ordinary solvents that renders it possible to identify a certain stain to be that of blood, after long periods of time. Dr. Tidy seems to have been able to obtain blood reactions from a stain which was supposed to be 100 years old. The crystals are of a dark-red colour, and present themselves in three forms, of which that of the rhombic prism is the most common (see fig.). But crystals like *b*, having six sides, also occur, and also crystals similar to *c*.

If the spot under examination has been scraped off an iron implement the hæmatin is not so easily extracted, but Dragendorff states that borax solution at 50° dissolves it, and separates it from the iron. Felletar has also extracted blood in combination with iron rust, by means of warm solution of caustic potash, and, after neutralisation with acetic acid, has precipitated the hæmin by means of tannin, and obtained from the tannin precipitate, by means of acetic acid, Teichmann's crystals. A little of the rust may also be placed in a test tube, powdered ammonium chloride added, also a little strong ammonia, and after a time filtered; a small quantity of the filtrate is placed on a slide with a crystal of sodium chloride and evaporated at a gentle heat, then glacial acetic acid added and allowed

[51] A. Welzel, *Centr. med. Wiss.*, xxvii. 732-734.

[52] *Compt. Rend. Soc. de Biol.*, v. 433.

[53] *Compt. Rend.*, cvi. 289.

to cool; in this way hæmin crystals have been obtained from a crowbar fifty days after having been blood-stained.[54]

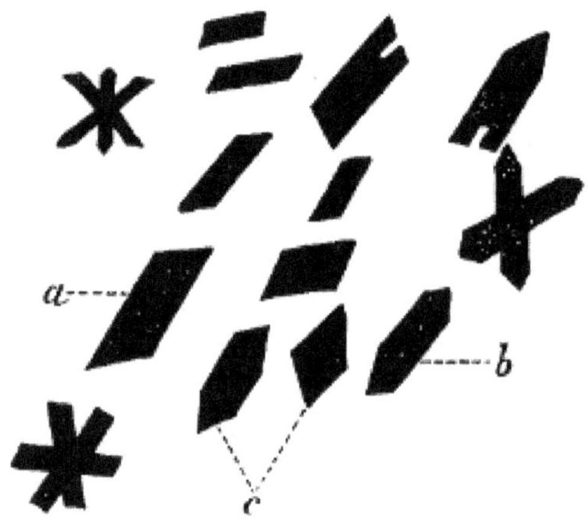

(3) **Guaiacum Test.**—This test depends upon the fact that a solution of hæmoglobin develops a beautiful blue colour, if brought into contact with fresh tincture of guaiacum and peroxide of hydrogen. The simplest way to obtain this reaction is to moisten the suspected stain with distilled water; after allowing sufficient time for the water to dissolve out some of the blood constituents, moisten a bit of filter-paper with the weak solution thus obtained; drop on to the moist space a single drop of tincture of guaiacum which has been prepared by digesting the inner portions of guaiacum resin in alcohol, and which has been already tested on known blood, so as to ascertain that it is really good and efficient for the purpose; and, lastly, a few drops of peroxide of hydrogen. Dragendorff uses his borax solution, and, after a little dilution with water, adds the tincture and then Heunefeld's turpentine solution, which is composed of equal parts of absolute alcohol, chloroform, and French turpentine, to which one part of acetic acid has been added. The chloroform separates, and, if blood was present, is of a blue colour.

§ 36. To prove by chemical and physical methods that a certain stain is that of blood, is often only one step in the inquiry, the next question being whether the blood is that of man or of animals. The blood-corpuscles of man are larger than those of any domestic animal inhabiting Europe. The diameter of the average red blood-corpuscle is about the $^1/_{126}$ of a millimetre, or 7.9 μ.[55] The corpuscles of man and of mammals, generally speaking, are round, those of birds and reptiles oval, so that there can be no confusion between man and birds, fishes or reptiles; if the corpuscles are circular in shape the blood will be that of a mammal. By careful measurements, Dr. Richardson, of Pennsylvania, affirms that it is quite possible to distinguish human blood from that of all common animals. He maintains, and it is true, that, by using very high magnifying powers and taking much trouble, an expert can satisfactorily identify human blood, if he has some half-dozen drops of blood from different animals—such as the sheep, goat, horse, dog, cat, &c., all fresh at hand for comparison, and *if the human blood is normal*. However, when we come to the blood of persons suffering from disease, there are changes in the diameter and even the form of the corpuscles which much complicate the matter; while, in blood-stains of any age, the blood-corpuscles, even with the most artfully-contrived solvent, are so distorted in shape that he would be a bold man who should venture on any definite conclusion as to whether the blood was certainly human, more especially if he had to give evidence in a criminal case.

Neumann affirms that the pattern which the fibrin or coagulum of the blood forms is peculiar to each animal, and Dr. Day, of Geelong, has independently confirmed his researches: this very interesting observation perhaps has not received the attention it merits.

When there is sufficient of the blood present to obtain a few milligrms. of ash, there is a means of distinguishing human blood from that of other common mammals, which has been neglected by authorities on the subject, and which may be found of real value. Its principle depends upon the relative amounts of potassium and sodium in the blood of man as compared with that in the blood of domestic animals. In the blood of the cow, sheep, fowl, pig, and

[54] *Brit. Med. Journ.*, Feb. 17, 1894.

[55] $^1/_{3200}$ of an inch; the Greek letter μ is the micro-millimetre, or 1000th of a millimetre, ·00003937 inch.

horse, the sodium very much exceeds the potassium in the ash; thus the proportion of sodium oxide to that of potassium oxide in the blood of the sheep is as K_2O .1 : Na_2O .6; in that of the cow, as 1 : 8; in that of the domestic fowl, as 1 : 16; while the same substances in human blood are sometimes equal, and vary from 1 : 1 to 1 : 4 as extremes, the mean numbers being as 1 : 2.2. The potassium is greater in quantity in the blood-corpuscles than in the blood serum; but, even in blood serum, the same marked differences between the blood of man and that of many animals is apparent. Thus, the proportion of potash to soda being as 1 : 10 in human blood, the proportion in sheep's blood is 1 to 15.7; in horse's serum as 1 to 16.4; and in the ox as 1 to 17. Since blood, when burnt, leaves from 6 to 7 per thousand of ash, it follows that a quantitative analysis of the relative amounts of potassium and sodium can only be satisfactorily effected when sufficient of the blood is at the analyst's disposal to give a weighable quantity of mineral matter. On the other hand, much work requires to be done before this method of determining that the blood is either human, or, at all events, not that of an herbivorous animal, can be relied on. We know but little as to the effect of the ingestion of sodium or potassium salts on either man or animals, and it is possible—nay, probable—that a more or less entire substitution of the one for the other may, on certain diets, take place. Bunge seems in some experiments to have found no sodium in the blood of either the cat or the dog.

The source from which the blood has emanated may, in a few cases, be conjectured from the discovery, by microscopical examination, of hair or of buccal, nasal, or vaginal epithelium, &c., mixed with the blood-stain.

Part III.—Poisonous Gases: Carbon Monoxide—Chlorine—Hydric Sulphide.

I.—Carbon Monoxide.

§ 37. Carbon monoxide, CO, is a colourless, odourless gas of 0.96709 sp. gravity. A litre weighs 1.25133 grm. It is practically insoluble in water. It unites with many metals, forming gaseous or volatile compounds, *e.g.*, nickel carbon oxide, $Ni(CO)_4$, is a fluid volatilising at 40°. These compounds have, so far as is known, the same effects as CO.

Whenever carbon is burned with an insufficient supply of air, CO in a certain quantity is produced. It is always present in ordinary domestic products of combustion, and must be exhaled from the various chimneys of a large city in considerable volumes. A "smoky" chimney or a defective flue will therefore introduce carbon monoxide into living-rooms. The vapour from burning coke or burning charcoal is rich in carbon monoxide. It is always a constituent of coal gas, in England the carbon monoxide in coal gas amounting to about 8 per cent. Poisoning by coal gas is practically poisoning by carbon monoxide. Carbon monoxide is also the chief constituent in water gas.

Carbon monoxide poisoning occurs far more frequently in France and Germany than in England; in those countries the vapour evolved from burning charcoal is a favourite method of suicide, on account of the supposed painlessness of the death. It has also occasionally been used as an instrument of murder. In this country carbon monoxide poisoning mainly takes place accidentally as the effect of breathing coal gas; possibly it is the secret and undetected cause of ill health where chimneys "smoke"; and it may have something to do with the sore throats and debility so often noticed when persons breathe for long periods air contaminated by small leakages of coal gas.

The large gas-burners (geysers) emit in burning under certain conditions much carbon monoxide. It has been proved by Gréhant[56] that a bunsen burner "lit below" also evolves large quantities of the same poisonous gas.

§ 38. **Symptoms.**—Nearly all the experience with regard to the symptoms produced by carbon monoxide is derived from breathing not the pure gas, but the gas diluted by air, by hydrogen or by carburetted hydrogen, as in coal gas, or mixed with large quantities of carbon dioxide. Two assistants of Christison breathed the pure gas: the one took from two to three inhalations; he immediately became giddy, shivered, had headache and then became unconscious. The second took a bigger dose, for, after emptying his lungs as much as possible, he took from three to four inhalations; he fell back paralysed, became unconscious and remained half-an-hour insensible and had the appearance of death, the pulse being almost extinguished. He was treated with inhalations of oxygen, but he remained for the rest of the day extremely ill; he had convulsive muscular movements, stupor, headache, and quick irregular pulse; on this passing away he still suffered from nausea, giddiness, alternate feeling of heat and chilliness, with some fever, and in the night had a restless kind of sleep. The chemist Chenot was accidentally poisoned by the pure gas, and is stated to have fell as if struck by lightning after a single inspiration, and remained for a quarter of an hour unconscious. Other recorded cases have shown very similar symptoms.

The pulse is at the onset large, full and frequent; it afterwards becomes small, slow and irregular. The temperature sinks from 1° to 3° C. The respiration at first slow, later becomes rattling. As vomiting occurs often when the sufferer is insensible, the vomited matters have been drawn by inspiration into the trachea and even into the bronchi, so that death takes place by suffocation.

The fatal coma may last even when the person has been removed from the gas from hours to days. Coma for three, four and five days from carbon monoxide has been frequently observed. The longest case on record is that of a person who was comatose for eight days, and died on the twelfth day after the fatal inhalation. Consciousness in this case returned, but the patient again fell into stupor and died.

The slighter kinds of poisoning by carbon monoxide, as in the Staffordshire case recorded by Dr. Reid, in which for a long time a much diluted gas has been breathed, produce pronounced headache and a general feeling of ill health and *malaise*, deepening, it may be, into a fatal slumber, unless the person is removed from the deadly

[56] *Compt. Rend. Soc. de Biol.*, ix. 779-780.

atmosphere. To the headache generally succeeds nausea, a feeling of oppression in the temples, a noise in the ears, feebleness, anxiety and a dazed condition deepening into coma. It is probably true that charcoal vapour is comparatively painless, for when larger amounts of the gas are breathed the insensibility comes on rapidly and the faces of those who have succumbed as a rule are placid. Vomiting, without being constant, is a frequent symptom, and in fatal cases the fæces and urine are passed involuntarily. There are occasional deviations from this picture; tetanic strychnine-like convulsions have been noticed and a condition of excitement in the non-fatal cases as if from alcohol; in still rarer cases temporary mania has been produced.

In non-fatal but moderately severe cases of poisoning sequelæ follow, which in some respects imitate the sequelæ seen on recovery from the infectious fevers. A weakness of the understanding, incapacity for rational and connected thought, and even insanity have been noticed. There is a special liability to local inflammations, which may pass into gangrene. Various paralyses have been observed. Eruptions of the skin, such as herpes, pemphigus and others. Sugar in the urine is an almost constant concomitant of carbon monoxide poisoning.

§ 39. The poisonous action of carbon monoxide is, without doubt, due to the fact that it is readily absorbed by the blood, entering into a definite chemical compound with the hæmoglobin; this combination is more stable than the similar compound with oxygen gas, and is therefore slow in elimination.

Hence the blood of an animal remaining in an atmosphere containing carbon monoxide is continually getting poorer in oxygen, richer in carbon monoxide. Gréhant has shown that if an animal breathes for one hour a mixture of 0.5 carbon monoxide to 1000 oxygen, the blood contains at the end of that time one-third less oxygen than normal, and contains 152 times more carbon monoxide than in the mixture. An atmosphere of 10 per cent. carbon monoxide changes the blood so quickly, that after from 10 to 25 seconds the blood contains 4 per cent. of carbon monoxide, and after from 75 to 90 seconds 18.4 per cent. Breathing even for half an hour an atmosphere containing from 0.07 to 0.12 per cent. carbon monoxide renders a fourth part of the red corpuscles of the blood incapable of uniting with oxygen.

The blood is, however, never saturated with carbon monoxide, for the animal dies long before this takes place.

The characteristics of the blood and its spectroscopic appearances are described earlier.

Besides the action on the blood there is an action on the nervous system. Kobert,[57] in relation to this subject, says:—"That CO has a direct action on the nervous system is shown in a marked manner when an atmosphere of oxygen, with at least 20 per cent. carbon oxide, is breathed; for in the first minute there is acute cramp or total paralysis of the limbs, when the blood in no way attains the saturation sufficiently great to account for such symptoms. Geppert has, through a special research, shown that an animal suffocated by withdrawal of oxygen, increases the number and depth of the respirations; but when the animal is submitted to CO, in which case there is quite as much a withdrawal of oxygen as in the former case, yet the animal is not in a condition to strengthen its respiratory movements; Geppert hence rightly concludes that CO must have a primary specific injurious action on the nerve centres. I (Kobert) am inclined to go a step further, and, on the ground of unpublished researches, to maintain that CO not only affects injuriously the ganglion cells of the brain, but also the peripheral nerves (*e.g.*, the phrenic), as well as divers other tissues, as muscles and glands, and that it causes so rapidly such a high degree of degeneration as not to be explained through simple slow suffocation; even gangrene may be caused."

It is this rapid degeneration which is the cause of the enormous increase of the products of the decomposition of albumin, found experimentally in animals.

§ 40. **Post-mortem Appearances.**—The face, neck, chest, abdomen are frequently covered with patches of irregular form and of clear rose-red or bluish-red colour; these patches are not noticed on the back, and thus do not depend upon the gravitation of the blood to the lower or most dependent part of the body; similar red patches have been noticed in poisoning by prussic acid; the cause of this phenomenon is ascribed to the paralysis of the small arteries of the skin, which, therefore, become injected with the changed blood. The blood throughout is generally fluid, and of a fine peculiar red colour, with a bluish tinge. The face is mostly calm, pale, and there is seldom any foam about the lips. Putrefaction is mostly remarkably retarded. There is nearly always a congestion of some of the internal organs; sometimes, and indeed usually, the membranes of the brain are strongly injected; sometimes the congestion is mainly in the lungs, which may be œdematous with effusion; and in a third class of cases the congestion is most marked in the abdominal cavity.

The right heart is commonly filled with blood, and the left side contains only a little blood.

Poisoning by a small dose of carbon monoxide may produce but few striking changes, and then it is only by a

[57] *Lehrbuch der Intoxicationen*, 526.

careful examination of the blood that evidence of the real nature of the case will be obtained.

§ 41. **Mass poisonings by Carbon Monoxide.**—An interesting series of cases of poisoning by water gas occurred at Leeds in 1889, and have been recorded by Dr. Thos. Stevenson.[58]

Water gas is made by placing coke in a vertical cylinder and heating the coke to a red heat. Through the red-hot coke, air is forced up from below for ten minutes; then the air is shut off and steam passes from above downwards for four minutes; the gas passes through a scrubber, and then through a ferric oxide purifier to remove SH_2. It contains about 50 per cent. of hydrogen and 40 per cent. of carbon monoxide, that is, about five times more carbon monoxide than coal gas.

On November 20, 1889, two men, R. French and H. Fenwick, both intemperate men, occupied a cabin at the Leeds Forge Works; the cabin was 540 c. feet in capacity, and was lighted by two burners, each burning 5.5 c. feet of water gas per hour; the cabin was warmed by a cooking stove, also burning water gas, the products of combustion escaping into the cabin. Both men went into the cabin after breakfast (8.30 A.M.). French was seen often going to and fro, and Fenwick was seen outside at 10.30 A.M. At 11.30 the foreman accompanied French to the cabin, and found Fenwick asleep, as he thought. At 12.30 P.M. French's son took the men their dinner, which was afterwards found uneaten. At that time French also appeared to be asleep; he was shaken by his son, upon which he nodded to his son to leave. The door of the cabin appears to have been shut, and all through the morning the lights kept burning; no smell was experienced. At 2.30 P.M. both the men were discovered dead. It was subsequently found that the stove was unlighted, and the water gas supply turned on.

What attracted most attention to this case was the strange incident at the *post-mortem* examination. The autopsies were begun two days after the death, November 22, in a room of 39,000 c. feet capacity. There were present Mr. T. Scattergood (senior), Mr. Arthur Scattergood (junior), Mr. Hargreaves, three local surgeons, Messrs. Brown, Loe and Jessop, and two assistants, Pugh and Spray. Arthur Scattergood first fainted, Mr. Scattergood, senior, also had some peculiar sensations, viz., tingling in the head and slight giddiness; then Mr. Pugh became faint and staggered; and Mr. Loe, Mr. Brown, and Mr. Spray all complained.

These symptoms were not produced, as was at first thought, by some volatile gas or vapour emanating from the bodies of the poisoned men, but, as subsequently discovered, admitted of a very simple explanation; eight burners in the room were turned partly on and not lighted, and each of the eight burners poured water gas into the room.

In 1891 occurred some cases of poisoning[59] by CO which are probably unique. The cases in question happened in January in a family at Darlaston. The first sign of anything unusual having happened to the family most affected was the fact that up to 9 A.M., Sunday morning, January 18, none of the family had been seen about. The house was broken into by the neighbours; and the father, mother, and three children were found in bed apparently asleep, and all efforts to rouse them utterly failed. The medical men summoned arrived about 10 A.M. and found the father and mother in a state of complete unconsciousness, and two of the children, aged 11 and 14 years, suffering from pain and sickness and diarrhœa; the third child had by this time been removed to a neighbouring cottage.

Dr. Partridge, who was in attendance, remained with the patients three hours, when he also began to suffer from headache; while others, who remained in the house longer, suffered more severely and complained of an indefinite feeling of exhaustion. These symptoms pointed to some exciting cause associated with the surroundings of the cottage; consequently, in the afternoon the two children were removed to another cottage, and later on the father and mother also. All the patients, with the exception of the mother, who was still four days afterwards suffering from the effects of an acute attack, had completely recovered. The opinion that the illness was owing to some local cause was subsequently strengthened by the fact that two canaries and a cat had died in the night in the kitchen of the cottage; the former in a cage and the latter in a cupboard, the door of which was open. Also in the same house on the opposite side of the road, the occupants of which had for some time suffered from headache and depression, two birds were found dead in their cage in the kitchen. It is important to notice that all these animals died in the respective kitchens of the cottages, and, therefore, on the ground floor, while the families occupied the first floor.

The father stated that for a fortnight or three weeks previous to the serious illness, he and the whole family had complained of severe frontal headache and a feeling of general depression. This feeling was continuous day and

[58] *Guy's Hospital Reports*, 1889.

[59] "Notes on cases of poisoning by the inhalation of carbon monoxide," by Dr. George Reid, Medical Officer of Health, County of Stafford. *Public Health*, vol. iii. 364.

night in the case of the rest of the family, but in his case, during the day, after leaving the house for his work, it gradually passed off, to return again during the night. The headaches were so intense that the whole family regularly applied vinegar rags to their heads, on going to bed each night during this period, for about three weeks. About two o'clock on Sunday morning the headaches became so severe that the mother got out of bed and renewed the application of vinegar and water all round, after which they all fell asleep, and, so far as the father and mother were concerned, remained completely unconscious until Monday morning.

A man who occupied the house opposite the house tenanted by the last-mentioned family informed the narrator (Dr. Reid) that on Sunday morning the family, consisting of four, were taken seriously ill with a feeling of sickness and depression accompanied by headache; and he also stated that for some time they had smelt what he termed a "fire stink" issuing from the cellar.

The cottage in which the family lived that had suffered so severely was situated about 20 or 30 yards from the shaft of a disused coal mine, and was the end house of a row of cottages. It had a cellar opening into the outer air, but this opening was usually covered over by means of a piece of wood. The adjoining house to this, the occupants of which had for some time suffered from headache, although to a less extent, had a cellar with a similar opening, but supplied with an ill-fitting cover. The house on the opposite side of the road, in which the two birds were found dead, had a cellar opening both at the front and the back; but both these openings, until a little before the occurrence detailed, had been kept closed. The cellars in all cases communicated with the houses by means of doors opening into the kitchens. According to the general account of the occupants, the cellars had smelled of "fire stink," which, in their opinion, proceeded from the adjoining mine.

The shaft of the disused mine communicated with a mine in working order, and, to encourage the ventilation in this mine, a furnace had for some weeks been lit and suspended in the shaft. This furnace had set fire to the coal in the disused mine and smoke had been issuing from the shaft for four weeks previously. Two days previous to the inquiry the opening of the shaft had been closed over with a view to extinguish the fire.

Dr. Reid considered, from the symptoms and all the circumstances of the case, that the illness was due to carbon monoxide gas penetrating into the cellars from the mine, and from thence to the living- and sleeping-rooms. A sample of the air yielded 0.015 per cent. of carbon monoxide, although the sample had been taken after the cellar windows had been open for twenty-four hours.

§ 42. **Detection of Carbon Monoxide.**—It may often be necessary to detect carbon monoxide in air and to estimate its amount. The detection in air, if the carbon monoxide is in any quantity, is easy enough; but traces of carbon monoxide are difficult. Where amounts of carbon monoxide in air from half a per cent. upwards are reasonably presumed to exist, the air is measured in a gas measuring apparatus and passed into an absorption pipette charged with alkaline pyrogallic acid, and when all the oxygen has been abstracted, then the residual nitrogen and gases are submitted to an ammoniacal solution of cuprous chloride.

The solution of cuprous chloride is prepared by dissolving 10.3 grms. of copper oxide in 150 c.c. of strong hydrochloric acid and filling the flask with copper turnings; the copper reduces the cupric chloride to cuprous chloride; the end of the reduction is known by the solution becoming colourless. The colourless acid solution is poured into some 1500 c.c. of water, and the cuprous chloride settles to the bottom as a precipitate. The supernatant fluid is poured off as completely as possible and the precipitate washed into a quarter litre flask, with 100 to 150 c.c. of distilled water and ammonia led into the solution until it becomes of a pale blue colour. The solution is made up to 200 c.c. so as to contain about 7.3 grms. per cent. of cuprous chloride.

Such a solution is an absorbent of carbon monoxide; it also absorbs ethylene and acetylene.

A solution of cuprous chloride which has absorbed CO gives it up on being treated with potassic bichromate and acid. It has been proposed by Wanklyn to deprive large quantities of air of oxygen, then to absorb any carbon monoxide present with cuprous chloride, and, lastly, to free the cuprous chloride from the last gas by treatment with acid bichromate, so as to be able to study the properties of a small quantity of pure gas.

By far the most reliable method to detect small quantities of carbon monoxide is, however, as proposed by Hempel, to absorb it in the lungs of a living animal.

A mouse is placed between two funnels joined together at their mouths by a band of thin rubber; one of the ends of the double funnel is connected with an aspirator, and the air thus sucked through, say for half an hour or more; the mouse is then killed by drowning, and a control mouse, which has not been exposed to a CO atmosphere, is also drowned; the bodies of both mice are cut in two in the region of the heart, and the blood collected. Each sample of blood is diluted in the same proportion and spectroscopically examined in the manner detailed earlier.

Winkler found that, when large volumes of gas were used (at least 10 litres), 0.05 per cent. of carbon monoxide could be readily detected.

II.—Chlorine.

§ 43. Chlorine is a yellow-green gas, which may, by cold and pressure, be condensed into a liquid. Its specific gravity is, as compared with hydrogen, 35.37; as compared with air, 2.45; a litre under standard conditions weighs 3.167 grms. It is soluble in water.

The usual method of preparation is the addition of hydrochloric acid to bleaching powder, which latter substance is hypochlorite of lime mixed with calcic chloride and, it may be, a little caustic lime. Another method is to treat manganese dioxide with hydrochloric acid or to act on manganese dioxide and common salt with sulphuric acid.

Accidents are liable to occur with chlorine gas from its extensive use as a disinfectant and also in its manufacture. In the "Weldon" process of manufacturing bleaching powder, a thick layer of lime is placed on the floor of special chambers; chlorine gas is passed into these chambers for about four days; then the gas is turned off; the unabsorbed gas is drawn off by an exhaust or absorbed by a lime distributor and the doors opened. Two hours afterwards the men go in to pack the powder. The packers, in order to be able to work in the chambers, wear a respirator consisting of about thirty folds of damp flannel; this is tightly bound round the mouth with the nostrils free and resting upon it. The men are obliged to inhale the breath through the flannel and exhale through the nostril, otherwise they would, in technical jargon, be "gassed." Some also wear goggles to protect their eyes. Notwithstanding these precautions they suffer generally from chest complaints.

§ 44. **Effects.** — Free chlorine, in the proportion of 0.04 to 0.06 per thousand, taken into the lungs is dangerous to life, since directly chlorine attacks a moist mucous membrane, hydrochloric acid is formed. The effects of chlorine can hardly be differentiated from hydrochloric acid gas, and Lehmann found that 1.5 per thousand of this latter gas affected animals, causing at once uneasiness, evidence of pain with great dyspnœa, and later coma. The eyes and the mucous membrane of the nose were attacked. Anatomical changes took place in the cornea, as evidenced by a white opacity.

In cases that recovered, a purulent discharge came from the nostrils with occasional necrosis of the mucous membrane. The symptoms in man are similar; there is great tightness of the breath, irritation of the nose and eyes, cough and, with small repeated doses, bronchitis with all its attendant evils. Bleaching powder taken by the mouth is not so deadly. Hertwig has given 1000 grms. to horses, 30 grms. to sheep and goats, and 15 grms. to dogs without producing death. The symptoms in these cases were quickening of the pulse and respiration, increased peristaltic action of the bowels and a stimulation of the kidney secretion. The urine smelt of chlorine.

§ 45. **Post-mortem Appearances.** — Hyperæmia of the lungs, with ecchymoses and pneumonic patches with increased secretion of the bronchial tubes. In the mucous membrane of the stomach, ecchymoses. The alkalescence of the blood is diminished and there may be external signs of bleaching. Only exceptionally has any chlorine smell been perceived in the internal organs.

§ 46. **Detection of Free Chlorine.** — The usual method of detection is to prepare a solution of iodide of potassium and starch and to soak strips of filter-paper in this solution. Such a strip, when moistened and submitted to a chlorine atmosphere, is at once turned blue, because chlorine displaces iodine from its combination with potassium. Litmus-paper, indigo blue or other vegetable colours are at once bleached.

To estimate the amount of chlorine a known volume of the air is drawn through a solution of potassium iodide, and the amount of iodine set free, determined by titration with sodic hyposulphite, as detailed earlier.

III.—Hydric Sulphide (Sulphuretted Hydrogen).

§ 47. Hydric sulphide, SH_2, is a colourless transparent gas of sp. gravity 1.178. It burns with a blue flame, forming water and sulphur dioxide, and is soluble in water; water absorbing about three volumes at ordinary temperatures. It is decomposed by either chlorine gas or sulphur dioxide.

It is a common gas as a constituent of the air of sewers or cesspools, and emanates from moist slag or moist earth containing pyrites or metallic sulphides; it also occurs whenever albuminous matter putrefies; hence it is a common constituent of the emanations from corpses of either man or animals. It has a peculiar and intense odour, generally compared to that of rotten eggs; this is really not a good comparison, for it is comparing the gas with itself, rotten eggs always producing SH_2; it is often associated with ammonium sulphide.

§ 48. **Effects.** — Pure hydric sulphide is never met with out of the chemist's laboratory, in which it is a common reagent either as a gas or in solution; so that the few cases of poisoning by the pure gas, or rather the pure gas mixed with ordinary air, have been confined to laboratories.

The greater number of cases have occurred accidentally to men working in sewers, or cleaning out cesspools and the like. In small quantities it is always present in the air of towns, as shown by the blackening of any silver ornament not kept bright by frequent use.

It is distinctly a blood poison, the gas uniting with the alkali of the blood, and the sulphide thus produced partly decomposing again in the lung and breathed out as SH_2. Lehmann[60] has studied the effects on animals; an atmosphere containing from 1 to 3 per thousand of SH_2 kills rabbits and cats within ten minutes; the symptoms are mainly convulsions and great dyspnœa. An atmosphere containing from 0.4 to 0.8 per thousand produces a local irritating action on the mucous membranes of the respiratory tract, and death follows from an inflammatory œdema of the lung preceded by convulsions; there is also a paralysis of the nervous centres. Lehmann has recorded the case of three men who breathed 0.2 per thousand of SH_2: within from five to eight minutes there was intense irritation of the eyes, nose, and throat, and after thirty minutes they were unable to bear the atmosphere any longer. Air containing 0.5 per thousand of SH_2 is, according to Lehmann, the utmost amount that can be breathed; this amount causes in half an hour smarting of the eyes, nasal catarrh, dyspnœa, cough, palpitation, shivering, great muscular weakness, headache and faintness with cold sweats. 0.7 to 0.8 per thousand is dangerous to human life, and from 1 to 1.5 per thousand destroys life rapidly. The symptoms may occur some little time after the withdrawal of the person from the poisonous atmosphere; for example, Cahn records the case of a student who prepared SH_2 in a laboratory and was exposed to the gas for two hours; he then went home to dinner and the symptoms first commenced in more than an hour after the first breathing of pure air. Taylor[61] records an unusual case of poisoning in 1857 at Cleator Moor. Some cottages had been built upon iron slag, the slag contained sulphides of calcium and iron; a heavy storm of rain washed through the slag and considerable volumes of SH_2 with, no doubt, other gases diffused during the night through the cottages and killed three adults and three children.

§ 49. **Post-mortem Appearances.**—The so-called apoplectic form of SH_2 poisoning, in which the sufferer dies within a minute or two, shows no special change. The most frequent change in slower poisoning is, according to Lehmann, œdema of the lungs. A green colour of the face and of the whole body is sometimes present, but not constant. A spectroscopic examination of the blood may also not lead to any conclusion, the more especially as the spectrum of sulphur methæmoglobin may occur in any putrid blood. The pupils in some cases have been found dilated; in others not so.

Chronic poisoning.—Chronic poisoning by SH_2 is of considerable interest in a public health point of view. The symptoms appear to be conjunctivitis, headache, dyspepsia and anæmia. A predisposition to boils has also been noted.

§ 50. **Detection.**—Both ammonium and hydric sulphides blacken silver and filter-paper moistened with acetate of lead solution. To test for hydric sulphide in air a known quantity may be aspirated through a little solution of lead acetate. To estimate the quantity a decinormal solution of iodine in potassium iodide[62] solution is used, and its exact strength determined by d.n. sodic hyposulphite solution[63]; the hyposulphite is run in from a burette into a known volume, *e.g.*, 50 c.c., of the d.n. iodine solution, until the yellow colour is almost gone; then a drop or two of fresh starch solution is added and the hyposulphite run in carefully, drop by drop, until the blue colour of the starch disappears. If now a known volume of air is drawn through 50 c.c. of the d.n. iodine solution, the reaction $I_2 + SH_2 = 2HI + S$ will take place, and for every 127 parts of iodine which have been converted into hydriodic acid 17 parts by weight of SH_2 will be necessary; hence on titrating the 50 c.c. of d.n. iodine solution, through which air containing SH_2 has been passed, less hyposulphite will be used than on the previous occasion, each c.c. of the hyposulphite solution being equal to 1.11 c.c. or to 1.7 mgrm. of SH_2.

[60] K. B. Lehmann, *Arch. f. Hygiene*, Bd. xiv., 1892, 135.

[61] *Principles and Practice of Medl. Jurisp.*, vol. ii. 122.

[62] 12.7 grms. of iodine, 16.6 grms. of potassium iodide, dissolved in a litre of water.

[63] 24.8 grms. of sodic hyposulphite, dissolved in a litre of water.

Part IV.—Acids and Alkalies.

SULPHURIC ACID—HYDROCHLORIC ACID—NITRIC ACID—ACETIC ACID—AMMONIA—POTASH—SODA—NEUTRAL SODIUM, POTASSIUM, AND AMMONIUM SALTS.

I.—Sulphuric Acid.

§ 51. Sulphuric acid (hydric sulphate, oil of vitriol, H_2SO_4) occurs in commerce in varying degrees of strength or dilution; the strong sulphuric acid of the manufacturer, containing 100 per cent. of real acid (H_2SO_4), has a specific gravity of 1.850. The ordinary brown acid of commerce, coloured by organic matter and holding in solution metallic impurities, chiefly lead and arsenic, has a specific gravity of about 1.750; and contains 67.95 of anhydrous SO_3 = 85.42 of hydric sulphate.

There are also weaker acids used in commerce, particularly in manufactories in which sulphuric acid is made, for special purposes without rectification. The British Pharmacopœia sulphuric acid is directed to be of 1.843 specific gravity, which corresponds to 78.6 per cent. sulphuric anhydride, or 98.8 per cent. of hydric sulphate. The dilute sulphuric acid of the pharmacopœia should have a specific gravity of 1.094, and is usually said to correspond to 10.14 per cent. of anhydrous sulphuric acid; but, if Ure's Tables are correct, such equals 11.37 per cent.

The general characters of sulphuric acid are as follows:—When pure, it is a colourless, or, when impure, a dark brown to black, oily liquid, without odour at common temperatures, of an exceedingly acid taste, charring most organic tissues rapidly, and, if mixed with water, evolving much heat. If 4 parts of the strong acid are mixed with 1 part of water at 0°, the mixture rises to a heat of 100°; a still greater heat is evolved by mixing 75 parts of acid with 27 of water.

Sulphuric acid is powerfully hygroscopic—3 parts will, in an ordinary atmosphere, increase to nearly 4 in twenty-four hours; in common with all acids, it reddens litmus, yellows cochineal, and changes all vegetable colours. There is another form of sulphuric acid, extensively used in the arts, known under the name of "Nordhausen sulphuric acid," "fuming acid," formula $H_2S_2O_4$. This acid is produced by the distillation of dry ferrous sulphate, at a nearly white heat—either in earthenware or in green glass retorts; the distillate is received in sulphuric acid. As thus manufactured, it is a dark fuming liquid of 1.9 specific gravity, and boiling at 53°. When artificially cooled down to 0°, the acid gradually deposits crystals, which consist of a definite compound of 2 atoms of anhydrous sulphuric acid and 1 atom of water. There is some doubt as to the molecular composition of Nordhausen acid; it is usually considered as hydric sulphate saturated with sulphur dioxide. This acid is manufactured chiefly in Bohemia, and is used, on a large scale, as a solvent for alizarine.

§ 52. **Sulphur Trioxide, or Sulphuric Anhydride** (SO_3), itself may be met with in scientific laboratories, but is not in commerce. Sulphur trioxide forms thin needle-shaped crystals, arranged in feathery groups. Seen in mass, it is white, and has something the appearance of asbestos. It fuses to a liquid at about 18°, boils at 35°, but, after this operation has been performed, the substance assumes an allotropic condition, and then remains solid up to 100°; above 100° it melts, volatilises, and returns to its normal condition. Sulphuric anhydride hisses when it is thrown into water, chemical combination taking place and sulphuric acid being formed. Sulphur trioxide is excessively corrosive and poisonous.

Besides the above forms of acid, there is an officinal preparation called "Aromatic Sulphuric Acid," made by digesting sulphuric acid, rectified spirit, ginger, and cinnamon together. It contains 10.19 per cent. of SO_3, alcohol, and principles extracted from cinnamon and ginger.

§ 53. Sulphuric acid, in the free state, may not unfrequently be found in nature. The author has had under examination an effluent water from a Devonshire mine, which contained more than one grain of free sulphuric acid per gallon, and was accused, with justice, of destroying the fish in a river. It also exists in large quantities in volcanic springs. In a torrent flowing from the volcano of Parcé, in the Andes, Boussingault calculated that 15,000 tons of sulphuric acid and 11,000 tons of hydrochloric acid were yearly carried down. In the animal and vegetable kingdom, sulphuric acid exists, as a rule, in combination with bases, but there is an exception in the saliva of the *Dolium galea*, a Sicilian mollusc.

§ 54. **Statistics.**—When something like 900,000 tons of sulphuric acid are produced annually in England alone, and when it is considered that sulphuric acid is used in the manufacture of most other acids, in the alkali trade, in the manufacture of indigo, in the soap trade, in the manufacture of artificial manure, and in a number of technical processes, there is no cause for surprise that it should be the annual cause of many deaths.

The number of deaths from sulphuric acid will vary, other things being equal, in each country, according to the manufactures in that country employing sulphuric acid. The number of cases of poisoning in England and Wales for ten years is given in the following table:—

DEATHS FROM SULPHURIC ACID IN ENGLAND AND WALES FOR THE TEN YEARS ENDING 1892.

Accident or Negligence.

Ages,	1-5	5-15	15-25	25-65	65 & upwards	Total
Males,	11	4	2	14	2	33
Females,	4	...	2	3	...	9
Totals,	15	4	4	17	2	42

Suicide.

Ages,	15-25	25-65	Total
Males,	4	25	29
Females,	5	19	24
Totals	9	44	53

During the ten years, no case of murder through sulphuric acid is on record; hence the total deaths, as detailed in the tables, amount to 95, or a little over 9 a year.

Falck,[64] in comparing different countries, considers the past statistics to show that in France sulphuric acid has been the cause of 4.5 to 5.5 per cent. of the total deaths from poison, and in England 5.9 per cent. In England, France, and Denmark, taken together, 10.8, Prussia 10.6; while in certain cities, as Berlin and Vienna, the percentages are much higher—Vienna showing 43.3 per cent., Berlin 90 per cent.

§ 55. **Accidental, Suicidal, and Criminal Poisoning.**—Deaths from sulphuric acid are, for the most part, accidental, occasionally suicidal, and, still more rarely, criminal. In 53 out of 113 cases collected by Böhm, in which the cause of the poisoning could, with fair accuracy, be ascertained, 45.3 per cent. were due to accident, 30.2 were suicidal, and 24.5 per cent. were cases of criminal poisoning, the victims being children.

The cause of the comparatively rare use of sulphuric acid by the poisoner is obvious. First of all, the acid can never be mixed with food without entirely changing its aspect; next, it is only in cases of insensibility or paralysis that it could be administered to an adult, unless given by force, or under very exceptional circumstances; and lastly, the stains on the mouth and garments would at once betray, even to uneducated persons, the presence of something wrong. As an agent of murder, then, sulphuric acid is confined in its use to young children, more especially to the newly born.

There is a remarkable case related by Haagan,[65] in which an adult man, in full possession of his faculties, neither paralysed nor helpless, was murdered by sulphuric acid. The wife of a day-labourer gave her husband drops of sulphuric acid on sugar, instead of his medicine, and finally finished the work by administering a spoonful of the acid. The spoon was carried well to the back of the throat, so that the man took the acid at a gulp. 11 grms. (171

[64] *Lehrbuch der praktischen Toxicologie*, p. 54.

[65] Gross: *Die Strafrechtspflege in Deutschland*, 4, 1861, Heft I. S. 181.

grains) of sulphuric acid, partly in combination with soda and potash, were separated from his stomach.

Accidental poisoning is most common among children. The oily, syrupy-looking sulphuric acid, when pure, may be mistaken for glycerin or for syrup; and the dark commercial acid might, by a careless person, be confounded with porter or any dark-looking medicine.

Serious and fatal mistakes have not unfrequently arisen from the use of injections. Deutsch[66] relates how a midwife, in error, administered to mother and child a sulphuric acid clyster; but little of the fluid could in either case have actually reached the rectum, for the mother recovered in eight days, and in a little time the infant was also restored to health. Sulphuric acid has caused death by injections into the vagina. H. C. Lombard[67] observed a case of this kind, in which a woman, aged thirty, injected half a litre of sulphuric acid into the vagina, for the purpose of procuring abortion. The result was not immediately fatal, but the subsequent inflammation and its results so occluded the natural passage that the birth became impossible, and a Cæsarean section extracted a dead child, the mother also dying.

An army physician prescribed for a patient an emollient clyster. Since it was late at night, and the apothecary in bed, he prepared it himself; but not finding linseed oil, woke the apothecary, who took a bottle out of one of the recesses and placed it on the table. The bottle contained sulphuric acid; a soldier noticed a peculiar odour and effervescence when the syringe was charged, but this was unheeded by the doctor. The patient immediately after the operation suffered the most acute agony, and died the following day; before his death, the bedclothes were found corroded by the acid, and a portion of the bowel itself came away.[68]

§ 56. **Fatal Dose.**—The amount necessary to kill an adult man is not strictly known; fatality so much depends on the concentration of the acid and the condition of the person, more especially whether the stomach is full or empty, that it will be impossible ever to arrive at an accurate estimate. Christison's case, in which 3.8 grms. (60 grains) of concentrated acid killed an adult, is the smallest lethal dose on record. Supposing that the man weighed 68½ kilo. (150 lbs.), this would be in the proportion of .05 grm. per kilo. There is also the case of a child of one year, recorded by Taylor, in which 20 drops caused death. If, however, it were asked in a court of law what dose of concentrated sulphuric acid would be dangerous, the proper answer would be: so small a quantity as from 2 to 3 drops of the strong undiluted acid might cause death, more especially if conveyed to the back of the throat; for if it is improbable that on such a supposition death would be sudden, yet there is a possibility of permanent injury to the gullet, with the result of subsequent contraction, and the usual long and painful malnutrition thereby induced. It may be laid down, therefore, that all quantities, even the smallest, of the *strong undiluted acid* come under the head of hurtful, noxious, and injurious.

§ 57. **Local Action of Sulphuric Acid.**—The action of the acid on living animal tissues has been studied of late by C. Ph. Falck and L. Vietor.[69] Concentrated acid precipitates albumen, and then redissolves it; fibrin swells and becomes gelatinous; but if the acid is weak (*e.g.*, 4 to 6 per cent.) it is scarcely changed. Muscular fibre is at first coloured amber-yellow, swells to a jelly, and then dissolves to a red-brown turbid fluid. When applied to the mucous membrane of the stomach, the mucous tissue and the muscular layer beneath are coloured white, swell, and become an oily mass.

When applied to a rabbit's ear,[70] the parenchyma becomes at first pale grey and semi-transparent at the back of the ear; opposite the drop of acid appear spots like grease or fat drops, which soon coalesce. The epidermis with the hair remains adherent; the blood-vessels are narrowed in calibre, and the blood, first in the veins, and then in the arteries, is coloured green and then black, and fully coagulates. If the drop, with horizontal holding of the ear, is dried in, an inflammatory zone surrounds the burnt spot in which the blood circulates; but there is complete stasis in the part to which the acid has been applied. If the point of the ear is dipped in the acid, the cauterised part rolls inwards; after the lapse of eighteen hours the part is brown and parchment-like, with scattered points of coagulated blood; then there is a slight swelling in the healthy tissues, and a small zone of redness; within fourteen days a bladder-like greenish-yellow scab is formed, the burnt part itself remaining dry. The vessels from the surrounding zone of redness gradually penetrate towards the cauterised spot, the fluid in the bleb becomes absorbed, and the destroyed tissues fall off in the form of a crust.

[66] *Preuss. Med. Vereins-Zeitung*, 1848, No. 13.

[67] *Journ. de Chim. Méd.*, tom. vii., 1831.

[68] Maschka's *Handbuch*, p. 86; *Journal de Chimie Médicale*, t. i. No. 8, 405, 1835.

[69] *Deutsche Klinik*, 1864, Mo. 1-32, and Vietor's *Inaugur.-Dissert.*, Marburg, 1803.

[70] Samuel, *Entzündung u. Brand, in Virchow's Archiv f. Path. Anat.*, Bd. 51, Hft. 1 u. 2, S. 41, 1870.

The changes that sulphuric acid cause in blood are as follows: the fibrin is at first coagulated and then dissolved, and the colouring matter becomes of a black colour. These changes do not require the strongest acid, being seen with an acid of 60 per cent.

§ 58. The action of the acid on various non-living matters is as follows: poured on all vegetable earth, there is an effervescence, arising from decomposition of carbonates; any grass or vegetation growing on the spot is blackened and dies; an analysis of the layer of earth, on which the acid is poured, shows an excess of sulphates as compared with a similar layer adjacent; the earth will only have an acid reaction, if there has been more than sufficient acid to neutralise all alkalies and alkaline earths.

Wood almost immediately blackens, and the spot remains moist.

Spots on paper become quickly dark, and sometimes exhibit a play of colours, such as reddish-brown; ultimately the spot becomes very black, and holes may be formed; even when the acid is dilute, the course is very similar, for the acid dries in, until it reaches a sufficient degree of concentration to attack the tissue. I found small drops of sulphuric acid on a brussels carpet, which had a red pattern on a dark green ground with light green flowers, act as follows: the spots on the red at the end of a few hours were of a dark maroon colour, the green was darkened, and the light green browned; at the end of twenty-four hours but little change had taken place, nor could any one have guessed the cause of the spots without a close examination. Spots of the strong acid on thin cotton fabrics rapidly blackened, and actual holes were formed in the course of an hour; the main difference to the naked eye, between the stains of the acid and those produced by a red-hot body, lay in the moistness of the spots. Indeed, the great distinction, without considering chemical evidence, between recent burns of clothing by sulphuric acid and by heat, is that in the one case—that of the acid—the hole or spot is very moist; in the other very dry. It is easy to imagine that this distinction may be of importance in a legal investigation.

Spots of acid on clothing fall too often under the observation of all those engaged in practical chemical work. However quickly a spot of acid is wiped off, unless it is immediately neutralised by ammonia, it ultimately makes a hole in the cloth; the spot, as a rule, whatever the colour of the cloth, is of a blotting-paper red.

Sulphuric acid dropped on iron, attacks it, forming a sulphate, which may be dissolved out by water. If the iron is exposed to the weather the rain may wash away all traces of the acid, save the corrosion; but it would be under those circumstances impossible to say whether the corrosion was due to oxidation or a solvent.

To sum up briefly: the characters of sulphuric acid spots on organic matters generally are black, brown, or red-coloured destructions of tissue, moisture, acid-reaction (often after years), and lastly the chemical evidence of sulphuric acid or sulphates in excess.

Caution necessary in judging of Spots, &c.—An important case, related by Maschka, shows the necessity of great caution in interpreting results, unless all the circumstances of a case be carefully collated. A live coal fell on the bed of a weakly infant, five months old. The child screamed, and woke the father, who was dozing by the fire; the man, in terror, poured a large pot of water on the child and burning bed. The child died the following day.

A *post-mortem* examination showed a burn on the chest of the infant 2 inches in length. The tongue, pharynx, and gullet were all healthy; in the stomach a patch of mucous membrane, about half an inch in extent, was found to be brownish, friable, and very thin. A chemical examination showed that the portion of the bed adjacent to the burnt place contained free sulphuric acid. Here, then, was the following evidence: the sudden death of a helpless infant, a carbonised bed-cover with free sulphuric acid, and, lastly, an appearance in the stomach which, it might be said, was not inconsistent with sulphuric acid poisoning. Yet a careful sifting of the facts convinced the judges that no crime had been committed, and that the child's death was due to disease. Afterwards, experiment showed that if a live coal fall on to any tissue, and be drenched with water, free sulphuric acid is constantly found in the neighbourhood of the burnt place.

§ 59. **Symptoms.**—The symptoms may be classed in two divisions, viz.:—1. External effects of the acid. 2. Internal effects and symptoms arising from its interior administration.

1. **External Effects.**—Of late years several instances have occurred in which the acid has been used criminally to cause disfiguring burns of the face. The offence has in all these cases been committed by women, who, from motives of revengeful jealousy, have suddenly dashed a quantity of the acid into the face of the object of their resentment. In such cases, the phenomena observed are not widely different from those attending scalds or burns from hot neutral fluids. There is destruction of tissue, not necessarily deep, for the acid is almost immediately wiped off; but if any should reach the eye, inflammation, so acute as to lead to blindness, is the probable consequence. The skin is coloured at first white, at a later period brown, and part of it may be, as it were, dissolved. If the tract or skin touched by the acid is extensive, death may result. The inflammatory processes in the skin are similar to those

noticed by Falck and Vietor in their experiments, already detailed.

Internal Effects of Acids generally.—It may not be out of place, before speaking of the internal effects of sulphuric acid, to make a few remarks upon the action of acids generally. This action differs according to the kind of animal; at all events, there is a great difference between the action of acids on the herb-eating animals and the carnivora; the latter bear large doses of acids well, the former ill. For instance, the rabbit, if given a dose of any acid not sufficient to produce local effects but sufficient to affect its functions, will soon become paralysed and lie in a state of stupor, as if dead; the same dose per kilo. will not affect the dog. The reason for this is that the blood of the dog is able to neutralise the acid by ammonia, and that the blood of the rabbit is destitute of this property. Man is, in this respect, nearer to the dog than to the plant-eaters. Stadelmann has shown that a man is able to ingest large relative doses of oxybutyric acid, to neutralise the acid by ammonia, and to excrete it by means of the kidneys as ammonium butyrate.

Acids, however, if given in doses too great to be neutralised, alike affect plant- and flesh-eaters; death follows in all cases before the blood becomes acid. Salkowsky[71] has, indeed, shown that the effect of lessening the alkalinity of the blood by giving a rabbit food from which it can extract no alkali produces a similar effect to the actual dosing with an acid.

2. **Internal Effects of Sulphuric Acid.**—When sulphuric acid is taken internally, the acute and immediate symptom is pain. This, however, is not constant, since, in a few recorded cases, no complaint of pain has been made; but these cases are exceptional; as a rule, there will be immediate and great suffering. The tongue swells, the throat is also swollen and inflamed, swallowing of saliva even may be impossible. If the acid has been in contact with the epiglottis and vocal apparatus, there may be spasmodic croup and even fatal spasm of the glottis.

The acid, in its passage down the gullet, attacks energetically the mucous membrane and also the lining of the stomach; but the action does not stop there, for Lesser found in eighteen out of twenty-six cases (69 per cent.) that the corrosive action extended as far as the duodenum. There is excessive vomiting and retching; the matters vomited are acid, bloody, and slimy; great pieces of mucous membrane may be in this way expelled, and the whole of the lining membrane of the gullet may be thrown up entire. The bowels are, as a rule, constipated, but exceptionally there has been diarrhœa; the urine is sometimes retained; it invariably contains an excess of sulphates and often albumen, with hyaline casts of the uriniferous tubes. The pulse is small and frequent, the breathing slow, the skin very cold and covered with sweat; the countenance expresses great anxiety, and the extremities may be affected with cramps or convulsions. Death may take place within from twenty-four to thirty-six hours, and be either preceded by dyspnœa or by convulsions; consciousness is, as a rule, maintained to the end.

There are also more rapid cases than the above; a large dose of sulphuric acid taken on an empty stomach may absolutely dissolve it, and pass into the peritoneum; in such a case there is really no difference in the symptoms between sudden perforation of the stomach from disease, a penetrating wound of the abdomen, and any other sudden fatal lesion of the organs in the abdominal cavity (for in all these instances the symptoms are those of pure collapse); the patient is ashen pale, with pulse quick and weak, and body bathed in cold sweat, and he rapidly dies, it may be without much complaint of local pain.

If the patient live longer than twenty-four hours, the symptoms are mainly those of inflammation of the whole mucous tract, from the mouth to the stomach; and from this inflammation the patient may die in a variable period, of from three to eleven days, after taking the poison. In one case the death occurred suddenly, without any immediately preceding symptoms rendering imminent death probable. If this second stage is passed, then the loss of substance in the gullet and in the stomach almost invariably causes impairment of function, leading to a slow and painful death. The common sequence is stricture of the gullet, combined with feeble digestion, and in a few instances stricture of the pylorus. A curious sequel has been recorded by Mannkopf, viz., obstinate intercostal neuralgia; it has been observed on the fourth, seventh, and twenty-second day.

§ 60. **Treatment of Acute Poisoning by the Mineral Acids.**—The immediate indication is the dilution and neutralisation of the acid. For this purpose, finely-divided chalk, magnesia, or sodic carbonate may be used, dissolved or suspended in much water. The use of the stomach-pump is inadvisable, for the mucous membrane of the gullet may be so corroded by the acid that the passage of the tube down will do injury; unless the neutralisation is *immediate*, but little good is effected; hence it will often occur that the bystanders, if at all conversant with the matter, will have to use the first thing which comes to hand, such as the plaster of a wall, &c.; and lastly, if even these rough antidotes are not to be had, the best treatment is enormous doses of water, which will dilute the acid

[71] Virchow's *Archiv*, Bd. 58, 1.

and promote vomiting. The treatment of the after-effects belongs to the province of ordinary medicine, and is based upon general principles.

§ 61. **Post-mortem Appearances.**[72] — The general pathological appearances to be found in the stomach and internal organs differ according as the death is rapid or slow; if the death takes place within twenty-four hours, the effects are fairly uniform, the differences being only in degree; while, on the other hand, in those cases which terminate fatally from the more remote effects of the acid, there is some variety. It may be well to select two actual cases as types, the one patient dying from acute poisoning, the other surviving for a time, and then dying from ulceration and contraction of the digestive tract.

A hatter, early in the morning, swallowed a large mouthful of strong sulphuric acid, a preparation which he used in his work—(whether the draught was taken accidentally or suicidally was never known). He died within two hours. The whole tongue was sphacelated, parts of the mucous membrane being dissolved; the inner surface of the gullet, as well as the whole throat, was of a grey-black colour; the mucous membrane of the stomach was coal-black, and so softened that it gave way like blotting-paper under the forceps, the contents escaping into the cavity of the abdomen. The peritoneum was also blackened as if burnt; probably there had been perforation of the stomach during life; the mucous membrane of the duodenum was swollen, hardened, and looked as if it had been boiled; while the blood was of a cherry-red colour, and of the consistence of a thin syrup. The rest of the organs were healthy; a chemical research on the fluid which had been collected from the stomach, gullet, and duodenum showed that it contained 87.25 grains of free sulphuric acid.[73]

This is, perhaps, the most extreme case of destruction on record; the cause of the unusually violent action is referable to the acid acting on an empty stomach. It is important to note that even with this extensive destruction of the stomach, life was prolonged for two hours.

The case I have selected to serve as a type of a chronic but fatal illness produced from poisoning by sulphuric acid is one related by Oscar Wyss. A cook, thirty-four years of age, who had suffered many ailments, drank, on the 6th of November 1867, by mistake, at eight o'clock in the morning, two mouthfuls of a mixture of 1 part of sulphuric acid and 4 of water. Pain in the stomach and neck, and vomiting of black masses, were the immediate symptoms, and two hours later he was admitted into the hospital in a state of collapse, with cold extremities, cyanosis of the face, &c. Copious draughts of milk were given, and the patient vomited much, the vomit still consisting of black pultaceous matters, in which, on a microscopical examination, could be readily detected columnar epithelium of the stomach and mucous tissue elements. The urine was of specific gravity 1.033, non-albuminous; on analysis it contained 3.388 grms. of combined sulphuric acid.

On the second day there was some improvement in the symptoms; the urine contained 1.276 grm. of combined sulphuric acid; on the third day 2.665 grms. of combined sulphuric acid; and on the tenth day the patient vomited up a complete cast of the mucous membrane of the gullet. The patient remained in the hospital, and became gradually weaker from stricture of the gullet and impairment of the digestive powers, and died, two months after taking the poison, on the 5th of January 1868.

The stomach was found small, contracted, with many adhesions to the pancreas and liver; it was about 12 centimetres long (4.7 inches), and from 2 to 2.5 centimetres (.7 to .9 inch) broad, contracted to somewhat the form of a cat's intestine; there were several transverse rugæ; the walls were thickened at the small curvature, measurements giving 5 mm. (.19 inch) in the middle, and beyond about 2.75 mm. (.11 inch); in the upper two-thirds the lumen was so contracted as scarcely to admit the point of the little finger. The inner surface was covered with a layer of pus, with no trace of mucous tissue, and was everywhere pale red, uneven, and crossed by cicatricial bands. In two parts, at the greater curvature, the mucous surface was strongly injected in a ring-like form, and in the middle of the ring was a deep funnel-shaped ulcer; a part of the rest of the stomach was strongly injected and scattered over with numerous punctiform, small, transparent bladders. The gullet was contracted at the upper part (just below the epiglottis) from 20 to 22 mm. (.78 to .86 inch) in diameter; it then gradually widened to measure about 12 mm. (.47 inch) at the diaphragm; in the neighbourhood of the last contraction the tissue was scarred, injected, and ulcerated; there were also small abscesses opening into this portion of the gullet.

E. Fraenkel and F. Reiche[74] have studied the effects of sulphuric acid on the kidney. In rapid cases they find a

[72] It has been observed that putrefaction in cases of death from sulphuric acid is slow. Casper suggests this may be due to the neutralisation of ammonia; more probably it is owing to the antiseptic properties all mineral acids possess.

[73] Casper, vol. ii. case 194.

[74] Virchow's *Archiv*, Bd. 131, f. 130.

wide-spread coagulation of the epithelium in the convoluted and straight urinary canaliculi, with destruction of the kidney parenchyma, but no inflammation.

§ 62. The museums of the different London hospitals afford excellent material for the study of the effects of sulphuric acid on the pharynx, gullet, and stomach; and it may be a matter of convenience to students if the more typical examples at these different museums be noticed in detail, so that the preparations themselves may be referred to.

In St. Bartholomew's Museum, No. 1942, is an example of excessive destruction of the stomach by sulphuric acid. The stomach is much contracted, and has a large aperture with ragged edges; the mucous membrane is thickened, charred, and blackened.

No. 1941, in the same museum, is the stomach of a person who died from a large dose of sulphuric acid. When recent, it is described as of a deep red colour, mottled with black; appearances which, from long soaking in spirit, are not true at the present time; but the rough, shaggy state of the mucous tissue can be traced; the gullet and the pylorus appear the least affected.

St. George's Hospital, ser. ix., 146, 11 and 43, e.—The pharynx and œsophagus of a man who was brought into the hospital in a state of collapse, after a large but unknown dose of sulphuric acid. The lips were much eroded, the mucous membrane of the stomach, pharynx, and œsophagus show an extraordinary shreddy condition; the lining membrane of the stomach is much charred, and the action has extended to the duodenum; the muscular coat is not affected.

Guy's Hospital, No. 1799.—A preparation showing the mucous membrane of the stomach entirely denuded. The organ looks like a piece of thin paper.

No. 1799^{20}. The stomach of a woman who poisoned herself by drinking a wine-glassful of acid before breakfast. She lived eleven days. The main symptoms were vomiting and purging, but there was no complaint of pain. There is extensive destruction of mucous membrane along the lesser curvature and towards the pyloric extremity; a portion of the mucous membrane is floating as a slough.

No. 1799^{25} is the gullet and stomach of a man who took about 3 drachms of the strong acid. He lived three days without much apparent suffering, and died unexpectedly. The lining membrane of the œsophagus has the longitudinal wrinkles or furrows so often, nay, almost constantly, met with in poisoning by the acids. The mucous tissue of the stomach is raised in cloudy ridges, and blackened.

No. 1799^{35} is a wonderfully entire cast of the gullet from a woman who swallowed an ounce of sulphuric acid, and is said, according to the catalogue, to have recovered.

University College.—In this museum will be found an exquisite preparation of the effects of sulphuric acid. The mucous membrane of the œsophagus is divided into small quadrilateral areas by longitudinal and transverse furrows; the stomach is very brown, and covered with shreddy and filamentous tissue; the brown colour is without doubt the remains of extravasated and charred blood.

No. 6201 is a wax cast representing the stomach of a woman who died after taking a large dose of sulphuric acid. A yellow mass was found in the stomach; there are two perforations, and the mucous membrane is entirely destroyed.

§ 63. **Chronic Poisoning by Sulphuric Acid.**—Weiske[75] has experimentally proved that lambs, given for six months small doses of sulphuric acid, grow thin, and their bones, with the exception of the bones of the head and the long bones, are poor in lime salts, the muscles also are poor in the same constituents. Kobert[76] thinks that drunkards on the continent addicted to "Schnaps," commonly a liquid acidified with sulphuric acid to give it a sharp taste, often show typical chronic sulphuric acid poisoning.

Detection and Estimation of Free Sulphuric Acid.

§ 64. The general method of separating the mineral acids is as follows: the tissues, or matters, are soaked in distilled water for some time. If no free acid is present, the liquid will not redden litmus-paper, or give an acid reaction with any of the numerous tinctorial agents in use by the chemist for the purposes of titration. After sufficient digestion in water, the liquid extract is made up to some definite bulk and allowed to subside. Filtration is unnecessary. A small fractional part (say, for example, should the whole be 250 c.c., $^1/_{100}$th or 2.5 c.c.) is taken, and using as an indicator cochineal or phenolphthalein, the total acidity is estimated by a decinormal solution of soda. By this preliminary operation, some guide for the conduct of the future more exact operations is obtained. Should

[75] H. Weiske, *Journ. f. Landwirthsch.*, 1887, 417.

[76] *Lehrbuch der Intoxicationen*, S. 210.

the liquid be very acid, a small quantity of the whole is to be now taken, but if the acidity is feeble, a larger quantity is necessary, and sufficient quinine then added to fix the acid—100 parts of sulphuric acid are saturated by 342 parts of quinine monohydrate. Therefore, on the supposition that all the free acid is sulphuric, it will be found sufficient to add 3.5 parts of quinine for every 1 part of acid, estimated as sulphuric, found by the preliminary rough titration; and as it is inconvenient to deal with large quantities of alkaloid, a fractional portion of the liquid extract (representing not more than 50 mgrms. of acid) should be taken, which will require 175 mgrms. of quinine.

On addition of the quinine, the neutralised liquid is evaporated to dryness, or to approaching dryness, and then exhausted by strong alcohol. The alcoholic extract is, after filtration, dried up, and the quinine sulphate, nitrate, or hydrochlorate, as the case may be, filtered off and extracted by boiling water, and precipitated by ammonia, the end result being quinine hydrate (which may be filtered off and used again for similar purposes) and a sulphate, nitrate or chloride of ammonia in solution. It therefore remains to determine the nature and quantity of the acids now combined with ammonia. The solution is made up to a known bulk, and portions tested for chlorides by nitrate of silver, and for nitrates by the copper or the ferrous sulphate test. If sulphuric acid is present, there will be a precipitate of barium sulphate, which, on account of its density and insolubility in nitric or hydrochloric acids, is very characteristic. For estimating the sulphuric acid thus found, it will only be necessary to take a known bulk of the same liquid, heat it to boiling after acidifying by hydrochloric acid, and then add a sufficient quantity of baric chloride solution. Unless this exact process is followed, the analyst is likely to get a liquid which refuses to filter clear, but if the sulphate be precipitated from a hot liquid, it usually settles rapidly to the bottom of the vessel, and the supernatant fluid can be decanted clear; the precipitate is washed by decantation, and ultimately collected on a filter, dried, and weighed.

The sulphate of baryta found, multiplied by .3434, equals the sulphuric anhydride.

The older process was to dissolve the free sulphuric acid out by alcohol. As is well known, mineral sulphates are insoluble in, and are precipitated by, alcohol, whereas sulphuric acid enters into solution. The most valid objection, as a quantitative process, to the use of alcohol, is the tendency which all mineral acids have to unite with alcohol in organic combination, and thus, as it were, to disappear; and, indeed, results are found, by experiment, to be below the truth when alcohol is used. This objection does not hold good if either merely qualitative evidence, or a fairly approximate quantation, is required. In such a case, the vomited matters, the contents of the stomach, or a watery extract of the tissues, are evaporated to a syrup, and then extracted with strong alcohol and filtered; a little phenolphthalein solution is added, and the acid alcohol exactly neutralised by an alcoholic solution of clear decinormal or normal soda. According to the acidity of the liquid, the amount used of the decinormal or normal soda is noted, and then the whole evaporated to dryness, and finally heated to gentle redness. The alkaline sulphate is next dissolved in very dilute hydrochloric acid, and the solution precipitated by chloride of barium in the usual way. The quantitative results, although low, would, in the great majority of cases, answer the purpose sufficiently.

A test usually enumerated, Hilger's test for mineral acid, may be mentioned. A liquid, which contains a very minute quantity of mineral acid, becomes of a blue colour (or, if 1 per cent. or above, of a green) on the addition of a solution of methyl aniline violet; but this test, although useful in examining vinegars (see "Foods," p. 519), is not of much value in toxicology, and the quinine method for this purpose meets every conceivable case, both for qualitative and quantitative purposes.

§ 65. **The Urine.**—Although an excess of sulphates is found constantly in the urine of persons who have taken large doses of sulphuric acid, the latter has never been found in that liquid in a free state, so that it will be useless to search for free acid. It is, therefore, only necessary to add HCl to filter the fluid, and precipitate direct with an excess of chloride of barium. It is better to operate in this manner than to burn the urine to an ash, for in the latter case part of the sulphates, in the presence of phosphates, are decomposed, and, on the other hand, any organic sulphur combinations are liable to be estimated as sulphates.

It may also be well to pass chlorine gas through the same urine which has been treated with chloride of barium, and from which the sulphate has been filtered off. The result of this treatment will be a second precipitate of sulphate derived from sulphur, in a different form of combination than that of sulphate.

The greatest amount of sulphuric acid as mineral and organic sulphate is separated, according to Mannkopf[77] and Schultzen,[78] within five hours after taking sulphuric acid; after three days the secretion, so far as total sulphates is concerned, is normal.

[77] "Toxicologie der Schwefelsäure," *Wiener med. Wochen.*, 1862, 1863.

[78] *Archiv. f. Anatom. u. Physiol.*, 1864.

The normal amount of sulphuric acid excreted daily, according to Thudichum, is from 1.5 to 2.5 grms., and organic sulphur up to .2 grm. in the twenty-four hours, but very much more has been excreted by healthy persons.

Lehmann made some observations on himself, and found that, on an animal diet, he excreted no less than 10.399 grms. of sulphuric acid per day, while on mixed food a little over 7 grms.; but, as Thudichum justly observes, this great amount must be referred to individual peculiarity. The amount of sulphates has a decided relation to diet. Animal food, although not containing sulphates, yet, from the oxidation of the sulphur-holding albumen, produces a urine rich in sulphate. Thus Vogel found that a person, whose daily average was 2.02 grms., yielded 7.3 on a meat diet. The internal use of sulphur, sulphides, and sulphates, given in an ordinary medicinal way, is traceable in the urine, increasing the sulphates. In chronic diseases the amount of sulphates is decreased, in acute increased.

Finally, it would appear that the determination of sulphates in the urine is not of much value, *save when the normal amount that the individual secretes is primarily known*. On the other hand, a low amount of sulphates in the urine of a person poisoned by sulphuric acid has not been observed within three days of the taking of the poison, and one can imagine cases in which such a low result might have forensic importance.

The presence of albumen in the urine has been considered by some a constant result of sulphuric acid poisoning, but although when looked for it is usually found, it cannot be considered constant. O. Smoler,[79] in eighteen cases of various degrees of sulphuric acid poisoning, found nothing abnormal in the urine. Wyss[80] found in the later stages of a case indican and pus. E. Leyden and Ph. Munn[81] always found blood in the urine, as well as albumen, with casts and cellular elements. Mannkopf[82] found albuminuria in three cases out of five; in two of the cases there were fibrinous casts; in two the albumen disappeared at the end of the second or third day, but in one it continued for more than twenty days. Bamberger[83] has observed an increased albuminuria, with separation of the colouring matter of the blood. In this case it was ascribed to the action of the acid on the blood.

§ 66. **The Blood.**—In Casper's case, No. 193, the vena cava of a child, who died within an hour after swallowing a large dose of sulphuric acid, was filled with a cherry-red, strongly acid-reacting blood. Again, Casper's case, No. 200, is that of a young woman, aged 19, who died from a poisonous dose of sulphuric acid. At the autopsy, four days after death, the following peculiarities of the blood were thus noted:—"The blood had an acid reaction, was dark, and had (as is usual in these cases) a syrupy consistence, while the blood-corpuscles were quite unchanged. The blood was treated with an excess of absolute alcohol, filtered, the filtrate concentrated on a water-bath, the residue exhausted with absolute alcohol, &c. It yielded a small quantity of sulphuric acid."

Other similar cases might be noted, but it must not for a moment be supposed that the mass of the blood contains any free sulphuric acid during life. The acidity of the blood in the vena cava may be ascribed to *post-mortem* endosmosis, the acid passing through the walls of the stomach into the large vessel.

§ 67. **Sulphates.**—If the acid swallowed should have been entirely neutralised by antidotes, such as chalk, &c., it becomes of the first importance to ascertain, as far as possible, by means of a microscopical examination, the nature of the food remaining in the stomach, and then to calculate the probable contents in sulphates of the food thus known to be eaten. It will be found that, with ordinary food, and under ordinary circumstances, only small percentages of combined sulphuric acid can be present.

As an example, take the ordinary rations of the soldier, viz.:—12 oz. of meat, 24 oz. of bread, 16 oz. of potatoes, 8 oz. of other vegetables; with sugar, salt, tea, coffee, and water. Now, if the whole quantity of these substances were eaten at a meal, they would not contain more than from 8 to 10 grains (.5 to .6 grm.) of anhydrous sulphuric acid, in the form of sulphates.

So far as the contents of the stomach are concerned, we have only to do with sulphates introduced in the food, but when once the food passes further along the intestinal canal, circumstances are altered, for we have sulphur-holding secretions, which, with ordinary chemical methods, yield sulphuric acid. Thus, even in the newly-born infant, according to the analyses of Zweifler, the mineral constituents of meconium are especially sulphate of lime, with a smaller quantity of sulphate of potash. The amount of bile which flows into the whole tract of the intestinal canal is estimated at about half a litre in the twenty-four hours; the amount of sulphur found in bile varies from .89 to 3 per cent., so that in 500 c.c. we might, by oxidising the sulphur, obtain from 2.2 to 7.5 grms. of sulphuric

[79] *Archiv der Heilkunde red. v.* E. Wagner, 1869, Hft. 2, S. 181.
[80] *Wiener Medicinal-Halle*, 1861, Jahr. 6, No. 46.
[81] Virchow's *Archiv f. path. Anat.*, 1861. Bd. 22, Hft. 3 u. 4, S. 237.
[82] *Wien. med. Wochenschrift*, 1862, Nro. 35; 1863, Nro. 5.
[83] *Wien. Med.-Halle*, 1864, Nro. 29, 30.

anhydride.

It is therefore certain that large quantities of organic sulphur-compounds may be found in the human intestinal canal, for with individuals who suffer from constipation, the residues of the biliary secretion accumulate for many days. Hence, if the analyst searches for sulphates in excretal matters, all methods involving destruction of organic substances, whether by fire or by fluid-oxidising agents, are wrong in principle, and there is nothing left save to separate soluble sulphates by dialysis, or to precipitate direct out of an aqueous extract.

Again, sulphate of magnesia is a common medicine, and so is sodic sulphate; a possible medicinal dose of magnesia sulphate might amount to 56.7 grms. (2 oz.), the more usual dose being half that quantity. Lastly, among the insane there are found patients who will eat plaster-of-Paris, earth, and similar matters, so that, in special cases, a very large amount of combined sulphuric acid may be found in the intestinal tract, without any relation to poisoning by the free acid; but in such instances it must be rare, indeed, that surrounding circumstances or pathological evidence will not give a clue to the real state of affairs.

II.—Hydrochloric Acid.

§ 68. *General Properties.*—Hydrochloric acid, otherwise called *muriatic acid, spirit of salt*, is, in a strictly chemical sense, a pure gas, composed of 97.26 per cent. of chlorine, and 2.74 per cent. of hydrogen; but, in an ordinary sense, it is a liquid, being a solution of the gas itself.

Hydrochloric acid is made on an enormous scale in the United Kingdom, the production being estimated at about a million tons annually.

The toxicology of hydrochloric acid is modern, for we have no evidence that anything was known of it prior to the middle of the seventeenth century, when Glauber prepared it in solution, and, in 1772, Priestley, by treating common salt with sulphuric acid, isolated the pure gas.

The common liquid hydrochloric acid of commerce has a specific gravity of from 1.15 to 1.20, and contains usually less than 40 parts of hydrochloric acid in the 100 parts. The strength of pure samples of hydrochloric acid can be told by the specific gravity, and a very close approximation, in default of tables, may be obtained by simply multiplying the decimal figures of the specific gravity by 200. For example, an acid of 1.20 gravity would by this rule contain 40 per cent. of real acid, for $.20 \times 200 = 40$.

The commercial acid is nearly always a little yellow, from the presence of iron derived from metallic retorts, and usually contains small quantities of chloride of arsenic,[84] derived from the sulphuric acid; but the colourless hydrochloric acid specially made for laboratory and medicinal use is nearly always pure.

The uses of the liquid acid are mainly in the production of chlorine, as a solvent for metals, and for medicinal and chemical purposes. Its properties are briefly as follows:

It is a colourless or faintly-yellow acid liquid, the depth of colour depending on its purity, and especially its freedom from iron. The liquid is volatile, and can be separated from fixed matters and the less volatile acids by distillation; it has a strong attraction for water, and fumes when exposed to the air, from becoming saturated with aqueous vapour. If exposed to the vapour of ammonia, extremely dense clouds arise, due to the formation of the solid ammonium chloride. The acid, boiled with a small quantity of manganese binoxide, evolves chlorine. Dioxide of lead has a similar action; the chlorine may be detected by its bleaching action on a piece of paper dipped in indigo blue; a little zinc foil immersed in the acid disengages hydrogen. These two tests—viz., the production of chlorine by the one, and the production of hydrogen by the other—separate and reveal the constituent parts of the acid. Hydrochloric acid, in common with chlorides, gives a dense precipitate with silver nitrate. The precipitate is insoluble in nitric acid, but soluble in ammonia; it melts without decomposition. Exposed to the light, it becomes of a purple or blackish colour. Every 100 parts of silver chloride are equal to 25.43 of hydrochloric acid, HCl, and to 63.5 parts of the liquid acid of specific gravity 1.20.

The properties of pure hydrochloric acid gas are as follows:—Specific gravity 1.262, consisting of equal volumes of hydrogen and chlorine, united without condensation. 100 cubic inches must therefore have a weight of 39.36 grains. The gas was liquefied by Faraday by means of a pressure of 40 atmospheres at 10°; it was colourless, and had a less refractive index than water.

Water absorbs the gas with avidity, 100 volumes of water absorbing 48,000 volumes of the gas, and becoming

[84] Some samples of hydrochloric acid have been found to contain as much as 4 per cent. of chloride of arsenic, but this is very unusual. Glenard found as a mean 2.5 grammes, As_2O_3 per kilogramme.

142 volumes. The solution has all the properties of strong hydrochloric acid, specific gravity 1.21. The dilute hydrochloric acid of the Pharmacopœia should have a specific gravity of 1.052, and be equivalent to 10.58 per cent. of HCl.

§ 69. **Statistics of Poisoning by Hydrochloric Acid.** — The following tables give the deaths, with age and sex distribution, due to hydrochloric acid for ten years (1883-92):

DEATHS FROM HYDROCHLORIC ACID IN ENGLAND AND WALES DURING THE TEN YEARS ENDING 1892.

Accident or Negligence.

Ages,	Under 1	1-5	5-15	15-25	25-65	65 and above	Total
Males,	1	16	2	...	26	3	48
Females,	...	8	...	...	9	1	18
Totals,	1	24	2	...	35	4	66

Suicide.

Ages,	5-15	15-25	25-65	65 and above	Total
Males,	...	2	73	8	83
Females,	1	8	42	65	116
Totals,	1	10	115	73	199

In 1889 a solitary case of the murder of a child is on record from hydrochloric acid; hence, with that addition, the total deaths from hydrochloric acid amount to 266 in the ten years, or about 26 a year.

§ 70. **Fatal Dose.**—The dose which destroys life is not known with any accuracy. In two cases, adults have been killed by 14 grms. (half an ounce) of the commercial acid; but, on the other hand, recovery is recorded when more than double this quantity has been taken. A girl, fifteen years of age, died from drinking a teaspoonful of the acid.[85]

§ 71. **Amount of Free Acid in the Gastric Juice.**—Hydrochloric acid exists in the gastric juice. This was first ascertained by Prout[86] in 1824; he separated it by distillation. The observation was afterwards confirmed by Gmelin,[87] Children,[88] and Braconnot.[89] On the other hand, Lehmann[90] pointed out that, as the stomach secretion contained, without doubt, lactic acid, the act of distillation, in the presence of this lactic acid, would set free hydrochloric acid from any alkaline chlorides. Blondlot and Cl. Bernard also showed that the gastric juice possessed no acid which would dissolve oxalate of lime, or develop hydrogen when treated with iron filings; hence there could not be free hydrochloric acid which, even in a diluted state, would respond to both these tests. Then followed the researches of C. Schmidt,[91] who showed that the gastric secretion of men, of sheep, and of dogs contained more hydrochloric acid than would satisfy the bases present; and he propounded the view that the gastric juice does not contain absolutely free hydrochloric acid, but that it is in loose combination with the pepsin.

The amount of acid in the stomach varies from moment to moment, and therefore it is not possible to say what

[85] *Brit. Med. Journ.*, March, 1871.

[86] *Philosophical Transactions*, 1824, p. 45.

[87] P. Tiedmann and L. Gmelin, *Die Verdauung nach Versuchen*, Heidelberg u. Leipsic, 1826, i.

[88] *Annals of Philosophy*, July, 1824.

[89] *Ann. de Chim.* t. lix. p. 348.

[90] *Journal f. prakt. Chemie*, Bd. xl. 47.

[91] Bidder u. Schmidt, *Verdauungs-Säfte*, &c.

the average acidity of gastric juice is. It has been shown that in the total absence of *free* hydrochloric acid digestion may take place, because hydrochloric acid forms a compound with pepsin which acts as a solvent on the food. The amount of physiologically active acid varies with the food taken. It is smallest when carbohydrates are consumed, greatest with meat. The maximum amount that Jaksch found in his researches, when meat was ingested, was .09 per cent. of hydrochloric acid. It is probable that anything above 0.2 per cent. of hydrochloric acid is either abnormal or owing to the recent ingestion of hydrochloric acid.

§ 72. **Influence of Hydrochloric Acid on Vegetation.**—Hydrochloric acid fumes, if emitted from works on a large scale, injure vegetation much. In former years, before any legal obligations were placed upon manufacturers for the condensing of the volatile products, the nuisance from this cause was great. In 1823, the duty on salt being repealed by the Government, an extraordinary impetus was given to the manufacture of hydrochloric acid, and since all the volatile products at that time escaped through short chimneys into the air, a considerable area of land round the works was rendered quite unfit for growing plants. The present law on the subject is, that the maximum quantity of acid escaping shall not exceed 2 grains per cubic foot of the air, smoke, or chimney gases; and, according to the reports of the alkali inspectors, the condensation by the improved appliances is well within the Act, and about as perfect as can be devised.

It appears from the reports of the Belgian Commission in 1855, when virtually no precautions were taken, that the gases are liable to injure vegetation to the extent of 2000 metres (2187 yards) around any active works; the more watery vapour the air contains, the quicker is the gas precipitated and carried to the earth. If the action of the vapour is considerable, the leaves of plants dry and wither; the chlorophyll becomes modified, and no longer gives the normal spectrum, while a thickening of the rind of trees has also been noticed. The cereals suffer much; they increase in stalk, but produce little grain. The leguminosæ become spotted, and have an air of dryness and want of vigour; while the potato, among plants utilised for food, appears to have the strongest resistance. Vines are very sensitive to the gas. Among trees, the alder seems most sensitive; then come fruit-trees, and last, the hardy forest-trees—the poplar, the ash, the lime, the elm, the maple, the birch, and the oak.[92]

§ 73. **Action upon Cloth and Manufactured Articles.**—On black cloth the acid produces a green stain, which is not moist and shows no corrosion. On most matters the stain is more or less reddish; after a little time no free acid may be detected, by simply moistening the spot; but if the stain is cut out and boiled with water, there may be some evidence of free acid. The absence of moisture and corrosion distinguishes the stain from that produced by sulphuric acid.

§ 74. **Poisonous Effects of Hydrochloric Acid Gas.**—Eulenberg[93] has studied the effects of the vapour of this acid on rabbits and pigeons. One of these experiments may be cited in detail. Hydrochloric acid gas, prepared by heating together common salt and sulphuric acid, was passed into a glass shade supported on a plate, and a rabbit was placed in the transparent chamber thus formed. On the entrance of the vapour, there was immediate blinking of the eyes, rubbing of the paws against the nostrils, and emission of white fumes with the expired breath, while the respiration was irregular (40 to the minute). After the lapse of ten minutes, the gas was again introduced, until the atmosphere was quite thick; the symptoms were similar to those detailed above, but more violent; and in fourteen minutes from the commencement, the rabbit sank down on its right side (respirations 32). When twenty-two minutes had elapsed, the gas was again allowed to enter. The rabbit now lay quiet, with closed eyes and laboured respiration, and, finally, after half-an-hour of intermittent exposure to the gas, the animal was removed.

The cornea were opalescent, and the eyes filled with water; there was frequent shaking of the head and working of the forepaws. After three minutes' exposure to the air, the respirations were found to be 128 per minute; this quickened respiration lasted for an hour, then gave place to a shorter and more superficial breathing. On the second day after the experiment, the rabbit suffered from laboured respiration (28 to the minute) and pain, and there was a rattling in the bronchial tubes. The animal died on the third day, death being preceded by slow respiration (12 to the

[92] Those who desire to study more closely the effect of acids generally on vegetation may consult the various papers of the alkali inspectors contained in the Local Government Reports. See also Schubarth, *Die saueren Gase, welche Schwefelsäure- und Soda-Fabriken verbreiten. Verhandlungen des Vereins zur Beförderung des Gewerbefleisses in Preussen*, 1857, S. 135. Dingler's *Journal*, Bd. 145, S. 374-427.

Christel, *Ueber die Einwirkung von Säuren-Dämpfen auf die Vegetation.*

Arch. f. Pharmacie, 1871, p. 252.

Vierteljahrsschrift für gerichtliche Medicin, 17 Bd. S. 404, 1872.

[93] *Gewerbe Hygiene*, Berlin, 1876, S. 51.

minute).

The appearances twenty-four hours after death were as follows:—The eyes were coated with a thick slime, and both cornea were opalescent; there was strong rigidity of the body. The pia mater covering the brain was everywhere hyperæmic, and at the hinder border of both hemispheres appeared a small clot, surrounded by a thin layer of bloody fluid. The *plex. venos spin.* was filled with coagulated blood, and there was also a thin extravasation of blood covering the medulla and pons. The lungs were mottled bright brown-red; the middle lobe of the right lung was dark brown, solid, and sank in water; the lower lobe of the same lung and the upper lobe of the left lung were nearly in a similar condition, but the edges were of a bright red. The parenchyma in the darker places on section did not crepitate. On the cut surface was a little dark, fluid, weakly-acid blood; the tracheal mucous membrane was injected. The heart was filled with thick coagulated blood; the liver was congested, of a reddish-brown colour, and rich in dark, fluid blood: in the vena cava inferior was coagulated blood. The kidneys were not hyperæmic; the intestines were superficially congested.

I think there can be little doubt that the symptoms during life, and the appearances after death, in this case are perfectly consistent with the following view:—The vapour acts first as a direct irritant, and is capable of exciting inflammation in the lung and bronchial tissues; but besides this, there is a secondary effect, only occurring when the gas is in sufficient quantity, and the action sufficiently prolonged—viz., a direct coagulation of the blood in certain points of the living vessels of the lungs. The consequence of this is a more or less general backward engorgement, the right side of the heart becomes distended with blood, and the ultimate cause of death is partly mechanical. The hyperæmia of the brain membranes, and even the hæmorrhages, are quite consistent with this view, and occur in cases where the obstruction to the circulation is of a coarser and more obvious character, and can therefore be better appreciated.

§ 75. **Effects of the Liquid Acid.**—There is one distinction between poisoning by hydrochloric and the other mineral acids—namely, the absence of corrosion of the skin. Ad. Lesser[94] has established, by direct experiment, that it is not possible to make any permanent mark on the skin by the application even of the strongest commercial acid (40 per cent.). Hence, in any case of suspected poisoning by acid, should there be stains on the lips and face as from an acid, the presumption will be rather against hydrochloric. The symptoms themselves differ very little from those produced by sulphuric acid. The pathological appearances also are not essentially different, but hydrochloric is a weaker acid, and the extensive disorganisation, solution, and perforation of the viscera, noticed occasionally with sulphuric acid, have never been found in hydrochloric acid poisoning. We may quote here the following case:

A woman, under the influence of great and sudden grief—not unmixed with passion—drew a bottle from her pocket, and emptied it very quickly. She immediately uttered a cry, writhed, and vomited a yellow-green fluid. The abdomen also became enlarged. Milk was given her, but she could not swallow it, and death took place, in convulsions, two hours after the drinking of the poison.

The *post-mortem* appearances were briefly as follows:—Mouth and tongue free from textural change: much gas in the abdomen, more especially in the stomach; the membranes of the brain congested; the lungs filled with blood. The stomach was strongly pressed forward, of a dark brown-red, and exhibited many irregular blackish spots, varying from two lines to half an inch in diameter (the spots were drier and harder than the rest of the stomach); the mucous membrane, internally, was generally blackened, and changed to a carbonised, shaggy, slimy mass, while the organ was filled with a blackish homogeneous pulp, which had no odour. The gullet was also blackened. A considerable quantity of hydrochloric acid was separated from the stomach.[95]

The termination in this instance was unusually rapid. In a case detailed by Casper,[96] in which a boy drank an unknown quantity of acid, death took place in seven hours. In Guy's Hospital museum, the duodenum and stomach are preserved of a patient who is said to have died in nine and a half hours from half an ounce of the acid. The same quantity, in a case related by Taylor, caused death in eighteen hours. From these and other instances, it may be presumed that death from acute poisoning by hydrochloric acid will probably take place within twenty-four hours. From the secondary effects, of course, death may take place at a remote period, *e.g.*, in a case recorded by Dr. Duncan (*Lancet*, April 12, 1890), a man drank about 1 oz. of HCl accidentally, was admitted to Charing Cross Hospital the same day, and treated with small quantities of sodium carbonate, and fed by the rectum. On the eighth day he brought up 34 oz. of blood; in a month he left apparently perfectly well, but was admitted again in about six

[94] Virchow's *Archiv f. path. Anat.*, Bd. 83, Hft. 2, S. 215, 1881.

[95] *Preuss. Med. Vereinszeit. u. Friederichs Blätter f. gerichtl. Anthropologie*, 1858, Hft. 6, S. 70.

[96] Case 230.—*Gerichtliche Medicin*, 6th Ed., Berlin, 1876.

weeks, and died of contraction of the stomach and stricture of the pylorus on the ninety-fourth day.

§ 76. **Post-mortem Appearances.**—The pathological appearances are very similar to those found in the case already detailed; though the skin of the face may not be eroded in any way by the acid, yet the more delicate mucous membrane of the mouth, gullet, &c., appears mostly to be changed, and is usually white or whitish-brown. There is, however, in the museum of the Royal College of Surgeons the stomach and gullet (No. 2386c.) of an infant thirteen months old; the infant drank a tea-cupful of strong hydrochloric acid, and died nine hours after the dose. The pharynx and the upper end of the gullet is quite normal, the corrosive action commencing at the lower end, so that, although the acid was concentrated, not the slightest effect was produced on the delicate mucous membrane of the throat and upper part of the gullet. The lower end of the gullet and the whole of the stomach were intensely congested; the rugæ of the latter were ecchymosed and blackened by the action of the acid. There were also small hæmorrhages in the lungs, which were ascribed to the action of the acid on the blood. Perforation of the stomach has not been noticed in hydrochloric acid poisoning.

In Guy's Hospital museum (prep. 1799[10]), the stomach and duodenum of the case mentioned exhibit the mucous membrane considerably injected, with extravasations of blood, which, at the time when the preparation was first arranged, were of various hues, but are now somewhat altered, through long keeping in spirit. In St. George's Hospital museum (ser. x. 43, d. 200) are preserved the stomach and part of the duodenum of a person who died from hydrochloric acid. The case is detailed in the *Medical Times and Gazette* for 1853, vol. ii. p. 513. The whole inner surface appears to be in a sloughing state, and the larynx and lung were also inflamed.

A preparation, presented by Mr. Bowman to King's College Hospital museum, exhibits the effects of a very large dose of hydrochloric acid. The gullet has a shrivelled and worm-eaten appearance; the stomach is injected with black blood, and was filled with an acid, grumous matter.[97]

Looking at these and other museum preparations illustrating the effects of sulphuric and hydrochloric acids, I was unable (in default of the history of the cases) to distinguish between the two, by the naked eye appearances, save in those cases in which the disorganisation was so excessive as to render hydrochloric acid improbable. On the other hand, the changes produced by nitric acid are so distinctive, that it is impossible to mistake its action for that of any other acid. The nitric acid pathological preparations may be picked out at a glance.

Detection and Estimation of Free Hydrochloric Acid.

§ 77. (1) **Detection.**—A large number of colouring reagents have been proposed as tests for the presence of free mineral acid; among the best is *methyl-aniline violet* decolorised by a large amount of hydrochloric acid; the violet turns to green with a moderate quantity, and to blue with a small quantity.

Tropæolin (00), in the presence of free mineral acid, strikes a ruby-red to a dark brown-red.

Congo-red is used in the form of paper dyed with the material; large amounts of free hydrochloric acid strike blue-black, small quantities blue.

Günzburg's test is 2 parts phloroglucin and 1 part vanillin, dissolved in 100 parts of alcohol. Fine red crystals are precipitated on the addition of hydrochloric acid. To test the stomach contents for free hydrochloric acid by means of this reagent, equal parts of the fluid and the test are evaporated to dryness in the water-bath in a porcelain dish. If free hydrochloric acid be present, the evaporated residue shows a red colour; 1 mgrm. of acid can by this test be detected. The reaction is not interfered with by organic acids, peptones, or albumin.

Jaksch speaks highly of *benzopurpurin* as a test. Filter-paper is soaked in a saturated aqueous solution of benzopurpurin 6 B (the variety 1 or 4 B is not so sensitive), and the filter-paper thus prepared allowed to dry. On testing the contents of the stomach with the reagent, if there is more than 4 parts per 1000 of hydrochloric acid the paper is stained intensely blue-black; but if the colour is brown-black, this is from butyric or lactic acids, or from a mixture of these acids with hydrochloric acid. If the paper is washed with pure ether, and the colour was due only to organic acids, the original hue of the paper is restored; if the colour produced was due to a mixture of mineral and organic acids, the brown-black colour is weakened; and, lastly, if due to hydrochloric acid alone, the colour is not altered by washing with ether. Acid salts have no action, nor is the test interfered with by large amounts of albumins and peptones.

A. Villiers and M. Favolle[98] have published a sensitive test for hydrochloric acid. The test consists of a saturated aqueous solution of colourless aniline, 4 parts; glacial acetic acid, 1 part; 0.1 mgrm. of hydrochloric acid strikes

[97] A drawing of parts of the gullet and stomach is given in Guy and Ferrier's *Forensic Medicine*.

[98] *Comptes Rend.*, cxviii.

with this reagent a blue colour, 1 mgrm. a black colour. The liquid under examination is brought by evaporation, or by the addition of water, to 10 c.c. and placed in a flask; to this is added 5 c.c. of a mixture of equal parts of sulphuric acid and water, then 10 c.c. of a saturated solution of potassic permanganate, and heated gently, conveying the gases into 3 to 5 c.c. of the reagent contained in a test-tube immersed in water. If, however, bromine or iodine (one or both) should be present, the process is modified as follows: — The hydracids are precipitated by silver nitrate; the precipitate is washed, transferred to a small flask, and treated with 10 c.c. of water and 1 c.c. of pure ammonia. With this strength of ammonia the chloride of silver is dissolved easily, the iodide not at all, and the bromide but slightly. The ammoniacal solution is filtered, boiled, and treated with SH_2; the excess of SH_2 is expelled by boiling, the liquid filtered, reduced to 10 c.c. by boiling or evaporation, sulphuric acid and permanganate added as before, and the gases passed into the aniline. The process is inapplicable to the detection of chlorides or hydrochloric acid if cyanides are present, and it is more adapted for traces of hydrochloric acid than for the quantities likely to be met with in a toxicological inquiry.

(2) **Quantitative estimation of Free Hydrochloric Acid.**—The contents of the stomach are diluted to a known volume, say 250 or 500 c.c. A fractional portion is taken, say 10 c.c., coloured with litmus or phenol-phthalein, and a decinormal solution of soda added drop by drop until the colour changes; this gives total acidity. Another 10 c.c. is shaken with double its volume of ether three times, the fluid separated from ether and titrated in the same way; this last titration will give the acidity due to mineral acids and acid salts;[99] if the only mineral acid present is hydrochloric acid the results will be near the truth if reckoned as such, and this method, although not exact for physiological research, is usually sufficient for the purpose of ascertaining the amount of hydrochloric acid or other mineral acids in a case of poisoning. It depends on the fact that ether extracts free organic acids, such as butyric and lactic acids, but does not extract mineral acids.

The free mineral acid, after extracting the organic acid by ether, can also be saturated with cinchonine; this hydrochlorate of cinchonine is extracted by chloroform, evaporated to dryness, and the residue dissolved in water acidified by nitric acid and precipitated by silver nitrate; the silver chloride produced is collected on a small filter, washed, and the filter, with its contents, dried and ignited in a porcelain crucible; the silver chloride, multiplied by 0.25426, equals HCl.

The best method of estimating free hydrochloric acid in the stomach is that of Sjokvist as modified by v. Jaksch;[100] it has the disadvantage of its accuracy being interfered with by phosphates; it also does not distinguish between actual free HCl and the loosely bound HCl with albuminous matters,—this in a toxicological case is of small importance, because the quantities of HCl found are likely to be large.

The method is based upon the fact that if carbonate of baryta be added to the contents of the stomach, the organic acids will decompose the barium carbonate, forming butyrate, acetate, lactate, &c., of barium; and the mineral acids, such as hydrochloric acid, will combine, forming salts of barium.

On ignition, chloride of barium will be unaffected, while the organic salts of barium will be converted into carbonate of barium, practically insoluble in carbonic acid free water.

The contents of the stomach are coloured with litmus, and barium carbonate added until the fluid is no longer acid (as shown by the disappearance of the red colour); then the contents are evaporated to dryness in a platinum dish, and ignited at a dull red heat; complete burning to an ash is not necessary. After cooling, the burnt mass is repeatedly exhausted with boiling water and filtered; the chloride of barium is precipitated from the filtrate by means of dilute sulphuric acid; the barium sulphate filtered off, washed, dried, and, after ignition, weighed; 233 parts of barium sulphate equal 73 parts of HCl.

A method somewhat quicker, but depending on the same principles, has been suggested by Braun.[101] A fractional part, say 10 c.c., of the fluid contents is coloured by litmus and titrated with decinormal soda. To the same

---

[99] To distinguish between acidity due to free acid and acid salts, or to acidity due to the combined action of acid salts and free acids, the method of Leo and Uffelmann is useful. A fractional portion of the contents of the stomach is triturated with pure calcium carbonate; if all the acidity is due to free acid, the fluid in a short time becomes neutral to litmus; if, on the other hand, the acidity is due entirely to acid salts, the fluid remains acid; or, if due to both acid and acid salts, there is a proportionate diminution of acidity due to the decomposition of the lime carbonate by the free acid. A quantitative method has been devised upon these principles. See Leo, *Diagnostik der Krankheiten der Verdauungsorgane*, Hirschwald, Berlin, 1890.

[100] *Klinische Diagnostik*, Dr. Rudolph v. Jaksch, Wien u. Leipzig, 1892. *Clinical Diagnosis*. English Translation, by Dr. Cagney. Second Edition. London: Charles Griffin & Co., Limited.

[101] *Op. cit.*, S. 157.

quantity is added 2 or 3 more c.c. of decinormal soda than the quantity used in the first titration; this alkaline liquid is evaporated to dryness and ultimately ignited. To the ash is now added exactly the quantity of decinormal sulphuric acid as the decinormal soda last used to make it alkaline—that is to say, if the total acidity was equal to 3.6 d.n. soda, and 5.0 d.n. soda was added to the 10 c.c. evaporated to dryness and burned, then 5.6 c.c. of d.n. sulphuric acid is added to the ash. The solution is now warmed to get rid of carbon dioxide, and, after addition of a little phenolphthalein, titrated with d.n. soda solution until the change of colour shows saturation, the number of c.c. used, multiplied by 0.00365, equals the HCl.

§ 78. In investigating the stains from hydrochloric acid on fabrics, or the leaves of plants, any free hydrochloric acid may be separated by boiling with water, and then investigating the aqueous extract. Should, however, the stain be old, all free acid may have disappeared, and yet some of the chlorine remain in organic combination with the tissue, or in combination with bases. Dr. Angus Smith has found weighed portions of leaves, &c., which had been exposed to the action of hydrochloric acid fumes, richer in chlorides than similar parts of the plants not thus exposed.

The most accurate method of investigation for the purpose of separating chlorine from combination with organic matters is to cut out the stained portions, weigh them, and burn them up in a combustion-tube, the front portion of the tube being filled with caustic lime known to be free from chlorides; a similar experiment must be made with the unstained portions. In this way a considerable difference may often be found; and it is not impossible, in some instances, to thus detect, after the lapse of many years, that certain stains have been produced by a chlorine-holding substance.

III.—Nitric Acid.

§ 79. **General Properties.**—Nitric acid—commonly known in England as *aqua fortis*, chemically as *nitric acid*, *hydric nitrate*, or *nitric monohydrate*—is a mono-hydrate of nitrogen pentoxide (N_2O_5), two equivalents, or 126 parts, of nitric acid containing 108 of N_2O_5, and 18 of H_2O. Anhydrous nitric acid, or nitrogen pentoxide, can be obtained by passing, with special precautions, dry chlorine over silver nitrate; the products are free oxygen and nitrogen pentoxide, according to the following equation:—

Silver Nitrate.		Chlorine.		Silver Chloride.		Nitrogen Pentoxide.		Oxygen.
Ag_2O,N_2O_5	+	2Cl	=	2AgCl	+	N_2O_5	+	O

By surrounding the receiver with a freezing mixture, the acid is condensed in crystals, which dissolve in water, with emission of much heat, forming nitric acid. Sometimes the crystals, though kept in sealed tubes, decompose, and the tube, from the pressure of the liberated gases, bursts with a dangerous explosion.

Pure nitric acid has a specific gravity of 1.52, and boils at 98°. Dr. Ure examined the boiling point and other properties of nitric acid very fully. An acid of 1.5 specific gravity boils at 98.8°; of specific gravity 1.45, at 115.5°; specific gravity 1.40, at 118.8°; of specific gravity 1.42, at 122.8°. The acid of specific gravity 1.42 is the standard acid of the British Pharmacopœia. It can always be obtained by distilling either strong or moderately weak nitric acid; for, on the one hand, the acid on distillation gets weaker until the gravity of 1.42 is reached, or, on the other, it becomes stronger.

There is little doubt that acid of 1.42 gravity is a definite hydrate, consisting of 1 atom of dry acid and 4 atoms of water; it corresponds to 75 per cent.[102] of the liquid acid HNO_3. There are also at least two other hydrates known—one an acid of 1.485 specific gravity, corresponding to 1 atom of dry acid and 2 of water, and an acid of specific gravity 1.334, corresponding to 1 atom of dry acid and 7 atoms of water.

In Germany the officinal acid is of 1.185 specific gravity, corresponding to about 30 per cent. of HNO_3. The dilute nitric acid of the Pharmacopœia is a colourless liquid, of specific gravity 1.101, and should contain about 17.4 per cent. of acid. The acids used in various industries are known respectively as *dyers'* and *engravers'* acid. *Dyers'* acid has a specific gravity of 1.33 to 1.34 (66° to 68° Twad.), that is, strength from 56 to 58 per cent. of HNO_3. *Engravers'* acid is stronger; being of 1.40 specific gravity (80° Twad.); and contains 70 per cent. of HNO_3. Although the *pure* acid of commerce is (and should be) almost colourless, most commercial specimens are of hues from yellow up to deep red. An acid saturated with red oxides of nitrogen is often known as "fuming nitric acid."

[102] The British Pharmacopœia states that the 1.42 acid equals 70 per cent. of HNO_3; but this is not in accordance with Ure's Tables, nor with the facts.

§ 80. **Use in the Arts.**—Nitric acid is employed very extensively in the arts and manufactures. The dyer uses it as a solvent for tin in the preparation of valuable mordants for calico and other fabrics; the engraver uses it for etching copper. It is an indispensable agent in the manufacture of gun-cotton, nitro-glycerin, picric acid, and sulphuric acid; it is also used in the manufacture of tallow, in preparing the felt for hats, and in the gilding trades. It is said to be utilised to make yellowish or fawn-coloured spots on cigar leaves, so as to give them the appearance of age and quality. It is also used as a medicine.

§ 81. **Statistics of Poisoning by Nitric Acid.**—In the ten years 1883-1892 no case of murder was ascribed to nitric acid, but it caused accidentally 25 deaths, and was used in 27 cases of suicide.

The following tables give the age and sex distribution of these deaths:—

DEATHS IN ENGLAND AND WALES DURING THE TEN YEARS ENDING 1892 FROM NITRIC ACID.

Accident or Negligence.

Ages,	1-5	5-15	15-25	25-65	65 and above	Total
Males,	6	2	1	9	...	18
Females,	3	...	...	4	...	7
Totals,	9	2	1	13	...	25

Suicide.

Ages,	15-25	25-65	65 and above	Total
Males,	3	14	1	18
Females,	1	8	...	9
Totals,	4	22	1	27

§ 82. **Fatal Dose.**—The dose which causes death has not been ascertained with any exactness. As in the case of sulphuric acid, we may go so far as to say that it is possible for a few drops of the strong acid to be fatal, for if brought into contact with the vocal apparatus, fatal spasm of the glottis might be excited. The smallest dose on record is 7.7 grms. (2 drachms), which killed a child aged 13.

§ 83. **Action of Nitric Acid on Vegetation.**—Nitric acid acts on plants injuriously in a two-fold manner—viz., by direct corrosive action, and also by decomposing the chlorides which all plants contain, thus setting free chlorine, which decomposes and bleaches the chlorophyll. The action is most intense on soft and delicate leaves, such as those of clover, the cabbage, and all the cruciferæ. The tobacco plant is particularly injured by nitric acid. Next to all herbaceous plants, trees, such as the apple, pear, and fruit trees, generally suffer. The coniferæ, whether from their impregnation with resin, or from some other cause, possess a considerable resisting-power against nitric acid vapours, and the same is true as regards the cereals; in the latter case, their siliceous armour acts as a preserving agent.

§ 84. **Nitric Acid Vapour.**—The action of nitric acid in a state of vapour, as evolved by warming potassic nitrate and sulphuric acid together, has been studied by Eulenberg. A rabbit was placed under a shade into which 63 grains of nitric acid in a state of vapour were introduced. From the conditions of the experiment, some nitric peroxide must also have been present. Irritation of the external mucous membranes and embarrassment in breathing were observed. The animal in forty-five minutes was removed, and suffered afterwards from a croupous bronchitis, from which, however, it completely recovered in eleven days. A second experiment with the same animal was followed by death. On inspection, there was found strong injection of the cerebral membranes, with small extravasations of blood; the lungs were excessively congested; the right middle lobe especially was of a liver-brown colour, and empty of air: it sank in water.

O. Lassar[103] has also made a series of researches on the influence of nitric acid vapour, from which he concludes that the acid is not absorbed by the blood, but acts only by its mechanical irritation, for he could not trace, by means of an examination of the urine, any evidence of such absorption.

There are a few instances on record of the vapour having been fatal to men; for example, the well-known case of Mr. Haywood, a chemist of Sheffield, may be cited. In pouring a mixture of nitric and sulphuric acids from a carboy of sixty pounds capacity, the vessel broke, and for a few minutes he inhaled the mixed fumes. He died eleven hours after the accident, although for the first three hours there were scarcely any symptoms of an injurious effect having been produced. On inspection, there was found intense congestion of the windpipe and bronchial tubes, with effusion of blood in the latter. The lining membrane of the heart and aorta was inflamed; unfortunately, the larynx was not examined.[104]

A very similar case happened in Edinburgh in 1863.[105] Two young men were carrying a jar of nitric acid; the jar broke, and they attempted to wipe up the acid from the floor. The one died ten hours after the accident, the other in less than twenty-four hours. The symptoms were mainly those of difficult breathing, and it is probable that death was produced from suffocation. Dr. Taylor relates also, that having accidentally inhaled the vapour in preparing gun-cotton, he suffered from severe constriction of the throat, tightness in the chest, and cough, for more than a week.[106]

§ 85. **Effects of Liquid Nitric Acid.**—Poisoning by nitric acid, though still rare, is naturally more frequent than formerly. At the beginning of this century, Tartra[107] wrote a most excellent monograph on the subject, and collated all the cases he could find, from the first recorded instances related by Bembo[108] in Venetian history, down to his own time. The number of deaths in those 400 years was but fifty-five, while, in our century, at least fifty can be numbered. Most of these (74 per cent.) are suicidal, a very few homicidal, the rest accidental. In one of Tartra's cases, some nitric acid was placed in the wine of a drunken woman, with fatal effect. Osenbrüggen[109] relates the case of a father murdering his six children by means of nitric acid; and C. A. Büchner[110] that of a soldier who poured acid into the mouth of his illegitimate infant. A curious case is one in which a man poisoned his drunken wife by pouring the acid into her right ear; she died after six weeks' illness. All these instances prove again, if necessary, that the acid is only likely to be used with murderous intent in the case of young children, or of sleeping, drunken, or otherwise helpless people.

As an example of the way in which accidents are brought about by heedlessness, may be cited the recent case of a woman who bought a small quantity of aqua fortis for the purpose of allaying toothache by a local application. She attempted to pour the acid direct from the bottle into the cavity of the tooth; the acid went down her throat, and the usual symptoms followed. She threw up a very perfect cast of the gullet (preserved in University College museum), and rapidly died. Nitric acid has been mistaken for various liquids, and has also been used by injection as an abortive, in every respect having a toxicological history similar to that of sulphuric acid.

§ 86. **Local Action.**—When strong nitric acid comes in contact with organic matters, there is almost constantly a development of gas. The tissue is first bleached, and then becomes of a more or less intense yellow colour. Nitric acid spots on the skin are not removed by ammonia, but become of an orange-red when moistened with potash and a solution of cyanide of potassium. The yellow colour seems to show that picric acid is one of the constant products of the reaction; sulphide of ammonium forms a sort of soap with the epidermis thus attacked, and detaches it.

§ 87. **Symptoms.**—The symptoms and course of nitric acid poisoning differ in a few details only from those of sulphuric acid. There is the same instant pain and frequent vomiting, destruction of the mucous membranes, and, in the less severe cases, after-contraction of the gullet, &c.

One of the differences in the action of nitric and sulphuric acids is the constant development of gas with the former. This, without doubt, adds to the suffering. Tartra made several experiments on dead bodies, and showed that very considerable distension of the intestinal canal, by gaseous products, was the constant result; the tissues were

[103] Hoppe-Seyler's *Zeitschrift f. physiol. Chemie*, Bd. i. S. 165-173, 1877-78.

[104] *Lancet*, April 15, 1854, p. 430.

[105] *Chemical News*, March 14, 1863, p. 132.

[106] *Principles and Practice of Medical Jurisprudence*, vol. i., 1873, p. 218.

[107] Tartra, A. E., Dr., *Traité de l'Empoisonnement par l'Acide Nitrique*, Paris, An. 10 (1802), pp. 300.

[108] *Bembo Cardinalis, Rerum Venetarium Historiæ*, lib. xii., lib. i. p. 12, Paris Ed., 1551.

[109] *Allgem.-Deutsche Strafrechtszeitung, herausgeg. v. Frz. v. Holtzendorff*, 5 Jahrg., 1865, Hft. 5, S. 273.

[110] Friederich's *Blätter f. ger. Med.*, 1866, Hft. 3, S. 187.

corroded and almost dissolved, being transformed, ultimately, into a sort of greasy paste. The vomited matters are of a yellow colour, unless mixed with blood, when they are of a dirty-brown hue, with shreds of yellow mucus, and have the strong acid reaction and smell of nitric acid. The teeth may be partially attacked from the solvent action of the acid on the enamel. The fauces and tongue, at first blanched, soon acquire a citron-yellow, or even a brown colour; the whole cavity may swell and inflame, rendering the swallowing of liquids difficult, painful, and sometimes impossible. The air passages may also become affected, and in one case tracheotomy was performed for the relief of the breathing.[111] The stomach rejects all remedies; there are symptoms of collapse; quick, weak pulse, frequent shivering, obstinate constipation, and death (often preceded by a kind of stupor) in from eighteen to twenty-four hours. The intellectual faculties remain clear, save in a few rare instances.

C. A. Wunderlich has recorded an unusual case, in which the symptoms were those of dysentery, and the large intestine was found acutely inflamed, while the small one was little affected. The kidneys had the same appearance as in Bright's disease.[112] The smallest fatal dose given by Taylor is from 2 drachms, which killed a child aged 13 years. Should the dose of nitric acid be insufficient to kill at once, or, what amounts to the same thing, should the acid be immediately diluted with water, or in some way be neutralised, the patient, as in the case of sulphuric acid, may yet die at a variable future time from stenosis of the gullet, impaired digestion, &c. For example, in an interesting case related by Tartra,[113] a woman, who had swallowed 42 grms. (1.5 oz.) of nitric acid, feeling acute pain, took immediately a quantity of water, and three hours afterwards was admitted into hospital, where she received appropriate treatment. At the end of a month she left, believing herself cured; but in a little while returned, and was re-admitted, suffering from marasmus, extreme weakness, and constant vomiting; ultimately she died. The *post-mortem* examination revealed extreme contraction of the intestinal canal throughout. The lumen would hardly admit a penholder. The stomach was no larger than an ordinary intestine, and adherent to adjacent organs; on its internal surface there were spots, probably cicatrices; there were also changes in the gullet, but not so marked. A somewhat similar case is related by the same author in his thirteenth observation. In the Middlesex Hospital there is preserved the stomach (No. 1363) of a man who died forty days after swallowing 2 ozs. of nitric acid diluted in a tumbler of water. The stomach is contracted, the mucous membrane of the lower part of the gullet, the lesser curvature, and the pyloric end of the stomach is extensively corroded, showing ulcerated patches commencing to cicatrize.

§ 88. **Post-mortem Appearances.**—The pathological changes in the tongue, gullet, and stomach can be readily studied from the preparations in the different museums. The staining by the nitric acid appears unchanged to the naked eye for many years; hence, most of the nitric acid preparations are in an excellent state of preservation. A very good example of the pathological changes is to be found in Nos. 1049 and 1050, University College museum.

No. 1049 presents the tongue, pharynx, and larynx of a man who had swallowed a tea-cupful of nitric acid. The epithelium of the œsophagus is for the most part wanting, and hangs in shreds; the dorsum of the tongue, in front of the circumvallate papillæ, is excavated, and over its central part superficially ulcerated; in other places the tongue is encrusted with a thick, loose, fawn-coloured layer, formed probably of desquamated epithelium. The whole of the mucous surface is stained of a dirty yellow.

No. 1050 is a preparation showing the tongue, gullet, and stomach of a person who died from the effects of nitric acid. The tongue in places is smooth and glazed; in others, slightly depressed and excavated. On the anterior wall and lower portion of the gullet two large sloughs exist.

Although perforation of the stomach is not so common with nitric as with sulphuric acid, such an accident may occur, as shown in a preparation at Guy's Hospital, in which there is a perforation at the cardiac end. All the mucous membrane has disappeared, and the inner surface is for the most part covered with flocculent shreds. Three ounces of nitric acid are said to have been swallowed, and the patient lived seventeen hours. There is the usual staining. There is also in the Middlesex Hospital (No. 1364) the œsophagus and stomach of a woman aged 30, who died six hours after swallowing 2 to 3 ozs. of strong nitric acid. The inner coats of the mucous membrane of the gullet and stomach are in part converted into opaque yellow and black eschars, and in part to a shreddy pulpy condition. At the most depending part of the stomach is a large ragged perforation, with pulpy margins, which allowed the contents of the stomach to escape into the peritoneal cavity.

In St. Bartholomew's museum, there is a very good specimen (No. 1870) of the appearances in the gullet and

---

[111] Arnott, *Med. Gaz.*, vol. xii. p. 220.

[112] *De Actionibus quibusdam Acidi Nitrici Caustico in Corpus Humanum immissi. Programma Academ.*, Lipsiæ, 1857, 4.

[113] *Op. cit.*

stomach after poisoning by nitric acid. The case is detailed in *St. Bartholomew's Hospital Reports*, vol. v. p. 247. A male died in fifteen hours after swallowing 1 oz. of nitric acid. The whole mucous membrane is wrinkled, or rather ploughed, into longitudinal furrows, the yellow discoloration stops abruptly, with an irregular border, at the commencement of the stomach, the epithelial and mucous coats of which are wanting—its surface being rough and of a brownish-red colour.

The following preparations are to be found in the museum of the London Hospital:—A. b. 1. and A. b. 8.—A. b. 1. shows the pharynx, œsophagus, larynx, and stomach of a young woman, who, after taking half an ounce of nitric acid, died in eight hours. The staining is very intense; as an unusual feature, it may be noted that the larynx is almost as yellow as the œsophagus. The abrasion or solution of the epithelium on the dorsum of the tongue has dissected out the circumvallate and fungiform papillæ, so that they project with unusual distinctness. The lining membrane of the gullet throughout is divided into minute squares by longitudinal and transverse furrows. The mucous membrane of the stomach appears wholly destroyed, and presents a woolly appearance.

A. b. 8. shows a very perfect cast of the œsophagus. The case was that of a woman, aged 35, who swallowed half an ounce of nitric acid. The symptoms for the first four days were the usual pain in the throat and stomach, which might be expected; the bowels were freely open, and the stools dark and offensive. On the sixth day, there was constant vomiting with offensive breath; on the ninth, the appearance of the patient was critical, and she threw up the cast preserved. She died on the tenth day after the taking of the acid. The gullet, stomach, trachea, and larynx were found after death much inflamed.

The following preparations are in St. Thomas' Hospital:—P. 5.—a stomach with gullet attached. The stomach is covered with yellowish-green patches of false membrane and deposit; the gullet has the usual longitudinal furrows so characteristic of corrosive fluids.

P. 6. is also from a case of nitric acid poisoning. It shows the lining membrane of the stomach partly destroyed and shreddy, yet but little discoloured, the hue being a sort of delicate fawn.

To these may be added a case described and figured by Lesser; to a baby, a few days old, an unknown quantity of fuming nitric acid was given; the child made a gurgling, choking sound, and died in a few minutes. The corpse, nine days after death, showed no signs of decomposition. The tongue and gums were yellow, the gullet less so, the stomach still less, and the small intestine had no yellow tint; the whole of the mouth, gullet, and stomach showed the corrosive action of the acid. The graduation of tint, Lesser remarks, is what is not seen when the yellow colour is due to poisoning by chromic acid or by strong solution of ferric perchloride; in such cases, wherever the liquid has gone, there is a yellowness.[114]

§ 89. **Detection and Estimation of Nitric Acid.**—The detection either of free nitric acid or of its salts is not difficult. Free nitric acid, after preliminary estimation of the total acidity by decinormal soda, may be separated by the cinchonine process. On precipitation by ammonia or soda solution, the nitrate of ammonia or soda (and, it may be, other similarly combined acids) remain in solution. If free nitric acid is present in small quantity only, it may be necessary to evaporate the filtrate from the quinine nearly to dryness, and to test the concentrated liquid for nitric acid. The ordinary tests are as follows:—

(1.) Nitrates, treated with mercury or copper and strong sulphuric acid, develop nitric oxide, recognised by red fumes, if mixed with air or oxygen.

(2.) A nitrate dissolved in a small quantity of water, with the addition of a crystal of ferrous sulphate (allowed to partially dissolve), and then of strong sulphuric acid—poured through a funnel with a long tube dipping to the bottom of the test-tube, so as to form a layer at the bottom—strikes a brown colour at the junction of the liquid. When the test is properly performed, there will be three layers—the uppermost being the nitrate solution, the middle ferrous sulphate, and the lowest sulphuric acid; the middle layer becomes of a smoky or black hue if a nitrate is present. Organic matter interferes much with the reaction.

(3.) Nitrates in solution, treated in the cold with a zinc copper couple, are decomposed first into nitrites, and then into ammonia. The nitrites may be detected by a solution of metaphenyldiamine, which strikes a red colour with an infinitesimal quantity. Hence, a solution which gives no red colour with metaphenyldiamine, when submitted to the action of a zinc copper couple, and tested from time to time, cannot contain nitrites; therefore, no nitrates were originally present.

(4.) Nitrates, on being treated with strong sulphuric acid, and then a solution of indigo carmine dropped in, decolorise the indigo; this is a useful test—not conclusive in itself, but readily applied, and if the cinchonine method

[114] A. Lesser, *Atlas der gerichtlichen Medicin*, Berlin, 1884, Tafel i. fig. 2.

of separation has been resorted to, with few sources of error.

There is a process of separating nitric acid direct from any organic tissue, which may sometimes be useful:—Place the substance in a strong, wide-mouthed flask, closed by a caoutchouc cork, and in the flask put a small, short test-tube, charged with a strong solution of ferrous chloride in hydrochloric acid. The flask is connected to the mercury pump (see fig.), and made perfectly vacuous by raising and lowering the reservoir. When this is effected, the tube SS'P is adjusted so as to deliver any gas evolved into a eudiometer, or other gas-measuring apparatus. By a suitable movement of the flask, the acid ferrous chloride is allowed to come in contact with the tissue, a gentle heat applied to the flask, and gases are evolved. These may be carbon dioxide, nitrogen, and nitric oxide. On the evolution of gas ceasing, the carbon dioxide is absorbed by passing up under the mercury a little caustic potash. When absorption is complete, the gas, consisting of nitrogen and nitric oxide, may be measured. A bubble or two of oxygen is now passed into the eudiometer; if nitric oxide is present, red fumes at once develop. On absorbing the excess of oxygen and the nitric peroxide by alkaline pyrogallate, and measuring the residual gas, it is easy to calculate how much nitric oxide was originally present, according to the principles laid down in "Foods," p. 587.

It is also obvious that, by treating nitric oxide with oxygen, and absorbing the nitric peroxide present by an alkaline liquid of known strength and free from nitrates or ammonia, the resulting solution may be dealt with by a zinc copper couple, and the ammonia developed by the action of the couple directly estimated by titration by a decinormal hydrochloric acid, if large in quantity, or by "*nesslerising*," if small in quantity. Crum's method of estimating nitrates ("Foods," p. 568) in the cases of minute stains on fabrics, &c., with a little modification, may be occasionally applicable.

IV.—Acetic Acid.

§ 90. In the ten years ending 1893 nine deaths (four males and five females) occurred in England and Wales from drinking, by mistake or design, strong acetic acid.

A few cases only have been recorded in medical literature although there have been many experiments on animals.

The symptoms in the human subject consist of pain, vomiting, and convulsions.

In animals it causes colic, paralysis of the extremities, bloody urine, and œdema of the lungs. The lethal dose for plant-eating animals is about 0.49 gramme per kilo.

There should be no difficulty in recognising acetic acid; the odour alone is, in most cases, strong and unmistakable. Traces are detected by distilling, neutralising the distillate by soda, evaporating to dryness, and treating the residue as follows:—A portion warmed with alcohol and sulphuric acid gives a smell of acetic ether. Another portion is heated in a small tube of hard glass with arsenious acid; if acetic acid is present, or an acetate, a smell of kakodyl is produced.

V.—Ammonia.

§ 91. Ammonia, (NH_3), is met with either as a vapour or gas, or as a solution of the pure gas in water.

Properties.—Pure ammonia gas is colourless, with a strong, irritating, pungent odour, forming white fumes of ammonic chloride, if exposed to hydric chloride vapour, and turning red moist litmus-paper strongly blue. By intense cold, or by a pressure of 6½ atmospheres at the ordinary temperature, the gas is readily liquefied; the liquid ammonia boils at 38°; its observed specific gravity is .731; it freezes at -57.1°. Ammonia is readily absorbed by water; at 0° water will take up 1000 times its own volume, and at ordinary temperatures about 600 times its volume. Alcohol also absorbs about 10 per cent. Ammonia is a strong base, and forms a number of salts. Ammonia is one of the constant products of the putrefaction of nitrogenous substances; it exists in the atmosphere in small proportions, and in everything that contains water. Indeed, water is the only compound equal to it in its universality of diffusion. The minute quantities of ammonia thus diffused throughout nature are probably never in the free state, but combinations of ammonia with hydric nitrate, carbon dioxide, &c.

§ 92. **Uses.**[115]—A solution of ammonia in water has many applications in the arts and industries; it is used in medicine, and is an indispensable laboratory reagent.

[115] Sir B. W. Richardson has shown that ammonia possesses powerful antiseptic properties.—*Brit. Med. Journal*, 1862.

The officinal caustic preparations of ammonia are—*ammoniæ liquor fortior* (*strong solution of ammonia*), which should contain 32.5 per cent. of ammonia, and have a specific gravity of .891.

Liquor ammoniæ (*solution of ammonia*), specific gravity .959, and containing 10 per cent. of ammonia. There is also a *liniment of ammonia*, composed of olive oil, 3 parts, and ammonia, 1 part.

Spiritus Ammoniæ Fœtidus (*fœtid spirit of ammonia*).—A solution of assafœtida in rectified spirit and ammonia solution, 100 parts by measure, contains 10 of strong solution of ammonia.

Strong solution of ammonia is an important ingredient in the "*linimentum camphoræ composita*" (*compound liniment of camphor*), the composition of which is as follows:—camphor, 2.5 parts; oil of lavender, .125; strong solution of ammonia, 5.0; and rectified spirit, 15 parts. Its content of strong solution of ammonia is then about 22.6 per cent. (equivalent to 7.3 of NH_3).[116]

The carbonate of ammonia is also caustic; it is considered to be a compound of acid carbonate of ammonium, NH_4HCO_3, with carbamate of ammonium, $NH_4NH_2CO_2$. It is in the form of colourless, crystalline masses; the odour is powerfully ammoniacal; it is strongly alkaline, and the taste is acrid. It completely volatilises with heat, is soluble in water, and somewhat soluble in spirit.

The officinal preparation is the "*spiritus ammoniæ aromaticus*," or aromatic spirit of ammonia. It is made by distilling in a particular way ammonic carbonate, 4 ozs.; strong solution of ammonia, 8 ozs.; rectified spirit, 120 ozs.; water, 60 ozs.; volatile oil of nutmeg, 4½ drms.; and oil of lemon, 6½ drms. Aromatic spirit of ammonia is a solution in a weak spirit of neutral carbonate, flavoured with oil of lemon and nutmeg; the specific gravity should be 0.896.

Smelling salts (*sal volatile*) are composed of carbonate of ammonia.

§ 93. **Statistics.**—Falck has found throughout literature notices of thirty cases of poisoning by ammonia, or some of its preparations. In two of these it was used as a poison for the purpose of murder, and in eight with suicidal intent; the remainder were all accidental. The two criminal cases were those of children, who both died. Six out of eight of the suicidal, and twelve of the twenty accidental cases also terminated fatally.

Ammonia was the cause of 64 deaths (39 male, 25 female) by accident and of 34 (18 male, 16 female) by suicide, making a total of 98 during the ten years 1883-1892 in England and Wales. At present it occupies the seventh place among poisons as a cause of accident, the ninth as a means of suicide.

§ 94. **Poisoning by Ammonia Vapour.**—Strong ammoniacal vapour is fatal to both animal and vegetable life. There are, however, but few instances of poisoning by ammonia vapour; these few cases have been, without exception, the result of accident. Two cases of death are recorded, due to an attempt to rouse epileptics from stupor, by an injudicious use of strong ammonia applied to the nostrils. In another case, when hydrocyanic acid had been taken, there was the same result. An instance is also on record of poisonous effects from the breaking of a bottle of ammonia, and the sudden evolution in this way of an enormous volume of the caustic gas. Lastly, a man employed in the manufacture of ice, by means of the liquefaction of ammonia (Carré's process), breathed the vapour, and had a narrow escape for his life.

§ 95. **Symptoms.**—The symptoms observed in the last case may well serve as a type of what may be expected to occur after breathing ammonia vapour. The man remained from five to ten minutes in the stream of gas; he then experienced a feeling of anxiety, and a sense of constriction in the epigastrium, burning in the throat, and giddiness. He vomited. The pulse was small and frequent, the face pale, the mouth and throat strongly reddened, with increased secretion. Auscultation and percussion of the chest elicited nothing abnormal, although during the course of four days he had from time to time symptoms of suffocation, which were relieved by emetics. He recovered by the eighth day.[117]

In experiments on animals, very similar symptoms are produced. There is increased secretion of the eyes, nose, and mouth, with redness. The cry of cats becomes remarkably hoarse, and they generally vomit. Great difficulty in breathing and tetanic convulsions are present. When the animal is confined in a small closed chamber, death takes place in about a quarter of an hour.

On section, the bronchial tubes, to the finest ramifications, are found to be filled with a tenacious mucus, and the air passages, from the glottis throughout, reddened. The lungs are emphysematous, but have not always any

---

[116] There is a common liniment for horses used in stables, and popularly known as "white oil." It contains 1 part of ammonia, and 4 parts of olive or rape oil; not unfrequently turpentine is added. Another veterinary liniment, called "egg oil," contains ammonia, oil of origanum, turpentine, and the yelks of eggs.

[117] Schmidt's *Jahrbuch*, 1872, i. S. 30.

special colour; the heart contains but little coagulated blood; the blood has a dark-red colour.

§ 96. The chronic effects of the gas, as shown in workmen engaged in manufactures in which the fumes of ammonia are frequent, appear to be an inflammation of the eyes and an affection of the skin. The latter is thought to be due to the ammonia uniting to form a soap with the oil of the lubricating skin glands. Some observers have also noticed deafness, and a peculiar colour of the skin of the nose and forehead, among those who work in guano manufactories. Its usual action on the body appears to be a diminution of the healthy oxidation changes, and a general lowering of bodily strength, with evident anæmia.

§ 97. **Ammonia in Solution.—Action on Plants.**—Solutions of strong ammonia, or solutions of the carbonate, act injuriously on vegetable life, while the neutral salts of ammonia are, on the contrary, excellent manures. A 30 per cent. solution of ammonic carbonate kills most plants within an hour, and it is indifferent whether the whole plant is watered with this solution, or whether it is applied only to the leaves. If, after this watering of the plant with ammonic carbonate water, the injurious salt is washed out as far as possible by distilled water, or by a weakly acidulated fluid, then the plant may recover, after having shed more or less of its leaves. These facts sufficiently explain the injurious effects noticed when urine is applied direct to plants, for urine in a very short time becomes essentially a solution of ammonic carbonate.

§ 98. **Action on Human Beings and Animal Life.**—The violence of the action of caustic solutions of ammonia almost entirely depends on the state of concentration.

The local action of the strong solution appears to be mainly the extraction of water and the saponifying of fat, making a soluble soap. On delicate tissues it has, therefore, a destructive action; but S. Samuel[118] has shown that ammonia, when applied to the unbroken epidermis, does not have the same intense action as potash or soda, nor does it coagulate albumen. Blood, whether exposed to ammonia gas, or mixed with solution of ammonia, becomes immediately dark-red; then, later, through destruction of the blood corpuscles, very dark, even black; lastly, a dirty brown-red. The oxygen is expelled, the hæmoglobin destroyed, and the blood corpuscles dissolved.

The albumen of the blood is changed to alkali-albuminate, and the blood itself will not coagulate. A more or less fluid condition of the blood has always been noticed in the bodies of those poisoned by ammonia.

Blood exposed to ammonia, when viewed by the spectroscope, shows the spectra of alkaline hæmatin, a weak absorption-band, in the neighbourhood of D; but if the blood has been acted on for some time by ammonia, then all absorption-bands vanish. These spectra, however, are not peculiar to ammonia, the action of caustic potash or soda being similar. The muscles are excited by ammonia, the functions of the nerves are destroyed.

When a solution of strong ammonia is swallowed, there are two main effects—(1) the action of the ammonia itself on the tissues it comes into contact with, and (2) the effects of the vapour on the air-passages. There are, therefore, immediate irritation, redness, and swelling of the tongue and pharynx, a burning pain reaching from the mouth to the stomach, with vomiting, and, it may be, nervous symptoms. The saliva is notably increased. In a case reported by Fonssagrives,[119] no less than 3 litres were expelled in the twenty-four hours. Often the glands under the jaw and the lymphatics of the neck are swollen.

Doses of from 5 to 30 grammes of the strong solution of ammonia may kill as quickly as prussic acid. In a case recorded by Christison,[120] death occurred in four minutes from a large dose, doubtless partly by suffocation. As sudden a result is also recorded by Plenk: a man, bitten by a rabid dog, took a mouthful of spirits of ammonia, and died in four minutes.

If death does not occur rapidly, there may be other symptoms—dependent not upon its merely local action, but upon its more remote effects. These mainly consist in an excitation of the brain and spinal cord, and, later, convulsive movements deepening into loss of consciousness. It has been noticed that, with great relaxation of the muscular system, the patients complain of every movement causing pain. With these general symptoms added to the local injury, death may follow many days after the swallowing of the fatal dose.

Death may also occur simply from the local injury done to the throat and larynx, and the patient may linger some time. Thus, in a case quoted by Taylor,[121] in which none of the poison appears actually to have been swallowed, the man died nineteen days after taking the poison from inflammation of the throat and larynx. As with the strong acids, so with ammonia and the alkalies generally, death may also be caused many weeks and even months

[118] Virchow's *Archiv f. path. Anat.*, Bd. 51, Hft. 1 u. 2, S. 41, &c., 1870.
[119] *L'Union Médicale*, 1857, No. 13, p. 49, No. 22, p. 90.
[120] Christison, 167.
[121] *Principles of Jurisprudence*, i. p. 235.

afterwards from the effects of contraction of the gullet, or from the impaired nutrition consequent upon the destruction, more or less, of portions of the stomach or intestinal canal.

§ 99. **Post-mortem Appearances.**—In recent cases there is an intense redness of the intestinal canal, from the mouth to the stomach, and even beyond, with here and there destruction of the mucous membrane, and even perforation. A wax preparation in the museum of University College (No. 2378) shows the effects on the stomach produced by swallowing strong ammonia; it is ashen-gray in colour, and most of the mucous membrane is, as it were, dissolved away; the cardiac end is much congested.

The contents of the stomach are usually coloured with blood; the bronchial tubes and glottis are almost constantly found inflamed—even a croup-like (or diphtheritic) condition has been seen. Œdema of the glottis should also be looked for: in one case this alone seems to have accounted for death. The blood is of a clear-red colour, and fluid. A smell of ammonia may be present.

If a sufficient time has elapsed for secondary effects to take place, then there may be other appearances. Thus, in the case of a girl who, falling into a fainting fit, was treated with a draught of undiluted spirits of ammonia, and lived four weeks afterwards, the stomach (preserved in St. George's Hospital museum, 43 b, ser. ix.) is seen to be much dilated and covered with cicatrices, and the pylorus is so contracted as hardly to admit a small bougie. It has also been noticed that there is generally a fatty degeneration of both the kidneys and liver.

It need scarcely be observed that, in such cases, no free ammonia will be found, and the question of the cause of death must necessarily be wholly medical and pathological.

§ 100. **Separation of Ammonia.**—Ammonia is separated in all cases by distillation, and if the organic or other liquid is already alkaline, it is at once placed in a retort and distilled. If neutral or acid, a little burnt magnesia may be added until the reaction is alkaline. It is generally laid down that the contents of the stomach in a putrid condition cannot be examined for ammonia, because ammonia is already present as a product of decomposition; but even under these circumstances it is possible to give an opinion whether ammonia *in excess* is present. For if, after carefully mixing the whole contents of the stomach, and then drying a portion and reckoning from that weight the total nitrogen (considering, for this purpose, the contents to consist wholly of albumen, which yields about 16 per cent. of nitrogen)—under these conditions, the contents of the stomach yield more than 16 per cent. of nitrogen as ammonia reckoned on the dry substance, it is tolerably certain that ammonia not derived from the food or the tissues is present.

If, also, there is a sufficient evolution of ammonia to cause white fumes, when a rod moistened with hydrochloric acid is brought near to the liquid, this is an effect never noticed with a normal decomposition, and renders the presence of extrinsic ammonia probable.

An alkaline-reacting distillate, which gives a brown colour with the "nessler" reagent, and which, when carefully neutralised with sulphuric acid, on evaporation to dryness by the careful heat of a water-bath, leaves a crystalline mass that gives a copious precipitate with platinic chloride, but is hardly at all soluble in absolute alcohol, can be no other substance than ammonia.

§ 101. **Estimation.**—Ammonia is most quickly estimated by distilling, receiving the distillate in decinormal acid, and then titrating back. It may also be estimated as the double chloride of ammonium and platinum $(NH_4Cl)_2PtCl_4$. The distillate is exactly neutralised by HCl, evaporated to near dryness, and an alcoholic solution of platinic chloride added in sufficient quantity to be always in slight excess, as shown by the yellow colour of the supernatant fluid. The precipitate is collected, washed with a little alcohol, dried, and weighed on a tared filter; 100 parts of the salt are equal to 7.6 of NH_3.

VI.—Caustic Potash and Soda.

§ 102. There is so little difference in the local effects produced by potash and soda respectively, that it will be convenient to treat them together.

Potash (potassa caustica).—Hydrate of potassium (KHO), atomic weight 56, specific gravity 2.1.

Properties.—Pure hydrate of potassium is a compact, white solid, usually met with in the form of sticks. When heated to a temperature a little under redness, it melts to a nearly colourless liquid; in this state it is intensely corrosive. It rapidly absorbs moisture from the air, and moist potash also absorbs with great avidity carbon dioxide; it is powerfully alkaline, changing red litmus to blue. It is soluble in half its weight of cold water, great heat being evolved during solution; it forms two definite hydrates—one, $KHO + H_2O$; the other, $KHO + 2H_2O$. It is sparingly soluble in ether, but is dissolved by alcohol, wood-spirit, fusel oil, and glycerin.

§ 103. **Pharmaceutical Preparations.**—Potassium hydrate, as well as the solution of potash, is officinal in all pharmacopœias. The *liquor potassæ*, or solution of potash, of the British Pharmacopœia, is a strongly alkaline, caustic liquid, of 1.058 specific gravity, and containing 5.84 per cent. by weight of KHO. It should, theoretically, not effervesce, when treated with an acid, but its affinity for CO_2 is so great that all solutions of potash, which have been in any way exposed to air, contain a little carbonate. Caustic sticks of potash and lime used to be officinal in the British Pharmacopœia. Filho's caustic is still in commerce, and is made by melting together two parts of potassium hydrate and one part of lime in an iron ladle or vessel; the melted mass is now moulded by pouring it into leaden moulds. Vienna paste is composed of equal weights of potash and lime made into a paste with rectified spirit or glycerin.

§ 104. **Carbonate of Potash** ($K_2CO_3 + 1\frac{1}{2}H_2O$), when pure, is in the form of small white crystalline grains, alkaline in taste and reaction, and rapidly deliquescing when exposed to moist air; it gives all the chemical reactions of potassium oxide, and carbon dioxide. Carbonate of potash, under the name of *salt of tartar*, or potashes, is sold by oilmen for cleansing purposes. They supply it either in a fairly pure state, or as a darkish moist mass containing many impurities.

§ 105. **Bicarbonate of Potash** ($KHCO_3$) is in the form of large transparent rhombic prisms, and is not deliquescent. The effervescing solution of potash (*liquor potassæ effervescens*) consists of 30 grains of $KHCO_3$ in a pint of water (3.45 grms. per litre), and as much CO_2 as the water will take up under a pressure of seven atmospheres.

§ 106. **Caustic Soda—Sodium Hydrate** (NaHO).—This substance is a white solid, very similar in appearance to potassium hydrate; it absorbs moisture from the air, and afterwards carbon dioxide, becoming solid again, for the carbonate is not deliquescent. In this respect, then, there is a great difference between potash and soda, for the former is deliquescent both as hydrate and carbonate; a stick of potash in a semi-liquid state, by exposure to the air, continues liquid, although saturated with carbon dioxide. Pure sodium hydrate has a specific gravity of 2.0; it dissolves in water with evolution of heat, and the solution gives all the reactions of sodium hydrate, and absorbs carbon dioxide as readily as the corresponding solution of potash. The *liquor sodæ* of the B.P. should contain 4.1 per cent. of NaHO.

§ 107. **Sodæ Carbonas—Carbonate of Soda**—($Na_2CO_3 10H_2O$).—The pure carbonate of soda for medicinal use is in colourless and transparent rhombic octahedrons; when exposed to air, the crystals effloresce and crumble. The *sodæ carbonas exsiccata*, or dried carbonate of soda, is simply the ordinary carbonate, deprived of its water of crystallisation, which amounts to 62.93 per cent.

§ 108. **Bicarbonate of Soda** ($NaHCO_3$) occurs in the form of minute crystals, or, more commonly, as a white powder. The *liquor sodæ effervescens* of the B.P. is a solution of the bicarbonate, 30 grains of the salt in 20 ozs. of water (3.45 grms. per litre), the water being charged with as much carbonic acid as it will hold under a pressure of seven atmospheres. *The bicarbonate of soda lozenges* (*trochisci sodæ bicarbonatis*) contain in each lozenge 5 grains (327 mgrms.) of the bicarbonate. The carbonate of soda sold for household purposes is of two kinds—the one, "seconds," of a dirty white colour and somewhat impure; the other, "best," is a white mass of much greater purity. *Javelle water* (*Eau de Javelle*) is a solution of hypochlorite of soda; its action is poisonous, more from the caustic alkali than from the chlorine, and may, therefore, be here included.

§ 109. **Statistics.**—Poisoning by the fixed alkalies is not so frequent as poisoning by ammonia. Falck has collected, from medical literature, 27 cases, 2 of which were the criminal administering of *Eau de Javelle*, and 5 were suicidal; 22, or 81.5 per cent., died—in 1 of the cases after twenty-four hours; in the others, life was prolonged for days, weeks, or months—in 1 case for twenty-seven months. In the ten years 1883-1892, in England and Wales, there were 27 deaths from poisoning by the fixed alkalies; 2 were suicidal (1 from potash, the other from soda); the remaining 25 were due to accident; of these, 7 (3 males and 4 females) were from caustic soda, and 18 (8 males and 10 females) from caustic potash.

§ 110. **Effects on Animal and Vegetable Life.**—The fixed alkalies destroy all vegetable life, if applied in strong solution or in substance, by dehydrating and dissolving the tissues. The effects on animal tissues are, in part, due also to the affinity of the alkalies for water. They extract water from the tissues with which they come in contact, and also attack the albuminous constituents, forming alkali-albuminate, which swells on the addition of water, and, in a large quantity, even dissolves. Cartilaginous and horny tissues are also acted upon, and strong alkalies will dissolve hair, silk, &c. The action of the alkali is by no means restricted to the part first touched, but has a remarkable faculty of spreading in all directions.

§ 111. **Local Effects.**—The effects of strong alkali applied to the epidermis are similar to, but not identical with, those produced by strong acids. S. Samuel[122] has studied this experimentally on the ear of the rabbit; a drop of a strong solution of caustic alkali, placed on the ear of a white rabbit, caused stasis in the arteries and veins, with first a greenish, then a black colour of the blood; the epidermis was bleached, the hair loosened, and there quickly followed a greenish coloration on the back of the ear, opposite to the place of application. Around the burned spot appeared a circle of anastomising vessels, a blister rose, and a slough separated in a few days. The whole thickness of the ear was coloured yellowish-green, and, later, the spot became of a rusty brown.

§ 112. **Symptoms.**—The symptoms observed when a person has swallowed a dangerous dose of caustic (fixed) alkali are very similar to those noticed with ammonia, with the important exception that there is no respiratory trouble, unless the liquid has come into contact with the glottis; nor has there been hitherto remarked the rapid death which has taken place in a few ammonia poisonings, the shortest time hitherto recorded being three hours, as related by Taylor, in a case in which a boy had swallowed 3 ozs. of a strong solution of carbonate of potash.

There is instant pain, extending from the mouth to the stomach, and a persistent and unpleasant taste; if the individual is not a determined suicide, and the poison (as is mostly the case) has been taken accidentally, the liquid is immediately ejected as much as possible, and water, or other liquid at hand, drunk freely. Shock may at once occur, and the patient die from collapse; but this, even with frightful destruction of tissue, appears to be rare. Vomiting supervenes; what is ejected is strongly alkaline, and streaked with blood, and has a soapy, frothy appearance. There may be diarrhœa, great tenderness of the abdomen, and quick pulse and fever. With caustic potash, there may be also noticed its toxic effects (apart from local action) on the heart; the pulse, in that case, is slow and weak, and loss of consciousness and convulsions are not uncommon. If the collapse and after-inflammation are recovered from, then, as in the case of the mineral acids, there is all the horrid sequence of symptoms pointing to contractions and strictures of the gullet or pylorus, and the subsequent dyspepsia, difficulty of swallowing, and not unfrequently actual starvation.

§ 113. **Post-mortem Appearances.**—In cases of recent poisoning, spots on the cheeks, lips, clothing, &c., giving evidence of the contact of the alkali, should be looked for; but this evidence, in the case of persons who have lived a few days, may be wanting. The mucous membrane of the mouth, throat, gullet, and stomach is generally more or less white—here and there denuded, and will be found in various stages of inflammation and erosion, according to the amount taken, and the concentration of the alkali. Where there is erosion, the base of the eroded parts is not brown-yellow, but, as a rule, pale red. The gullet is most affected at its lower part, and it is this part which is mostly subject to stricture. Thus Böhm[123] found that in 18 cases of contraction of the gullet, collected by him, 10 of the 18 showed the contraction at the lower third.

The changes which the stomach may present if the patient has lived some time, are well illustrated by a preparation in St. George's museum (43 a. 264, ser. ix.). It is the stomach of a woman, aged 44, who had swallowed a concentrated solution of carbonate of potash. She vomited immediately after taking it, and lived about two months, during the latter part of which she had to be nourished by injections. She died mainly from starvation. The gullet in its lower part is seen to be much contracted, its lining membrane destroyed, and the muscular coats exposed. The coats of the stomach are thickened, but what chiefly arrests the attention is a dense cicatrix at the pylorus, with an aperture so small as only to admit a probe.

The colour of the stomach is generally bright red, but in that of a child, preserved in Guy's Hospital museum (No. 1798[24]), the mucous membrane is obliterated, the rugæ destroyed, and a dark-brown stain is a noticeable feature. The stomach is not, however, necessarily affected. In a preparation in the same museum (No. 1798[20]) the mucous membrane of the stomach of a child who swallowed soap-lees is seen to be almost healthy, but the gullet is much discoloured. The action on the blood is to change it into a gelatinous mass; the blood corpuscles are destroyed, and the whole colour becomes of a dirty blackish-red; the spectroscopic appearances are identical with those already described.

The question as to the effects of chronic poisoning by the alkalies or their carbonates may arise. Little or nothing is, however, known of the action of considerable quantities of alkalies taken daily. In a case related by Dr. Tunstall,[124] a man for eighteen years had taken daily 2 ozs. of bicarbonate of soda for the purpose of relieving indigestion. He died suddenly, and the stomach was found extensively diseased; but since the man, before taking the alkali, had complained of pain, &c., it is hardly well, from this one case, to draw any conclusion.

---

[122] Virchow's *Archiv. f. path. Anat.*, Bd. 51, Hft. 1 u. 2, 1870.

[123] *Centralblatt für die Med. Wiss.*, 1874.

[124] *Med. Times*, Nov. 30, 1850, p. 564.

It is important to observe that the contents of the stomach may be acid, although the death has been produced by caustic alkali. A child, aged 4, drank from a cup some 14 per cent. soda lye. He vomited frequently, and died in fifteen hours. The stomach contained 80 c.c. of sour-smelling turbid fluid, the reaction of which was acid. There were hæmorrhagic patches in the stomach, and signs of catarrhal inflammation; there was also a similarly inflamed condition of the duodenum.[125]

§ 114. **Chemical Analysis.**—The tests for potassium or sodium are too well known to need more than enumeration. The intense yellow flame produced when a sodium salt is submitted to a Bunsen flame, and the bright sodium-line at D when viewed by the spectroscope, is a delicate test; while potassium gives a dull red band in the red, and a faint but very distinct line in the violet. Potassium salts are precipitated by tartaric acid, while sodium salts do not yield this precipitate; potassium salts also give a precipitate with platinic chloride insoluble in strong alcohol, while the compound salt with sodium is rapidly dissolved by alcohol or water. This fact is utilised in the separation and estimation of the two alkalies.

§ 115. **Estimation of the Fixed Alkalies.**—To detect a fixed alkali in the contents of the stomach, a convenient process is to proceed by dialysis, and after twenty-four hours, to concentrate the outer liquid by boiling, and then, if it is not too much coloured, to titrate directly with a decinormal sulphuric acid. After exact neutralisation, the liquid is evaporated to dryness, carbonised, the alkaline salts lixiviated out with water, the sulphuric acid exactly precipitated by baric chloride, and then, after separation of the sulphate, the liquid treated with milk of lime. The filtrate is treated with a current of CO_2 gas, boiled, and any precipitate filtered off; the final filtrate will contain only alkalies. The liquid may now be evaporated to dryness with either hydrochloric or sulphuric acids, and the total alkalies weighed as sulphates or chlorides. Should it be desirable to know exactly the proportion of potassium to sodium, it is best to convert the alkalies into chlorides—dry gently, ignite, and weigh; then dissolve in the least possible quantity of water, and precipitate by platinic chloride, which should be added so as to be a little in excess, but not much. The liquid thus treated is evaporated nearly to dryness, and then extracted with alcohol of 80 per cent., which dissolves out any of the double chloride of platinum and sodium. Finally, the precipitate is collected on a tared filter and weighed, after drying at 100°. In this way the analyst both distinguishes between the salts of sodium and potassium, and estimates the relative quantities of each. It is hardly necessary to observe that, if the double chloride is wholly soluble in water or alcohol, sodium alone is present. This, however, will never occur in operating on organic tissues and fluids, for both alkalies are invariably present. A correction must be made when complex organic fluids are in this way treated for alkalies which may be naturally in the fluid. Here the analyst will be guided by his preliminary titration, which gives the total free alkalinity. In cases where the alkali has been neutralised by acids, of course no free alkali will be found, but the corresponding salt.

VII.—Neutral Sodium, Potassium, and Ammonium Salts.

§ 116. The neutral salts of the alkalies are poisonous, if administered in sufficient doses, and the poisonous effect of the sulphate, chloride, bromide, iodide, tartrate, and citrate appears to depend on the specific action of the alkali metal, rather than on the acid, or halogen in combination. According to the researches of Dr. Ringer and Dr. Harrington Sainsbury,[126] with regard to the relative toxicity of the three, as shown by their effect on the heart of a frog—first, the potassium salts were found to exert the most poisonous action, next come the ammonium, and, lastly, the sodium salts. The highest estimate would be that sodium salts are only one-tenth as poisonous as those of ammonium or potassium; the lowest, that the sodium salts are one-fifth: although the experiments mainly throw light upon the action of the alkalies on one organ only, yet the indications obtained probably hold good for the organism as a whole, and are pretty well borne out by clinical experience.

There appear to be four cases on record of poisoning by the above neutral salts; none of them belong to recent times, but lie between the years 1837-1856. Hence, the main knowledge which we possess of the poisonous action of the potassium salts is derived from experiments on animals.

§ 117. **Sodium Salts.**—Common salt in such enormous quantity as half a pound to a pound has destroyed human life, but these cases are so exceptional that the poisonous action of sodium salts is of scientific rather than practical interest.

§ 118. **Potassium Salts.**—Leaving for future consideration the nitrate and the chlorate of potassium, potassic

---

[125] Lesser, *Atlas d. gericht. Med.*, Tafel ii.

[126] *Lancet*, June 24, 1882.

sulphate and tartrate are substances which have destroyed human life.

Potassic Sulphate (K_2SO_4) is in the form of colourless rhombic crystals, of bitter saline taste. It is soluble in 10 parts of water.

Hydropotassic Tartrate ($KHC_4H_4O_6$), when pure, is in the form of rhombic crystals, tasting feebly acid. It is soluble in 210 parts of water at 17°.

§ 119. **Action on the Frog's Heart.**—Both excitability and contractility are affected to a powerful degree. There is a remarkable slowing of the pulsations, irregularity, and, lastly, cessation of pulsation altogether.

§ 120. **Action on Warm-Blooded Animals.**—If a sufficient quantity of a solution of a potassic salt is injected into the blood-vessels of an animal, there is almost immediate death from arrest of the heart's action. Smaller doses, subcutaneously applied, produce slowing of the pulse, dyspnœa, and convulsions, ending in death. Small doses produce a transitory diminution of the force of arterial pressure, which quickly passes, and the blood-pressure rises. There is at first, for a few seconds, increase in the number of pulsations, but later a remarkable slowing of the pulse. The rise in the blood-pressure occurs even after section of the spinal cord. Somewhat larger doses cause rapid lowering of the blood-pressure, and apparent cessation of the heart's action; but if the thorax be then opened, the heart is seen to be contracting regularly, making some 120-160 rhythmic movements in the minute. If the respiration be now artificially maintained, and suitable pressure made on the walls of the chest, so as to empty the heart of blood, the blood-pressure quickly rises, and natural respiration may follow. An animal which lay thirty-six minutes apparently dead was in this way brought to life again (*Böhm*). The action of the salts of potassium on the blood is the same as that of sodium salts. The blood is coloured a brighter red, and the form of the corpuscles changed; they become shrivelled through loss of water. Voluntary muscle loses quickly its contractility when a solution of potash is injected into its vessels. Nerves also, when treated with a 1 per cent. solution of potassic chloride, become inexcitable.

§ 121. **Elimination.**—The potassium salts appear to leave the body through the kidneys, but are excreted much more slowly than the corresponding sodium salts. Thus, after injection of 4 grms. of potassic chloride—in the first sixteen hours .748 grm. of KCl was excreted in the urine, and in the following twenty-four hours 2.677 grms.

§ 122. **Nitrate of Potash** (KNO_3).—Pure potassic nitrate crystallises in large anhydrous hexagonal prisms with dihedral summits; it does not absorb water, and does not deliquesce. Its fusing point is about 340°; when melted it forms a transparent liquid, and loses a little of its oxygen, but this is for the most part retained by the liquid given off when the salt solidifies. At a red-heat it evolves oxygen, and is reduced first to nitrite; if the heat is continued, potassic oxide remains. The specific gravity of the fused salt is 2.06. It is not very soluble in cold water, 100 parts dissolving only 26 at 15.6°; but boiling water dissolves it freely, 100 parts dissolving 240 of the salt.

A solution of nitrate of potash, when treated with a zinc couple (see "Foods," p. 566), is decomposed, the nitrate being first reduced to nitrite, as shown by its striking a red colour with metaphenylene-diamine, and then the nitrite farther decomposing, and ammonia appearing in the liquid. If the solution is alkalised, and treated with aluminium foil, hydrogen is evolved, and the same effect produced. As with all nitrates, potassic nitrate, on being heated in a test-tube with a little water, some copper filings, and sulphuric acid, evolves red fumes of nitric peroxide.

§ 123. **Statistics.**—Potassic nitrate, under the popular name of "*nitre*," is a very common domestic remedy, and is also largely used as a medicine for cattle. There appear to be twenty cases of potassic nitrate poisoning on record—of these, eight were caused by the salts having been accidentally mistaken for magnesic sulphate, sodic sulphate, or other purgative salt; two cases were due to a similar mistake for common salt. In one instance, the nitrate was used in strong solution as an enema, but most of the cases were due to the taking of too large an internal dose.

§ 124. **Uses in the Arts**, &c.—Both sodic and potassic nitrates are called "nitre" by the public indiscriminately. Sodic nitrate is imported in large quantities from the rainless districts of Peru as a manure. Potassic nitrate is much used in the manufacture of gunpowder, in the preservation of animal substances, in the manufacture of gun cotton, of sulphuric and nitric acids, &c. The maximum medicinal dose of potassium nitrate is usually stated to be 30 grains (1.9 grm.).

§ 125. **Action of Nitrates of Sodium and Potassium.**—Both of these salts are poisonous. Potassic nitrate has been taken with fatal result by man; the poisonous nature of sodic nitrate is established by experiments on animals. The action of the nitrates of the alkalies is separated from that of the other neutral salts of potassium, &c., because in this case the toxic action of the combined nitric acid plays no insignificant part. Large doses, 3-5 grms. (46.3-77.2 grains), of potassic nitrate cause considerable uneasiness in the stomach and bowels; the digestion is disturbed; there may be vomiting and diarrhœa, and there is generally present a desire to urinate frequently. Still larger doses, 15-30 grms. (231.5-463 grains), rapidly produce all the symptoms of acute gastro-enteritis—great pain, frequent vomiting (the ejected matters being often bloody), with irregularity and slowing of the pulse; weakness, cold sweats, painful cramps in single muscles (especially in the calves of the legs); and, later, convulsions, aphonia, quick collapse, and death.

In the case of a pregnant woman, a handful of "nitre" taken in mistake for Glauber's salts produced abortion after half-an-hour. The woman recovered. Sodic nitrate subcutaneously applied to frogs kills them, in doses of .026 grm. (.4 grain), in about two hours; there are fibrillar twitchings of single groups of muscles and narcosis. The heart dies last, but after ceasing to beat may, by a stimulus, be made again to contract. Rabbits, poisoned similarly by sodic nitrate, exhibit also narcotic symptoms; they lose consciousness, lie upon their side, and respond only to the sharpest stimuli. The breathing, as well as the heart, is "slowed," and death follows after a few spasmodic inspirations.

Sodic nitrite was found by Barth to be a more powerful poison, less than 6 mgrms. (.1 grain) being sufficient to kill a rabbit of 455.5 grms. (7028 grains) weight, when subcutaneously injected. The symptoms were very similar to those produced by the nitrate.

§ 126. The *post-mortem* appearances from potassic nitrate are as follows:—An inflamed condition of the stomach, with the mucous membrane dark in colour, and readily tearing; the contents of the stomach are often mixed with blood. In a case related by Orfila, there was even a small perforation by a large dose of potassic nitrate, and a remarkable preservation of the body was noted.

It is believed that the action of the nitrates is to be partly explained by a reduction to nitrites, circulating in the blood as such. To detect nitrites in the blood, the best method is to place the blood in a dialyser, the outer liquid being alcohol. The alcoholic solution may be evaporated to dryness, extracted with water, and then tested by metaphenylene-diamine.

§ 127. **Potassic Chlorate** ($KClO_3$).—Potassic chlorate is in the form of colourless, tabular crystals with four or six sides. About 6 parts of the salt are dissolved by 100 of water at 15°, the solubility increasing with the temperature, so that at 100° nearly 60 parts dissolve; if strong sulphuric acid be dropped on the crystals, peroxide of chlorine is evolved; when rubbed with sulphur in a mortar, potassic chlorate detonates. When the salt is heated strongly, it first melts, and then decomposes, yielding oxygen gas, and is transformed into the perchlorate. If the heat is continued, this also is decomposed, and the final result is potassic chloride.

§ 128. **Uses.**—Potassic chlorate is largely used as an oxidiser in calico printing, and in dyeing, especially in the preparation of aniline black. A considerable quantity is consumed in the manufacture of lucifer matches and fireworks; it is also a convenient source of oxygen. Detonators for exploding dynamite are mixtures of fulminate of mercury and potassic chlorate. It is employed as a medicine both as an application to inflamed mucous membranes, and for internal administration; about 2000 tons of the salt for these various purposes are manufactured yearly in the United Kingdom.

§ 129. **Poisonous Properties.**—The facility with which potassic chlorate parts with its oxygen by the aid of heat, led to its very extensive employment in medicine. No drug, indeed, has been given more recklessly, or on a less scientific basis. Wherever there were sloughing wounds, low fevers, and malignant sore throats, especially those of a diphtheritic character, the practitioner administered potassic chlorate in colossal doses. If the patient died, it was ascribed to the malignity of the disease—if he recovered, to the oxygen of the salt; and it is possible, from the light which of recent years has been thrown on the action of potassic chlorate, that its too reckless use has led to many unrecorded accidents.

§ 130. **Experiments on Animals.**—F. Marchand[127] has studied the effects of potassic chlorate on animals, and on blood. If either potassic chlorate or sodic chlorate is mixed with fresh blood, it shows after a little while peculiar changes; the clear red colour at first produced passes, within a few hours, into a dark red-brown, which gradually becomes pure brown. This change is produced by a 1 per cent. solution, in from fifteen to sixteen hours; and a 4 per cent. solution at 15° destroys every trace of oxyhæmoglobin within four hours. Soon the blood takes a syrupy consistence, and, with a 2-4 per cent. solution of the salt, passes into a jelly-like mass. The jelly has much permanence, and resists putrefactive changes for a long time.

Marchand fed a dog of 17 kilos. in weight with 5 grms. of potassic chlorate for a week. As there were no apparent symptoms, the dose was doubled for two days; and as there was still no visible effect, lastly, 50 grms. of sodic chlorate were given in 5 doses. In the following night the dog died. The blood was found after death to be of a sepia-brown colour, and remained unaltered when exposed to the air. The organs were generally of an unnatural

[127] *Virchow's Archiv. f. path. Anat.*, Bd. 77, Hft. 3, S. 455, 1879.

brown colour; the spleen was enormously enlarged; the kidneys were swollen, and of a dark chocolate brown—on section, almost black-brown, the colour being nearly equal, both in the substance and in the capsule. A microscopical examination of the kidney showed the canaliculi to be filled with brownish cylinders consisting of altered blood. A spectroscopic examination of the blood showed weak hæmoglobin bands, and a narrow band in the red. With farther dilution, the hæmoglobin bands vanished, but the band in the red remained. The diluted blood, when exposed to the light, still remained of a coffee-brown colour; and on shaking, a white-brown froth was produced on the surface.

A second experiment in which a hound of from 7-8 kilos. in weight was given 3-5 grm. doses of potassic chlorate in sixteen hours, and killed by bleeding seven to eight hours after the last dose, showed very similar appearances. The kidneys were intensely congested, and the peculiar brown colour was noticeable.

§ 131. **Effects on Man.**—I find in literature thirty-nine cases recorded, in which poisonous symptoms were directly ascribed to the action of chlorate of potassium; twenty-eight of these terminated fatally. A quadruple instance of poisoning, recorded by Brouardel and L'Hôte,[128] illustrates many of the points relative to the time at which the symptoms may be expected to commence, and the general aspect of potassic chlorate poisoning. The "*supérieure*" of a religious institution was in the habit of giving, for charitable purposes, a potion containing 15 grms. (3.8 drms.) of potassic chlorate, dissolved in 360 c.c. (about 12½ ozs.) of a vegetable infusion.

This potion was administered to four children—viz., David, aged 2½; Cousin, aged 3½; Salmont, 2½; and Guérin, 2½. David took the whole in two and a half hours, the symptoms commenced after the potion was finished, and the child died five and a half hours after taking the first dose; there were vomiting and diarrhœa. Cousin took the medicine in seven hours; the symptoms also commenced after the last spoonful, and the death took place eight and a half hours from the first spoonful. The symptoms were mainly those of great depression; the lips were blue, the pulse feeble, there was no vomiting, no diarrhœa. Salmont took the medicine in nine hours, and died in twelve. There was some diarrhœa, the stools were of a green colour. Guérin took the whole in two hours, the symptoms commenced in four hours; the lips were very pale, the gums blue. Death took place in four days.

There was an autopsy in the case of David only. The stomach showed a large ecchymosis on its mucous membrane, as if it had been burnt by an acid; the spleen was gorged with blood, and its tissue friable; the kidneys do not seem to have been thoroughly examined, but are said to have been tumefied. Potassic chlorate was discovered by dialysis. In the cases of the children just detailed, the symptoms appear to be a mixture of the depressing action of the potassium, and irritant action of the chlorate.

§ 132. In adults, the main symptoms are those of nephritis, and the fatal dose for an adult is somewhere about an ounce (28.3 grms.), but half this quantity would probably be dangerous, especially if given to a person who had congestion or disease of the kidneys.

Dr. Jacobi[129] gives the following cases.

Dr. Fountain in 1858, experimenting on himself, took 29.2 grms. (8.7 drms.) of potassic chlorate; he died on the seventh day from nephritis. A young lady swallowed 30 grms. (8.5 drms.), when using it as a gargle; she died in a few days from nephritis. A man, thirty years of age, died in four days after having taken 48 grms. (12.3 drms.) of sodic chlorate in six hours. The *shortest time* in which I can find the salt to have been fatal, is a case related by Dr. Manouvriez, in which a woman took 45 grms., and died in five hours. The *smallest dose* which has proved fatal is one in which an infant three years old was killed by 3 grms. (46.3 grains).

Jacobi considers that the maximum dose to be given in divided doses during the twenty-four hours, to infants under three, should be from 1-1.5 grm. (15.4-23.1 grains), to children from three years old, up to 2 grms. (30.8 grains); and adults from 6-8 grms. (92.6-123.4 grains).

§ 133. **Elimination.**—Potassic chlorate is quickly absorbed by mucous membranes, and by the inflamed skin, and rapidly separated from the body by the action of the kidneys. Wöhler, as early as 1824, recognised that it in great part passed out of the body unchanged, and, lately, Isambert, in conjunction with Hirne,[130] making quantitative estimations, recovered from the urine no less than 95 per cent. of the ingested salts. Otto Hehner has also made several auto-experiments, and taking 2½ drms., found that it could be detected in the urine an hour and a half afterwards. At that time 17.23 per cent. of the salt had been excreted, and, by the end of eleven hours, 93.8 per cent. was recovered. It is then difficult to believe that the salt gives any oxygen to the tissues, for though it is true that in

[128] *Annales d'Hygiène publique*, 1881, p. 232.

[129] *Amer. Med. Times*, 1860.

[130] *Gaz. Méd. de Paris*, 1875, Nro. 17, 35, 41, 43.

all the investigations a small percentage remains to be accounted for, and also that Binz,[131] making experiments by mixing solutions of potassic chlorate with moist organic substances, such as pus, yeast, fibrin, &c., has declared that, at a blood heat the chlorate is rapidly reduced, and is no longer recognisable as chlorate—yet it may be affirmed that potassic chlorate is recovered from the urine as completely as anything which is ever excreted by the body, and that deductions drawn from the changes undergone by the salt in solutions of fibrin, &c., have only an indirect bearing on the question.

§ 134. The essential action of potassic chlorate seems to be that it causes a peculiar change in the blood, acting on the colouring matter and corpuscles; the latter lose their property as oxygen carriers; the hæmoglobin is in part destroyed; the corpuscles dissolved. The decomposed and altered blood-corpuscles are crowded into the kidneys, spleen, &c.; they block up the uriniferous canaliculi, and thus the organs present the curious colouring seen after death, and the kidneys become inflamed.

Detection and Estimation of Potassic Chlorate.

§ 135. Organic fluids are best submitted to dialysis; the dialysed fluid should then be concentrated and qualitative tests applied. One of the best tests for the presence of a chlorate is, without doubt, that recommended by Fresenius. The fluid to be tested is acidulated with a few drops of sulphuric acid; sulphate of indigo added sufficient to colour the solution blue, and finally a few drops of sulphurous acid. In presence of potassic or sodic chlorate, the blue colour immediately vanishes. This method is capable of detecting 1 part in 128,000; provided the solution is not originally coloured, and but little organic matter is present.

The urine can be examined direct, but if it contain albumen, the blue colour may disappear and yet chlorate be present; if too much sulphurous acid be also added, the test may give erroneous results. These are but trivial objections, however, for if the analyst obtains a response to the test, he will naturally confirm or disprove it by the following process:—

The liquid under examination, organic or otherwise, is divided into two equal parts. In the one, all the chlorine present is precipitated as chloride by silver nitrate in the usual way, and the chloride of silver collected and weighed. In the other, the liquid is evaporated to dryness and well charred by a dull red heat, the ash dissolved in weak nitric acid, and the chlorides estimated as in the first case. If chlorates were present, there will be a difference between the two estimations, proportionate to the amount of chlorates which have been converted into chlorides by the carbonisation, and the first silver chloride subtracted from the second will give an argentic chloride which is to be referred to chlorate. In this way also the amount present may be quantitatively estimated, 100 parts of silver chloride equalling 85.4 of potassic chlorate.

Toxicological Detection of Alkali Salts.

§ 136. Sodium, in combination, especially with chlorine, and also with sulphuric, carbonic, and phosphoric acids, is found in the plasma of the blood, in the urinary secretion, in the pancreatic juice, in human bile, and in serous transudations, &c. Potassium, in combination, is especially found in the red blood-corpuscles, in the muscles, in the nervous tissues, and in milk. Ammonia, in combination with acids, is naturally found in the stomach, in the contents of the intestine; it is also a natural constituent of the blood in small traces, and in a corpse is copiously evolved from putrefactive changes.

It hence follows, that mere qualitative tests for these elements in the tissues or fluids of the body are of not the slightest use, for they are always present during the life of the healthiest individual, and can be found after death in persons dying from any malady whatever. To establish the fact of a person having taken an unusual dose of any of the alkali salts, by simply chemical evidence, it must be proved that the alkalies are present in unusual quantities or in an abnormal state of combination.

In cases of rapid death, caused by sodic or potassic salts, they will be found in such quantity in the contents of the stomach, or in matters vomited, that there will probably be no difficulty in coming to a direct conclusion; but if some time has elapsed, the analyst may not find a sufficient ground for giving a decided judgment, the excretion of the alkali salts being very rapid.

In most cases, it will be well to proceed as follows:—The contents of the stomach are, if necessary, diluted with distilled water, and divided into three parts, one of which is submitted to dialysis, and then the dialysed liquid evaporated to a small bulk and examined qualitatively, in order to ascertain whether a large amount of the alkaline

[131] *Berlin klin. Wochenschr.*, xi. 10, S. 119, 1874.

salts is present, and in what form. In this way, the presence or absence of nitrate of potassium or sodium may be proved, or the iodide, bromide, sulphate, and chlorate detected.

To find, in this way, nitrate of potassium, a coarse test is preferable to the finer tests dependent upon conversion of the nitrate into nitrites or into ammonia, for these tests are so delicate, that nitrates may be detected in traces; whereas, in this examination, to find traces is of no value. Hence, the old-fashioned test of treating the concentrated liquid in a test-tube with copper filings and then with sulphuric acid, and looking for the red fumes, is best, and will act very well, even should, as is commonly the case, some organic matters have passed through the dialyser.

Chlorates are indicated if the liquid is divided into two parts and tested in the manner recommended at already. If present in any quantity, chlorates or nitrates may be indicated by the brilliant combustion of the organic matter when heated to redness, as also by the action of strong sulphuric acid on the solid substances—in the one case, yellow vapours of peroxide of chlorine being evolved—in the other, the red fumes already mentioned of nitric peroxide.

With regard to a substance such as the hydro-potassic tartrate, its insolubility in water renders it not easy of detection by dialysis; but its very insolubility will aid the analyst, for the contents of the stomach may be treated with water, and thus all soluble salts of the alkalies extracted. On now microscopically examining the insoluble residue, crystals of bitartrate, if present, will be readily seen. They may be picked up on a clean platinum wire and heated to redness in a Bunsen flame, and spectroscopically examined. After heating, the melted mass will have an alkaline reaction, and give a precipitate with platinic chloride. All other organic salts of potassium are soluble, and a white crystal giving such reaction must be hydro-potassic tartrate.

Ammonium Salts.—If the body is fresh, and yet the salts of ammonium present in large amount, it is safe to conclude that they have an external origin; but there might be some considerable difficulty in criminal poisoning by a neutral salt of ammonium, and search for it in a highly putrid corpse. Probably, in such an exceptional case, there would be other evidence. With regard to the quantitative separation and estimation of the fixed alkalies in the ash of organic substances, the reader is referred to the processes given in "Foods," p. 99, *et seq.*, and in the present work.

PART V.—MORE OR LESS VOLATILE POISONOUS SUBSTANCES CAPABLE OF BEING SEPARATED BY DISTILLATION FROM NEUTRAL OR ACID LIQUIDS.

HYDROCARBONS—CAMPHOR—ALCOHOL—AMYL NITRITE—ETHER—CHLOROFORM AND OTHER ANÆSTHETICS—CHLORAL—CARBON DISULPHIDE—CARBOLIC ACID—NITRO-BENZENE—PRUSSIC ACID—PHOSPHORUS.

I.—Hydrocarbons.

1. PETROLEUM.

§ 137. Petroleum is a general term for a mixture of hydrocarbons of the paraffin series, which are found naturally in certain parts of the world, and are in commerce under liquid and solid forms of various density. Crude petroleum is not imported into England, the original substance having previously undergone more or less rectification. The lighter and more volatile portions are known under the name of cymogene, rhigolene, gasolene, and naphtha.

§ 138. **Cymogene** has a specific gravity of .590, and boils at 0°. It has been employed in refrigerating machines. It appears to consist chiefly of butane (C_4H_{10}).

§ 139. **Rhigolene** is now used in medicine in the form of spray to produce local anæsthesia. It boils at 18°, and has a density of .650.

§ 140. **Gasolene** has a density of .680-.688; it has received technical applications in the "naphthalising" of air and gas.

§ 141. **Benzoline (mineral naphtha, petroleum naphtha, petroleum spirit, petroleum ether)** is a mixture of the lighter series of hydro-carbons; the greater part consists of heptane, and there is also a considerable quantity of pentane (C_7H_{16}) present. The specific gravity varies from .69 to .74. It is very inflammable, and is used in sponge lamps, and also as a solvent for gutta-percha, naphthalene, paraffin, wax, and many other bodies. By the practical chemist it is much employed.

The similarity of the terms *benzoline* and *benzene* has caused benzoline to be often confused with *benzol* or *benzene*, the leading constituent of coal-tar naphtha (C_6H_6). Mr Allen[132] gives in the following table a summary of the chief points of distinction, both between petroleum naphtha, shale naphtha, and coal-tar naphtha. The table is founded upon the examination of particular samples, and commercial samples may present a few minor deviations.

TABLE OF THE VARIETIES OF NAPHTHA.

Petroleum Naphtha.	Shale Naphtha.	Coal-tar Naphtha.
Contains at least 75 per cent. of heptane, C_7H_{16}, and other hydrocarbons of the marsh gas or paraffin series; the remainder apparently olefins, C_nH_{2n}, with distinct traces of benzene and its homologues.	Contains at least 60 to 70 per cent. of heptylene, C_7H_{14}, and other hydrocarbons of the olefin series; the remainder paraffins. No trace of benzene or its homologues.	Consists almost wholly of benzene, C_6H_6, and other homologous hydrocarbons, with a small percentage of light hydrocarbons in some samples.
Specific gravity at 15°, .600.	Specific gravity at 15°, .718.	Specific gravity .876.
Distils between 65° and 100°.	Distils between 65° and 100°.	Distils between 80° and 120°.

[132] *Commercial Organic Analysis*, vol. ii. p. 31.

Dissolves coal-tar pitch, but slightly; liquid, but little coloured even after prolonged contact.	Behaves similarly to petroleum naphtha with regard to the solution of pitch.	Readily dissolves pitch, forming a deep brown solution.
On shaking three measures of the sample with one measure of fused crystals of absolute carbolic acid, no solution. Liquids not miscible.	When treated with fused carbolic acid crystals, the liquids mix perfectly.	The liquids form a homogeneous mixture when treated with fused carbolic acid crystals.
Combines with 10 per cent. of its weight of bromine in the cold.	Combines with upwards of 90 per cent. of its weight of bromine.	Combines slowly with 30-40 per cent. of its weight of bromine.

§ 142. **Paraffin Oil** (or **kerosine, mineral oil, photogen**, &c.) is the chief product resulting from the distillation of American petroleum—the usual specific gravity is about .802—it is a mixture of hydrocarbons of the paraffin series. It should be free from the more volatile constituents, and hence should not take fire when a flame is applied near the surface of the cold liquid.

§ 143. **Effects of Petroleum.**—Since we have here to deal with a commercial substance of such different degrees of purity, and various samples of which are composed of such various proportions of different hydrocarbons, its action can only be stated in very general terms. Eulenberg[133] has experimented with the lighter products obtained from the distillation of Canadian petroleum. This contained sulphur products, and was extremely poisonous, the vapour killing a rabbit in a short time, with previous insensibility and convulsions. The autopsy showed a thin extravasation of blood on the surface of each of the bulbi, much coagulated blood in the heart, congested lungs, and a bloody mucus covering the tracheal mucous membrane. An experiment made on a cat with the lighter petroleum (which had no excess of sulphur) in the state of vapour, showed that it was an anæsthetic, the anæsthesia being accompanied by convulsions, which towards the end were tetanic and violent. The evaporation of 1.5 grm. in a close chamber killed the animal in three hours. The lungs were found congested, but little else was remarkable. Much petroleum vapour is breathed in certain factories, especially those in which petroleum is refined.[134] From this cause there have been rather frequent toxic symptoms among the workmen. Eulenberg[135] describes the symptoms as follows:—A person, after breathing an overdose of the vapour, becomes very pale, the lips are livid, the respiration slow, the heart's action weak and scarcely to be felt. If he does not immediately go into the open air away from the poisonous vapour, these symptoms may pass on to insensibility, convulsions, and death. It often occasions a condition of the voluntary muscles similar to that induced by drunkenness, and on recovery the patient is troubled by singing in the ears and noises in the head. The smell and taste of the poison may remain for a long time.

§ 144. Poisoning by taking light petroleum into the stomach is not common. In a case recorded by Taylor,[136] a woman, for the purpose of suicide, swallowed a pint of petroleum, There followed a slight pain in the stomach, and a little febrile disturbance, and a powerful smell of petroleum remained about the body for six days; but she completely recovered. In August 1870 a sea-captain drank a quantity of paraffin, that is, lighting petroleum, and died in a few hours in an unconscious state. A child, 2 years old, was brought to King's College Hospital within ten minutes after taking a teaspoonful of paraffin. It was semi-comatose and pale, with contracted pupils; there was no vomiting or purging. Emetics of sulphate of zinc were administered, and the child recovered in twenty-four hours. In another case treated at the same hospital, a child had swallowed an unknown quantity of paraffin. It fell into a comatose state, which simulated tubercular meningitis, and lasted for nearly three weeks.[137] In a case recorded by Mr. Robert Smith,[138] a child, 4 years of age, had swallowed an unknown quantity of paraffin. A few minutes

[133] *Gewerbe-Hygiene.*

[134] The vapour most likely to rise at the ordinary temperature, and mix with the atmosphere, is that of the lighter series, from cymogene to benzoline.

[135] *Op. cit.*

[136] *Poisons*, p. 656.

[137] *Brit. Med. Journ.*, Sept. 16, 1876, p. 365.

[138] *Brit. Med. Journ.*, Oct. 14, 1876.

afterwards, the symptoms commenced; they were those of suffocation, with a constant cough; there was no expectoration; the tongue, gums, and cheeks were blanched and swollen where the fluid touched them; recovery followed. A woman, aged 32, who had taken a quarter of a pint of paraffin, was found unconscious and very cold; the stomach-pump was used, and she recovered.[139] Hence it is tolerably certain, from the above instances, that should a case of petroleum poisoning occur, the expert will not have to deal with infinitesimal quantities; but while the odour of the oil will probably be distinctly perceptible, there will be also a sufficient amount obtained either from matters vomited, or the contents of the stomach, &c., so that no difficulty will be experienced in identifying it.

§ 145. In order to separate petroleum from any liquid, the substances under examination must be carefully distilled in the manner recommended under "*Ether*." The lighter petroleums will distil by the aid of a water-bath; but the heavier require a stronger heat; redistillation of the distillate may be necessary. The odour of the liquid, its inflammable character, and its other properties, will be sufficient for identification.

2. COAL-TAR-NAPHTHA—BENZENE.

§ 146. Coal-tar-naphtha in its crude state, is an extremely complex liquid, of a most disagreeable smell. Much benzene (C_6H_6) is present with higher homologues of the benzene series. Toluene (C_7H_8), naphthalene ($C_{10}H_8$), hydrocarbons of the paraffin series, especially hexane (C_6H_{14}), and hydrocarbons of the olefin series, especially pentylene, hexylene, and heptylene (C_5H_{10}, C_6H_{12} and C_7H_{14}). Besides these, there are nitrogenised bases, such as aniline, picoline, and pyridine; phenols, especially carbolic acid; ammonia, ammonium sulphide, carbon disulphide, and probably other sulphur compounds; acetylene and aceto-nitrile. By distillation and fractional distillation are produced what are technically known "*once run*" *naphtha*, *90 per cent. benzol*, *50 and 90 per cent. benzol*,[140] *30 per cent. benzol*, *solvent naphtha*, and residue known as "*last runnings*."

§ 147. Taylor[141] records a case in which a boy, aged 12, swallowed about 3 ozs. of naphtha, the kind usually sold for burning in lamps, and died with symptoms of narcotic poisoning. The child, after taking it, ran about in wild delirium, he then sank into a state of collapse, breathing stertorously, and the skin became cold and clammy. On vomiting being excited, he rejected about two tablespoonfuls of the naphtha, and recovered somewhat, but again fell into collapse with great muscular relaxation. The breathing was difficult; there were no convulsions; the eyes were fixed and glassy, the pupils contracted; there was frothing at the mouth. In spite of every effort to save him, he died in less than three hours after taking the poison. The body, examined three days after death, smelt strongly of naphtha, but the *post-mortem* appearances were in no way peculiar, save that the stomach contained a pint of semi-fluid matter, from which a fluid, having the characteristics of impure benzene, was separated.

§ 148. The effects of the vapour of benzene have been studied by Eulenberg in experiments on cats and rabbits, and there are also available observations on men[142] who have been accidentally exposed to its influence. From these sources of information, it is evident that the vapour of benzene has a distinctly narcotic effect, while influencing also in a marked degree the spinal cord. There are, as symptoms, noises in the head, convulsive trembling and twitchings of the muscles, with difficulty of breathing.

DETECTION AND SEPARATION OF BENZENE.

§ 149. Benzene is separated from liquids by distillation, and may be recognised by its odour, and by the properties described earlier. The best process of identification, perhaps, is to purify and convert it into nitro-benzene, and then into aniline, in the following manner:—

1. **Purification.**—The liquid is agitated with a solution of caustic soda; this dissolves out of the benzene any bodies of an acid character, such as phenol, &c. The purified liquid should again be distilled, collecting that portion of the distillate which passes over between 65° and 100°; directly the thermometer attains nearly the 100°, the distillation should be stopped. The distillate, which contains all the benzene present, is next shaken with concentrated sulphuric acid in the cold; this will dissolve out all the hydrocarbons of the ethylene and acetylene series. On removing the layer of benzene from the acid, it must be again shaken up with dilute soda, so as to remove any trace of acid. The benzene is, by this rather complicated series of operations, obtained in a very fair state of

[139] *Pharm. Journ.*, Feb. 12, 1875; also for other cases see *Brit. Med. Journ.*, Nov. 4, 1876; and Köhler's *Physiol. Therap.*, p. 437.

[140] Or $^{50}/_{90}$ benzol, this indicates that 50 per cent. distils over below 100°; and 40, making in all 90, below 120°.

[141] *Op. cit.*, p. 657.

[142] Dr. Stone, *Med. Gaz.*, 1848, vol. xii. p. 1077.

purity, and may be converted into nitro-benzene, as follows:—

2. **Conversion into Nitro-Benzene.**—The oily liquid is placed in a flask, and treated with four times its volume of fuming nitric acid. The flask must be furnished with an upright condenser; a vigorous action mostly takes place without the application of heat, but if this does not occur, the flask may be warmed for a few minutes.

After the conversion is over, the liquid, while still warm, must be transferred into a burette furnished with a glass tap, or to a separating funnel, and all, except the top layer, run into cold water; if benzene was originally present, either oily drops of nitro-benzene will fall, or if the benzene was only in small quantity, a fine precipitate will gradually settle down to the bottom of the vessel, and a distinct bitter-almond smell be observed; but, if there be no benzene in the original liquid, and, consequently, no nitro-benzene formed, no such appearance will be observed.

3. **Conversion into Aniline.**—The nitro-benzene may itself be identified by collecting it on a wet filter, dissolving it off the filter by alcohol, acidifying the alcoholic solution by hydrochloric acid, and then boiling it for some time with metallic zinc. In this way aniline is formed by reduction. On neutralising and diluting the liquid, and cautiously adding a little clear solution of bleaching-powder, a blue or purple colour passing to brown is in a little time produced.

3. TERPENES—ESSENTIAL OILS—OIL OF TURPENTINE.

§ 150. The terpenes are hydrocarbons of the general formula C_nH_{2n-4}. The natural terpenes are divided into three classes:—

1. **The true terpenes,** *formula* ($C_{10};H_{16}$)—a large number of essential oils, such as those of turpentine, orange peel, nutmeg, caraway, anise, thyme, &c., are mainly composed of terpenes.

2. **The cedrenes,** *formula* ($C_{15}H_{24}$)—the essential oil of cloves, rosewood, cubebs, calamus, cascarilla, and patchouli belong to this class.

3. **The colophene hydrocarbons,** *formula* ($C_{20}H_{32}$), represented by colophony.

Of all these, oil of turpentine alone has any toxicological significance; it is, however, true that all the essential oils, if taken in considerable doses, are poisonous, and cause, for the most part, vascular excitement and complex nervous phenomena, but their action has not been very completely studied. They may all be separated by distillation, but a more convenient process for recovering an essential oil from a liquid is to shake it up with petroleum ether, separating the petroleum and evaporating spontaneously; by this means the oil is left in a fair state of purity.

4. OIL OF TURPENTINE—SPIRIT OF TURPENTINE—"TURPS."

§ 151. Various species of pine yield a crude turpentine, holding in solution more or less resin. The turpentine may be obtained from this exudation by distillation, and when the first portion of the distillate is treated with alkali, and then redistilled, the final product is known under the name of "rectified oil of turpentine," and is sometimes called "camphene." It mainly consists of terebenthene. Terebenthene obtained from French turpentine differs in some respects from that obtained from English or American turpentine. They are both mobile, colourless liquids, having the well-known odour of turpentine and highly refractive; but the French terebenthene turns a ray of polarised light to the left -40.3° for the sodium ray, and the English to the right +21.5°; the latter terebenthene is known scientifically as austra-terebenthene. This action on polarised light is retained in the various compounds and polymers of the two turpentine oils.

The specific gravity of turpentine oil is .864; its boiling point, when consisting of pure terebenthene, 156°, but impurities may raise it up to 160°; it is combustible and burns with a smoky flame. Oil of turpentine is very soluble in ether, petroleum ether, carbon disulphide, chloroform, benzene, fixed and essential oils, and by the use of these solvents it is conveniently separated from the contents of the stomach. It is insoluble in water, glycerin, and dilute alkaline and acid solutions; and very soluble in absolute alcohol, from which it may be precipitated by the addition of water.

It is polymerised by the action of strong sulphuric acid, the polymer, of course, boiling at a higher temperature than the original oil. With water it forms a crystalline hydrate ($C_{10}H_{20}O_2,H_2O$). On passing nitrosyl chloride gas into the oil, either pure or diluted with chloroform or alcohol, the mixture being cooled by ice, a white crystalline body is deposited, of the formula $C_{10}H_{16}(NOCl)$. By treating this compound with alcoholic potash, the substitution product ($C_{10}H_{16}NO$) is obtained. By treating turpentine with an equal bulk of warm water, and shaking it in a large bottle with air, camphoric acid and peroxide of hydrogen are formed. When turpentine oil is left in contact with concentrated hydrochloric acid, there is formed terebenthene dihydrochloride ($C_{10}H_{16}2HCl$), which forms rhombic plates, insoluble in water, and decomposable by boiling alcoholic potash, with formation of terpinol, $(C_{10}H_{17})_2O$. The dihydrochloride gives a colour-reaction with ferric chloride. This is an excellent test—not, it is true, confined to oil of turpentine—but common to the dihydrochlorides of all the terpenes. A few drops of the oil are stirred in a porcelain capsule with a drop of hydrochloric acid, and one of ferric chloride solution; on gently heating, there is produced first a rose colour, then a violet-red, and lastly a blue.

§ 152. **Effects of the Administration of Turpentine.**—L. W. Liersch[143] exposed animals to the vapour of turpentine, and found that a cat and a rabbit died within half an hour. There was observed uneasiness, reeling, want of power in the limbs (more especially in the hinder extremities), convulsions partial, or general, difficulty of respiration; and the heart's action was quickened. Death took place, in part, from asphyxia, and in part was attributable to a direct action on the nervous centres. The autopsy showed congestion of the lungs, ecchymoses of the kidney, and much blood in the liver and spleen. Small doses of turpentine-vapour cause (according to Sir B. W. Richardson)[144] giddiness, deficient appetite, and anæmia. From half an ounce to an ounce is frequently prescribed in the country as a remedy for tape-worm; in smaller quantities it is found to be a useful medicine in a great variety of ailments. The larger doses produce a kind of intoxication with giddiness, followed often by purging and strangury, not unfrequently blood and albumen (or both) is found in the urine. When in medical practice I have given the oil, and seen it given by others, in large doses for tape-worm to adults, in perhaps 40 cases, but in no one instance were the symptoms severe; the slight intoxication subsided quickly, and in a few hours the patients recovered completely. Nevertheless it has been known to destroy the lives of children, and cause most serious symptoms in adults. Two fatal cases are mentioned by Taylor; one was that of a child who died fifteen hours after taking half an ounce of the oil; in another an infant, five months old, died rapidly from a teaspoonful. The symptoms in these fatal cases were profound coma and slight convulsions; the pupils were contracted, and there was slow and irregular breathing. Turpentine is eliminated in a changed form by the kidneys, and imparts an odour of violet to the urine; but the nature of the odoriferous principle has not yet been investigated.

II.—Camphor.

§ 153. A great many essential oils deposit, after exposure to air, camphors produced by oxidation of their terpenes. Ordinary camphor is imported in the rough state from China and Japan, and is prepared by distilling with water the wood of *Camphora officinarum*; it is resublimed in England. The formula of camphor is $C_{10}H_{10}O$; it has a density of .986 to .996; melts at 175°, and boils at 205°. It is readily sublimed, especially in a vacuum, and is indeed so volatile at all temperatures, that a lump of camphor exposed to the air wastes away. It is somewhat insoluble in water (about 1 part in 1000), but this is enough to impart a distinct taste to the water; it is insoluble in chloroform, ether, acetone, acetic acid, carbon disulphide, and oils. It has a fragrant odour and a burning taste. A 10 per cent. solution in alcohol turns a ray of polarised light to the right +42.8°. By distillation with zinc chloride, cymene and other products are produced. By prolonged treatment with nitric acid, camphor is oxidised to camphoric acid ($C_{10}H_{16}O_4$). Camphor unites with bromine to form a crystalline, unstable dibromide, which splits up on distillation into hydrobromic acid and monobrom-camphor ($C_{10}H_{15}BrO$). The latter is used in medicine; it crystallises in prisms fusible at 76°, and is readily soluble in alcohol.

§ 154. **Pharmaceutical Preparations.**—The preparations officinal in the British Pharmacopœia are *camphor water*—water saturated with camphor, containing about one part per thousand.

Camphor Liniment.—A solution of camphor in olive oil, strength 25 per cent.

Compound Camphor Liniment.—Composed of camphor, oil of lavender, strong solution of ammonia and alcohol; strength in camphor about 11 per cent.

Spirit of Camphor.—A solution of camphor in spirit; strength, 10 per cent.

Camphor is also a constituent of the *compound tincture of camphor*; but in this case it may be considered only a flavouring agent. There is a homœopathic solution of camphor in spirit (Rubini's Essence of Camphor). The solution is made by saturating alcohol with camphor; it is, therefore, very strong—about half the bulk consisting of camphor. Camphor is used in veterinary medicine, both externally and internally.

§ 155. **Symptoms.**—Camphor acts energetically on the brain and nervous system, especially if it is given in

[143] Clarus in Schmidt's *Jahrbücher*, Bd. cxvii., i. 1863; and *Vierteljahrsschr. für ger. Med.*, xxii., Oct. 1862.
[144] *Brit. and For. Med.-Chir. Review*, April 1863.

strong alcoholic solution, and thus placed under conditions favouring absorption. Some years ago, Dr. G. Johnson[145] published a series of cases arising from the injudicious use of "homœopathic solution of camphor," from 7 to 40 drops of Rubini's homœopathic camphor taken for colds, sore throat, &c., having produced coma, foaming at the mouth, convulsions, and partial paralysis. All the patients recovered, but their condition was for a little time alarming.

The cases of fatal poisoning by camphor are very rare. A woman, aged 46, pregnant four months, took 12 grms. (about 184 grains) in a glass of brandy for the purpose of procuring abortion. In a very short time the symptoms commenced; she had intolerable headache, the face was flushed, and there was a sensation of burning in the stomach. In eight hours after taking the dose, she had strangury and vomiting, and the pain in the epigastrium was intense. These symptoms continued with more or less severity until the third day, when she became much worse. Her face was pale and livid, the eyes hollow, the skin cold and insensible, pulse weak and thready, breathing laboured. There were violent cramps in the stomach and retention of urine for twenty-four hours, and then coma. The patient lingered on yet another three days, aborted, and died.[146]

Dr. Schaaf[147] has recorded three cases of poisoning—one of which was fatal. A woman gave about half a teaspoonful of a camphor solution to each of her three children, the ages being respectively five and three years and fifteen months. The symptoms noted were pallor of the face, a burning pain in the throat, thirst, vomiting, purging, convulsions, and afterwards coma. The youngest child died in seven hours; the others recovered. The smallest dose known to have produced violent symptoms in an adult is 1.3 grm. (20 grains); the largest dose known to have been recovered from is 10.4 grms. (160 grains).[148]

§ 156. **Post-mortem Appearances.**—The bodies of animals or persons dying from poisoning by camphor, smell strongly of the substance. The mucous membrane of the stomach has been found inflamed, but there seem to be no characteristic lesions.

§ 157. **Separation of Camphor from the Contents of the Stomach.**—The identification of camphor would probably in no case present any difficulty. It may be readily dissolved out from organic fluids by chloroform. If dissolved in fixed oils, enough for the purposes of identification may be obtained by simple distillation. It is precipitated from its alcoholic solution by the addition of water.

III.—Alcohols.

1. ETHYLIC ALCOHOL.

§ 158. The chemical properties of ordinary alcohol are fully described, with the appropriate tests, in "Foods," pp. 369-384, and the reader is also referred to the same volume for the composition and strength of the various alcoholic drinks.

Statistics.—If we were to include in one list the deaths indirectly due to chronic, as well as acute poisoning by alcohol, it would stand first of all poisons in order of frequency, but the taking of doses so large as to cause death in a few hours is rare. The deaths from alcohol are included by the English registrar-general under two heads, viz., those returned as dying from *delirium tremens*, and those certified as due directly to intemperance.

During the twenty-five years, from 1868 to 1892, 30,219 deaths have been registered as due to intemperance, which gives an average of 1209 per year. The rate per million has varied during the period from 29 to 71; and the figures taken as a whole show that deaths from intemperance appear to be increasing; the increase may be only apparent, not real, for it is a significant circumstance that deaths registered under liver diseases show a corresponding decrease; it is, therefore, not unlikely that deaths which formerly would be ascribed to liver disease, are more often now stated to be the effects of intemperance.

Deaths directly due to large doses of alcohol are not uncommon; during the ten years ending 1892, 105 deaths (81 males and 24 females) were ascribed under the head of "accident or negligence" directly to alcohol.

[145] *Brit. Med. Journ.*, Feb. 27, 1878, p. 272; see also *ibid.*, Feb. 1875.
[146] *Journ. de Chim. Méd.*, May 1860.
[147] *Journ. de Chim. Méd.*, 1850, p. 507.
[148] Taylor on *Poisons*, 3rd ed., 661.

CHART SHEWING DEATHS PER MILLION PERSONS LIVING, FROM INTEMPERANCE & FROM LIVER DISEASES.

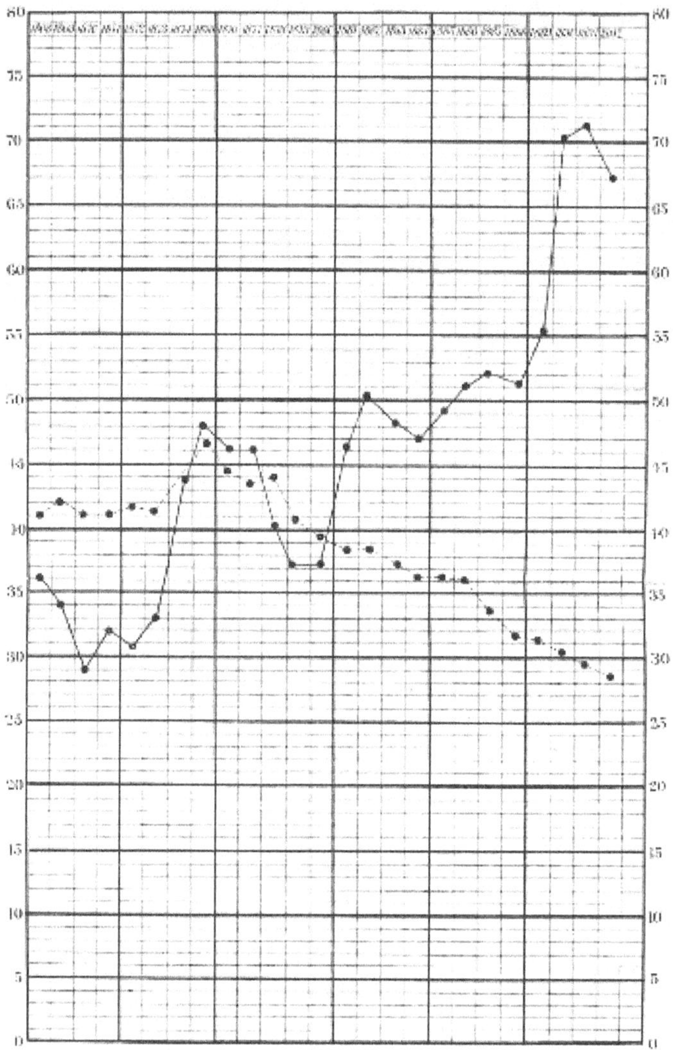

THE MEDICAL "OFFICERS OF HEALTH" CHART. ENT. AT STA. HALL.

Notes.

Intemperance ————

Liver disease ·· — — — — –

The Scale for Intemperance is as printed.

That for Liver diseases is 10 times larger.

§ 159. **Criminal or Accidental Alcoholic Poisoning.**—Suicide by alcohol, in the common acceptation of the term, is rare, and murder still rarer, though not unknown. In the ten years ending 1892, only three deaths from alcohol (1 male and 2 females) are recorded as suicidal. Perhaps the most common cause of fatal acute poisoning by alcohol is either a foolish wager, by which a man bets that he can drink so many glasses of spirits without bad effect; or else the drugging of a person already drunk by his companions in a sportive spirit.

§ 160. **Fatal Dose.**—It is difficult to say what would be likely to prove a lethal dose of alcohol, for a great deal depends, without doubt, on the dilution of the spirit, since the mere local action of strong alcohol on the mucous membranes of the stomach, &c., is severe (one may almost say corrosive), and would aid the more remote effects.

In Maschka's case,[149] a boy of nine years and a girl of five, died from about two and a half ounces of spirit of 67 per cent. strength, or 48.2 c.c. (1.7 oz.) of absolute alcohol.

In a case related by Taylor, a child, seven years old, died from some quantity of brandy, probably about 113.4 c.c. (4 ozs.), which would be equal to at least 56.7 c.c. (2 ozs.) of absolute alcohol. From other cases in which the quantity of absolute alcohol can be, with some approximation to the truth, valued, it is evident that, for any child below ten or twelve, quantities of from 28.3 to 56.6 c.c. (1-2 ozs.) of absolute alcohol contained in brandy, gin, &c., would be a highly dangerous and probably fatal dose; while the toxic dose for adults is somewhere between 71.8-141.7 c.c. (2.5-5 ozs.).

§ 161. **Symptoms.**—In the cases of rapid poisoning by a large dose of alcohol, which alone concern us, the preliminary, and too familiar excitement of the drunkard, may be hardly observable; but the second stage, that of depression, rapidly sets in; the unhappy victim sinks down to the ground helpless, the face pale, the eyes injected and staring, the pupils dilated, acting sluggishly to light, and the skin remarkably cold. Fräntzel[150] found, in a case in which the patient survived, a temperature of only 24.6° in the rectum, and in that of another person who died, a temperature of 23.8°. The mucous membranes are of a peculiar dusky blue; the pulse, which at first is quick, soon becomes slow and small; the respiration is also slowed, intermittent, and stertorous; there is complete loss of consciousness and motion; the breath smells strongly of the alcoholic drink, and if the coma continues there may be vomiting and involuntary passing of excreta. Death ultimately occurs through paralysis of the respiratory centres. Convulsions in adults are rare, in children frequent. Death has more than once been immediately caused, not by the poison, but by accidents dependent upon loss of consciousness. Thus food has been sucked into the air-tubes, or the person has fallen, so that the face was buried in water, ordure, or mud; here suffocation has been induced by mechanical causes.

A remarkable course not known with any other narcotic is that in which the symptoms remit, the person wakes up, as it were, moves about and does one or more rational acts, and then suddenly dies. In this case also, the death is not directly due to alcohol, but indirectly—the alcohol having developed œdema, pneumonia, or other affection of the lungs, which causes the sudden termination when the first effect of the poison has gone off. The time that may elapse from the commencement of coma till death varies from a few minutes to days; death has occurred after a quarter of an hour, half an hour, and an hour. It has also been prolonged to three, four, and six days, during the whole of which the coma has continued. The average period may, however, be put at from six to ten hours.

§ 162. **Post-mortem Appearances.**—Cadaveric rigidity lasts tolerably long. Casper has seen it still existing nine days after death, and Seidel[151] seven days (in February). Putrefaction is retarded in those cases in which a very large dose has been taken, but this is not a very noticeable or constant characteristic. The pupils are mostly dilated. The smell of alcohol should be watched for; sometimes it is only present in cases where but a short time has elapsed between the taking of the poison and death; putrefaction may also conceal it, but under favourable circumstances, especially if the weather is cold, the alcoholic smell may remain a long time. Alcohol may cause the most intense redness and congestion of the stomach. The most inflamed stomach I ever saw, short of inflammation by the corrosive poisons, was that of a sailor, who died suddenly after a twenty-four hours' drinking bout: all the organs of the body were fairly healthy, the man had suffered from no disease; analysis could detect no poison but alcohol; and the history of the case, moreover, proved clearly that it was a pure case of alcoholic poisoning.

In a case related by Taylor, in which a child drank 4 ozs. of brandy and died, the mucous membrane of the

[149] Recorded by Maschka (*Gutachten der Prager Facultät*, iv. 239; see also Maschka's *Handbuch der gericht. Medicin*, Band. ii. p. 384). The following is a brief summary:—Franz. Z., nine years old, and Caroline Z., eight years old, were poisoned by their stepfather with spirit of 67 per cent. strength taken in small quantities by each—at first by persuasion, and the remainder administered by force. About one-eighth of a pint is said to have been given to each child. Both vomited somewhat, then lying down, stertorous breathing at once came on, and they quickly died. The autopsy, three days after death, showed dilatation of the pupils; *rigor mortis* present in the boy, not in the girl; and the membranes of the brain filled with dark fluid blood. The smell of alcohol was perceptible on opening the chest; the mucous membrane of the bronchial tubes and gullet was normal, both lungs œdematous, the fine tubes gorged with a bloody frothy fluid, and the mucous membrane of the whole intestinal canal was reddened. The stomach was not, unfortunately, examined, being reserved for chemical analysis. The heart was healthy; the pericardium contained some straw-coloured fluid. Chemical analysis gave an entirely negative result, which must have been from insufficient material having been submitted to the analyst, for I cannot see how the vapours of alcohol could have been detected by the smell, and yet have evaded chemical processes.

[150] *Temperaturerniedrigung durch Alcoholintoxication, Charité Annalen*, i. 371.

[151] Seidel, Maschka's *Handbuch*, Bd. ii. p. 380.

stomach presented patches of intense redness, and in several places was thickened and softened, some portions being actually detached and hanging loose, and there were evident signs of extravasations of blood. The effect may not be confined to the stomach, but extend to the duodenum and even to the whole intestinal canal. The blood is generally dark and fluid, and usually the contents of the skull are markedly hyperæmic, the pia very full of blood, the sinuses and plexus gorged; occasionally, the brain-substance shows signs of unusual congestion; serum is often found in the ventricles. The great veins of the neck, the lungs, and the right side of the heart, are very often found full of blood, and the left side empty. Œdema of the lungs also occurs with tolerable frequency. The great veins of the abdomen are also filled with blood, and if the coma has been prolonged, the bladder will be distended with urine. A rare phenomenon has also been noticed—namely, the occurrence of blebs on the extremities, &c., just as if the part affected had been burnt or scalded. Lastly, with the changes directly due to the fatal dose may be included all those degenerations met with in the chronic drinker, provided the case had a history of previous intemperance.

§ 163. **Excretion of Alcohol.**—Alcohol, in the diluted form, is quickly absorbed by the blood-vessels of the stomach, &c., and circulates in the blood; but what becomes of it afterwards is by no means settled. I think there can be little doubt that the lungs are the main channels through which it is eliminated; with persons given up to habits of intemperance, the breath has constantly a very peculiar ethereal odour, probably dependent upon some highly volatile oxidised product of alcohol.

Alcohol is eliminated in small proportion only by the kidneys. Thudichum, in an experiment[152] by which 4000 grms. of absolute alcohol were consumed by thirty-three men, could only find in the collected urine 10 grms. of alcohol. The numerous experiments by Dupré also establish the same truth, that but a fraction of the total alcohol absorbed is excreted by the kidneys. According to Lallemand, Perrin, and Duroy the content of the brain in alcohol is more than that of the other organs. I have found also that the brain after death has a wonderful attraction for alcohol, and yields it up at a water-heat very slowly and with difficulty. In one experiment, in which a finely-divided portion of brain, which had been soaking in alcohol for many weeks, was submitted to a steam heat of 100°, twenty-four hours' consecutive heating failed to expel every trace of spirit.

It is probable that true alcoholates of the chemical constituents of the brain are formed. In the case of vegetable colloidal bodies, such, for example, as the pulp of cherries, a similar attraction has been observed, the fruit condensing, as it were, the alcohol in its own tissues, and the outer liquid being of less alcoholic strength than that which can be expressed from the steeped cherries. Alcohol is also excreted by the sweat, and minute fractions have been found in the fæces.

§ 164. **Toxicological Detection of Alcohol** (see "Foods," pp. 406-419).—The living cells of the body produce minute quantities of alcohol, as also some of the bacteria normally inhabiting the small intestine produce small quantities of alcohol, and it is often found in traces in putrefying fluids. Hence, mere qualitative proofs of the presence of alcohol are insufficient on which to base an opinion as to whether alcohol had been taken during life or not, and it will be necessary to estimate the quantity accurately by some of the processes detailed in "Foods," p. 409, *et seq.* In those cases in which alcohol is found in quantity in the stomach, there can, of course, be no difficulty; in others, the whole of the alcohol may have been absorbed, and chemical evidence, unless extremely definite, must be supplemented by other facts.

2. AMYLIC ALCOHOL.

§ 165. **Amylic Alcohol**—*Formula*, $C_5H_{11}HO$.—There is more than one amylic alcohol according to theory; eight isomers are possible, and seven are known. The amylic alcohols are identical in their chemical composition, but differ in certain physical properties, primary amylic alcohol boiling at 137°, and iso-amyl alcohol at 131.6°. The latter has a specific gravity of .8148, and is the variety produced by fermentation and present in fusel oil.

§ 166. The experiments of Eulenberg[153] on rabbits, Cross[154] on pigeons, Rabuteau[155] on frogs, and Furst on rabbits, with those of Sir B. W. Richardson[156] on various animals, have shown it to be a powerful poison, more especially if breathed in a state of vapour.

Richardson, as the result of his investigations, considers that amyl alcohol when breathed sets up quite a peculiar

[152] See Thudichum's *Pathology of the Urine*, London, 1877, in which both his own and Dr. Dupré's experiments are summarised.
[153] *Gewerbe Hygiene*, 1876, p. 440.
[154] *De l'Alcohol Amylique et Méthyl sur l'Organisme (Thèse)*, Strasburg, 1863.
[155] "Ueber die Wirkung des Aethyl, Butyl u. Amyl Alcohols," *L'Union*, Nos. 90, 91, 1870. Schmidt's *Jahrb.*, Bd. 149, p. 263.
[156] *Trans. Brit. Association*, 1864, 1865, and 1866. Also, *Brit. and Foreign Med. Chir. Rev.*, Jan. 7, 1867, p. 247.

class of symptoms which last for many hours, and are of such a character, that it might be thought impossible for the animal to recover, although they have not been known to prove fatal. There is muscular paralysis with paroxysms of tremulous convulsions; the spasms are excited by touching the animal, breathing upon it, or otherwise subjecting it to trifling excitation.

§ 167. Hitherto, neither the impure fusel oil, nor the purer chemical preparation, has had any toxicological importance. Should it be necessary at any time to recover small quantities from organic liquids, the easiest way is to shake the liquid up with chloroform, which readily dissolves amylic alcohol, and on evaporation leaves it in a state pure enough to be identified. Amyl alcohol is identified by the following tests:—(1) Its physical properties; (2) if warmed with twice its volume of strong sulphuric acid, a rose or red colour is produced; (3) heated with an acetate and strong sulphuric acid, *amyl acetate*, which has the odour of the jargonelle pear, is formed; (4) heated with sulphuric acid and potassic dichromate, valeric aldehyde is first produced, and then valeric acid is formed; the latter has a most peculiar and strong odour.

§ 168. **Amyl Nitrite, Iso-amyl Ester Nitrite** ($C_5H_{11}NO_2$).—Boiling point 97° to 99°, specific gravity .877. Amyl nitrite is a limpid, and, generally, slightly yellow liquid; it has a peculiar and characteristic odour. On heating with alcoholic potash, the products are nitrite of potash and amylic alcohol; the amylic alcohol may be distilled off and identified. The presence of a nitrite in the alkaline solution is readily shown by the colour produced, by adding a few drops of a solution of meta-phenylenediamine.

Sir B. W. Richardson and others have investigated the action of amyl nitrite, as well as that of the acetate and iodide; they all act in a similar manner, the nitrite being most potent. After absorption, the effects of amyl nitrite are especially seen on the heart and circulation: the heart acts violently, there is first dilatation of the capillaries, then this is followed by diminished action of the heart and contraction of the capillaries.

According to Richardson, it suspends the animation of frogs. No other substance known will thus suspend a frog's animation for so long a time without killing it. Under favourable circumstances, the animal will remain apparently dead for many days, and yet recover. Warm-blooded animals may be thrown by amyl nitrite into a cataleptic condition. It is not an anæsthetic, and by its use consciousness is not destroyed, unless a condition approaching death be first produced. When this occurs there is rarely recovery, the animal passes into actual death.

Post-Mortem Appearances.—If administered quickly, the lungs and all the other organs are found blanched and free from blood, the right side of the heart gorged with blood, the left empty, the brain being free from congestion. If administered slowly, the brain is found congested, and there is blood both on the left and right sides of the heart.

IV.—Ether.

§ 169. **Ether, Ethylic Ether, Ethyl Oxide,** $(C_2H_5)_2O$.—Ethylic ether is a highly mobile liquid of peculiar penetrating odour and sweetish pungent taste. It is perfectly colourless, and evaporates so rapidly, that when applied in the form of spray to the skin, the latter becomes frozen, and is thus deprived of sensibility.

Pure ether has a density of .713, its boiling-point is 35°, but commercial samples, which often contain water (1 part of water is soluble in 35 of ether), may have a higher gravity, and also a higher boiling-point. The readiest way to know whether an ether is anhydrous or not, is to shake it up with a little carbon disulphide. If it is hydrous, the mixture is milky. Methylated ether is largely used in commerce; its disagreeable odour is due to contamination by methylated compounds; otherwise the ether made from methylated spirit is ethylic ether, for methylic ether is a gas which escapes during the process. Hence the term "methylated" ether is misleading, for it contains no methylic ether, but is essentially a somewhat impure ethylic ether.

§ 170. **Ether as a Poison.**—Ether has but little toxicological importance. There are a few cases of death from its use as an anæsthetic, and a few cases of suicide. Ether is used by some people as a stimulant, but ether drinkers are uncommon. It causes an intoxication very similar to that of alcohol, but of brief duration. In a case of chronic ether-taking recorded by Martin,[157] in which a woman took daily doses of ether for the purpose of allaying a gastric trouble, the patient suffered from shivering or trembling of the hands and feet, muscular weakness, cramp in the calves of the legs, pain in the breast and back, intermittent headaches, palpitation, singing in the ears, vomitings, and wakefulness; the ether being discontinued, the patient recovered. In one of Orfila's experiments, half an ounce

[157] Virchow's *Jahresber.*, 1870.

of ether was administered to a dog. The animal died insensible in three hours. The mucous membrane of the stomach was found highly inflamed, the inflammation extending somewhat into the duodenum; the rest of the canal was healthy. The lungs were gorged with fluid blood.

§ 171. **Fatal Dose.**—The fatal dose of ether, when taken as a liquid, is not known. 4 grms. (1.28 drms.) cause toxic symptoms, but the effect soon passes. Buchanan has seen a brandy-drinker consume 25 grms. (7 drms.) and yet survive. It is probable that most adults would be killed by a fluid ounce (28.4 c.c.).

§ 172. **Ether as an Anæsthetic.**—Ether is now much used as an anæsthetic, and generally in conjunction with chloroform. Anæsthesia by ether is said to compare favourably with that produced by chloroform. In 92,000 cases of operations performed under ether, the proportion dying from the effects of the anæsthetic was only .3 per 10,000 (Morgan), while chloroform gives a higher number. The mortality in America, again, from a mixture of chloroform and ether in 11,000 cases is reckoned at 1.7 per 10,000; but this proportion is rather above some of the calculations relative to the mortality from pure chloroform, so that the question can hardly be considered settled. The symptoms of ether narcosis are very similar to those produced by chloroform. The chief point of difference appears to be its action on the heart. Ether, when first breathed, stimulates the heart's action, and the after-depression that follows never reaches so high a grade as with chloroform. Ether is said to kill by paralysing the respiration, and in cases which end fatally the breathing is seen to stop suddenly: convulsions have not been noticed. The *post-mortem* appearances, as in the case of chloroform, are not characteristic.

§ 173. **Separation of Ether from Organic Fluids, &c.**—Despite the low boiling-point of ether, it is by no means easy to separate it from organic substances *so as to recover the whole of the ether present*. The best way is to place the matters in a flask connected with an ordinary Liebig's condenser, the tube of the latter at its farther end fitting closely into the doubly perforated cork of a flask. Into the second perforation is adapted an upright tube about 2 feet long, which may be of small diameter, and must be surrounded by a freezing mixture of ice and salt. The upper end of this tube is closed by a thistle-head funnel with syphon, and in the bend of the syphon a little mercury serves as a valve. Heat is now applied to the flask by means of a water-bath, and continued for several hours; the liquid which has distilled over is then treated with dry calcic chloride and redistilled exactly in the same way. To this distillate again a similar process may be used, substituting dry potassic carbonate for the calcic chloride. It is only by operating on these principles that the expert can recover in an approximate state of anhydrous purity such a volatile liquid. Having thus obtained it pure, it may be identified (1) by its smell, (2) by its boiling-point, (3) by its inflammability, and (4) by its reducing chromic acid. The latter test may be applied to the vapour. An asbestos fibre is soaked in a mixture of strong sulphuric acid and potassic dichromate, and then placed in the tube connected with the flask—the ethereal (or alcoholic) vapour passing over the fibre, immediately reduces the chromic acid to chromic oxide, with the production of a green colour.

V.—Chloroform.

CHLOROFORM, TRICHLOROMETHANE OR METHENYL CHLORIDE ($CHCl_3$).

§ 174. Chloroform appears to have been discovered independently by Soubeiran and Liebig, about 1830. It was first employed in medicine by Simpson, of Edinburgh, as an anæsthetic. Pure chloroform has a density of 1.491 at 17°, and boils at 60.8°; but commercial samples have gravities of from 1.47 to 1.491. It is a colourless liquid, strongly refracting light; it cannot be ignited by itself, but, when mixed with alcohol, burns with a smoky flame edged with green. Its odour is heavy, but rather pleasant; the taste is sweet and burning.

Chloroform sinks in water, and is only slightly soluble in that fluid (.44 in 100 c.c.), it is perfectly neutral in reaction, and very volatile. When rubbed on the skin, it should completely evaporate, leaving no odour. Pure absolute chloroform gives an opaline mixture if mixed with from 1 to 5 volumes of alcohol, but with any quantity above 5 volumes the mixture is clear; it mixes in all proportions with ether. Chloroform coagulates albumen, and is an excellent solvent for most organic bases—camphor, caoutchouc, amber, opal, and all common resins. It dissolves phosphorus and sulphur slightly—more freely iodine and bromine. It floats on hydric sulphate, which only attacks it at a boiling heat.

Chloroform is frequently impure from faulty manufacture or decomposition. The impurities to be sought are alcohol, methylated chloroform,[158] dichloride of ethylene ($C_2H_4Cl_2$), chloride of ethyl (C_2H_5Cl), aldehyde, chlorine, hydrochloric, hypochlorous, and traces of sulphuric acid: there have also been found chlorinated oils. One of the best tests for contamination by alcohol, wood spirit, or ether, is that known as Roussin's; dinitrosulphide of iron[159] is added to chloroform. If it contain any of these impurities, it acquires a dark colour, but if pure, remains bright and colourless.

The presence of alcohol or ether, or both, may also be discovered by the bichromate test, which is best applied as follows:—A few milligrammes of potassic bichromate are placed at the bottom of a test-tube with four or five drops of sulphuric acid, which liberates the chromic acid; next, a very little water is added to dissolve the chromic acid; and lastly, the chloroform. The whole is now shaken, and allowed to separate. If the chloroform is pure, the mass is hardly tinged a greenish-yellow, and no layer separates. If, however, there is anything like 5 per cent. of alcohol or ether present, the deep green of chromium chloride appears, and there is a distinct layer at the bottom of the tube.

Another way to detect alcohol in chloroform, and also to make an approximate estimation of its quantity, is to place 20 c.c. of chloroform in a burette, and then add 80 c.c. of water. On shaking violently, pure chloroform will sink to the bottom in clear globules, and the measurement will be as nearly as possible the original quantity; but if anything like a percentage of alcohol be present, the chloroform is seen to be diminished in quantity, and its surface is opalescent, the diminution being caused by the water dissolving out the alcohol. The addition of a few drops of potash solution destroys the meniscus, and allows of a close reading of the volume. The supernatant water may be utilised for the detection of other impurities, and tested for sulphuric acid by baric chloride, for free chlorine and hypochlorous acid by starch and potassic iodide, and for hydrochloric acid by silver nitrate.[160] Fuchsine, proposed by Stœdeler, is also a delicate reagent for the presence of alcohol in chloroform, the sample becoming red in the presence of alcohol, and the tint being proportionate to the quantity present. The most delicate test for alcohol is, however, the iodoform test fully described in "Foods," p. 375.[161] Dichloride of ethylene is detected by shaking up the chloroform with dry potassic carbonate, and then adding metallic potassium. This does not act on pure chloroform, but only in presence of ethylene dichloride, when the gaseous chlor-ethylene (C_2H_3Cl) is evolved. Ethyl-chloride is detected by distilling the chloroform and collecting the first portions of the distillate; it will have a distinct odour of ethyl-chloride should it be present. Methyl compounds and empyreumatic oils are roughly detected by allowing the chloroform to evaporate on a cloth. If present, the cloth, when the chloroform has evaporated, will have a peculiar disagreeable odour. Aldehyde is recognised by its reducing action on argentic nitrate; the mineral acids by the reddening of litmus paper, and the appropriate tests. Hypochlorous acid first reddens, and then bleaches, litmus-paper.

Dr. Dott, *Pharm. Journ.*, 1894, p. 629, gives the following tests:—Specific gravity, 1.490 to 1.495. On allowing ½ fluid drm. to evaporate from a clean surface, no foreign odour is perceptible at any stage of the evaporation. When 1 fluid drm. is agitated with an equal volume of solution of silver nitrate, no precipitate or turbidity is produced after standing for five minutes. On shaking up the chloroform with half its volume of distilled water, the water should not redden litmus-paper. When shaken with an equal volume of sulphuric acid, little or no colour should be imparted to the acid.

§ 175. The ordinary method of manufacturing chloroform is by distilling alcohol with chlorinated lime; but another mode is now much in use—viz., the decomposition of chloral hydrate. By distilling it with a weak alkali, this process yields such a pure chloroform, that, for medicinal purposes, it should supersede every other.

Poisonous Effects of Chloroform.

1. AS A LIQUID.

[158] Methylated chloroform is that which is prepared from methylated spirit. It is liable to more impurities than that made from pure alcohol, but, of course, its composition is the same, and it has recently been manufactured from this source almost chemically pure.

[159] Made by slowly adding ferric sulphate to a boiling solution of ammonic sulphide and potassic nitrite, as long as the precipitate continues to redissolve, and then filtering the solution.

[160] Neither an alcoholic nor an aqueous solution of silver nitrate causes the slightest change in pure chloroform.

[161] An attempt has been made by Besnou to estimate the amount of alcohol by the specific gravity. He found that a chloroform of 1.4945 gravity, mixed with 5 per cent. of alcohol, gave a specific gravity of 1.4772; 10 per cent., 1.4602; 20 per cent., 1.4262; and 25 per cent., 1.4090. It would, therefore, seem that every percentage of alcohol lowers the gravity by .0034.

§ 176. **Statistics.**—Falck finds recorded in medical literature 27 cases of poisoning by chloroform having been swallowed—of these 15 were men, 9 were women, and 3 children. Eighteen of the cases were suicidal, and 10 of the 18 died; the remainder took the liquid by mistake.

§ 177. **Local Action of Chloroform.**—When applied to the skin or mucous membranes in such a way that the fluid cannot evaporate—as, for example, by means of a cloth steeped in chloroform laid on the bare skin, and covered over with some impervious material—there is a burning sensation, which soon ceases, and leaves the part anæsthetised, while the skin, at the same time, is reddened and sometimes even blistered.

§ 178. Chloroform added to blood, or passed through it in the state of vapour, causes it to assume a peculiar brownish colour owing to destruction of the red corpuscles and solution of the hæmoglobin in the plasma. The change does not require the presence of atmospheric air, but takes place equally in an atmosphere of hydrogen. It has been shown by Schmiedeberg that the chloroform enters in some way into a state of combination with the blood-corpuscles, for the entire quantity cannot be recovered by distillation; whereas the plasma, similarly treated, yields the entire quantity which has in the first place been added. Schmiedeberg also asserts that the oxygen is in firmer combination with the chloroformised blood than usual, as shown by its slow extraction by stannous oxide. Muscle, exposed to chloroform liquid by arterial injection, quickly loses excitability and becomes rigid. Nerves are first stimulated, and then their function for the time is annihilated; but on evaporation of the chloroform, the function is restored.

§ 179. **General Effects of the Liquid.**—However poisonous in a state of vapour, chloroform cannot be considered an extremely active poison when taken into the stomach as a liquid, for enormous quantities, relatively, have been drunk without fatal effect. Thus, there is the case recorded by Taylor, in which a man, who had swallowed 113.4 grms. (4 ozs.), walked a considerable distance after taking the dose. He subsequently fell into a state of coma, with dilated pupils, stertorous breathing, and imperceptible pulse. These symptoms were followed by convulsions, but the patient recovered in five days.

In a case related by Burkart,[162] a woman desired to kill herself with chloroform, and procured for that purpose 50 grms. (a little less than one ounce and a half); she drank some of it, but the burning taste and the sense of heat in the mouth, throat, and stomach, prevented her from taking the whole at once. After a few moments, the pain passing off, she essayed to drink the remainder, and did swallow the greater portion of it, but was again prevented by the suffering it caused. Finally, she poured what remained on a cloth, and placing it over her face, soon sank into a deep narcosis. She was found lying on the bed very pale, with blue lips, and foaming a little at the mouth; the head was rigidly bent backwards, the extremities were lax, the eyes were turned upwards and inwards, the pupils dilated and inactive, the face and extremities were cold, the body somewhat warmer, there was no pulse at the wrist, the carotids beat feebly, the breathing was deep and rattling, and after five or six inspirations ceased. By the aid of artificial respiration, &c., she recovered in an hour.

A still larger dose has been recovered from in the case of a young man, aged 23,[163] who had swallowed no less than 75 grms. (2.6 ozs.) of chloroform, but yet, in a few hours, awoke from the stupor. He complained of a burning pain in the stomach; on the following day he suffered from vomiting, and on the third day symptoms of jaundice appeared,—a feature which has been several times noticed as an effect of chloroform.

On the other hand, even small doses have been known to destroy life. In a case related by Taylor, a boy, aged 4, swallowed 3.8 grms. (1 drm.) of chloroform and died in three hours, notwithstanding that every effort was used for his recovery.

§ 180. The smallest dose that has proved fatal *to an adult* is 15 grms. (a little over 4 drms.).

From twenty-two cases in which the quantity taken had been ascertained with some degree of accuracy, Falck draws the following conclusions:—In eight of the cases the dose was between 4 and 30 grms., and one death resulted from 15 grms. As for the other fourteen persons, the doses varied from 35 to 380 grms., and eight of these patients died—two after 40, two after 45, one after 60, 90, 120, and 180 grms. respectively. Hence, under conditions favouring the action of the poison, 15 grms. (4.3 drms.) may be fatal to an adult, while doses of 40 grms. (11.3 drms.) and upwards will almost certainly kill.

§ 181. **Symptoms.**—The symptoms can be well gathered from the cases quoted. They commence shortly after the taking of the poison; and, indeed, the local action of the liquid immediately causes first a burning sensation, followed by numbness.

[162] *Vierteljahrsschr. für ger. Med.*, 1876.

[163] *Brit. Med. Journ.*, 1879.

Often after a few minutes, precisely as when the vapour is administered, a peculiar, excited condition supervenes, accompanied, it may be, by delirium. The next stage is narcosis, and the patient lies with pale face and livid lips, &c., as described earlier; the end of the scene is often preceded by convulsions. Sometimes, however, consciousness returns, and the irritation of the mucous membranes of the gastro-intestinal canal is shown by bloody vomiting and bloody stools, with considerable pain and general suffering. In this way, a person may linger several days after the ingestion of the poison. In a case observed by Pomeroy, the fatal malady was prolonged for eight days. Among those who recover, a common *sequela*, as before mentioned, is jaundice.

A third form of symptoms has been occasionally observed, viz.:—The person awakes from the coma, the breathing and pulse become again natural, and all danger seems to have passed, when suddenly, after a longer or shorter time, without warning, a state of general depression and collapse supervenes, and death occurs.

§ 182. **Post-mortem Appearances.**—The *post-mortem* appearances from a fatal dose of liquid chloroform mainly resolve themselves into redness of the mucous membrane of the stomach, though occasionally, as in Pomeroy's case, there may be an ulceration. In a case recorded by Hoffman,[164] a woman, aged 30, drank 35 to 40 grms. of chloroform and died within the hour. Almost the whole of the chloroform taken was found in the stomach, as a heavy fluid, coloured green, through the bile. The epithelium of the pharynx, epiglottis, and gullet was of a dirty colour, partly detached, whitened, softened, and easily stripped off. The mucous membrane of the stomach was much altered in colour and consistence, and, with the duodenum, was covered with a tenacious grey slime. There was no ecchymosis.

2. THE VAPOUR OF CHLOROFORM.

§ 183. **Statistics.**—Accidents occur far more frequently in the use of chloroform vapour for anæsthetic purposes than in the use of the liquid.

Most of the cases of death through chloroform vapour, are those caused accidentally in surgical and medical practice. A smaller number are suicidal, while for criminal purposes, its use is extremely infrequent.

The percentage of deaths caused by chloroform administered during operations is unaccountably different in different years, times, and places. The diversity of opinion on the subject is partly (though not entirely) explicable, by the degrees of purity in the anæsthetic administered, the different modes of administration, the varying lengths of time of the anæsthesia, and the varying severity of the operations.

During the Crimean War, according to Baudens and Quesnoy, 30,000 operations were done under chloroform, but only one death occurred attributable to the anæsthetic. Sansom[165] puts the average mortality at .75 per 10,000, Nussbaum at 1.3, Richardson at 2.8,[166] Morgan[167] at 3.4. In the American war of secession, in 11,000 operations, there were seven deaths—that is, 6.3 per 10,000, the highest number on a large scale which appears to be on record. In the ten years 1883-1892, 103 deaths are attributed to chloroform in England and Wales, viz., 88 deaths (57 males, 31 females) from accidents (no doubt in its use as a general anæsthetic), 14 (9 males, 5 females) from suicide, and a solitary case of murder.

§ 184. **Suicidal and Criminal Poisoning by Chloroform.**—Suicidal poisoning by chloroform will generally be indicated by the surrounding circumstances; and in no case hitherto reported has there been any difficulty or obscurity as to whether the narcosis was self-induced or not. An interesting case is related by Schauenstein,[168] in which a physician resolved to commit suicide by chloroform, a commencing amaurosis having preyed upon his mind, and his choice having been determined by witnessing an accidental death by this agent. He accordingly plugged his nostrils, fitted on to the face an appropriate mask, and fastened it by strips of adhesive plaster. In such an instance, there could be no doubt of the suicidal intent, and the question of accident would be entirely out of the question.

A dentist in Potsdam,[169] in a state of great mental depression from embarrassed circumstances, killed his wife, himself, and two children by chloroform. Such crimes are fortunately very rare.

There is a vulgar idea that it is possible, by holding a cloth saturated with chloroform to the mouth of a sleeping

[164] *Lehrbuch der ger. Medicin*, 2te Aufl.

[165] *Chloroform: its Action, &c.*, London, 1865.

[166] *Med. Times and Gazette*, 1870.

[167] *Med. Soc. of Virginia*, 1872.

[168] Maschka: *Handbuch der gerichtlich. Medicin*, p. 787, Tübingen, 1882.

[169] Casper: *Handbuch der ger. Med.*

person (or one, indeed, perfectly awake), to produce *sudden* insensibility; but such an occurrence is against all experimental and clinical evidence. It is true that a nervous person might, under such circumstances, faint and become insensible by mere nervous shock; but a true sudden narcosis is impossible.

Dolbeau has made some interesting experiments in order to ascertain whether, under any circumstances, a sleeping person might be anæsthetised. The main result appears to answer the question in the affirmative, at least with certain persons; but even with these, it can only be done by using the greatest skill and care, first allowing the sleeper to breathe very dilute chloroform vapour, and then gradually exhibiting stronger doses, and taking the cloth or inhaler away on the slightest symptom of approaching wakefulness. In 75 per cent. of the cases, however, the individuals awoke almost immediately on being exposed to the vapour. This cautious and scientific narcosis, then, is not likely to be used by the criminal class, or, if used, to be successful.

§ 185. **Physiological Effects.**—Chloroform is a protoplasmic poison. According to Jumelle, plants can even be narcotised, ceasing to assimilate and no longer being sensitive to the stimulus of light. Isolated animal cells, like leucocytes, lose through chloroform vapour their power of spontaneous movement, and many bacteria cease to multiply if in contact with chloroform water. According to Binx, chloroform narcosis in man is to be explained through its producing a weak coagulation of the cerebral ganglion cells. As already mentioned, chloroform has an affinity for the red blood-corpuscles. Chloroform stimulates the peripheral ends of the nerves of sensation, so that it causes irritation of the skin or mucous membranes when locally applied. Flourens considers that chloroform first affects the cerebrum, then the cerebellum, and finally the spinal cord; the action is at first stimulating, afterwards paralysing. Most anæsthetics diminish equally the excitability of the grey and the white nervous substance of the brain, and this is the case with chloroform, ether, and morphine; but apparently this is not the case with chloral hydrate, which only diminishes the conductivity of the cortical substance of the brain, and leaves the grey substance intact. Corresponding to the cerebral paralysis, the blood pressure sinks, and the heart beats slower and weaker.[170] The Hyderabad Commission made 735 researches on dogs and monkeys, and found that in fatal narcosis, so far as these animals are concerned, the respiration ceased before the heart, and this may be considered the normal mode of death; but it is probably going too far to say that it is the exclusive form of death in man, for there have been published cases in which the heart failed first.

§ 186. **Symptoms.**—There is but little outward difference between man and animals, in regard to the symptoms caused by breathing chloroform; in the former we have the advantage that the sensations preceding narcosis can be described by the individual.

The action of chloroform is usually divided into three more or less distinct stages. In the *first* there is a "drunken" condition, changes in the sense of smell and taste, and it may be hallucinations of vision and hearing; there are also often curious creeping sensations about the skin, and sometimes excessive muscular action, causing violent struggles. I have also seen epileptiform convulsions, and delirium is almost always present. The face during this stage is generally flushed, covered with perspiration, and the pupils contracted. The first stage may last from one minute to several, and passes into the *second stage*, or that of depression. Spontaneous movements cease, sensibility to all external stimuli vanishes, the patient falls into a deep sleep, the consciousness is entirely lost, and reflex movements are more and more annihilated. The temperature is less than normal, the respirations are slow, and the pulse is full and slow. The pupils in this stage are usually dilated, all the muscles are relaxed, and the limbs can be bent about in any direction. If now the inhalation of chloroform is intermitted, the patient wakes within a period which is usually from twenty to forty minutes, but may be several hours, after the last inhalation.

The *third stage* is that of paralysis; the pulse becomes irregular, the respirations superficial, there is a cyanotic colouring of the lips and skin, while the pupils become widely dilated. Death follows quickly through paralysis of the respiratory centre, the respirations first ceasing, then the pulse; in a few cases, the heart ceases first to beat.

According to Sansom's facts,[171] in 100 cases of death by chloroform, 44.6 per cent. occurred before the full narcosis had been attained, that is in the first stage, 34.7 during the second stage, and 20.6 shortly after. So, also, Kappeler has recorded that in 101 cases of death from chloroform, 47.7 per cent. occurred before the full effect, and 52.2 during the full effect. This confirms the dictum of Billroth, that in all stages of anæsthesia by chloroform, death may occur. The *quantity* of chloroform, which, when inhaled in a given time, will produce death, is unknown; for all depends upon the greater or less admixture of air, and probably on other conditions. It has been laid down, that the inhalation of chloroform should be so managed as to insure that the air breathed shall never contain more than

[170] Kobert's *Lehrbuch der Intoxicationen.*
[171] *Op. cit.*

3.9 per cent. of chloroform. Fifteen drops have caused death, but Taylor, on the other hand, records a case of tetanus, treated at Guy's Hospital, in which no less a quantity than 700 grms. (22.5 ozs.) was inhaled in twenty-four hours. Frequent breathing of chloroform in no way renders the individual safe from fatal accident. A lady[172] having repeatedly taken chloroform, was anæsthetised by the same agent merely for the purpose of having a tooth extracted. About 6 grms. (1.5 drm.) were poured on a cloth, and after nine to ten inspirations, dangerous symptoms began—rattling breathing and convulsive movements—and, despite all remedies, she died.

§ 187. Chronic chloroform poisoning is not unknown. It leads to various ailments, and seems to have been in one or two instances the cause of insanity.

Buchner records the case of an opium-eater, who afterwards took to chloroform; he suffered from periodic mania. In a remarkable case related by Meric, the patient, who had also first been a morphine-eater, took 350 grms. of chloroform in five days by inhalation; as often as he woke he would chloroform himself again to sleep. In this case, there was also mental disturbance, and instances in which chloroform produced marked mental aberration are recorded by Böhm[173] and by Vigla.[174]

§ 188. **Post-mortem Appearances.**—The lesions found on section are neither peculiar to, nor characteristic of, chloroform poisoning. It has been noted that bubbles of gas are, from time to time, to be observed after death in the blood of those poisoned by chloroform, but it is doubtful whether the bubbles are not merely those to be found in any other corpse—in 189 cases, only eighteen times were these gas-bubbles observed,[175] so that, even if they are characteristic, the chances in a given case that they will *not* be seen are greater than the reverse. The smell of chloroform may be present, but has been noticed very seldom.

§ 189. **The detection and estimation of chloroform** from organic substances is not difficult, its low boiling-point causing it to distil readily. Accordingly (whatever may be the ultimate modifications, as suggested by different experimenters), the first step is to bring the substances, unless fluid, into a pulp with water, and submit this pulp to distillation by the heat of a water-bath. If the liquid operated upon possesses no particular odour, the chloroform may in this way be recognised in the distillate, which, if necessary, may be redistilled in the same manner, so as to concentrate the volatile matters in a small compass.

There are four chief tests for the identification of chloroform:—

(1.) The final distillate is tested with a little aniline, and an alcoholic solution of soda or potash lye; either immediately, or upon gently warming the liquid, there is a peculiar and penetrating odour of phenylcarbylamine, C_6H_5NC; it is produced by the following reaction:—

$$CHCl_3 + 3KOH + C_6H_5NH_2 = C_6H_5NC + 3KCl + 3H_2O.$$

Chloral, trichloracetic acid, bromoform and iodoform also give the same reaction; on the other hand, ethylidene chloride does not yield under these circumstances any carbylamine (isonitrile).

(2.) Chloroform reduces Fehling's alkaline copper solution, *when applied to a distillate*, thus excluding a host of more fixed bodies which have the same reaction; it is a very excellent test, and may be made quantitative. The reaction is as follows:—

$$CHCl_3 + 5KHO + 2CuO = Cu_2O + K_2CO_3 + 3KCl + 3H_2O;$$

thus, every 100 parts of cuprous oxide equals 83.75 of chloroform.

(3.) The fluid to be tested (which, if acid, should be neutralised), is distilled in a slow current of hydrogen, and the vapour conducted through a short bit of red-hot combustion-tube containing platinum gauze. Under these circumstances, the chloroform is decomposed and hydrochloric acid formed; hence, the issuing vapour has an acid reaction to test-paper, and if led into a solution of silver nitrate, gives the usual precipitate of argentic chloride. Every 100 parts of silver chloride equal 27.758 of chloroform.

(4.) The fluid is mixed with a little thymol and potash; if chloroform be present, a reddish-violet colour is developed, becoming more distinct on the application of heat.[176]

§ 190. For the quantitative estimation of chloroform the method recommended by Schmiedeberg[177] is, however,

---

[172] *Edin. Med. Journ.*, 1855.

[173] Ziemssen's *Handbuch*, Bd. 15.

[174] *Med. Times*, 1855.

[175] Schauenstein (*Op. cit.*).

[176] S. Vidali in *Deutsch-Amerikan. Apoth.-Zeitung*, vol. iij., Aug. 15, 1882.

[177] *Ueber die quantitative Bestimmung des Chloroforms im Blute.* Inaug. Dissert., Dorpat, 1866.

the best. A combustion-tube of 24 to 26 cm. long, and 10 to 12 mm. in diameter, open at both ends, is furnished at the one end with a plug of asbestos, while the middle part, to within 5-6 cm. of the other end, is filled with pieces of caustic lime, from the size of a lentil to that of half a pea. The lime must be pure, and is made by heating a carbonate which has been precipitated from calcic nitrate. The other end of the tube is closed by a cork, carrying a silver tube, 16-18 cm. long, and 4 mm. thick. The end containing the asbestos plug is fitted by a cork to a glass tube. The combustion-tube thus prepared is placed in the ordinary combustion-furnace; the flask containing the chloroform is adapted, and the distillation slowly proceeded with. It is best to add a tube, bent at right angles and going to the bottom of the flask, to draw air continuously through the apparatus. During the whole process, the tube containing the lime is kept at a red heat. The chloroform is decomposed, and the chlorine combines with the lime. The resulting calcic chloride, mixed with much unchanged lime, is, at the end of the operation, cooled, dissolved in dilute nitric acid, and precipitated with silver nitrate. Any silver chloride is collected and weighed and calculated into chloroform.[178]

VI.—Other Anæsthetics.

§ 191. When chlorine acts upon marsh-gas, the hydrogen can be displaced atom by atom; and from the original methane (CH_4) can be successively obtained chloromethane or methyl chloride (CH_3Cl), dichloromethane, or methene dichloride, methylene dichloride (CH_2Cl_2), trichloromethane, or chloroform ($CHCl_3$), already described, and carbon tetrachloride (CCl_4). All these are, more or less, capable of producing anæsthesia; but none of them, save chloroform, are of any toxicological importance.

Methene dichloride, recommended by Sir B. W. Richardson as an anæsthetic, has come somewhat into use. It is a colourless, very volatile liquid, of specific gravity 1.360, and boiling at 41°. It burns with a smoky flame, and dissolves iodine with a brown colour.

§ 192. **Pentane** (C_5H_{12}).—There are three isomers of pentane; that which is used as an anæsthetic is normal pentane, CH_3-CH_2-CH_2-CH_2-CH_3; its boiling-point is 37-38°. It is one of the constituents of petroleum ether.

Under the name of "Pental" it is used in certain hospitals extensively, for instance, at the Kaiser Friederich's Children's Hospital, Berlin.[179] It is stated to have no action on the heart.

One death[180] has been recorded from its use:—A lad, aged 14, was put under pental for the purpose of having two molars painlessly extracted. He was only a minute or two insensible, and 4-5 grms. of pental was the quantity stated to have been inhaled. The boy spat out after the operation, then suddenly fainted and died. The *post-mortem* showed œdema of the lungs; the right side of the heart was empty. The organs of the body smelled strongly of pental.

§ 193. **Aldehyde** (Acetaldehyde), 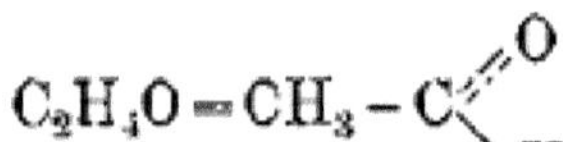, a fluid obtained by the careful oxidation of alcohol (boiling-point, 20.8°), is in large doses toxic; in smaller, it acts as a narcotic.

Metaldehyde $(C_2H_4O_2)_2$, obtained by treating acetaldehyde at a low temperature with hydrochloric acid. It occurs in the form of prisms, which sublime at about 112°; it is also poisonous.

§ 194. **Paraldehyde** ($C_6H_{12}O_3$) is a colourless fluid, boiling at 124°; specific gravity .998 at 15°. By the action of cold it may be obtained in crystals, the melting point of which is 10.5°. It is soluble in eight parts of water at 13°; in warm water it is less soluble; hence, on warming a solution, it becomes turbid. Paraldehyde acts very similarly to chloral; it causes a deep sleep, and (judging by experiments on animals) produces no convulsive movements.

[178] S. Vidali has made the ingenious suggestion of developing hydrogen in the usual way, by means of zinc and sulphuric acid, in the liquid supposed to contain chloroform, to ignite the hydrogen, as in Marsh's test, when it issues from the tube, and then to hold in the flame a clean copper wire. Since any chloroform is burnt up in the hydrogen flame to hydrochloric acid, the chloride of copper immediately volatilises and colours the flame green.

[179] *Zeit. f. Kinderheilk.*, Bd. iii.-iv., 1893.

[180] Dr. Bremme, *Vierteljahrsschr. f. gerichtliche Medicin*, Bd. v., 1893.

VII.—Chloral.

§ 195. **Chloral Hydrate** ($C_2H_3Cl_3O_2$) is made by mixing equivalent quantities of anhydrous chloral[181] and water. The purest chloral is in the form of small, granular, sugar-like crystals. When less pure, the crystals are larger. These melt into a clear fluid at from 48° to 49°, and the melted mass solidifies again at 48.9°. Chloral boils at 97.5°; it is not very soluble in cold chloroform, requiring four times its weight. The only substance with which chloral hydrate may well be confused is chloral alcoholate ($C_4H_7Cl_3O_2$), but chloral alcoholate melts at a lower temperature (45°), and boils at a higher (113.5°); it is easily soluble in cold chloroform, and inflames readily, whereas chloral scarcely burns.

Chloral hydrate completely volatilises, and can be distilled in a vacuum without change. If, however, boiled in air, it undergoes slow decomposition, the first portions of the distillate being overhydrated, the last underhydrated; the boiling-point, therefore, undergoes a continuous rise. The amount of hydration of a commercial sample is of practical importance; if too much water is present, the chloral deliquesces, especially in warm weather; if too little, it may become acid, and in part insoluble from the formation of meta-chloral ($C_6H_3Cl_9O_3$). Chloral hydrate, by the action of the volatile or fixed alkalies, is decomposed, an alkaline formiate and chloroform resulting thus—

$C_2HCl_3O,H_2O + NaHO = NaCHO_2 + H_2O + CHCl_3$.

Trichlor-acetic acid is decomposed in a similar manner.

Statistics.—Chloral caused, during the ten years 1883-1892 in England and Wales, 127 deaths—viz., 111 (89 males, 22 females) accidentally, 15 (14 males, 1 female) from suicide, and a case in which chloral was the agent of murder.

§ 196. **Detection.**—It is, of course, obvious that after splitting up chloral into chloroform, the latter can be detected by distillation and applying the tests given earlier and *seq.* Chloral hydrate is soluble in one and a half times its weight of water; the solution should be perfectly neutral to litmus. It is also soluble in ether, in alcohol, and in carbon disulphide. It may be extracted from its solution by shaking out with ether. There should be no cloudiness when a solution is tested with silver nitrate in the cold; if, however, to a boiling solution nitrate of silver and a little ammonia are added, there is a mirror of reduced silver.

§ 197. The assay of chloral hydrate in solutions is best effected by distilling the solution with slaked lime; the distillate is received in water contained in a graduated tube kept at a low temperature. The chloroform sinks to the bottom, and is directly read off; the number of c.c. multiplied by 2.064 equals the weight of the chloral hydrate present.

Another method, accurate but only applicable to the fairly pure substance, is to dissolve 1 to 2 grms. in water, remove any free acid by baric carbonate, and then treat the liquid thus purified by a known volume of standard soda. The soda is now titrated back, using litmus as an indicator, each c.c. of normal alkali neutralised by the sample corresponds to 0.1655 grm. of chloral hydrate. Small quantities of chloral hydrate may be conveniently recovered from complex liquids by shaking them up with ether, and removing the ethereal layer, in the tube represented in the figure.[182] The ether must be allowed to evaporate spontaneously; but there is in this way much loss of chloral. The best method of estimating minute quantities is to alkalise the liquid, and slowly distil the vapour through a red-hot

[181] Anhydrous chloral (C_2HCl_3O) is an oily liquid, of specific gravity 1.502 at 18°; it boils at 97.7°. It is obtained by the prolonged action of chlorine on absolute alcohol.

[182] The figure is from "Foods"; the description may be here repeated:—A is a tube of any dimensions most convenient to the analyst. Ordinary burette size will perhaps be the most suitable for routine work; the tube is furnished with a stopcock and is bent at B, the tube at K having a very small but not quite capillary bore. The lower end is attached to a length of pressure-tubing, and is connected with a small reservoir of mercury, moving up and down by means of a pulley. To use the apparatus: Fill the tube with mercury by opening the clamp at H, and the stopcock at B, and raising the reservoir until the mercury, if allowed, would flow out of the beak. Now, the beak is dipped into the liquid to be extracted with the solvent, and by lowering the reservoir, a strong vacuum is created, which draws the liquid into the tube; in the same way the ether is made to follow. Should the liquid be so thick that it is not possible to get it in by means of suction, the lower end of the tube is disconnected, and the syrupy mass worked in through the wide end. When the ether has been sucked into the apparatus, it is emptied of mercury by lowering the reservoir, and then firmly clamped at H, and the stopcock also closed. The tube may now be shaken, and then allowed to stand for the liquids to separate. When there is a good line of demarcation, by raising the reservoir after opening the clamp and stopcock, the whole of the light solvent can be run out of the tube into a flask or beaker, and recovered by distillation. For heavy solvents (such as chloroform), which sink to the bottom, a simple burette, with a fine exit tube is preferable; but for petroleum ether, ordinary ether, &c., the apparatus figured is extremely useful.

combustion-tube charged with pure lime, as in the process described earlier. A dilute solution of chloral may also be treated with a zinc-copper couple, the nascent hydrogen breaks the molecule up, and the resulting chloride may be titrated, as in water analyses, by silver nitrate and potassic chromate.

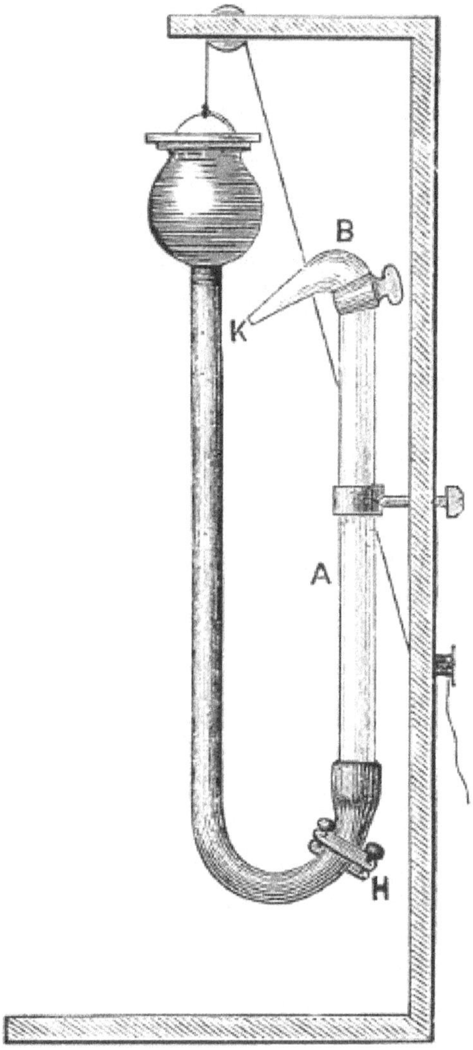

§ 198. **Effects of Chloral Hydrate on Animals.**—Experiments on animals have taught us all that is known of the physiological action of chloral. It has been shown that the drug influences very considerably the circulation, at first exciting the heart's action, and then paralysing the automatic centre. The heart, as in animals poisoned by atropine, stops in diastole, and the blood-pressure sinks in proportion to the progressive paralysis of the cardiac centre. At the same time, the respiration is slowed and finally ceases, while the heart continues to beat. The body temperature of the warm-blooded animals is very remarkably depressed, according to Falck, even to 7.6°. Vomiting has been rather frequently observed with dogs and cats, even when the drug has been taken into the system by subcutaneous injection.

The secretion of milk, according to Röhrig, is also diminished. Reflex actions through small doses are intensified; through large, much diminished. .025-.05 grm. (.4-.7 grain), injected subcutaneously into frogs, causes a slowing of the respiration, a diminution of reflex excitability, and lastly, its complete cessation; this condition lasts several hours; at length the animal returns to its normal state. If the dose is raised to .1 grm. (1.5 grain) after the cessation of reflex movements, the heart is paralysed—and a paralysis not due to any central action of the vagus, but to a direct action on the cardiac ganglia. Rabbits of the ordinary weight of 2 kilos. are fully narcotised by the subcutaneous injection of 1 grm.; the sleep is very profound, and lasts several hours; the animal wakes up spontaneously, and is apparently none the worse. If 2 grms. are administered, the narcotic effects, rapidly developed, are much prolonged. There is a remarkable diminution of temperature, and the animal dies, the respiration ceasing without convulsion or other sign. Moderate-sized dogs require 6 grms. for a full narcosis, and the symptoms are similar; they also wake after many hours, in apparent good health.[183]

§ 199. Liebreich considered that the action of chloral was due to its being broken up by the alkali of the blood, and the system being thus brought into a state precisely similar to its condition when anæsthetised by chloroform vapour. This view has, however, been proved to be erroneous. Chloral hydrate can, it is true, be decomposed in some degree by the blood at 40°; but the action must be prolonged for several hours. A 1 per cent. solution of alkali does not decompose chloral at a blood-heat in the time within which chloral acts in the body; and since narcotic effects are commonly observed when, in the fatty group, hydrogen has been displaced by chlorine, it is more probable that chloral hydrate is absorbed and circulates in the blood as such, and is not broken up into chloroform and an alkaline formiate.

§ 200. **Effects of Chloral Hydrate on Man.**—Since the year 1869, in which chloral was first introduced to medicine, it has been the cause of a number of accidental and other cases of poisoning. I find, up to the year 1884, recorded in medical literature, thirty-one cases of poisoning by chloral hydrate. This number is a small proportion only of the actual number dying from this cause. In nearly all the cases the poison was taken by the mouth, but in one instance the patient died in three hours, after having injected into the rectum 5.86 grms. of chloral hydrate. There is also on record a case in which, for the purpose of producing surgical anæsthesia, 6 grms. of chloral were injected into the veins; the man died in as many minutes.[184]

§ 201. **Fatal Dose.**—It is impossible to state with any exactness the precise quantity of chloral which may cause death. Children bear it better, in proportion, than adults, while old persons (especially those with weak hearts, and those inclined to apoplexy) are likely to be strongly affected by very small doses. A dose of .19 grm. (3 grains) has been fatal to a child a year old in ten hours. On the other hand, according to Bouchut's observations on 10,000 children, he considers that the full therapeutic effect of chloral can be obtained safely with them in the following ratio:—

Children of 1 to 3 years,	dose 1 to 1.5 grm.	(15.4 to 23.1 grains	)
,, 3 ,, 5 ,,	,, 2 ,, 3 ,,	(30.8 ,, 46.3 ,,	)
,, 5 ,, 7 ,,	,, 3 ,, 4 ,,	(46.3 ,, 61.7 ,,	)

These quantities being dissolved in 100 c.c. of water.

These doses are certainly too high, and it would be dangerous to take them as a guide, since death has occurred in a child, aged 5, from a dose of 3 grms. (46.3 grains). Medical men in England consider 20 grains a very full dose for a child of four years old, and 50 for an adult, while a case is recorded in which a dose of 1.9 grm. (30 grains) proved fatal in thirty-five hours to a young lady aged 20. On the other hand, we find a case[185] in which, to a patient suffering from epileptic mania, a dose of 31.1 grms. (1.1 oz.) of chloral hydrate was administered; she sank into a deep sleep in five minutes. Subcutaneous injections of strychnine were applied, and after sleeping for forty-eight hours, there was recovery. On the third day a vivid scarlatinal rash appeared, followed by desquamation. The examples quoted—the fatal dose of 1.9 grm., and recovery from 31 grms.—are the two extremes for adults. From other cases, it appears tolerably plain that most people would recover, especially with appropriate treatment, from a single dose under 8 grms., but anything above that quantity taken at one time would be very dangerous, and doses

[183] C. Ph. Falck has divided the symptoms into (1) Preliminary hypnotic; (2) an adynamic state; and (3) a comatose condition.

[184] This dangerous practice was introduced by M. Ore. In a case of traumatic tetanus, in which M. Ore injected into the veins 9 grms. of chloral in 10 grms. of water, there was profound insensibility, lasting eleven hours, during which time a painful operation on the thumb was performed. The next day 10 grms. were injected, when the insensibility lasted eight hours; and 9 grms. were injected on each of the two following days. The man recovered. In another case, Ore anæsthetised immediately a patient by plunging the subcutaneous needle of his syringe into the radial vein, and injected 10 grms. of chloral hydrate with 30 of water. The patient became insensible before the whole quantity was injected with "*une immobilité rappellant celle du cadavre.*" On finishing the operation, the patient was roused immediately by the application of an electric current, one pole on the left side of the neck, the other on the epigastrium. *Journ. de Pharm. et de Chimie.*, t. 19, p. 314.

[185] *Chicago Medical Review*, 1882.

of 10 grms. and above, almost always fatal. If, however, 8 grms. were taken in divided doses during the twenty-four hours, it could (according to Sir B. W. Richardson) be done with safety. The time from the taking of the poison till death varies considerably, and is in part dependent on the dose.

In seven cases of lethal poisoning, three persons who took the small doses of 1.25, 2.5, and 1.95 grms. respectively, lived from eight to ten hours; two, taking 4 and 5 grms. respectively, died very shortly after the administration of the chloral. In a sixth case, related by Brown, in which 3.12 grms. had been taken, the patient lived an hour; and in another, after a dose of 5 grms., recorded by Jolly, death took place within a quarter of an hour.

§ 202. **Symptoms.**—With moderate doses there are practically no symptoms, save a drowsiness coming on imperceptibly, and followed by heavy sleep. With doses up to 2 grms. (30.8 grains), the hypnotic state is perfectly under the command of the will, and if the person chooses to walk about or engage in any occupation, he can ward off sleep; but with those doses which lead to danger, the narcosis is completely uncontrollable, the appearance of the sleeper is often strikingly like that of a drunken person. There is great diminution of temperature commencing in from five to twenty minutes after taking the dose—occasionally sleep is preceded by a delirious state. During the deep slumber the face is much flushed, and in a few cases the sleep passes directly into death without any marked change. In others, symptoms of collapse appear, and the patient sinks through exhaustion.

§ 203. With some persons doses, which, in themselves, are insufficient to cause death, yet have a peculiar effect on the mental faculties. A case of great medico-legal interest is described by the patient himself, Dr. Manjot.[186] He took in three doses, hourly, 12 grms. of chloral hydrate. After the first dose the pain, for which he had recourse to chloral, vanished; but Manjot, although he had all the appearance of being perfectly conscious, yet had not the slightest knowledge of what he was doing or speaking. He took the other two doses, and sank into a deep sleep which lasted twelve hours. He then awoke and answered questions with difficulty, but could not move; he lay for the next twelve hours in a half slumber, and the following night slept soundly—to wake up recovered.

§ 204. The treatment of acute chloral poisoning which has been most successful is that by strychnine injections, and the application of warmth to counteract the loss of temperature which is so constant a phenomenon. As an illustration of the treatment by strychnine, an interesting case recorded by Levinstein[187] may be quoted.

A man, thirty-five years old, took at one dose, for the purpose of suicide, 24 grms. of chloral hydrate. In half an hour afterwards he was found in a deep sleep, with flushed face, swollen veins, and a pulse 160 in the minute. After a further half hour, the congestion of the head was still more striking; the temperature was 39.5°; the pulse hard and bounding 92; the breathing laboured, at times intermittent.

Artificial respiration was at once commenced, but in spite of this, in about another half hour, the face became deadly pale, the temperature sank to 32.9°. The pupils contracted, and the pulse was scarcely to be felt; 3 mgrms. (.04 grain) of strychnine were now injected subcutaneously; this caused tetanic convulsions in the upper part of the body and trismus. The heart's action again became somewhat stronger, the temperature rose to 33.3°, and the pupils dilated; but soon followed, again, depression of the heart's action, and the respiration could only be kept going by faradisation. Two mgrms. (.03 grain) of strychnine were once more injected, and the heart's action improved. During the succeeding six hours the respiration had to be assisted by faradisation. The temperature gradually rose to 36.5°; ten hours after taking the dose the patient lay in a deep sleep, breathing spontaneously and reacting to external stimuli with a temperature of 38.5°. Eighteen hours from the commencement, the respiration again became irregular, and the galvanic current was anew applied. The last application aroused the sleeper, he took some milk and again slept; after twenty-seven hours he could be awakened by calling, &c., but had not full consciousness; he again took some milk and sank to sleep. It was not until thirty-two hours had elapsed from the ingestion of the poison that he awoke spontaneously; there were no after effects.

§ 205. **Chronic Poisoning by Chloral Hydrate.**—An enormous number of people habitually take chloral hydrate. The history of the habit is usually that some physician has given them a chloral prescription for neuralgia, for loss of sleep, or other cause, and finding that they can conjure sleep, oblivion, and loss (it may be) of suffering whenever they choose, they go on repeating it from day to day until it becomes a necessity of their existence. A dangerous facility to chloral-drinking is the existence of patent medicines, advertised as sleep-producers, and containing chloral as the active ingredient. A lady, aged 35, died in 1876, at Exeter, from an overdose of "Hunter's solution of chloral, or sedative draught and sleep producer." Its strength was stated at the inquest to be 25 grains to

[186] *Gaz. des Hôp.*, 1875.

[187] *Vierteljahrsschr. f. ger. Med.*, Bd. xx., 1874.

the drachm (41.6 per cent.).[188]

The evil results of this chloral-drinking are especially to be looked for in the mental faculties, and the alienists have had since 1869 a new insanity-producing factor. In the asylums may usually be found several cases of melancholia and mania referred rightly (or wrongly) to chloral-drinking. Symptoms other than cerebral are chilliness of the body, inclination to fainting, clonic convulsions, and a want of co-ordination of the muscles of the lower extremities. In a case recorded by Husband,[189] a lady, after twelve days' treatment by chloral hydrate, in doses of from 1 to 2 grms. (15.4 to 30.8 grains), suffered from a scarlatina-like rash, which was followed by desquamation. Among the insane, it has also been noticed that its use has been followed by nettle-rash and petechiæ (Reimer and others).

§ 206. **Excretion of Chloral.**—Chloral hydrate is separated in the urine partly as urochloral acid ($C_8H_{11}Cl_3O_7$). Butylchloral is separated as butyl urochloral acid ($C_{10}H_{15}Cl_2O_7$). Urochloral acid is crystalline, soluble in water, in alcohol, and in ether, reduces copper from Fehling's solution, and rotates a ray of polarised light to the left. Urochloral acid, on boiling with either dilute sulphuric or hydrochloric acid, splits up into trichlorethyl alcohol and glycuronic acid—

$$C_8H_{11}Cl_3O_7 + H_2O = C_2H_3Cl_3O + C_6H_{10}O_7.$$

Trichloralcohol is an oily fluid (boiling-point 150°-152°); it yields by oxidation trichloracetic acid.

Urobutyl chloral acid gives on treatment with mineral acids trichlorbutyl alcohol and glycuronic acid.

To separate urochloral acid from the urine the following process has been found successful:—

The urine is evaporated to a syrup at the heat of the water-bath, and then strongly acidulated with sulphuric acid and repeatedly shaken out in a separating tube with a mixture of 3 vols. of ether and 1 vol. of alcohol. The ether-alcohol is separated and distilled off, the acid residue is neutralised with KHO, or potassic carbonate, and evaporated; the dry mass is then taken up with 90 per cent. alcohol, the filtrate precipitated with ether, and the precipitate washed with ether and absolute alcohol.

Next the precipitate is boiled with absolute alcohol and filtered hot. On cooling, the potassium salt of urochloral acid separates out in tufts of silky needles. The crystals are dried over sulphuric acid and again washed several times with absolute alcohol and ether to remove impurities.

To obtain the free acid, the potassium salt is dissolved in a little water and acidulated with hydrochloric acid; the liquid is then shaken out in a separating tube, with a mixture of 8 vols. of ether and 1 of alcohol. The ether-alcohol is distilled off, the residue treated with moist silver oxide until no farther separation of silver chloride occurs, the silver chloride is separated by filtration, the soluble silver salt decomposed by SH_2, and the filtrate carefully evaporated to a syrup; after a few hours, the acid crystallises in stars of needles.

Urobutylchloral acid can be obtained in quite a similar way.[190]

§ 207. **Separation of Chloral from Organic Matters.**—It will be most convenient to place the organic fluid or pulped-up solid, mixed with water, in a retort, to acidify with tartaric acid, and to distil.

Chloral hydrate distils over from a liquid acidified with tartaric acid; to obtain the whole of the chloral requires distillation in a vacuum almost to dryness.

The distillation will, unless there is also some partly decomposed chloral, not smell of chloroform, and yet give chloroform reactions.

To identify it, to the distillate should be added a little burnt magnesia, and the distillate thus treated boiled for half an hour in a flask connected with an inverted condenser; in this way the chloral hydrate is changed into chloroform and magnesium formate—

$$2CCl_3CH(OH)_2 + MgO = 2CHCl_3 + (HCOO)_2Mg + H_2O.$$

The fluid may now be tested for formic acid: it will give a black precipitate with solution of silver nitrate—

$$(HCOO)_2Mg + 4AgNO_3 = 4Ag + Mg(NO_3)_2 + 2CO_2 + 2HNO_3.$$

It will give a white precipitate of calomel when treated with mercuric chloride solution—

$$(HCOO)_2Mg + 4HgCl_2 = 2Hg_2Cl_2 + MgCl_2 + 2HCl + 2CO_2.$$

Chloral (or chloroform), when boiled with resorcinol and the liquid made strongly alkaline with NaHO, gives a red colour, which disappears on acidifying and is restored by alkalies. If, on the other hand, there is an excess of resorcinol and only a very small quantity of NaHO used, the product shows a yellowish-green fluorescence; $\frac{1}{10}$ of

[188] *Exeter and Plymouth Gazette*, Jan. 12, 1876.

[189] *Lancet*, 1871.

[190] V. Mering u. Musculus, *Ber.*, viii. 662; v. Mering, *ibid.*, xv. 1019; E. Kulz, *Ber.*, xv., 1538.

a milligramme of chloral hydrate gives this reaction distinctly when boiled with 50 mgrms. of resorcinol and 5 drops of a normal solution of sodium hydrate.[191]

Dr. Frank Ogston[192] has recommended sulphide of ammonium to be added to any liquid as a test for chloral. The contents of the stomach are filtered or submitted to dialysis, and the test applied direct. If chloral is present, there is first an orange-yellow colour; on standing, the fluid becomes more and more brown, then troubled, an amorphous precipitate falls to the bottom, and a peculiar odour is developed. With 10 mgrms. of chloral in 1 c.c. of water, there is an evident precipitate, and the odour can readily be perceived; with 1 mgrm. dissolved in 1 c.c. of water, there is an orange-yellow colour, and also the odour, but no precipitate; with .1 mgrm. in 1 c.c. of water, there is a weak, pale, straw-yellow colour, which can scarcely be called characteristic. The only substance giving in neutral solutions the same reactions is antimony; but, on the addition of a few drops of acid, the antimony falls as an orange-yellow precipitate, while, if chloral alone is present, there is a light white precipitate of sulphur.

VIII.—Bisulphide of Carbon.

§ 208. Bisulphide of carbon—*carbon disulphide, carbon sulphide* (CS_2)—is a colourless, volatile fluid, strongly refracting light. Commercial samples have a most repulsive and penetrating odour, but chemically pure carbon sulphide has a smell which is not disagreeable. The boiling-point is 47°; the specific gravity at 0° is 1.293. It is very inflammable, burning with a blue flame, and evolving sulphur dioxide; is little soluble in water, but mixes easily with alcohol or ether. Bisulphide of carbon, on account of its solvent powers for sulphur, phosphorus, oils, resins, caoutchouc, gutta-percha, &c., is in great request in certain industries. It is also utilised for disinfecting purposes, the liquid being burnt in a lamp.

§ 209. **Poisoning by Carbon Bisulphide.**—In spite of the cheapness and numerous applications of this liquid, poisoning is very rare. There appears to be a case on record of attempted self-destruction by this agent, in which a man took 2 ozs. (56.7 c.c.) of the liquid, but without a fatal result. The symptoms in this case were pallor of the face, wide pupils, frequent and weak pulse, lessened bodily temperature, and spasmodic convulsions. Carbon disulphide was detected in the breath by leading the expired air through an alcoholic solution of triethyl-phosphin, with which it struck a red colour. It could also be found in the urine in the same way. An intense burning in the throat, giddiness, and headache lasted for several days.

§ 210. Experiments on animals have been frequent, and it is found to be fatal to all forms of animal life. There is, indeed, no more convenient agent for the destruction of various noxious insects, such as moths, the weevils in biscuits, the common bug, &c., than bisulphide of carbon. It has also been recommended for use in exterminating mice and rats.[193] Different animals show various degrees of sensitiveness to the vapour; frogs and cats being less affected by it than birds, rabbits, and guinea-pigs. It is a blood poison; methæmoglobin is formed, and there is disintegration of the red blood corpuscles. There is complete anæsthesia of the whole body, and death occurs through paralysis of the respiratory centre, but artificial respiration fails to restore life.

§ 211. **Chronic Poisoning.**—Of some importance is the chronic poisoning by carbon disulphide, occasionally met with in manufactures necessitating the daily use of large quantities for dissolving caoutchouc, &c. When taken thus in the form of vapour daily for some time, it gives rise to a complex series of symptoms which may be divided into two principal stages—viz., a stage of excitement and one of depression. In the first phase, there is more or less permanent headache, with considerable indigestion, and its attendant loss of appetite, nausea, &c. The sensitiveness of the skin is also heightened, and there are curious sensations of creeping, &c. The mind at the same time in some degree suffers, the temper becomes irritable, and singing in the ears and noises in the head have been noticed. In one factory a workman suffered from an acute mania, which subsided in two days upon removing him from the noxious vapour (*Eulenberg*). The sleep is disturbed by dreams, and, according to Delpech,[194] there is considerable sexual excitement, but this statement has in no way been confirmed. Pains in the limbs are a constant phenomenon, and the French observers have noticed spasmodic contractions of certain groups of muscles.

The stage of depression begins with a more or less pronounced anæsthesia of the skin. This is not confined to the outer skin, but also affects the mucous membranes; patients complain that they feel as if the tongue were covered

[191] C. Schwarz, *Pharm. Zeit.*, xxxiii. 419.

[192] *Vierteljahrsschrift f. gerichtl. Medicin*, 1879, Bd. xxx. Hft. 1, S. 268.

[193] Cloëz, *Compt. Rend.*, t. 63, 85.

[194] *Mémoire sur les Accidents que développe chez les ouvrières en caoutchouc du sulfure de carb. en vapeur*, Paris, 1856.

with a cloth. The anæsthesia is very general. In a case recorded by Bernhardt,[195] a girl, twenty-two years old, who had worked six weeks in a caoutchouc factory, suffered from mental weakness and digestive troubles; there was anæsthesia and algesis of the whole skin. In these advanced cases the mental debility is very pronounced, and there is also weakness of the muscular system. Paralysis of the lower limbs has been noted, and in one instance a man had his right hand paralysed for two months. It seems uncertain how long a person is likely to suffer from the effects of the vapour after he is removed from its influence. If the first stage of poisoning only is experienced, then recovery is generally rapid; but if mental and muscular weakness and anæsthesia of the skin have been developed, a year has been known to elapse without any considerable improvement, and permanent injury to the health may be feared.

§ 212. **Post-mortem Appearances.**—The pathological appearances found after sudden death from disulphide of carbon are but little different to those found after fatal chloroform breathing.

§ 213. **Detection and Separation of Carbon Disulphide.**—The extreme volatility of the liquid renders it easy to separate it from organic liquids by distillation with reduced pressure in a stream of CO_2. Carbon disulphide is best identified by (1) Hofman's test, viz., passing the vapour into an ethereal solution of triethyl-phosphin, $(C_2H_5)_3P$. Carbon disulphide forms with triethyl-phosphin a compound which crystallises in red scales. The crystals melt at 95° C., and have the following formula—$P(C_2H_5)_3CS_2$. This will detect 0.54 mgrm. Should the quantity of bisulphide be small, no crystals may be obtained, but the liquid will become of a red colour. (2) CS_2 gives, with an alcoholic solution of potash, a precipitate of potassic xanthate, $CS_2C_2H_5OK$.

§ 214. **Xanthogenic acid or ethyloxide-sulphocarbonate** ($CS_2C_2H_5OH$) is prepared by decomposing potassic xanthogenate by diluted hydrochloric or sulphuric acid. It is a colourless fluid, having an unpleasant odour, and a weakly acid and rather bitter taste. It burns with a blue colour, and is easily decomposed at 24°, splitting up into ethylic alcohol and hydric sulphide. It is very poisonous, and has an anæsthetic action similar to bisulphide of carbon. Its properties are probably due to CS_2 being liberated within the body.

§ 215. **Potassic xanthogenate** ($CS_2C_2H_5OK$) and **potassic xanthamylate** ($CS_2C_5H_{11}OK$) (the latter being prepared by the substitution of amyl alcohol for ethyl alcohol), both on the application of a heat below that of the body, develop CS_2, and are poisonous, inducing symptoms very similar to those already detailed.

IX.—The Tar Acids—Phenol—Cresol.

§ 216. **Carbolic Acid. Syn. Phenol, Phenyl Alcohol, Phenylic Hydrate; Phenic Acid; Coal-Tar Creasote.**—The formula for carbolic acid is C_6H_5HO. The pure substance appears at the ordinary temperature as a colourless solid, crystallising in long prisms; the fusibility of the crystals is given variously by different authors: from my own observation, the pure crystals melt at 40°-41°, any lower melting-point being due to the presence of cresylic acid or other impurity; the crystals again become solid about 15°. Melted carbolic acid forms a colourless limpid fluid, sinking in water. It boils under the ordinary pressure at 182°, and distils without decomposition; it is very readily and completely distilled in a vacuum at about the temperature of 100°. After the crystals have been exposed to the air, they absorb water, and a hydrate is formed containing 16.07 per cent. of water. The hydrate melts at 17°, any greater hydration prevents the crystallisation of the acid; a carbolic acid, containing about 27 per cent. of water, and probably corresponding to the formula $C_6H_6O,2H_2O$, is obtained by gradually adding water to carbolic acid so long as it continues to be dissolved. Such a hydrate dissolves in 11.1 times its measure of water, and contains 8.56 per cent. of real carbolic acid. Carbolic acid does not redden litmus, but produces a greasy stain on paper, disappearing on exposure to the air; it has a peculiar smell, a burning numbing taste, and in the fluid state it strongly refracts light. Heated to a high temperature it takes fire, and burns with a sooty flame.

When an aqueous solution of carbolic acid is shaken up with ether, benzene, carbon disulphide, or chloroform, it is fully dissolved by the solvent, and is thus easily separated from most solutions in which it exists in the free state. Petroleum ether, on the other hand, only slightly dissolves it in the cold, more on warming. Carbolic acid mixes in all proportions with glycerin, glacial or acetic acid, and alcohol. It coagulates albumen, the precipitate being soluble in an excess of albumen; it also dissolves iodine, without changing its properties. It dissolves many resins, and also sulphur, but, on boiling, sulphuretted hydrogen is disengaged. Indigo blue is soluble in hot carbolic acid, and may be obtained in crystals on cooling. Carbolic acid is contained in castoreum, a secretion derived from the beaver, but it has not yet been detected in the vegetable kingdom. The source of carbolic acid is at present coal-

[195] *Ber. klin. Wochenschrift*, No. 32, 1866.

tar, from which it is obtained by a process of distillation. There are, however, a variety of chemical actions in the course of which carbolic acid is formed.

§ 217. The common disinfecting carbolic acid is a dark reddish liquid, with a very strong odour; at present there is very little phenol in it; it is mainly composed of meta- and para-cresol. It is officinal in Germany, and there must contain at least 50 per cent. of the pure carbolic acid. The pure crystallised carbolic acid is officinal in our own and all the continental pharmacopœias. In the British Pharmacopœia, a solution of carbolic acid in glycerin is officinal; the proportions are 1 part of carbolic acid and 4 parts of glycerin, that is, strength by measure = 20 per cent. The Pharmacopœia Germanica has a *liquor natri carbolici*, made with 5 parts carbolic acid, 1 caustic soda, and 4 of water; strength in carbolic acid = 50 per cent. There is also a strongly alkaline crude sodic carbolate in use as a preservative of wood.

There are various disinfecting fluids containing amounts of carbolic acid, from 10 per cent. upwards. Many of these are somewhat complex mixtures, but, as a rule, any poisonous properties they possess are mainly due to their content of phenol or cresol. A great variety of disinfecting powders, under various names, are also in commerce, deriving their activity from carbolic acid. Macdougall's disinfecting powder is made by adding a certain proportion of impure carbolic acid to a calcic sulphite, which is prepared by passing sulphur dioxide over ignited limestone.

Calvert's carbolic acid powder is made by adding carbolic acid to the siliceous residue obtained from the manufacture of aluminic sulphate from shale. There are also various carbolates which, by heating or decomposing with sulphuric acid, give off carbolic acid.

Carbolic acid soaps are also made on a large scale—the acid is free, and some of the soaps contain as much as 10 per cent. In the inferior carbolic acid soaps there is little or no carbolic acid, but cresylic takes its place. Neither the soaps nor the powders have hitherto attained any toxicological importance, but the alkaline carbolates are very poisonous.

§ 218. **The chief uses** of carbolic acid are indicated by the foregoing enumeration of the principal preparations used in medicine and commerce. The bulk of the carbolic acid manufactured is for the purposes of disinfection. It is also utilised in the preparation of certain colouring matters or dyes, and during the last few years has had another application in the manufacture of salicylic acid. In medicine it is administered occasionally internally, while the antiseptic movement in surgery, initiated by Lister, has given it great prominence in surgical operations.

§ 219. **Statistics.**—The tar acids, *i.e.*, pure carbolic acid and the impure acids sold under the name of carbolic acid, but consisting (as stated before) mainly of cresol, are, of all powerful poisons, the most accessible, and the most recklessly distributed. We find them at the bedside of the sick, in back-kitchens, in stables, in public and private closets and urinals, and, indeed, in almost all places where there are likely to be foul odours or decomposing matters. It is, therefore, no wonder that poisoning by carbolic acid has, of late years, assumed large proportions. The acid has become vulgarised, and quite as popularly known, as the most common household drugs or chemicals.[196] This familiarity is the growth of a very few years, since it was not discovered until 1834, and does not seem to have been used by Lister until about 1863. It was not known to the people generally until much later. At present it occupies the third place in fatality of all poisons in England. The following table shows that, in the past ten years, carbolic acid has killed 741 people, either accidentally or suicidally; there is also one case of murder by carbolic acid within the same period, bringing the total up to 742:—

DEATHS FROM CARBOLIC ACID IN ENGLAND AND WALES DURING THE TEN YEARS ENDING 1892.

Accident or Negligence.

Ages,	0-1	1-5	5-15	15-25	25-65	65 and above	Total
Males,	2	39	13	5	83	8	150
Females,	2	21	7	13	51	7	101
Totals,	4	60	20	18	134	15	251

[196] Although this is so, yet much ignorance still prevails as to its real nature. In a case reported in the *Pharm. Journ.*, 1881, p. 334, a woman, thirty years of age, drank two-thirds of an ounce of liquid labelled "*Pure Carbolic Acid*" by mistake, and died in two hours. She read the label, and a lodger also read it, but did not know what it meant.

Suicide.

Ages,	15-25	25-65	65 and above	Total
Males,	26	186	7	219
Females,	72	194	5	271
Totals,	98	380	12	490

Falck has collected, since the year 1868, no less than 87 cases of poisoning from carbolic acid recorded in medical literature. In one of the cases the individual died in nine hours from a large dose of carbolate of soda; in a second, violent symptoms were induced by breathing for three hours carbolic acid vapour; in the remaining 85, the poisoning was caused by the liquid acid. Of these 85 persons, 7 had taken the poison with suicidal intent, and of the 7, 5 died; 39 were poisoned through the medicinal use of carbolic acid, 27 of the 39 by the antiseptic treatment of wounds by carbolic acid dressings, and of these 8 terminated fatally; in 8 cases, symptoms of poisoning followed the rubbing or painting of the acid on the skin for the cure of scabies, favus, or psoriasis, and 6 of these patients died. In 4 cases, carbolic acid enemata, administered for the purpose of dislodging ascarides, gave rise to symptoms of poisoning, and in one instance death followed.

The substitution of carbolic acid for medicine happened as follows:—

	Cases.
Taken instead of Tincture of Opium,	1
,, ,, Infusion of Senna,	3
,, ,, Mineral Water,	2
,, ,, other Mixtures,	3
,, inwardly instead of applied outwardly,	3
	12

Of these 12, 8 died.

Again, 10 persons took carbolic acid in mistake for various alcoholic drinks, such as schnapps, brandy, rum, or beer, and 9 of the 10 succumbed; 17 persons drank carbolic acid simply "by mistake," and of these 13 died. Thus, of the whole 85 cases, no less than 51 ended fatally—nearly 60 per cent.

It must be always borne in mind that, with regard to statistics generally, the term "carbolic acid" is not used by coroners, juries, or medical men, in a strictly chemical sense, the term being made to include disinfecting fluids which are almost wholly composed of the cresols, and contain scarcely any phenol. In this article, with regard to symptoms and pathological appearances, it is only occasionally possible to state whether the pure medicinal crystalline phenol or a mixture of tar-acids was the cause of poisoning.

§ 220. **Fatal Dose.**—The minimum fatal dose for cats, dogs, and rabbits, appears to be from .4 to .5 grm. per kilogram. Falck has put the minimum lethal dose for man at 15 grms. (231.5 grains), which would be about .2 per kilo., basing his estimate on the following reasoning. In 33 cases he had a fairly exact record of the amount of acid taken, and out of the 33, he selects only those cases which are of use for the decision of the question. Among adults, in 5 cases the dose was 30 grms., and all the 5 cases terminated by death, in times varying from five minutes to an hour and a half. By other 5 adults a dose of 15 grms. was taken; of the 5, 3 men and a woman died, in times varying from forty-five minutes to thirty hours, while 1 woman recovered. Doses of 11.5, 10.8, and 9 grms. were taken by different men, and recovered from; on the other hand, a suicide who took one and a half teaspoonful (about 6 grms.) of the concentrated acid, died in fifty minutes. Doses of .3 to 3 grms. have caused symptoms of poisoning, but the patients recovered, while higher doses than 15 grms. in 12 cases, with only one exception, caused death. Hence, it may be considered tolerably well established, that 15 grms. (231.5 grains) may be taken as representing the minimum lethal dose.

The largest dose from which a person appears to have recovered is, I believe, that given in a case recorded by Davidson, in which 150 grms. of crude carbolic acid had been taken. It must, however, be remembered that, as this was the impure acid, probably only half of it was really carbolic acid. The German Pharmacopœia prescribes as a maximum dose .05 grm (.7 grain) of the crystallised acid, and a daily maximum quantity given in divided doses of .15 grm. (2.3 grains).

§ 221. **Effects on Animals.**—Carbolic acid is poisonous to both animal and vegetable life.

Infusoria.—One part of the acid in 10,000 parts of water rapidly kills ciliated animalcules,—the movements become sluggish, the sarcode substance darker, and the cilia in a little time cease moving.

Fish.—One part of the acid in 7000 of water kills dace, minnows, roach, and gold fish. In this amount of dilution the effect is not apparent immediately; but, at the end of a few hours, the movements of the fish become sluggish, they frequently rise to the surface to breathe, and at the end of twenty-four hours are found dead. Quantities of carbolic acid, such as 1 part in 100,000 of water, appear to affect the health of fish, and render them more liable to be attacked by the fungus growth which is so destructive to fish-life in certain years.

Frogs.—If .01 to .02 grm. of carbolic acid be dissolved in a litre of water in which a frog is placed, there is almost immediately signs of uneasiness in the animal, showing that pain from local contact is experienced; a sleepy condition follows, with exaltation of reflex sensibility; convulsions succeed, generally, though not always; then reflex sensibility is diminished, ultimately vanishes, and death occurs; the muscles and nerves still respond to the electric current, and the heart beats, but slowly and weakly, for a little after the respiration has ceased.

§ 222. **Warm-blooded Animals.**—For a rabbit of the average weight of 2 kilos., .15 grm. is an active dose, and .3 a lethal dose (that is .15 per kilo.). The sleepy condition of the frog is not noticed, and the chief symptoms are clonic convulsions with dilatation of the pupils, the convulsions passing into death, without a noticeable paralytic stage. The symptoms observed in poisoned dogs are almost precisely similar, the dose, according to body-weight, being the same. It has, however, been noticed that with doses large enough to produce convulsions, a weak condition has supervened, causing death in several days. There appears to be no cumulative action, since equal toxic doses can be given to animals for some time, and the last dose has no greater effect than the first or intermediate ones. The pathological appearances met with in animals poisoned by the minimum lethal doses referred to are not characteristic; but there is a remarkable retardation of putrefaction.

§ 223. **Symptoms in Man, external application.**—A 5 per cent. solution of carbolic acid, applied to the skin, causes a peculiar numbness, followed, it may be, by irritation. Young subjects, and those with sensitive skins, sometimes exhibit a pustular eruption, and concentrated solutions cause more or less destruction of the skin. Lemaire[197] describes the action of carbolic acid on the skin as causing a slight inflammation, with desquamation of the epithelium, followed by a very permanent brown stain, but this he alone has observed. Applied to the mucous membrane, carbolic acid turns the epithelial covering white; the epithelium, however, is soon thrown off, and the place rapidly heals; there is the same numbing, aconite-like feeling before noticed. The vapour of carbolic acid causes redness of the conjunctivæ, and irritation of the air-passages. If the application is continued, the mucous membrane swells, whitens, and pours out an abundant secretion.

Dr. Whitelock, of Greenock, has related two instances in which children were treated with carbolic acid lotion (strength 2½ per cent.) as an application to the scalp for ringworm; in both, symptoms of poisoning occurred—in the one, the symptoms at once appeared; in the other they were delayed some days. In order to satisfy his mind, the experiment was repeated twice, and each time gastric and urinary troubles followed.

Nussbaum, of Munich, records a case[198] in which symptoms were induced by the forcible injection of a solution of carbolic acid into the cavity of an abscess.

Macphail[199] gives two cases of poisoning by carbolic acid from external use. In the one, a large tumour had been removed from a woman aged 30, and the wound covered with gauze steeped in a solution of carbolic acid, in glycerin, strength 10 per cent.; subsequently, there was high fever, with diminished sulphates in the urine, which smelt strongly of carbolic acid, and was very dark. On substituting boracic acid, none of these troubles were observed. The second case was that of a servant suffering from axillary abscess; the wound was syringed out with carbolic acid solution, of strength 2½ per cent., when effects were produced similar to those in the first case. It was noted that in both these cases the pulse was slowed. Scattered throughout surgical and medical literature, there are many other cases recorded, though not all so clear as those cited. Several cases are also on record in which poisonous symptoms (and even death) have resulted from the application of carbolic acid lotion as a remedy for scabies or

[197] Lemaire, Jul., "*De l'Acide phénique*," Paris, 1864.

[198] *Leitfaden zur antiseptischer Wundbehandlung*, 141.

[199] "Carbolic Acid Poisoning (Surgical)," by S. Rutherford Macphail, M.B., *Ed. Med. Journal*, cccxiv., Aug. 1881, p. 134.

itch.

A surgeon prescribed for two joiners who suffered from scabies a lotion, which was intended to contain 30 grms. of carbolic acid in 240 c.c. of water; but the actual contents of the flasks were afterwards from analysis estimated by Hoppe-Seyler to be 33.26 grms., and the quantity used by each to be equal to 13.37 grms. (206 grains) of carbolic acid. One of the men died; the survivor described his own symptoms as follows:—He and his companion stood in front of the fire, and rubbed the lotion in; he rubbed it into his legs, breast, and the front part of his body; the other parts were mutually rubbed. Whilst rubbing his right arm, and drying it before the fire, he felt a burning sensation, a tightness and giddiness, and mentioned his sensations to his companion, who laughed. This condition lasted from five to seven minutes, but he did not remember whether his companion complained of anything, nor did he know what became of him, nor how he himself came to be in bed. He was found holding on to the joiner's bench, looking with wide staring eyes, like a drunken man, and was delirious for half an hour. The following night he slept uneasily and complained of headache and burning of the skin. The pulse was 68, the appearance of the urine, appetite, and sense of taste were normal; the bowels confined. He soon recovered.

The other joiner seems to have died as suddenly as if he had taken prussic acid. He called to his mother, "*Ich habe einen Rausch*," and died with pale livid face, after taking two deep, short inspirations.

The *post-mortem* examination showed the sinuses filled with much fluid blood, and the vessels of the pia mater congested. Frothy, dark, fluid blood was found in the lungs, which were hyperæmic; the mucous tissues of the epiglottis and air-tubes were reddened, and covered with a frothy slime. Both ventricles—the venæ cavæ and the vessels of the spleen and kidneys—were filled with dark fluid blood. The muscles were very red; there was no special odour. Hoppe-Seyler recognised carbolic acid in the blood and different organs of the body.[200]

In another case, a child died from the outward use of a 2 per cent. solution of carbolic acid. It is described as follows:—An infant of seven weeks old suffered from varicella, and one of the pustules became the centre of an erysipelatous inflammation. To this place a 2 per cent. solution of carbolic acid was applied by means of a compress steeped in the acid; the following morning the temperature rose from 36.5° (97.7° F.) to 37° (98.6° F.), and poisonous symptoms appeared. The urine was coloured dark. There were sweats, vomitings, and contracted pupils, spasmodic twitchings of the eyelids and eyes, with strabismus, slow respiration, and, lastly, inability to swallow. Under the influence of stimulating remedies the condition temporarily improved, but the child died twenty-three and a half hours after the first application. An examination showed that the vessels of the brain and the tissue of the lungs were abnormally full of blood. The liver was softer than natural, and exhibited a notable yellowishness in the centre of the acini. Somewhat similar appearances were noticed in the kidneys, the microscopic examination of which showed the *tubuli contorti* enlarged and filled with fatty globules. In several places the epithelium was denuded, in other places swollen, and with the nuclei very visible.

In an American case,[201] death followed the application of carbolic acid to a wound. A boy had been bitten by a dog, and to the wound, at one o'clock in the afternoon, a lotion, consisting of nine parts of carbolic acid and one of glycerin, was applied. At seven o'clock in the evening the child was unconscious, and died at one o'clock the following day.

§ 224. **Internal Administration.**—Carbolic acid may be taken into the system, not alone by the mouth, but by the lungs, as in breathing carbolic acid spray or carbolic acid vapour. It is also absorbed by the skin when outwardly applied, or in the dressing or the spraying of wounds with carbolic acid. Lastly, the ordinary poisonous effects have been produced by absorption from the bowel, when administered as an enema. When swallowed undiluted, and in a concentrated form, the symptoms may be those of early collapse, and speedy death. Hence, the course is very similar to that witnessed in poisoning by the mineral acids.

If lethal, but not excessive doses of the diluted acid are taken, the symptoms are—a burning in the mouth and throat, a peculiarly unpleasant persistent taste, and vomiting. There is faintness with pallor of the face, which is covered by a clammy sweat, and the patient soon becomes unconscious, the pulse small and thready, and the pupils sluggish to light. The respiration is profoundly affected; there is dyspnœa, and the breathing becomes shallow. Death occurs from paralysis of the respiratory apparatus, and the heart is observed to beat for a little after the respiration has ceased. All these symptoms may occur from the application of the acid to the skin or to mucous membranes, and have been noticed when solutions of but moderate strength have been used—e.g., there are cases in gynæcological practice in which the mucous membrane (perhaps eroded) of the uterus has been irrigated with

---

[200] R. Köhler, *Würtem. Med. Corr. Bl.*, xlii., No. 6, April 1872; H. Abelin, *Schmidt's Jahrbücher*, 1877, Bd. 173, S. 163.

[201] *American Journal of Pharmacy*, vol. li., 4th Ser.; vol. ix., 1879, p. 57.

carbolic acid injections. Thus, Küster[202] relates a case in which, four days after confinement, the uterus was washed out with a 2 per cent. solution of carbolic acid without evil result. Afterwards a 5 per cent. solution was used, but it at once caused violent symptoms of poisoning, the face became livid, clonic convulsions came on, and at first loss of consciousness, which after an hour returned. The patient died on the ninth day. There was intense diphtheria of the uterus and vagina. Several other similar cases (although not attended with such marked or fatal effects) are on record.[203]

§ 225. The symptoms of carbolic acid poisoning admit of considerable variation from those already described. The condition is occasionally that of deep coma. The convulsions may be general, or may affect only certain groups of muscles. Convulsive twitchings of the face alone, and also muscular twitchings only of the legs, have been noticed. In all cases, however, a marked change occurs in the urine. Subissi[204] has noted the occurrence of abortion, both in the pig and the mare, as a result of carbolic acid, but this effect has not hitherto been recorded in the human subject.

It has been experimentally shown by Küster, that previous loss of blood, or the presence of septic fever, renders animals more sensitive to carbolic acid. It is also said that children are more sensitive than adults.

The course of carbolic acid poisoning is very rapid. In 35 cases collected by Falck, in which the period from the taking of the poison to the moment of death was accurately noted, the course was as follows:—12 patients died within the first hour, and in the second hour 3; so that within two hours 15 died. Between the third and the twelfth hour, 10 died; between the thirteenth and the twenty-fourth hour, 7 died; and between the twenty-fifth and the sixtieth hour, only 3 died. Therefore, slightly over 71 per cent. died within twelve hours, and 91.4 per cent. within the twenty-four hours.

§ 226. **Changes in the Urine.**—The urine of patients who have absorbed in any way carbolic acid is dark in colour, and may smell strongly of the acid. It is now established—chiefly by the experiments and observations of Baumann[205]—that carbolic acid, when introduced into the body, is mainly eliminated in the form of phenyl-sulphuric acid, $C_6H_5HSO_4$, or more strictly speaking as potassic phenyl-sulphate, $C_6H_5KSO_4$, a substance which is not precipitated by chloride of barium until it has been decomposed by boiling with a mineral acid. Cresol is similarly excreted as cresol-sulphuric acid, $C_6H_4CH_3HSO_4$, ortho-, meta-, or para-, according to the kind of cresol injected; a portion may also appear as hydro-tolu-chinone-sulphuric acid. Hence it is that, with doses of phenol or cresol continually increasing, the amount of sulphates naturally in the urine (as estimated by simply acidifying with hydrochloric acid, and precipitating in the cold with chloride of barium) continually decreases, and may at last vanish, for all the sulphuric acid present is united with the phenol. On the other hand, the precipitate obtained by prolonged boiling of the strongly acidified urine, after filtering off any $BaSO_4$ thrown down in the cold, is ever increasing.

Thus, a dog voided urine which contained in 100 c.c., .262 grm. of precipitable sulphuric acid, and .006 of organically-combined sulphuric acid; his back was now painted with carbolic acid, and the normal proportions were reversed, the precipitable sulphuric acid became .004 grm., while the organically-combined was .190 in 100 c.c. In addition to phenyl-sulphuric acid, it is now sufficiently established[206] that hydroquinone ($C_6H_4{}^{OH}_{OH}$) (paradihydroxyl phenol) and pyrocatechin ($C_6H_4{}^{OH}_{OH}$) (orthodihydroxyl phenol) are constant products of a portion of the phenol. The hydroquinone appears in the urine, in the first place, as the corresponding ether-sulphuric acid, which is colourless; but a portion of it is set free, and this free hydroquinone (especially in alkaline urine) is quickly oxidised to a brownish product, and hence the peculiar colour of urine. Out of dark coloured carbolic acid urine the

[202] *Centralblatt. f. Gynäkologie*, ii. 14, 1878.

[203] A practitioner in Calcutta injected into the bowel of a boy, aged 5, an enema of diluted carbolic acid, which, according to his own statement, was 1 part in 60, and the whole quantity represented 144 grains of the acid. The child became insensible a few minutes after the operation, and died within four hours. There was no *post-mortem* examination; the body smelt strongly of carbolic acid.—*Lancet*, May 19, 1883.

[204] *L'Archivio della Veterinaria Ital.*, xi., 1874.

[205] *Pflüger's Archiv*, 13, 1876, 289.

[206] E. Baumann and C. Preuss, *Zeitschrift f. phys. Chemie*, iii. 156; *Anleitung zur Harn-Analyse*, W. F. Löbisch, Leipzig, 1881, pp. 142, 160; Schmiedeberg, *Chem. Centrbl.* (3), 13, 598.

hydroquinone and its products of decomposition can be obtained by shaking with ether; on separation of the ether, an extract is obtained, reducing alkaline silver solution, and developing quinone on warming with ferric chloride.

To separate pyro-catechin, 200 c.c. of urine may be evaporated to an extract, the extract treated with strong alcohol, the alcoholic liquid evaporated, and the extract then treated with ether. On separation and evaporation of the ether, a yellowish mass is left, from which the pyro-catechin may be extracted by washing with a small quantity of water. This solution will reduce silver solution in the cold, or, if treated with a few drops of ferric chloride solution, show a marked green colour, changing on being alkalised by a solution of sodic hydro-carbonate to violet, and then on being acidified by acetic acid, changing back again to green. According to Thudichum,[207] the urine of men and dogs, after the ingestion of carbolic acid, contains a blue pigment.

§ 227. **The Action of Carbolic Acid considered physiologically.**—Researches on animals have elucidated, in a great measure, the mode in which carbolic acid acts, and the general sequence of effects, but there is still much to be learnt.

E. Küster[208] has shown that the temperature of dogs, when doses of carbolic acid in solution are injected subcutaneously, or into the veins, is immediately, or very soon after the operation, raised. With small and moderate doses, this effect is but slight—from half to a whole degree—on the day after the injection the temperature sinks below the normal point, and only slowly becomes again natural. With doses that are just lethal, first a rise and then a rapid sinking of temperature are observed; but with those excessive doses which speedily kill, the temperature at once sinks without a preliminary rise. The action on the heart is not very marked, but there is always a slowing of the cardiac pulsations; according to Hoppe-Seyler the arteries are relaxed. The respiration is much quickened; this acceleration is due to an excitement of the vagus centre, since Salkowsky has shown that section of the vagus produces a retardation of the respiratory wave. Direct application of the acid to muscles or nerves quickly destroys their excitability without a previous stage of excitement. The main cause of the lethal action of carbolic acid—putting on one side those cases in which it may kill by its local corrosive action—appears to be paralysis of the respiratory nervous centres. The convulsions arise from the spinal cord. On the cessation of the convulsions, the superficial nature of the breathing assists other changes by preventing the due oxidation of the blood.

§ 228. Carbolic acid is separated from the body in the forms already mentioned, a small portion is also excreted by the skin. Salkowsky considers that, with rabbits, he has also found oxalic acid in the urine as an oxidation product. According to the researches of Binnendijk,[209] the separation of carbolic acid by the urine commences very quickly after its ingestion; and, under favourable circumstances, it may be completely excreted within from twelve to sixteen hours. It must be remembered that normally a small amount of phenol may be present in the animal body, as the result of the digestion of albuminous substances or of their putrefaction. The amount excreted by healthy men when feeding on mixed diet, Engel,[210] by experiment, estimates to be in the twenty-four hours 15 mgrms.

§ 229. **Post-mortem Appearances.**—No fact is better ascertained from experiments on animals than the following:—That with lethal doses of carbolic acid, administered by subcutaneous injection, or introduced by the veins, no appearances may be found after death which can be called at all characteristic. Further, in the cases in which death has occurred from the outward application of the acid for the cure of scabies, &c., no lesion was ascertained after death which could—apart from the history of the case and chemical evidence—with any confidence be ascribed to a poison.

On the other hand, when somewhat large doses of the acid are taken by the mouth, very coarse and appreciable changes are produced in the upper portion of the alimentary tract. There may be brownish, wrinkled spots on the cheek or lips; the mucous membrane of the mouth, throat, and gullet is often white, and if the acid was concentrated, eroded. The stomach is sometimes thickened, contracted, and blanched, a condition well shown in a pathological preparation (ix. 206, 43 *f*) in St. George's Hospital. The mucous membrane, indeed, may be quite as much destroyed as if a mineral acid had been taken. Thus, in Guy's Hospital museum (1799[40]), there is preserved the stomach of a child who died from taking accidentally carbolic acid. It looks like a piece of paper, and is very white, with fawn-coloured spots; the rugæ are absent, and the mucous membrane seems to have entirely vanished. Not unfrequently the stomach exhibits white spots with roundish edges. The duodenum is often affected, and the action is not always limited to the first part of the intestine.

[207] *On the Pathology of the Urine*, Lond., 1877, p. 198.
[208] *Archiv f. klin. Chirurgie*, Bd. 23, S. 133, 1879.
[209] *Journal de Pharmacie et de Chimie.*
[210] *Annal. de Chimie et de Physique*, 5 Sér. T. 20, p. 230, 1880.

The respiratory passages are often inflamed, and the lungs infiltrated and congested. As death takes place from an asphyxiated condition, the veins of the head and brain, and the blood-vessels of the liver, kidney and spleen, are gorged with blood, and the right side of the heart distended, while the left is empty. On the other hand, a person may die of sudden nervous shock from the ingestion of a large quantity of the acid, and in such a case the *post-mortem* appearances will not then exhibit precisely the characters just detailed. Putrefaction is retarded according to the dose, and there is often a smell of carbolic acid.[211] If any urine is contained in the bladder, it will probably be dark, and present the characters of carbolic urine, detailed earlier.

Tests for Carbolic Acid.

§ 230. 1. **The Pinewood Test.**—Certain pinewood gives a beautiful blue colour when moistened first with carbolic acid, and afterwards with hydrochloric acid, and exposed to the light. Some species of pine give a blue colour with hydrochloric acid alone, and such must not be used; others do not respond to the test for carbolic acid. Hence it is necessary to try the chips of wood first, to see how they act, and with this precaution the test is very serviceable, and, in cautious hands, no error will be made.

2. **Ammonia and Hypochlorite Test.**—If to a solution containing even so small a quantity as 1 part of carbolic acid in 5000 parts of water, first, about a quarter of its volume of ammonia hydrate be added, and then a small quantity of sodic hypochlorite solution, avoiding excess, a blue colour appears, warming quickens the reaction: the blue is permanent, but turns to red with acids. If there is a smaller quantity than the above proportion of acid, the reaction may be still produced feebly after standing for some time.

3. **Ferric Chloride.**—One part of phenol in 3000 parts of water can be detected by adding a solution of ferric chloride; a fine violet colour is produced. This is also a very good test, when applied to a distillate; but if applied to a complex liquid, the disturbing action of neutral salts and other substances may be too great to make the reaction under those circumstances of service.

4. **Bromine.**—The most satisfactory test of all is treatment of the liquid by bromine-water. A precipitate of tri-bromo-phenol ($C_6H_3Br_3O$) is rapidly or slowly formed, according to the strength of the solution; in detecting very minute quantities the precipitate must be given time to form. According to Allen,[212] a solution containing but $^1/_{60000}$ of carbolic acid gave the reaction after standing twenty-four hours.

The properties of the precipitate are as follows:—It is crystalline, and under the microscope is seen to consist of fine stars of needles; its smell is peculiar; it is insoluble in water and acid liquids, but soluble in alkalies, ether, and absolute alcohol; a very minute quantity of water suffices to precipitate it from an alcoholic solution; it is therefore essential to the success of the test that the watery liquid to be examined is either neutral or acid in reaction.

§ 231. Tri-bromo-phenol may be used for the quantitative estimation of carbolic acid, 100 parts of tri-bromo-phenol are equal to 29.8 of carbolic acid; by the action of sodium amalgam, tri-bromo-phenol is changed back into carbolic acid.

That bromine-water precipitates several volatile and fixed alkaloids from their solutions is no objection to the bromine test, for it may be applied to a distillation product, the bases having been previously fixed by sulphuric acid. Besides, the properties of tri-bromo-phenol are distinct enough, and therefore there is no valid objection to the test. It is the best hitherto discovered. There are also other reactions, such as that Millon's reagent strikes a red—molybdic acid, in concentrated sulphuric acid, a blue—and potassic dichromate, with sulphuric acid, a brown colour—but to these there are objections. Again, we have the *Euchlorine* test, in which the procedure is as follows:—A test-tube is taken, and concentrated hydrochloric acid is allowed to act therein upon potassic chlorate. After the gas has been evolved for from 30 to 40 seconds, the liquid is diluted with 1½ volume of water, the gas removed by blowing through a tube, and solution of strong ammonia poured in so as to form a layer on the top; after blowing out the white fumes of ammonium chloride, a few drops of the sample to be tested are added. In the presence of carbolic acid, a rose-red, blood-red, or red-brown tint is produced, according to the quantity present. Carbolic acid may be confounded with *cresol* or with *creasote*, but the distinction between pure carbolic acid, pure cresol, and creasote is plain.

§ 232. **Cresol (Cresylic Acid, Methyl-phenol),** $C_6H_4\langle{}^{OH}_{CH_3}$—There are three cresols—ortho-, meta-, and

[211] In order to detect this odour, it is well to open the head first, lest the putrefaction of the internal viscera be so great as to mask the odour.

[212] *Commercial Organic Analysis*, vol. i. p. 306.

para-. Ordinary commercial cresol is a mixture of the three, but contains but little ortho-cresol; the more important properties of the pure cresols are set out in the following table:—

	Melting-point.	Boiling-point.	Converted by fusion with Potash into—
Ortho-,	31-31.5° C.	188.0°	Salicylic Acid (Ortho-oxybenzoic acid).
Meta-,	Fluid at ordinary temperature.	201.0°	Meta-oxybenzoic acid.
Para-,	36°	198°	Para-oxybenzoic acid.

Pure ortho-, meta-, or para-cresol have been obtained by synthetical methods; they cannot be said to be in ordinary commerce.

Commercial cresol is at ordinary temperatures a liquid, and cannot be obtained in a crystalline state by freezing. Its boiling-point is from 198° to 203°; it is almost insoluble in strong ammonia, and, when 16 volumes are added, it then forms crystalline scales. On the other hand, carbolic acid is soluble in an equal volume of ammonia, and is then precipitated by the addition of 1½ volume of water. Cresol is insoluble in small quantities of pure 6 per cent. soda solution; with a large excess, it forms crystalline scales; while carbolic acid is freely soluble in small or large quantities of alkaline solutions.

Cold petroleum spirit dissolves cresol, but no crystalline scales can be separated out by a freezing mixture. Carbolic acid, on the contrary, is but sparingly soluble in cold petroleum, and a solution of carbolic acid in hot petroleum, when exposed to sudden cold produced by a freezing mixture, separates out crystals from the upper layer of liquid. Cresol is miscible with glycerin of specific gravity 1.258 in all proportions; 1 measure of glycerin mixed with 1 measure of cresol is completely precipitated by 1 measure of water. Carbolic acid, under the same circumstances, is not precipitated. The density of cresol is about 1.044. It forms with bromine a tri-bromo-cresol, but this is liquid at ordinary temperatures, while tri-bromo-phenol is solid. On the other hand, it resembles carbolic acid in its reactions with ferric chloride and with nitric and sulphuric acid.

§ 233. **Creasote** or **Kreozote** is a term applied to the mixture of crude phenols obtained from the distillation of wood-tar. It consists of a mixture of substances of which the chief are guaiacol or oxycresol ($C_7H_8O_2$), boiling at 200°, and creasol ($C_8H_{10}O_2$), boiling at 217°; also in small quantities phlorol ($C_8H_{10}O$), methyl creasol ($C_9H_{12}O_2$), and other bodies. Morson's English creasote is prepared from Stockholm tar, and boils at about 217°, consisting chiefly of creasol; it is not easy, by mere chemical tests, to distinguish creasote from cresylic acid. Creasote, in its reactions with sulphuric and nitric acid, bromine and gelatin, is similar to carbolic and cresylic acids, and its solubility in most solvents is also similar. It is, however, distinguished from the tar acids by its insolubility in Price's glycerin, specific gravity 1.258, whether 1, 2, or 3 volumes of glycerin be employed. But the best test is its action on an ethereal solution of nitro-cellulose. Creasote mixes freely with the B.P. collodium, while cresylic acid or carbolic acid at once coagulates the latter. With complicated mixtures containing carbolic acid, cresol, and creasote, the only method of applying these tests with advantage is to submit the mixture to fractional distillation.

Flückiger[213] tests for small quantities of carbolic acid in creasote, by mixing a watery solution of the sample with one-fourth of its volume of ammonia hydrate, wetting the inside of a porcelain dish with this solution, and then carefully blowing bromine fumes on to the surface. A fine blue colour appears if carbolic acid is present, but if the sample consists of creasote only, then it is dirty green or brown. Excess of bromine spoils the reaction.[214]

---

[213] *Arch. der Pharmacie*, cxiii. p. 30.

[214] Creasote is, without doubt, poisonous, though but little is known of its action, and very few experiments are on record in which pure creasote has been employed. Eulenberg has studied the symptoms in rabbits, by submitting them to vaporised creasote—*i.e.*, the vapour from 20 drops of creasote diffused through a glass shade under which a rabbit was confined. There was at once great uneasiness, with a watery discharge from the eyes, and after seven minutes the rabbit fell on its side, and was slightly convulsed. The cornea was troubled, and the eyes prominent; a white slime flowed from the mouth and eyes. After fifteen minutes there was narcosis, with lessened reflex action; the temperature was almost normal. There was rattling breathing, and in half an hour the animal died, the respiration ceasing, and fluid blood escaping from the nose. Section after death showed the

§ 234. **Carbolic Acid in Organic Fluids or in the Tissues of the Body.**—If the routine process given earlier, where the organic fluid is distilled in a vacuum after acidifying with tartaric acid, is employed, phenol or cresol, if present, will certainly be found in the distillate. If, however, a special search be made for the acids, then the fluid must be well acidified with sulphuric acid, and distilled in the usual way. The distillation should be continued as long as possible, and the distillate shaken up with ether in the apparatus figured earlier. On separation and evaporation of the ether, the tar acids, if present, will be left in a pure enough form to show its reactions. The same process applies to the tissues, which, in a finely-divided state, are boiled and distilled with dilute sulphuric acid, and the distillate treated as just detailed.

Like most poisons, carbolic acid has a selective attraction for certain organs, so that, unless all the organs are examined, it is by no means indifferent which particular portion is selected for the inquiry. Hoppe-Seyler applied carbolic acid to the abdomen and thighs of dogs, and when the symptoms were at their height bled them to death, and separately examined the parts. In one case, the blood yielded .00369 per cent.; the brain, .0034 per cent.; the liver, .00125; and the kidneys, .00423 per cent. of their weight of carbolic acid. The liver then contains only one-third of the quantity found in an equal weight of blood, and, therefore, the acid has no selective affinity for that organ. On the other hand, the nervous tissue, and especially the kidneys, appear to concentrate it.

§ 235. **Examination of the Urine for Phenol or Cresol.**—It has been previously stated that the urine will not contain these as such, but as compounds—viz., phenyl or cresyl sulphate of potassium. By boiling with a mineral acid, these compounds may be broken up, and the acids obtained, either by distillation or by extraction with ether. To detect very minute quantities, a large quantity of the urine should be evaporated down to a syrup, and treated with hydrochloric acid and ether. On evaporating off the ether, the residue should be distilled with dilute sulphuric acid, and this distillate then tested with bromine-water, and the tri-bromo-phenol or cresol collected, identified, and weighed.

Thudichum[215] has separated crystals of potassic phenyl-sulphate itself from the urine of patients treated endermically by carbolic acid, as follows:—

The urine was evaporated to a syrup, extracted with alcohol of 90 per cent., treated with an alcoholic solution of oxalic acid as long as this produced a precipitate, and then shaken with an equal volume of ether. The mixture was next filtered, neutralised with potassic carbonate, evaporated to a small bulk, and again taken up with alcohol. Some oxalate and carbonate of potassium were separated, and, on evaporation to a syrup, crystals of potassic phenyl-sulphate were obtained. They gave to analysis 46.25 per cent. H_2SO_4, and 18.1 K—theory requiring 46.2 of H_2SO_4 and 18.4 of K. Alkaline phenyl-sulphates strike a deep purple colour with ferric chloride. To estimate the amount of phenyl-sulphate or cresol-sulphate in the urine, the normal sulphates may be separated by the addition of chloride of barium in the cold, first acidifying with hydrochloric acid. On boiling the liquid a second crop of sulphate is obtained, due to the breaking up of the compound sulphate, and from this second weight the amount of acid can be obtained, *e.g.*, in the case of phenol—$C_6H_5HSO_4 : BaSO_4 :: 174 : 233$.

§ 236. **Assay of Disinfectants, Carbolic Acid Powders, &c.**—For the assay of crude carbolic acid, Mr. Charles Lowe[216] uses the following process:—A thousand parts of the sample are distilled without any special condensing arrangement; water first comes over, and is then followed by an oily fluid. When a hundred parts of the latter, as measured in a graduated tube, have been collected, the receiver is changed. The volume of water is read off. If the oily liquid floats on the water, it contains light oil of tar; if it is heavier than the water, it is regarded as hydrated acid, containing 50 per cent. of real carbolic acid. The next portion consists of anhydrous cresylic and carbolic acids, and 625 volumes are distilled over; the remainder in the retort consists wholly of cresylic acid and the higher homologues. The relative proportions of carbolic and cresylic acids are approximately determined by taking the solidifying point, which should be between 15.5° and 24°, and having ascertained this temperature, imitating it by making mixtures of known proportions of carbolic and cresylic acids.

E. Waller[217] has recommended the following process for the estimation of carbolic acid. It is based on the

brain to be hyperæmic, the mucous membranes of the air-passages to be covered with a thin layer of fluid blood, and the lungs to be congested; the right side of the heart was gorged with fluid blood.

The *post-mortem* appearances and the symptoms generally are, therefore, closely allied to those produced by carbolic acid. A dark colour of the urine has also been noticed.

[215] *Pathology of the Urine*, p. 193.

[216] *Allen's Commercial Organic Analysis*, vol. i. p. 311.

[217] *Chem. News*, April 1, 1881, p. 152.

precipitation of the tar acids by bromine, and, of course, all phenols precipitated in this way will be returned as carbolic acid. The solutions necessary are—

1. A solution containing 10 grms. of pure carbolic acid to the litre; this serves as a standard solution.
2. A solution of bromine in water.
3. Solution of alum in dilute sulphuric acid. A litre of 10 per cent. sulphuric acid is shaken with alum crystals until saturated.

The actual process is as follows:—10 grms. of the sample are weighed out and run into a litre flask, water added, and the mixture shaken. The flask being finally filled up to the neck, some of the solution is now filtered through a dry filter, and 10 c.c. of this filtrate is placed in a 6 or 8-ounce stoppered bottle, and 30 c.c. of the alum solution added. In a similar bottle 10 c.c. of the standard solution of carbolic acid are placed, and a similar quantity of alum solution is added, as in the first bottle. The bromine-water is now run into the bottle containing the standard solution of carbolic acid from a burette until there is no further precipitate; the bottle is stoppered and shaken after every addition. Towards the end of the reaction the precipitate forms but slowly, and when the carbolic acid is saturated, the slight excess of bromine-water gives the solution a pale yellow tint. The solution from the sample is treated in the same way, and from the amount of bromine-water used, the percentage of the sample is obtained by making the usual calculations. Thus, supposing that 5 c.c. of the standard required 15 c.c. of the bromine-water for precipitation, and 10 c.c. of the solution of the sample required 17 c.c., the calculation would be $15 \times 2 : 17 = 100 : x$ per cent. With most samples of crude carbolic acid, the precipitate does not readily separate. It is then best to add a little of the precipitate already obtained by testing the standard solution, which rapidly clears the liquid.

Koppeschaar's volumetric method is more exact, but also more elaborate, than the one just described. Caustic normal soda is treated with bromine until permanently yellow, and the excess of bromine is then driven off by boiling. The liquid now contains $5NaBr + NaBrO_3$, and on adding this to a solution containing carbolic acid, and a sufficient quantity of hydrochloric acid to combine with the sodium, the following reactions occur:—

(1.) $5NaBr + NaBrO_3 + 6HCl = 6NaCl + 6Br + 3H_2O$;

and

(2.) $C_6H_6O + 6Br = C_6H_3Br_3O + 3HBr$.

Any excess of bromine liberated in the first reaction above that necessary for the second, will exist in the free state, and from the amount of bromine which remains free the quantity of carbolic acid can be calculated, always provided the strength of the bromine solution is first known. The volumetric part of the analysis, therefore, merely amounts to the determination of free bromine, which is best found by causing it to react on potassium iodide, and ascertaining the amount of free iodine by titration with a standard solution of sodium thiosulphate. In other words, titrate in this way the standard alkaline bromine solution, using as an indicator starch paste until the blue colour disappears. Another method of indicating the end of the reaction is by the use of strips of paper first soaked in starch solution, and dried, and then the same papers moistened with zinc iodide, and again dried; the least excess of bromine sets free iodine, and strikes a blue colour.

Colorimetric Method of Estimation.—A very simple and ever-ready way of approximately estimating minute quantities of the phenols consists in shaking up 10 grms. of the sample with water, allowing any tar or insoluble impurities to subside. Ten c.c. of the clear fluid are then taken, and half a c.c. of a 5 per cent. solution of ferric chloride added. The colour produced is imitated by a standard solution of carbolic acid, and a similar amount of the reagent, on the usual principles of colorimetric analysis.

§ 237. **Carbolic Acid Powders.**—Siliceous carbolic acid powders are placed in a retort and distilled. Towards the end the heat may be raised to approaching redness. The distillate separates into two portions—the one aqueous, the other consisting of the acids—and the volume may be read off, if the distillate be received in a graduated receiver. Carbolic acid powders, having lime as a basis, may be distilled in the same way, after first decomposing with sulphuric acid. The estimation of the neutral tar oils in the distillate is easily performed by shaking the distillate with caustic soda solution, which dissolves completely the tar acids. The volume of the oils may be directly read off if the receiver is a graduated tube. Allen[218] has suggested the addition of a known volume of petroleum to the distillate, which dissolves the tar oils, and easily separates, and thus the volume may be more accurately determined, a correction being of course made by subtracting the volume of petroleum first added.

§ 238. **Carbolic Acid Soap.**—A convenient quantity of soap is carefully weighed, and dissolved in a solution of caustic soda by means of heat. A saturated solution of salt is next added, sufficient to precipitate entirely the soap,

[218] *Op. cit.*, i. p. 310.

which is filtered off; the filtrate is acidified with hydrochloric acid, and bromine water added. The precipitated tribromo-phenol is first melted by heat, then allowed to cool, and the mass removed from the liquid, dried, and weighed.

X.—Nitro-Benzene.

§ 239.—Nitro-benzene is the product resulting from the action of strong nitric acid on benzene. Its chemical formula is $C_6H_5NO_2$. When pure, it is of a pale yellow colour, of a density of 1.186, and boils at from 205° to 210°. It may be obtained in prismatic crystals by exposure to a temperature of 3°. Its smell is exactly the same as that from the oil or essence of bitter almonds; and it is from this circumstance, under the name of "essence of mirbane," much used in the preparation of perfumes and flavouring agents.

In commerce there are three kinds of nitro-benzene—the purest, with the characters given above; a heavier nitro-benzene, boiling at 210° to 220°; and a very heavy variety, boiling at 222° to 235° The last is specially used for the preparation of aniline, or aniline blue. Nitro-benzene has been used as an adulterant of bitter almond oil, but the detection is easy (see "Foods," p. 551). Nitro-benzene was first discovered by Mitscherlich in 1834, and its poisonous properties were first pointed out by Casper[219] in 1859. Its technical use in perfumes, &c., dates from about 1848, and in the twenty-eight years intervening between that date and 1876, Jübell[220] has collected 42 cases of poisoning by this agent, 13 of which were fatal. One of these cases was suicidal, the rest accidental.

§ 240. **Effects of Poisoning by Nitro-benzene.**—Nitro-benzene is a very powerful poison, whether taken in the form of vapour or as a liquid. The action of the vapour on animals has been studied by Eulenberg[221] and others. One experiment will serve as an illustration. Fifteen grms. of nitro-benzene were evaporated on warm sand under a glass shade, into which a cat was introduced. There was immediately observed in the animal much salivation, and quickened and laboured breathing. After thirty minutes' exposure, on removing the shade to repeat the dose of 15 grms., the cat for the moment escaped. On being put back there was again noticed the salivation and running at the eyes, with giddiness, and repeated rising and falling. The animal at last, about one hour and forty minutes after the first dose, succumbed with dyspnœa, and died with progressive paralysis of the respiration. The membranes of the brain were found gorged with blood, the lungs liver-coloured, the mucous membrane of the trachea—to the finest sub-divisions of the bronchia—reddened, inflamed, and clothed with a fine frothy mucus. The left side of the heart was filled with thick black blood. The bladder contained 8 grms. of clear urine, in which aniline was discovered. There was a notable smell of bitter almonds.

§ 241. The effects of the vapour on man are somewhat different in their details to those just described. In a remarkable case related by Dr. Letheby, a man, aged 42, had spilt some nitro-benzene over his clothes. He went about several hours breathing an atmosphere of nitro-benzene, he then became drowsy, his expression was stupid, and his gait unsteady, presenting all the appearances of intoxication. The stupor suddenly deepened into coma, and the man died; the fatal course being altogether about nine hours—viz., four hours before coma, and five hours of total insensibility.

An interesting case of poisoning by the vapour is recorded by Taylor.[222] A woman, aged 30, tasted a liquid used for flavouring pastry, which was afterwards chemically identified as pure nitro-benzene. She immediately spat it out, finding that it had an acrid taste, and probably did not swallow more than a drop. In replacing the bottle, however, she spilt about a tablespoonful, and allowed it to remain for some minutes; it was a small room, and the vapour rapidly pervaded it, and caused illness in herself as well as in a fellow-servant. She had a strange feeling of numbness in the tongue, and in three hours and a quarter after the accident was seen by a medical man; she then presented all the appearances of prussic acid poisoning. The eyes were bright and glassy, the features pale and ghastly, the lips and nails purple, as if stained with blackberries, the skin clammy, and the pulse feeble, but the mind was then clear. An emetic was administered, but she suddenly became unconscious; the emetic acted, and brought up a fluid with an odour of nitro-benzene. The stomach-pump was also used, but the liquid obtained had scarcely any odour of nitro-benzene. In about eleven hours consciousness returned, and in about seventeen hours she partially recovered, but complained of flashes of light and strange colours before her eyes. Recovery was not complete for

[219] *Vierteljahrsschrift für ger. Med.*, 1859, Bd. xvi. p. 1.
[220] *Die Vergiftungen mit Blausäure u. Nitro-benzol in forensischer Beziehung*, Erlangen, 1876.
[221] *Gewerbe Hygiene*, S. 607, Berlin, 1876.
[222] *Poisons*, Third Edition, p. 665.

weeks. In this case the small quantity swallowed would probably of itself have produced no symptoms, and the effects are to be mainly ascribed to the breathing of the vapour.

§ 242. The liquid, when swallowed, acts almost precisely in the same way as the vapour, and the symptoms resemble very much those produced by prussic acid. The great distinction between prussic acid and nitro-benzene poisoning is that, in the latter, there is an interval between the taking of the poison and its effects. This is, indeed, one of the strangest phenomena of nitro-benzene poisoning, for the person, after taking it, may appear perfectly well for periods varying from a quarter of an hour to two or three hours, or even longer, and then there may be most alarming symptoms, followed by rapid death. Poisoning by nitro-benzene satisfies the ideal of the dramatist, who requires, for the purposes of his plot, poisons not acting at once, but with an interval sufficiently prolonged to admit of lengthy rhapsodies and a complicated *dénouement*. On drinking the poison there is a burning taste in the mouth, shortly followed by a very striking blueness or purple appearance of the lips, tongue, skin, nails, and even the conjunctivæ. This curious colour of the skin has, in one or two instances, been witnessed an hour before any feeling of illness manifested itself; vomiting then comes on, the vomited matter smelling of nitro-benzene. The skin is cold, there is great depression, and the pulse is small and weak. The respiration is affected, the breathing being slow and irregular, the breath smelling strongly of the liquid, and the odour often persisting for days. A further stage is that of loss of consciousness, and this comes on with all the suddenness of a fit of apoplexy. The coma is also similar in appearance to apoplectic coma, but there have frequently been seen trismus and convulsions of the extremities. The pupils are dilated and do not react to light, and reflex sensibility is sometimes completely extinguished. Cases vary a little in their main features; in a few the blue skin and the deep sleep are the only symptoms noted. Death, for the most part, occurs after a period of from eight to twenty-four hours (occasionally as soon as four or five hours) after taking the poison.

From the following remarkable train of symptoms in a dog, it is probable, indeed, that nitro-benzene, taken by a human being, might produce death, after a rather prolonged period of time, by its secondary effects:—To a half-bred greyhound[223] were administered 15 grms. of nitro-benzene, when shortly after there were noticed much salivation, shivering, and muscular twitchings. The same dose was repeated at the end of five, of seven, and of eight hours respectively, so that the dog altogether took 60 grms., but with no other apparent symptom than the profuse salivation. On the following day, the dog voided a tapeworm; vomiting supervened; the heart's action was quickened, and the breathing difficult; convulsions followed, and the pupils were seen to be dilated. For eight days the dog suffered from dyspnœa, quickened pulse, shivering of the legs or of the whole body, tetanic spasms, bloody motions, great thirst and debility. The temperature gradually sank under 25°, and the animal finally died. The autopsy showed, as the most striking change, the whole mucous membrane of the intestinal tract covered with a yellow layer, which chemical analysis proved to be caused by picric acid, and in the urine, liver, and lungs, aniline was discovered.

§ 243. **Fatal Dose.**—It is probable, from recorded cases, that 1 grm. (15.4 grains) would be quite sufficient to kill an adult, and, under favourable circumstances, less than that quantity. It would seem that spirituous liquids especially hasten and intensify the action of nitro-benzene, so that a drunken person, *cæteris paribus*, taking the poison with spirits, would be more affected than taking it under other conditions.

In a case related by Stevenson,[224] in which so small a quantity as 1.74 grm. was taken in seven doses, spread

[223] Eulenberg, *Gewerbe Hygiene*, S. 607.

[224] This case is not uninteresting. Through a mistake in reading an extremely illegible prescription, M. S. S., æt. 21, was supplied by a druggist with the following mixture:—

℞. Benzole-Nit., ʒiij.
Ol. Menth, pep., ʒss.
Ol. Olivæ, ʒx.
gutt. xxx., t. ds.

He took on sugar seven doses, each of 20 minims, equalling in all 23 min. (or by weight 27.1 grains, 1.74 grm.) of nitro-benzene—viz., three doses on the first day, three on the second, and one on the morning of the third day. The first two days he was observed to be looking pale and ill, but went on with his work until the seventh dose, which he took on the third day at 9 A.M. About 2 P.M. (or six hours after taking the seventh dose), he fell down insensible, the body pale blue, and with all the symptoms already described in the text, and usually seen in nitro-benzene poisoning. With suitable treatment he recovered. The next morning, from 8 ounces of urine some nitro-benzene was extracted by shaking with chloroform.—Thos. Stevenson, M.D., in *Guy's Hospital Reports*, MS., vol. xxi., 1876.

over more than forty-eight hours; there were yet extremely alarming symptoms, and the patient seems to have had a narrow escape. On the other hand, a woman admitted into the General Hospital, Vienna, took 100 grms. (about 3½ ozs.) and recovered; on admission she was in a highly cyanotic condition, with small pulse, superficial respiration, and dribbling of urine, which contained nitro-benzol. Artificial respiration was practised, and camphor injections were administered. Under this treatment consciousness was restored, and the patient recovered. On the fourth day the urine resembled that of a case of cystitis (*Lancet*, Jan. 16, 1894). The quantity of nitro-benzene which would be fatal, if breathed, is not known with any accuracy.

§ 244. **Pathological Appearances.**—The more characteristic appearances seem to be, a dark brown or even black colour of the blood, which coagulates with difficulty (an appearance of the blood that has even been noticed during life), venous hyperæmia of the brain and its membranes, and general venous engorgement. In the stomach, when the fluid has been swallowed, the mucous membrane is sometimes reddened diffusely, and occasionally shows ecchymoses of a punctiform character.

§ 245. **The essential action of nitro-benzene** is of considerable physiological interest. The blood is certainly in some way changed, and gives the spectrum of acid hæmatin.[225] Filehne has found that the blood loses, in a great degree, the power of carrying and imparting oxygen to the tissues, and its content of carbon dioxide is also increased. Thus, the normal amount of oxygen gas which the arterial blood of a hound will give up is 17 per cent.; but in the case of a dog which had been poisoned with nitro-benzene, it sank to 1 per cent. During the dyspnœa from which the dog suffered, the carbon dioxide exhaled was greater than the normal amount, and the arterial blood (the natural content of which should have been 30 per cent. of this gas), only gave up 9 per cent. Filehne seeks to explain the peculiar colour of the skin by the condition of the blood, but the explanation is not altogether satisfactory. Some part of the nitro-benzene, without doubt, is reduced to aniline in the body—an assertion often made, and as often contradicted—but it has been found in too many cases to admit of question. It would also seem from the experiment on the dog, that a conversion into picric acid is not impossible. A yellow colour of the skin and conjunctivæ, as if picric-acid-stained, has been noticed in men suffering under slow poisoning by nitro-benzene.

§ 246. **Detection and Separation of Nitro-Benzene from the Animal Tissues.**—It is evident from the changes which nitro-benzene may undergo that the expert, in any case of suspected nitro-benzene poisoning, must specially look (1) for nitro-benzene, (2) for aniline, and (3) for picric acid. The best general method for the separation of nitro-benzene is to shake up the liquid (or finely-divided solid) with light benzoline (petroleum ether), which readily dissolves nitro-benzene. On evaporation of the petroleum ether, the nitro-benzene is left, perhaps mixed with fatty matters. On treating with cold water, the fats rise to the surface, and the nitro-benzene sinks to the bottom; so that, by means of a separating funnel, the nitro-benzene may be easily removed from animal fats. The oily drops, or fine precipitate believed to be nitro-benzene, may be dissolved in spirit and reduced to aniline by the use of nascent hydrogen, developed from iron filings by hydrochloric acid, and the fluid tested with bleaching powder, or, the aniline itself may be recovered by alkalising the fluid, and shaking up with ether in the separation-tube, the ether dissolves the aniline, and leaves it, on spontaneous evaporation, as an oily yellowish mass, which, on the addition of a few drops of sodic hypochlorite, strikes a blue or violet-blue—with acids, a rose-red—and with bromine, a flesh-red. It gives alkaloidal reactions with such general reagents as platinum chloride, picric acid, &c. Aniline itself may be extracted from the tissues and fluids of the body by petroleum ether, but in any special search it will be better to treat the organs as in Stas' process—that is, with strong alcohol, acidified with sulphuric acid. After a suitable digestion in this menstruum, filter, and then, after evaporating the alcohol, dissolve the alcoholic extract in water; alkalise the aqueous solution, and extract the aniline by shaking it up with light benzoline. On separating the benzoline, the aniline will be left, and may be dissolved in feebly-acid water, and the tests before enumerated tried.

Malpurgo[226] recommends the following test for nitro-benzene:—2 drops of melted phenol, 3 drops of water, and a fragment of caustic potash are boiled in a small porcelain dish, and to the boiling liquid the aqueous solution to be tested is added. On prolonged boiling, if nitro-benzene is present, a crimson ring is produced at the edges of the liquid; this crimson colour, on the addition of a little bleaching powder, turns emerald-green.

Oil of bitter almonds may be distinguished from nitro-benzene by the action of manganese dioxide and sulphuric acid; bitter almond oil treated in this way loses its odour, nitro-benzene is unaltered. To apply the test, the liquid must be heated on the water-bath for a little time.

---

[225] Filehne, W., "*Ueber die Gift-Wirkungen des Nitrobenzols,*" *Arch. für exper. Pathol. u. Pharm.*, ix. 329.

[226] *Zeit. anal. Chem.*, xxxii. 235.

XI.—Dinitro-benzol.

§ 247. **Dinitro-benzol**, $C_6H_4(NO_2)_2$ (ortho-, meta-, para-).—The ortho-compound is produced by the action of nitric acid on benzol, aided by heat in the absence of strong sulphuric acid to fix water. Some of the para-dinitro-benzol is at the same time produced. The meta-compound is obtained by the action of fuming nitric acid on nitro-benzol at a boiling temperature.

The physical properties of the three dinitro-benzols are briefly as follows:—

Ortho-d. is in the form of needles; m.p. 118°.

Meta-d. crystallises in plates; m.p. 90°.

Para-d. crystallises, like the ortho-compound, in needles, but the melting-point is much higher, 171° to 172°.

Just as nitro-benzol by reduction yields aniline, so do the nitro-benzols on reduction yield ortho-, meta-, or para-phenylene diamines.

Meta-phenylene diamine is an excellent test for nitrites; and, since the commercial varieties of dinitro-benzol either consist mainly or in part of meta-dinitro-benzol, the toxicological detection is fairly simple, and is based upon the conversion of the dinitro-benzol into meta-phenylene-diamine.

Dinitro-benzol is at present largely employed in the manufacture of explosives, such as roburite, sicherheit, and others. It has produced much illness among the workpeople in the manufactures, and amongst miners whose duty it has been to handle such explosives.

§ 248. **Effects of Dinitro-benzol.**—Huber[227] finds that if dinitro-benzol is given to frogs by the mouth in doses of from 100 to 200 mgrms., death takes place in a few hours. Doses of from 2.5 to 5 mgrms. cause general dulness and ultimately complete paralysis, and death in from one to six days.

Rabbits are killed by doses of 400 mgrms., in time varying from twenty-two hours to four days.

In a single experiment on a small dog, the weight of which was 5525 grms., the dog died in six hours after a dose of 600 mgrms.

It is therefore probable that a dose of 100 mgrms. per kilo would kill most warm-blooded animals.

A transient exposure to dinitro-benzol vapours in man causes serious symptoms; for instance, in one of Huber's cases, a student of chemistry had been engaged for one hour and a half only in preparing dinitro-benzol, and soon afterwards his comrades remarked that his face was of a deep blue colour. On admission to hospital, on the evening of the same day, he complained of slight headache and sleeplessness; both cheeks, the lips, the muscles of the ear, the mucous membrane of the lips and cheeks, and even the tongue, were all of a more or less intense blue-grey colour. The pulse was dicrotic, 124; T. 37.2°. The next morning the pulse was slower, and by the third day the patient had recovered.

Excellent accounts of the effects of dinitro-benzol in roburite factories have been published by Dr. Ross[228] and Professor White,[229] of Wigan. Mr. Simeon Snell[230] has also published some most interesting cases of illness, cases which have been as completely investigated as possible. As an example of the symptoms produced, one of Mr. Snell's cases may be here quoted.

C. F. W., aged 38, consulted Mr. Snell for his defective sight on April 9, 1892. He had been a mixer at a factory for the manufacture of explosives. He was jaundiced, the conjunctiva yellow, and the lips blue. He was short of breath, and after the day's work experienced aching of the forearms and legs and tingling of the fingers. The urine was black in colour, of sp. gr. 1024; it was examined spectroscopically by Mr. MacMunn, who reported the black colour as due neither to indican, nor to blood, nor bile, but to be caused by some pigment belonging to the aromatic series. The patient's sight had been failing since the previous Christmas. Vision in the right eye was $6/24$, left $6/36$, both optic papillæ were somewhat pale. In each eye there was a central scotoma for red, and contraction of the field (see diagram). The man gradually gave up the work, and ultimately seems to have recovered. It is, however, interesting to note that, after having left the work for some weeks, he went back for a single day to the "mixing," and was taken very ill, being insensible and delirious for five hours.

§ 249. **The Blood in Nitro-benzol Poisoning.**—The effect on the blood has been specially studied by Huber.[231]

[227] "*Beiträge zur Giftwirkung des Dinitrobenzols*," A. Huber, Virchow's *Archiv*, 1891, Bd. 126, S. 240.

[228] *Medical Chronicle*, 1889, 89.

[229] *Practitioner*, 1889, ii. 15.

[230] *Brit. Med. Journ.*, March 3, 1894.

[231] *Op. cit.*

The blood of rabbits poisoned by dinitro-benzol is of a dark chocolate colour, and the microscope shows destruction of the red corpuscles; the amount of destruction may be gathered from the following:—the blood corpuscles of a rabbit before the experiment numbered 5,588,000 per cubic centimetre; a day after the experiment 4,856,000; a day later 1,004,000; on the third day the rabbit died.

In one rabbit, although the corpuscles sank to 1,416,000, yet recovery took place.

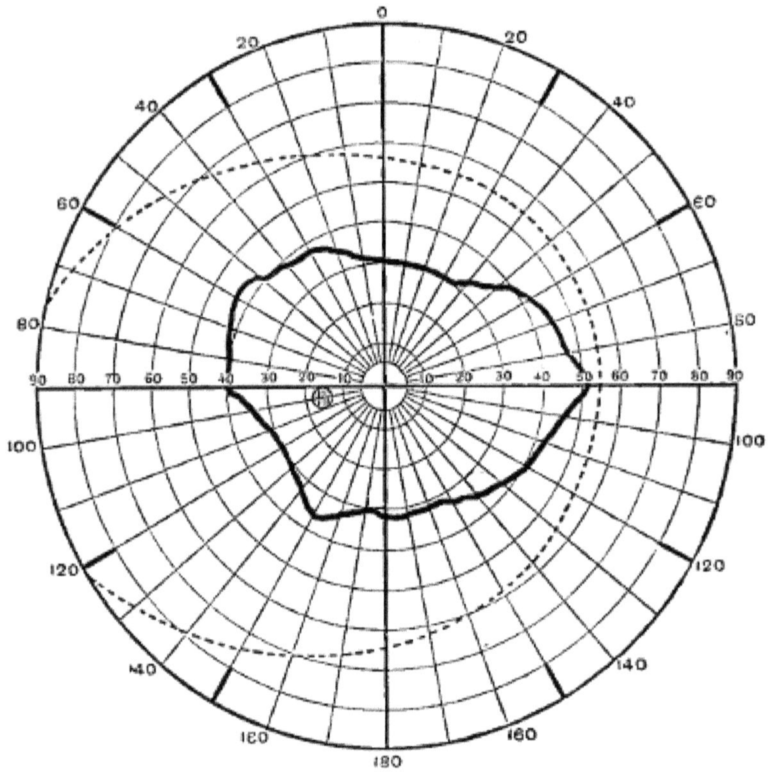

Diagram of Visual Field.

Dr. MacMunn[232] has examined specimens of blood from two of Mr. Snell's patients; he found a distinct departure from the normal; the red corpuscles were smaller than usual, about 5 or 6 μ in diameter, and the appearances were like those seen in pernicious anæmia. Huber, in some of his experiments on animals, found a spectroscopic change in the blood, viz., certain absorption bands, one in the red between C and D, and two in the green between D and E; the action of reducing agents on this dinitro-benzol blood, as viewed in a spectroscope provided with a scale in which C = 48, D = 62, and E = 80.5, was as follows:—

	Dinitro-Bands. In Red.	In Green.	
	50-52	62-66	70-77
After NH_4SO_4,	53-55	62-66	70-77
„ NH_3,	54-58	60-65	70-77
„ $NH_4SO_4 + NH_3$,	52-55	60-65	70-77

Taking the symptoms as a whole, there has been noted:—a blue colour of the lips, not unfrequently extending over the whole face, and even the conjunctivæ have been of a marked blue colour, giving the sufferer a strange livid

[232] *Op. cit.*

appearance. In other cases there have been jaundice, the conjunctivæ and the skin generally being yellow, the lips blue. Occasionally gastric symptoms are present. Sleeplessness is common, and not unfrequently there is some want of muscular co-ordination, and the man staggers as if drunk. In more than one case there has been noticed sudden delirium. There is in chronic cases always more or less anæmia, and the urine is remarkable in its colour, which ranges from a slightly dark hue up to positive blackness. In a large proportion of cases there is ophthalmic trouble, the characteristics of which (according to Mr. Snell) are "failure of sight, often to a considerable degree, in a more or less equal extent on the two sides; concentric attraction of visual field with, in many cases, a central colour scotoma; enlargement of retinal vessels, especially the veins; some blurring, never extensive, of edges of disc, and a varying degree of pallor of its surface—the condition of retinal vessels spoken of being observed in workers with the dinitro-benzol, independently of complaints of defective sight. Cessation of work leads to recovery."

§ 250. **Detection of Dinitro-benzol.**—Dinitro-benzol may be detected in urine, in blood, and in fluids generally, by the following process:—Place tinfoil in the fluid, and add hydrochloric acid to strong acidity, after allowing the hydrogen to be developed for at least an hour, make the fluid alkaline by caustic soda, and extract with ether in a separating tube; any metaphenylene-diamine will be contained in the ether; remove the ether into a flask, and distil it off; dissolve the residue in a little water.

Acidify a solution of sodium nitrite with dilute sulphuric acid; on adding the solution, if it contains metaphenylene-diamine, a yellow to red colour will be produced, from the formation of Bismarck brown (triamido-phenol).

XII.—Hydrocyanic Acid.

§ 251. **Hydrocyanic Acid (hydric cyanide)**—specific gravity of liquid 0.7058 at 18° C., boiling-point 26.5° (80° F.), HCy = 27.—The anhydrous acid is not an article of commerce, and is only met with in the laboratory. It is a colourless, transparent liquid, and so extremely volatile that, if a drop fall on a glass plate, a portion of it freezes. It has a very peculiar peach-blossom odour, and is intensely poisonous. It reddens litmus freely and transiently, dissolves red oxide of mercury freely, forms a white precipitate of argentic cyanide when treated with silver nitrate, and responds to the other tests described hereafter.

§ 252. **Medicinal Preparations of Prussic Acid.**—The B.P. acid is a watery solution of prussic acid; its specific gravity should be 0.997, and it should contain 2 per cent. of the anhydrous acid, 2 per cent. is also the amount specified in the pharmacopœias of Switzerland and Norway, and in that of Borussica (VI. ed.); the latter ordains, however, a spirituous solution, and the Norwegian an addition of 1 per cent. of concentrated sulphuric acid. The French prussic acid is ordered to be prepared of a strength equalling 10 per cent.

The adulterations or impurities of prussic acid are hydrochloric, sulphuric,[233] and formic acids. Traces of silver may be found in the French acid, which is prepared from cyanide of silver. Tartaric acid is also occasionally present. Hydrochloric acid is most readily detected by neutralising with ammonia, and evaporating to dryness in a water-bath; the ammonium cyanide decomposes and volatilises, leaving as a saline residue chloride of ammonium. This may easily be identified by the precipitate of chloride of silver, which its solution gives on testing with silver nitrate, and the deep brown precipitate with Nessler solution. Sulphuric acid is, of course, detected by chloride of barium; formic acid by boiling a small quantity with a little mercuric oxide; if present, the oxide will be reduced, and metallic mercury fall as a grey precipitate. Silver, tartaric acid, and any other fixed impurities are detected by evaporating the acid to dryness, and examining any residue which may be left. It may be well to give the various strengths of the acids of commerce in a tabular form:—

		Per cent.
British Pharmacopœia, Switzerland, and Bor. (vj),		2
France,		10
Vauquelin's	Acid,	3 .3
Scheele's	„	4 to 5[234]

[233] A trace of sulphuric or hydrochloric acid should not be called an *adulteration*, for it greatly assists the preservation, and therefore makes the acid of greater therapeutic efficiency.

[234] Strength very uncertain.

Riner's	„	10	
Robiquet's	„	50	
Schraeder's	„	1	.5
Duflos'	„	9	
Pfaff's	„	10	
Koller's	„	25	

In English commerce, the analyst will scarcely meet with any acid stronger than Scheele's 5 per cent.

Impure oil of bitter almonds contains hydric cyanide in variable quantity, from 5 per cent. up to 14 per cent. There is an officinal preparation obtained by digesting cherry-laurel leaves in water, and then distilling a certain portion over. This *Aqua Lauro-cerasi* belongs to the old school of pharmacy, and is of uncertain strength, but varies from .7 to 1 per cent. of HCN.

§ 253. **Poisoning by Prussic Acid.**—Irrespective of suicidal or criminal poisoning, accidents from prussic acid may occur—

1. From the use of the cyanides in the arts.

2. From the somewhat extensive distribution of the acid, or rather of prussic-acid producing substances in the vegetable kingdom.

1. **In the Arts.**—The galvanic silvering[235] and gilding of metals, photography, the colouring of black silks, the manufacture of Berlin blue, the dyeing of woollen cloth, and in a few other manufacturing processes, the alkaline cyanides are used, and not unfrequently fumes of prussic acid developed.

2. **In the Animal Kingdom.**—One of the myriapods (*Chilognathen*) contains glands at the roots of the hairs, which secrete prussic acid; when the insect is seized, the poisonous secretion is poured out from the so-called *foramina repugnatoria*.

3. **In the Vegetable Kingdom.**—A few plants contain cyanides, and many contain amygdalin, or bodies formed on the type of amygdalin. In the presence of emulsin (or similar principles) and water, this breaks up into prussic acid and other compounds—an interesting reaction usually represented thus—

$C_{20}H_{27}NO_{11} + 2H_2O = CNH + C_7H_6O + 2C_6H_{12}O_6$.

1 equivalent of amygdalin—*i.e.*, 457 parts—yielding 1 equivalent of CNH or 27 parts; in other words, 100 parts of amygdalin yield theoretically 5.909 parts of prussic acid,[236] so that, the amount of either being known, the other can be calculated from it.

Greshoff[237] has discovered an amygdalin-like glucoside in the two tropical trees *Pygeum parriflorum* and *P. latifolium*. The same author states that the leaves of *Gymnema latifolium*, one of the Asclepiads, yields to distillation benzaldehyde hydrocyanide. Both *Lasia* and *Cyrtosperma*, plants belonging to the natural family of the Orontads, contain in their flowers potassic cyanide. *Pangium edule*, according to Greshoff, contains so much potassic cyanide that he was able to prepare a considerable quantity of that salt from one sample of the plant. An Indian plant (*Hydnocarpus inebrians*) also contains a cyanide, and has been used for the purpose of destroying fish. Among the Tiliads, Greshoff found that *Echinocarpus Sigun* yielded hydrocyanic acid on distillation. Even the common linseed contains a glucoside which breaks up into sugar, prussic acid, and a ketone.

The following plants, with many others, all yield, by appropriate treatment, more or less prussic acid:—Bitter almonds (*Amygdalus communis*); the *Amygdalus persica*; the cherry laurel (*Prunus laurocerasus*); the kernels of the plum (*Prunus domestica*); the bark, leaves, flowers, and fruit of the wild service-tree (*Prunus padus*); the kernels of the common cherry and the apple; the leaves of the *Prunus capricida*; the bark of the *Pr. virginiana*; the flowers and kernels of the *Pr. spinosa*; the leaves of the *Cerasus acida*; the bark and almost all parts of the *Sorbus aucuparia*,

[235] The preparation used for the silvering of copper vessels is a solution of cyanide of silver in potassic cyanide, to which is added finely powdered chalk. Manipulations with this fluid easily develop hydrocyanic acid fumes, which, in one case related by Martin (*Aerztl. Intelligenzbl.*, p. 135, 1872), were powerful enough to produce symptoms of poisoning.

[236] According to Liebig and Wöhler, 17 grms. of amygdalin yield 1 of prussic acid (*i.e.*, 5.7 per cent.) and 8 of oil of bitter almonds. Thirty-four parts of amygdalin, mixed with 66 of emulsin of almonds, give a fluid equalling the strength of acid of most pharmacopœias, viz., 2 per cent.

[237] M. Greshoff—*Erster Bericht über die Untersuchung von Pflanzenstoffen Niederländisch-Indiens. Mittheilungen aus dem chemisch-pharmakologischen Laboratorium des botan. Gartens des Staates*, vii., Batavia, 1890, Niederländisch. Dr. Greshoff's research indicates that there are several other cyanide-yielding plants than those mentioned in the text.

S. hybrida, and *S. torminalis*; the young twigs of the *Cratægus oxyacantha*; the leaves and partly also the flowers of the shrubby *Spiræaceæ*, such as *Spiræa aruncus*, *S. sorbifolia*, and *S. japonica*;[238] together with the roots of the bitter and sweet *Cassava*.

In only a few of these, however, has the exact amount of either prussic acid or amygdalin been determined; 1 grm. of bitter almond pulp is about equal to 2½ mgrms. of anhydrous prussic acid. The kernels from the stones of the cherry, according to Geiseler, yield 3 per cent. of amygdalin; therefore, 1 grm. equals 1.7 mgrm. of HCN.

§ 254. The wild service-tree (*Prunus padus*) and the cherry-laurel (*Prunus Laurocerasus*) contain, not amygdalin but a compound of amygdalin with amygdalic acid; to this has been given the name of laurocerasin. It was formerly known as amorphous amygdalin; its formula is $C_{40}H_{55}NO_{24}$; 933 parts are equivalent to 27 of hydric cyanide—that is, 100 parts equal to 2.89.

In the bark of the service-tree, Lehmann found .7 per cent. of laurocerasin (= .02 HCN), and in the leaves of the cherry-laurel 1.38 per cent. (= 0.39 HCN).

Francis,[239] in a research on the prussic acid in cassava root, gives as the mean in the sweet cassava .0168 per cent., in the bitter .0275 per cent., the maximum in each being respectively .0238 per cent., and .0442 per cent. The bitter-fresh cassava root has long been known as a very dangerous poison; but the sweet has hitherto been considered harmless, although it is evident that it also contains a considerable quantity of prussic acid.

The kernels of the peach contain about 2.85 per cent. amygdalin (= .17 HCN); those of the plum .96 per cent. (= .056 HCN); and apple pips .6 per cent. (= .035 per cent. HCN).

It is of great practical value to know, even approximately, the quantity of prussic acid contained in various fruits, since it has been adopted as a defence in criminal cases that the deceased was poisoned by prussic acid developed in substances eaten.

§ 255. **Statistics.**—Poisoning by the cyanides (prussic acid or cyanide of potassium) occupies the third place among poisons in order of frequency in this country, and accounts for about 40 deaths annually.

In the ten years ending 1892 there were recorded no less than 395 cases of accidental, suicidal, or homicidal poisoning by prussic acid and potassic cyanide. The further statistical details may be gathered from the following tables:—

DEATHS IN ENGLAND AND WALES DURING THE TEN YEARS 1883-1892 FROM PRUSSIC ACID AND POTASSIC CYANIDE.

Prussic Acid (Accident or Negligence).

Ages,	0-1	1-5	5-15	15-25	25-65	65 and above	Total
Males,	...	1	1	1	12	1	16
Females,	1	1	...	2	7	...	11
Totals,	1	2	1	3	19	1	27

Cyanide of Potassium (Accident or Negligence).

Ages,	1-5	5-15	15-25	25-65	65 and above	Total
Males,	1	1	4	1	...	7
Females,	1	...	...	3	...	4
Totals,	2	1	4	4	...	11

Prussic Acid (Suicide).

[238] The bark and green parts of the *Prunus avium*, L., *Prunus mahaleb*, L., and herbaceous *Spiræa* yield no prussic acid.
[239] "On Prussic Acid from Cassava," *Analyst*, April 1877, p. 5.

Ages,	15-25	25-65	65 and above	Total
Males,	23	156	23	202
Females,	5	13	1	19
Totals,	28	169	24	221

Potassium Cyanide (Suicide).

Ages,	5-15	15-25	25-65	65 and above	Total
Males,	1	6	88	5	100
Females,	...	6	15	1	22
Totals,	1	12	103	6	122

To these figures must be added 10 cases of murder (2 males and 8 females) by prussic acid, and 4 cases of murder (3 males and 1 female) by potassic cyanide.

In order to ascertain the proportion in which the various forms of commercial cyanides cause death, and also the proportion of accidental, suicidal, and criminal deaths from the same cause, Falck collated twelve years of statistics from medical literature with the following result:—

In 51 cases of cyanide poisoning, 29 were caused by potassic cyanide, 9 by hydric cyanide, 5 by oil of bitter almonds, 3 by peach stones (these 3 were children, and are classed as "domestic," that is, taking the kernels as a food), 3 by bitter almonds (1 of the 3 suicidal and followed by death, the other 2 "domestic"), 1 by tartaric acid and potassic cyanide (a suicidal case, an apothecary), and 1 by ferro-cyanide of potassium and tartaric acid. Of the 43 cases first mentioned, 21 were suicidal, 7 criminal, 8 domestic, and 7 medicinal; the 43 patients were 24 men, 14 children, and 5 women.

The cyanides are very rarely used for the purpose of murder: a poison which has a strong smell and a perceptible taste, and which also kills with a rapidity only equalled by deadly bullet or knife-wounds, betrays its presence with too many circumstances of a tragic character to find favour in the dark and secret schemes of those who desire to take life by poison. In 793 poisoning cases of a criminal character in France, 4 only were by the cyanides.

Hydric and potassic cyanides were once the favourite means of self-destruction employed by suicidal photographers, chemists, scientific medical men, and others in positions where such means are always at hand; but, of late years, the popular knowledge of poisons has increased, and self-poisoning by the cyanides scarcely belongs to a particular class. A fair proportion of the deaths are also due to accident or unfortunate mistakes, and a still smaller number to the immoderate or improper use of cyanide-containing vegetable products.

§ 256. **Accidental and Criminal Poisoning by Prussic Acid.**—The poison is almost always taken by the mouth into the stomach, but occasionally in other ways—such, for example, as in the case of the illustrious chemist, Scheele, who died from inhalation of the vapour of the acid which he himself discovered, owing to the breaking of a flask. There is also the case related by Tardieu, in which cyanide of potassium was introduced under the nails; and that mentioned by Carrière,[240] in which a woman gave herself, with suicidal intent, an enema containing cyanide of potassium. It has been shown by experiments, in which every care was taken to render it impossible for the fumes to be inhaled, that hydrocyanic acid applied to the eye of warm-blooded animals may destroy life in a few minutes.[241]

With regard to errors in dispensing, the most tragic case on record is that related by Arnold:[242]—A pharmaceutist had put in a mixture for a child potassic cyanide instead of potassic chlorate, and the child died after the first dose: the chemist, however, convinced that he had made no mistake, to show the harmlessness of the preparation, drank some of it, and there and then died; while Dr. Arnold himself, incautiously tasting the draught, fell insensible, and was unconscious for six hours.

§ 257. **Fatal Dose.**—Notwithstanding the great number of persons who in every civilised country fall victims

[240] "*Empoisonnement par le cyanure de potassium,—guérison,*" *Bullet. général de Thérap.*, 1869, No. 30.
[241] N. Gréhant, *Compt. rend. Soc. Biol.* [9], xi. 64, 65.
[242] Arnold, A. B., "Case of Poisoning by the Cyanide of Potassium," *Amer. Journ. of Med. Scien.*, 1869.

to the cyanides, it is yet somewhat doubtful what is the minimum dose likely to kill an adult healthy man. The explanation of this uncertainty is to be sought mainly in the varying strength of commercial prussic acid, which varies from 1.5 (Schraeder's) to 50 per cent. (Robiquet's), and also in the varying condition of the person taking the poison, more especially whether the stomach be full or empty. In by far the greater number, the dose taken has been much beyond that necessary to produce death, but this observation is true of most poisonings.

The dictum of Taylor, that a quantity of commercial prussic acid, equivalent to 1 English grain (65 mgrm.) of the anhydrous acid, would, under ordinary circumstances, be sufficient to destroy adult life, has been generally accepted by all toxicologists. The minimum lethal dose of potassic cyanide is similarly put at 2.41 grains (.157 grm.). As to bitter almonds, if it be considered that as a mean they contain 2.5 per cent. of amygdalin, then it would take 45 grms., or about 80 almonds, to produce a lethal dose for an adult; with children less—in fact, 4 to 6 bitter almonds are said to have produced poisoning in a child.

§ 258. **Action of Hydric and Potassic Cyanides on Living Organisms.**—Both hydric cyanide and potassic cyanide are poisonous to all living forms, vegetable or animal, with the exception of certain fungi. The cold-blooded animals take a larger relative dose than the warm-blooded, and the mammalia are somewhat more sensitive to the poisonous action of the cyanides than birds; but all are destroyed in a very similar manner, and without any essential difference of action. The symptoms produced by hydric and potassic cyanide are identical, and, as regards general symptoms, what is true as to the one is also true as to the other. There is, however, one important difference in the action of these two substances, if the mere local action is considered, for potassic cyanide is very alkaline, possessing even caustic properties. I have seen, *e.g.*, the gastric mucous membrane of a woman, who had taken an excessive dose of potassic cyanide on an empty stomach, so inflamed and swollen, that its state was similar to that induced by a moderate quantity of solution of potash. On the other hand, the acid properties of hydric cyanide are very feeble, and its effect on mucous membranes or the skin in no way resembles that of the mineral acids.

It attacks the animal system in two ways: the one, a profound interference with the ordinary metabolic changes; the other, a paralysis of the nervous centres. Schönbein discovered that it affected the blood corpuscles in a peculiar way; normal blood decomposes with great ease hydrogen peroxide into oxygen and water. If to normal venous blood a little peroxide of hydrogen be added, the blood at once becomes bright red; but if a trace of prussic acid be present, it is of a dark brown colour. The blood corpuscles, therefore, lose their power of conveying oxygen to all parts of the system, and the phenomena of asphyxia are produced. Geppert[243] has proved that this is really the case by showing, in a series of researches, that, under the action of hydric cyanide, less oxygen is taken up, and less carbon dioxide formed than normal, even if the percentage of oxygen in the atmosphere breathed is artificially increased. The deficiency of oxygen is in part due to the fact that substances like lactic acid, the products of incomplete combustion, are formed instead of CO_2.

At the same time the protoplasm of the tissues is paralysed, and unable to take up the loosely bound oxygen presented. This explains a striking symptom which has been noticed by many observers, that is, if hydrocyanic acid be injected into an animal, the venous blood becomes of a bright red colour; in warm-blooded animals this bright colour is transitory, but in cold-blooded animals, in which the oxidation process is slower, the blood remains bright red.

§ 259. **Symptoms observed in Animals.**—The main differences between the symptoms induced in cold-blooded and warm-blooded animals, by a fatal dose of hydric cyanide, are as follows:—

The respiration in frogs is at first somewhat dyspnœic, then much slowed, and at length it ceases. The heart, at first slowed, later contracts irregularly, and at length gradually stops; but it may continue to beat for several minutes after the respiration has ceased. But all these progressive symptoms are without convulsion. Among warm-blooded animals, on the contrary, convulsions are constant, and the sequence of the symptoms appears to be—dyspnœa, slowing of the pulse, giddiness, falling down, then convulsions with expulsion of the urine and fæces; dilatation of the pupils, exophthalmus, and finally cessation of the pulse and breathing. The convulsions also frequently pass into general paralysis, with loss of reflex movements, weak, infrequent breathing, irregular, quick, and very frequent pulse, and considerable diminution of temperature.

The commencement of the symptoms in animals is extremely rapid, the rapidity varying according to the dose and the concentration of the acid. It was formerly thought that the death from a large dose of the concentrated acid followed far more quickly than could be accounted for by the blood carrying the poison to the nervous centres; but Blake was among the first to point out that this doubt was not supported by facts carefully observed, since there is

[243] Geppert, *Ueber das Wesen der CNH-Vergift; mit einer Tafel*, Berlin, 1889; *Sep.-Abdr. aus Ztschr. f. klin. Med.*, Bd. xv.

always a sufficient interval between the entry of the poison into the body and the first symptoms, to support the theory that the poison is absorbed in the usual manner. Even when Preyer injected a cubic centimetre of 60 per cent. acid into the jugular vein of a rabbit, twenty-nine seconds elapsed before the symptoms commenced. Besides, we have direct experiments showing that the acid—when applied to wounds in limbs, the vessels of which are tied, while the free nervous communication is left open—only acts when the ligature is removed. Magendie describes, in his usual graphic manner, how he killed a dog by injecting into the jugular vein prussic acid, and "*the dog died instantly, as if struck by a cannon ball*," but it is probable that the interval of time was not accurately noted. A few seconds pass very rapidly, and might be occupied even by slowly pressing the piston of the syringe down, and in the absence of accurate measurements, it is surprising how comparatively long intervals of time are unconsciously shortened by the mind. In any case, this observation by Magendie has not been confirmed by the accurate tests of the more recent experimenters; and it is universally acknowledged that, although with strong doses of hydric cyanide injected into the circulation—or, in other words, introduced into the system—in the most favourable conditions for its speediest action, death occurs with appalling suddenness, yet that it takes a time sufficiently long to admit of explanation in the manner suggested. This has forensic importance, which will be again alluded to. Experiments on animals show that a large dose of a dilute acid kills quite as quickly as an equivalent dose of a stronger acid, and in some cases it even seems to act more rapidly. If the death does not take place within a few minutes, life may be prolonged for hours, and even, in rare cases, days, and yet the result be death. Coullon poisoned a dog with prussic acid; it lived for nineteen days, and then died; but this is quite an exceptional case, and when the fatal issue is prolonged beyond an hour, the chance of recovery is considerable.

§ 260. The length of time dogs poisoned by fatal doses survive, generally varies from two to fifteen minutes. The symptoms are convulsions, insensibility of the cornea, cessation of respiration, and, finally, the heart stops—the heart continuing to beat several minutes after the cessation of the respirations.[244] When the dose is short of a fatal one, the symptoms are as follows:—Evident giddiness and distress; the tongue is protruded, the breath is taken in short, hurried gasps, there is salivation, and convulsions rapidly set in, preceded, it may be, by a cry. The convulsions pass into paralysis and insensibility. After remaining in this state some time, the animal again wakes up, as it were, very often howls, and is again convulsed; finally, it sinks into a deep sleep, and wakes up well.

Preyer noticed a striking difference in the symptoms after section of the vagus in animals, which varied according to whether the poison was administered by the lungs, or subcutaneously. In the first case, if the dose is small, the respirations are diminished in frequency; then this is followed by normal breathing; if the dose is larger, there is an increase in the frequency of the respirations. Lastly, if a very large quantity is introduced into the lungs, death quickly follows, with respirations diminished in frequency. On the other hand, when the poison is injected subcutaneously, small doses have no influence on the breathing; but with large doses, there is an increase in the frequency of the respirations, which sink again below the normal standard.

§ 261. **Symptoms in Man.**—When a fatal but not excessive dose of either potassic or hydric cyanide is taken, the sequence of symptoms is as follows:—Salivation, with a feeling of constriction in the throat, nausea, and occasionally vomiting. After a few minutes a peculiar constricting pain in the chest is felt, and the breathing is distinctly affected. Giddiness and confusion of sight rapidly set in, and the person falls to the ground in convulsions similar to those of epilepsy. The convulsions are either general, or attacking only certain groups of muscles; there is often true trismus, and the jaws are so firmly closed that nothing will part them. The respiration is peculiar, the inspiration is short, the expiration prolonged,[245] and between the two there is a long interval ever becoming more protracted as death is imminent. The skin is pale, or blue, or greyish-blue; the eyes are glassy and staring, with dilated pupils; the mouth is covered with foam, and the breath smells of the poison; the pulse, at first quick and small, sinks in a little while in frequency, and at length cannot be felt. Involuntary evacuation of fæces, urine, and semen is often observed, and occasionally there has been vomiting, and a portion of the vomit has been aspirated into the air-passages. Finally, the convulsions pass into paralysis, abolition of reflex sensibility, and gradual ceasing of the respiration. With large doses these different stages may occur, but the course is so rapid that they are merged the one into the other, and are undistinguishable. The shortest time between the taking of the acid and the commencement of the symptoms may be put at about ten seconds. If, however, a large amount of the vapour is

[244] N. Gréhant, *Compt. rend.*, t. 109, pp. 502, 503.

[245] In a case quoted by Seidel (Maschka's *Handbuch*, p. 321), a man, 36 years of age, four or five minutes after swallowing 150 mgrms. anhydrous HCN in spirits, lay apparently lifeless, without pulse or breathing. After a few minutes was noticed an extraordinary deep expiration, by which the ribs were drawn in almost to the spine, and the chest made quite hollow.

inhaled at once, this period may be rather lessened. The interval of time is so short that any witnesses generally unintentionally exaggerate, and aver that the effects were witnessed *before* the swallowing of the liquid—"As the cup was at his lips"—"He had hardly drunk it," &c. There is probably a short interval of consciousness, then come giddiness, and, it may be, a cry for assistance; and lastly, there is a falling down in convulsions, and a speedy death. Convulsions are not always present, the victim occasionally appears to sink lifeless at once. Thus, in a case related by Hufeland, a man was seen to swallow a quantity of acid, equivalent to 40 grains of the pure acid—that is, about forty times more than sufficient to kill him. He staggered a few paces, and then fell dead, without sound or convulsion.

§ 262. The very short interval that may thus intervene between the taking of a dose of prussic acid and loss of consciousness, may be utilised by the sufferer in doing various acts, and thus this interval becomes of immense medico-legal importance. The question is simply this:—What can be done by a person in full possession of his faculties in ten seconds? I have found from experiment that, after drinking a liquid from a bottle, the bottle may be corked, the individual can get into bed, and arrange the bedclothes in a suitable manner; he may also throw the bottle away, or out of the window; and, indeed, with practice, in that short time a number of rapid and complicated acts may be performed. This is borne out both by experiments on animals and by recorded cases.

In Mr. Nunneley's numerous experiments on dogs, one of the animals, after taking poison, "went down three or four steps of the stairs, saw that the door at the bottom was closed, and came back again." A second went down, came up, and went again down the steps of a long winding staircase, and a third retained sufficient vigour to jump over another dog, and then leap across the top of a staircase.

In a remarkable case related by Dr. Guy,[246] in which a young man, after drinking more wine than usual, was seized by a sudden impulse to take prussic acid, and drank about 2 drachms, producing symptoms which, had it not been for prompt treatment, would, in all probability, have ended fatally—the interval is again noteworthy. After taking the poison in bed, he rose, walked round the foot of a chest of drawers, standing within a few yards of the bedside, placed the stopper firmly in the bottle, and then walked back to bed with the intention of getting into it; but here a giddiness seized him, and he sat down on the edge, and became insensible.

A case related by Taylor is still stronger. A woman, after swallowing a fatal dose of essence of almonds, went to a well in the yard, drew water, and drank a considerable quantity. She then ascended two flights of stairs and called her child, again descended a flight of stairs, fell on her bed, and died within half an hour from the taking of the poison.

Nevertheless, these cases and similar ones are exceptional, and only show what is possible, not what is usual, the rule being that after fatal doses no voluntary act of significance—save, it may be, a cry for assistance—is performed.[247]

§ 263. **Chronic poisoning by hydric cyanide** is said to occur among photographers, gilders, and those who are engaged daily in the preparation or handling of either hydric or potassic cyanides. The symptoms are those of feeble poisoning, headache, giddiness, noises in the ears, difficult respiration, pain over the heart, a feeling of constriction in the throat, loss of appetite, nausea, obstinate constipation, full pulse, with pallor and offensive breath. Koritschoner[248] has made some observations on patients who were made to breathe at intervals, during many weeks, prussic acid vapour, with the idea that such a treatment would destroy the tubercle bacilli. Twenty-five per cent. of those treated in this way suffered from redness of the pharynx, salivation, headache, nausea, vomiting, slow pulse, and even albuminuria.

§ 264. **Post-mortem Appearances.**[249]—If we for the moment leave out of consideration any changes which may be seen in the stomach after doses of potassic cyanide, then it may be affirmed that the pathological changes produced by hydric and potassic cyanides mainly coincide with those produced by suffocation. The most striking appearance is the presence of bright red spots; these bright red spots or patches are confined to the surface of the body, the blood in the deeper parts being of the ordinary venous hue, unless, indeed, an enormous dose has been

[246] *Forensic Medicine*, 4th ed., p. 615.

[247] Dr. J. Autal, a Hungarian chemist, states that cobalt nitrate is an efficacious antidote to poisoning by either HCN or KCN. The brief interval between the taking of a fatal dose and death can, however, be rarely utilised.—*Lancet*, Jan. 16, 1894.

[248] *Wiener klin. Woch.*, 1891.

[249] Hydric cyanide has, according to C. Brame, a remarkable antiseptic action, and if administered in sufficient quantity to animals, preserves them after death for a month. He considers that there is some more or less definite combination with the tissues.

taken; in that case the whole mass of blood may be bright red; this bright colour is due, according to Kobert, to the formation of cyanmethæmoglobin. The lungs and right heart are full of blood, and there is a backward engorgement produced by the pulmonic block. The veins of the neck and the vessels of the head generally are full of blood, and, in like manner, the liver and kidneys are congested. In the mucous membrane of the bronchial tubes there is a bloody foam, the lungs are gorged, and often œdematous in portions; ecchymoses are seen in the pleura and other serous membranes; and everywhere, unless concealed by putrefaction, or some strong-smelling ethereal oil, there is an odour of hydric cyanide.

Casper has rightly recommended the head to be opened and examined first, so as to detect the odour, if present, in the brain. The abdominal and chest cavities usually possess a putrefactive smell, but the brain is longer conserved, so that, if this course be adopted, there is a greater probability of detecting the odour.

The stomach in poisoning by hydric cyanide is not inflamed, but if alcohol has been taken at the same time, or previously, there may be more or less redness.

In poisoning by potassic cyanide, the appearances are mainly the same as those just detailed, with, it may be, the addition of caustic local action. I have, however, seen, in the case of a gentleman who drank accidentally a considerable dose of potassic cyanide just after a full meal, not the slightest trace of any redness, still less of corrosion. Here the contents of the stomach protected the mucous membrane, or possibly the larger amount of acid poured out during digestion sufficiently neutralised the alkali. Potassic cyanide, in very strong solution, may cause erosions of the lips, and the caustic effect may be traced in the mouth, throat, gullet, to the stomach and duodenum; but this is unusual, and the local effects are, as a rule, confined to the stomach and duodenum. The mucous membrane is coloured blood-red, reacts strongly alkaline,[250] is swollen, and it may be even ulcerated. The upper layers of the epithelium are also often dyed with the colouring-matter of the blood, which has been dissolved out by the cyanide. This last change is a *post-mortem* effect, and can be imitated by digesting the mucous membrane of a healthy stomach in a solution of cyanide. The intensity of these changes are, of course, entirely dependent on the dose and emptiness of the stomach. If the dose is so small as just to destroy life, there may be but little redness or swelling of the stomach, although empty at the time of taking the poison. In those cases in which there has been vomiting, and a part of the vomit has been drawn into the air-passages, there may be also inflammatory changes in the larynx. If essence of almonds has been swallowed, the same slight inflammation may be seen which has been observed with other essential oils, but no erosion, no strong alkaline reaction, nor anything approaching the effects of the caustic cyanide.

In poisoning by bitter almonds no inflammatory change in the mucous membrane of the coats of the stomach would be anticipated, yet in one recorded case there seems to have been an eroded and inflamed patch.

§ 265. **Tests for Hydrocyanic Acid and Cyanide of Potassium.**—(1.) The addition of silver nitrate to a solution containing prussic acid, or a soluble cyanide,[251] produces a precipitate of argentic cyanide. 100 parts of argentic cyanide are composed of 80.60 Ag and 19.4 CN, equivalent to 20.1 HCN. It is a white anhydrous precipitate, soluble either in ammonia or in a solution of cyanide of potassium. It is soluble in hot dilute nitric acid, but separates on cooling. A particle of silver cyanide, moistened with strong ammonia, develops needles; silver chloride treated similarly, octahedral crystals. It is insoluble in water. Upon ignition it is decomposed into CN and metallic silver, mixed with a little paracyanide of silver.

A very neat process for the identification of cyanide of silver is the following:—Place the perfectly dry cyanide in a closed or sealed tube, containing a few crystals of iodine. On heating slightly, iodide of cyanogen is sublimed in beautiful needles. These crystals again may be dissolved in a dilute solution of potash, a little ferrous sulphate added, and hydrochloric acid, and in this way Prussian blue produced. If the quantity to be tested is small, the vapour of the acid may be evolved in a very short test-tube, the mouth of which is closed by the ordinary thin discs of microscopic glass, the under surface of which is moistened with a solution of nitrate of silver; the resulting crystals of silver cyanide are very characteristic, and readily identified by the microscope.

[250] The following case came under my own observation:—A stout woman, 35 years of age, the wife of a French polisher, drank, in a fit of rage, a solution of cyanide of potassium. It was estimated that about 15 grains of the solid substance were swallowed. She died within an hour. The face was flushed, the body not decomposed; the mouth smelt strongly of cyanide; the stomach had about an ounce of bloody fluid in it, and was in a most intense state of congestion. There was commencing fatty degeneration of the liver, the kidneys were flabby, and the capsule adherent. The contents of the stomach showed cyanide of potassium, and the blood was very fluid. The woman was known to be of intemperate habits.

[251] In the case of testing in this way for the alkaline cyanides, the solution must contain a little free nitric acid.

(2.) If, instead of silver nitrate, the disc be moistened with a solution of sulphate of iron (to which has been added a little potash), and exposed to the vapour a short time, and then some dilute hydrochloric acid added, the moistened surface first becomes yellow, then green, lastly, and permanently, blue. No other blue compound of iron (with the exception of Prussian blue) is insoluble in dilute hydrochloric acid.

(3.) A third, and perhaps the most delicate of all, is the so-called sulphur test. A yellow sulphide of ammonium, containing free sulphur, is prepared by saturating ammonia by SH_2, first suspending in the fluid a little finely-precipitated sulphur (or an old, ill-preserved solution of sulphide of ammonium may be used). Two watch-glasses are now taken; in the one the fluid containing prussic acid is put, and the second (previously moistened with the sulphide of ammonium described) is inverted over it. The glasses are conveniently placed for a few minutes in the water-oven; the upper one is then removed, the moist surface evaporated to dryness in the water-bath, a little water added, and then a small drop of solution of chloride of iron. If hydrocyanic acid is present, the sulphocyanide of iron will be formed of a striking blood-red colour.

(4.) The reaction usually called Schönbein's, or Pagenstecher and Schönbein's[252] (but long known,[253] and used before the publication of their paper), consists of guaiacum paper, moistened with a very dilute solution of sulphate of copper (1 : 2000). This becomes blue if exposed to the vapour of hydrocyanic acid. Unfortunately, the same reaction is produced by ammonia, ozone, nitric acid, hypochlorous acid, iodine, bromine, chromate of potash, and other oxidising agents, so that its usefulness is greatly restricted.

(5.) A very delicate test for prussic acid is as follows:—About one-half centigrm. of ammonia, ferrous sulphate (or other pure ferrous salt), and the same quantity of uranic nitrate, are dissolved in 50 c.c. of water, and 1 c.c. of this test-liquid is placed in a porcelain dish. On now adding a drop of a liquid containing the smallest quantity of prussic acid, a grey-purple colour, or a distinct purple precipitate is produced.[254]

(6.) A hot solution of potassic cyanide, mixed with picric acid, assumes a blood-red colour, due to the formation of picro-cyanic acid. Free HCN does not give this reaction, and therefore must first be neutralised by an alkali.

(7.) **Schönbein's Test.**—To a few drops of defibrinated ox-blood are added a few drops of the carefully-neutralised distillate supposed to contain prussic acid, and then a little neutral peroxide of hydrogen is added. If the distillate contains no prussic acid, then the mixture becomes of a bright pure red and froths strongly; if, on the other hand, a trace of prussic acid be present, the liquid becomes brown and does not froth, or only slightly does so.

(8.) **Kobert's Test.**—A 1-4 per cent. solution of blood, to which a trace of ferridcyanide of potassium is added, is prepared, and the neutralised distillate added to this solution. If hydric cyanide be present, then the liquid becomes of a bright red colour, and, examined spectroscopically, instead of the spectrum of methæmoglobin, will be seen the spectrum of cyanmethæmoglobin. Kobert proposes to examine the blood of the poisoned, for the purpose of diagnosis, during life. A drop of blood from a healthy person, and a drop of blood from the patient, are examined side by side, according to the process just given.

§ 266. **Separation of Hydric Cyanide or Potassic Cyanide from Organic Matters, such as the Contents of the Stomach, &c.**—It is very necessary, before specially searching for hydric cyanide in the contents of the stomach, to be able to say, by careful and methodical examination, whether there are or are not any fragments of bitter almonds, of apples, peaches, or other substance likely to produce hydric cyanide. If potassic cyanide has been taken, simple distillation will always reveal its presence, because it is found partly decomposed into hydric cyanide by the action of the gastric acids. Nevertheless, an acid should always be added, and if, as in the routine process given earlier, there is reasonable doubt for suspecting that there will be no cyanide present, it will be best to add tartaric acid (for this organic acid will in no way interfere with subsequent operations), and distil, as recommended, in a vacuum. If, however, from the odour and from the history of the case, it is pretty sure to be a case of poisoning by hydric or potassic cyanide, then the substances, if fluid, are at once placed in a retort or flask, and acidified with a suitable quantity of sulphuric acid, or if the tissues or other solid matters are under examination, they are finely divided, or pulped, and distilled, after acidifying with sulphuric acid as before. It may be well here, as a caution, to remark that the analyst must not commit the unpardonable error of first producing a cyanide by reagents acting on animal matters, and then detecting as a poison the cyanide thus manufactured. If, for example, a healthy liver is carbonised by nitric acid, saturated with potash, and then burnt up, cyanide of potassium is always one of the

[252] *Neues Repert. de Pharm.*, 18, 356.

[253] This reaction (with tincture of guaiacum and copper) has been long known. "I remember a pharmaceutist, who attended my father's laboratory, showing me this test in 1828 or 1829."—Mohr's *Toxicologie*, p. 92.

[254] M. Carey Lea, *Amer. Journ. of Science* [3], ix. pp. 121-123; *J. C. Society*, 1876, vol. i. p. 112.

products; and, indeed, the ashes of a great variety of nitrogenous organic substances may contain cyanides—cyanides not pre-existing, but manufactured by combination. By the action of nitric acid even on sugar,[255] hydric cyanide is produced.

The old method of distillation was to distil by the gentle heat of a water-bath, receiving the distillate in a little weak potash water, and not prolonging the process beyond a few hours. The experiments of Sokoloff, however, throw a grave doubt on the suitability of this simple method for quantitative results.

N. Sokoloff[256] recommends the animal substances to be treated by water strongly acidified with hydric sulphate, and then to be distilled in the water-bath for from two to three days; or to be distilled for twenty-four hours, by the aid of an oil-bath, at a high temperature. He gives the following example of quantitative analysis by the old process of merely distilling for a few hours, and by the new:—

Old Process.—(1.) Body of a hound—age, 2 years; weight, 5180 grms.; dose administered, 57 mgrms. HCN; death in fifteen minutes. After five days there was found in the saliva 0.6 mgrm., stomach 3.2 mgrms., in the rest of the intestines 2.6 mgrms., in the muscles 4.1—total, 10.5.

(2.) Weight of body, 4000 grms.; dose given, 38 mgrms.; death in eleven minutes. After fifteen days, in the saliva 0.8, in the stomach 7.2, in the rest of the intestines 2.2, in the muscles 3.2—total, 13.4.

New Process.—Weight of body, 5700 grams; dose, 57 mgrms.; death in twenty-four minutes. After fifteen days, in the saliva 1.1 mgrm., in the stomach 2.6, in the rest of the intestines 9.6, in the muscles 31.9, and in the whole, 45.2 mgrms. Duration of process, thirteen hours.

From a second hound, weighing 6800 grms.; dose, 67 mgrms.; 25.1 mgrms. were separated three days after death.

From a third hound, weighing 5920 grms.; dose, 98 mgrms.; after forty days, by distillation on a sand-bath, there were separated 2.8 mgrms. from the saliva, 4.8 from the stomach, 16.8 from the intestines, 23.6 from the muscles—total, 48 mgrms.

It would also appear that he has separated 51.2 mgrms. of anhydrous acid from the corpse of a dog which had been poisoned by 57 mgrms. of acid, and buried sixty days.[257]

From another canine corpse, three days laid in an oven, and left for twenty-seven days at the ordinary temperature, 5.1 mgrms. were recovered out of a fatal dose of 38 mgrms.

The estimation was in each case performed by titrating the distillate with argentic nitrate, the sulphur compounds having been previously got rid of by saturating the distillate with KHO, and precipitating by lead acetate.

Venturoli[258] has, on the contrary, got good quantitative results without distillation at all. A current of pure hydrogen gas is passed through the liquid to be tested and the gas finally made to bubble through silver nitrate. He states that the whole of the hydric cyanide present is carried over in an hour. Metallic cyanides must be decomposed by sulphuric acid or tartaric acid. Mercury cyanide must be decomposed with SH_2, the solution acidified with tartaric acid, neutralised with freshly precipitated calcic carbonate to fix any ferro- or ferri-cyanides present, and hydrogen passed in and the issuing gases led first through a solution of bismuth nitrate to remove SH_2 and then into the silver solution.

§ 267. **How long after Death can Hydric or Potassic Cyanides be Detected?**—Sokoloff appears to have separated prussic acid from the body of hounds at very long periods after death—in one case sixty days. Dragendorff recognised potassic cyanide in the stomach of a hound after it had been four weeks in his laboratory,[259] and in man eight days after burial. Casper also, in his 211th case, states that more than 18 mgrms. of anhydrous prussic acid were obtained from a corpse eight days after death.[260] Dr. E. Tillner[261] has recognised potassic cyanide in a corpse four months after death. Lastly, Struve[262] put 300 grms. of flesh, 400 of common water, and 2.378 of KCy in a flask, and then opened the flask after 547 days. The detection was easy, and the estimation agreed with the amount placed

[255] *Chemical News*, 68, p. 75.

[256] *Ber. d. deutsch. chem. Gesellsch.*, Berlin, ix. p. 1023.

[257] Without wishing to discredit the statements of M. Sokoloff, we may point out that a loss of half-a-dozen mgrms. only appears rather extraordinary.

[258] L'Orosi. xv. 85-88.

[259] Dragendorff, G., *Beitr. zur gericht. Chem.*, p. 59.

[260] Casper's *Pract. Handbuch der gerichtlichen Medicin*, p. 561.

[261] *Vierteljahr. f. gerichtl. Med.*, Berlin, 1881, p. 193.

[262] *Zeitschrift f. anal. Chemie*, von Fresenius, 1873, xii. p. 4.

there at first. So that, even in very advanced stages of putrefaction, and at periods after death extending beyond many months, the detection of prussic acid cannot be pronounced impossible.

§ 268. **Estimation of Hydrocyanic Acid or Potassic Cyanide.**—In all cases, the readiest method of estimating prussic acid (whether it be in the distillate from organic substances or in aqueous solution) is to saturate it with soda or potash, and titrate the alkaline cyanide thus formed with nitrate of silver. The process is based on the fact that there is first formed a soluble compound (KCy, AgCy), which the slightest excess of silver breaks up, and the insoluble cyanide is at once precipitated. If grains are used, 17 grains of nitrate of silver are dissolved in water, the solution made up to exactly 1000 grain measures, each grain measure equalling .0054 grain of anhydrous hydrocyanic acid. If grammes are employed, the strength of the nitrate of silver solution should be 1.7 grm. to the litre, each c.c. then = .0054 hydrocyanic acid, or .01302 grm. of potassic cyanide.

Essential oil of bitter almonds may also be titrated in this way, provided it is diluted with sufficient spirit to prevent turbidity from separation of the essential oil. If hydrocyanic acid is determined gravimetrically (which is sometimes convenient, when only a single estimation is to be made), it is precipitated as cyanide of silver, the characters of which have been already described.

§ 269. **Case of Poisoning by Bitter Almonds.**—Instances of poisoning by bitter almonds are very rare. The following interesting case is recorded by Maschka:—

A maid-servant, 31 years of age, after a quarrel with her lover, ate a quantity of bitter almonds. In a few minutes she sighed, complained of being unwell and faint; she vomited twice, and, after about ten minutes more had elapsed, fell senseless and was convulsed. An hour afterwards, a physician found her insensible, the eyes rolled upwards, the thumb clenched within the shut fists, and the breathing rattling, the pulse very slow. She died within an hour-and-a-half from the first symptoms.

The autopsy showed the organs generally healthy, but all, save the liver, exhaling a faint smell of bitter almonds. The right side of the heart was full of fluid dark blood, the left was empty. Both lungs were rich in blood, which smelt of prussic acid. The stomach was not inflamed—it held 250 grms. of a yellow fluid, containing white flocks smelling of bitter almond oil. In the most dependent portion of the stomach there was a swollen patch of mucous membrane, partially denuded of epithelium. The mucous membrane of the duodenum was also swollen and slightly red. The contents of the stomach were acid, and yielded, on distillation, hydride of benzole and hydric cyanide. Residues of the almonds themselves were also found, and the whole quantity taken by the woman from various data was calculated to be 1200 grains of bitter almonds, equal to 43 grains of amygdalin, or 2.5 grains of pure hydric cyanide.

Poisonous Cyanides other than Hydric and Potassic Cyanides.

§ 270. The action of both *sodic and ammonic cyanides* is precisely similar to that of potassic cyanide. With regard to ammonic cyanide, there are several experiments by Eulenberg,[263] showing that its vapour is intensely poisonous.

A weak stream of ammonic cyanide vapour was passed into glass shades, under which pigeons were confined. After a minute, symptoms of distress commenced, then followed convulsions and speedy death. The *post-mortem* signs were similar to those produced by prussic acid, and this substance was separated from the liver and lungs.

§ 271. With regard to the *double cyanides*, all those are poisonous from which hydric cyanide can be separated through dilute acids, while those which, like potassic ferro-cyanide, do not admit of this decomposition, may be often taken with impunity, and are only poisonous under certain conditions.

Sonnenschein records the death of a colourist, after he had taken a dose of potassic ferro-cyanide and then one of tartaric acid; and Volz describes the death of a man, who took potassic ferro-cyanide and afterwards equal parts of nitric and hydrochloric acids. In this latter case, death took place within the hour, with all the symptoms of poisoning by hydric cyanide; so that it is not entirely true, as most text-books declare, that ferro-cyanide is in no degree poisonous. Carbon dioxide will decompose potassic ferro-cyanide at 72°-74°, potass ferrous cyanide being precipitated—$K_2Fe_2(CN)_6$. A similar action takes place if ferro-cyanide is mixed with a solution of peptone and casein, and digested at blood heat[264] (from 37° to 40° C.), so that it is believed that when ferro-cyanide is swallowed HCN is liberated, but the quantity is usually so small at any given moment that no injury is caused: but there are

[263] *Gewerbe Hygiene*, p. 385.

[264] Autenrieth, *Arch. Pharm.*, 231, 99-109.

conditions in which it may kill speedily.[265]

Mercuric cyanide, it has been often said, acts precisely like mercuric chloride (corrosive sublimate), and a poisonous action is attributed to it not traceable to cyanogen; but this is erroneous teaching. Bernard[266] declares that it is decomposed by the gastric juice, and hydric cyanide set free; while Pelikan puts it in the same series as ammonic and potassic cyanides. Lastly, Tolmatscheff,[267] by direct experiment, has found its action to resemble closely that of hydric cyanide.[268]

Silver cyanide acts, according to the experiments of Nunneley, also like hydric cyanide, but very much weaker.

Hydric sulphocyanide in very large doses is poisonous.

Potassic sulphocyanide, according to Dubreuil and Legros,[269] if subcutaneously injected, causes first local paralysis of the muscles, and later, convulsions.

Cyanogen chloride (CNCl) and also the compound ($C_3N_3Cl_3$)—the one a liquid, boiling at 15°, the other a solid, which may be obtained in crystals—are both poisonous, acting like hydric cyanide.

Methyl cyanide is a liquid obtained by distillation of a mixture of calcic methyl sulphate and potassic cyanide. It boils at 77°, and is intensely poisonous. Eulenberg[270] has made with this substance several experiments on pigeons. An example of one will suffice:—A young pigeon was placed under a glass shade, into which methyl cyanide vapour, developed from calcic methyl sulphate and potassic cyanide, was admitted. The pigeon immediately became restless, and the fæces were expelled. In forty seconds it was slightly convulsed, and was removed after a few minutes' exposure. The pupils were then observed not to be dilated, but the respiration had ceased; the legs were feebly twitching; the heart still beat, but irregularly; a turbid white fluid dropped out of the beak, and after six minutes life was extinct.

The pathological appearances were as follows:—In the beak much watery fluid; the membranes covering the brain weakly injected; the *plexus venosus spinalis* strongly injected; in the region of the cervical vertebra a small extravasation between the dura mater and the bone; the right lung of a clear cherry-red colour, and the left lung partly of the same colour, the parenchyma presented the same hue as the surface; on section of the lungs a whitish froth exuded from the cut surface. In the cellular tissue of the trachea, there were extravasations 5 mm. in diameter; the mucous membrane of the air-passages was pale; the right ventricle and the left auricle of the heart were filled with coagulated and fluid dark red blood; liver and kidneys normal; the blood dark red and very fluid, becoming bright cherry-red on exposure to the air; blood corpuscles unchanged. Cyanogen was separated, and identified from the lungs and the liver.

Cyanuric acid ($C_3O_3N_3H_3$), one of the decomposition products obtained from urea, is poisonous, the symptoms and pathological effects closely resembling those due to hydric cyanide. In experiments on animals, there has been no difficulty in detecting prussic acid in the lungs and liver after poisoning by cyanuric acid.

---

[265] The presence of ferro-cyanide is easily detected. The liquid is, if necessary, filtered and then acidified with hydrochloric acid and a few drops of ferric chloride added; if the liquid contains ferro-cyanide, there is immediate production of Prussian blue. It may happen that potassic or sodic cyanide has been taken as well as ferro-cyanide, and it will be necessary then to devise a process by which only the prussic acid from the simple cyanide is distilled over. According to Autenrieth, if sodium hydrocarbonate is added to the liquid in sufficient quantity and the liquid distilled, the hydric cyanide that comes over is derived wholly from the sodium or potassium cyanide. Should mercury cyanide and ferro-cyanide be taken together, then this process requires modification; bicarbonate of soda is added as before, and then a few c.c. of water saturated with hydric sulphide; under these circumstances, only the hydric cyanide derived from the mercury cyanide distils over. If the bicarbonate of soda is omitted, the distillate contains hydric cyanide derived from the ferro-cyanide.

[266] *Substances Toxiques*, pp. 66-103.

[267] "*Einige Bemerkungen über die Wirkung von Cyanquecksilber*," in Hoppe-Seyler's *Med. Chem. Untersuchungen*, 2 Heft, p. 279.

[268] Mercury cyanide may be detected in a liquid after acidifying with tartaric acid, and adding a few c.c. of SH_2 water and then distilling. S. Lopes suggests another process: the liquid is acidified with tartaric acid, ammonium chloride added in excess, and the liquid is distilled. A double chloride of ammonium and mercury is formed, and HCN distils over with the steam.—*J. Pharm.*, xxvii. 550-553.

[269] *Compt. rend.*, t. 64, 1867, p. 561.

[270] *Gewerbe Hygiene*, p. 392.

XIII.—Phosphorus.

§ 272. **Phosphorus.**—Atomic weight 31, specific gravity 1.77 to 1.840. Phosphorus melts at from 44.4° to 44.5° to a pale yellow oily fluid. The boiling-point is about 290°.

The phosphorus of commerce is usually preserved under water in the form of waxy, semi-transparent sticks; if exposed to the air white fumes are given off, luminous in the dark, with a peculiar onion-like odour. On heating phosphorus it readily inflames, burning with a very white flame.

At 0° phosphorus is brittle; the same quality may be imparted to it by a mere trace of sulphur. Phosphorus may be obtained in dodecahedral crystals by slowly cooling large melted masses. It may also be obtained crystalline by evaporating a solution in bisulphide of carbon or hot naphtha in a current of carbon dioxide. It is usually stated to be absolutely insoluble in water, but Julius Hartmann[271] contests this, having found in some experiments that 100 grms. of water digested with phosphorus for sixty-four hours at 38.5° dissolved .000127 grm. He also investigated the solvent action of bile, and found that 100 grms. of bile under the same conditions, dissolved .02424 grm., and that the solubility of phosphorus rose both in water and bile when the temperature was increased. Phosphorus is somewhat soluble in alcohol and ether, and also, to some extent, in fatty and ethereal oils; but the best solvent is carbon disulphide.

The following is the order of solubility in certain menstrua, the figures representing the number of parts by weight of the solvent required to dissolve 1 part of phosphorus:—

Carbon Disulphide,	4
Almond Oil,	100
Concentrated Acetic Acid,[272]	100
Ether,	250
Alcohol, specific gravity .822,	400
Glycerin,	588

Phosphorus exists in, or can be converted into, several allotropic modifications, of which the red or amorphous phosphorus is the most important. This is effected by heating it for some time, in the absence of air, from 230° to 235°. It is not poisonous.[273] Commercial red phosphorus does, however, contain very small quantities of unchanged or ordinary phosphorus—according to Fresenius, from .6 per cent. downwards; it also contains phosphorous acid, and about 4.6 per cent. of other impurities, among which is graphite.[274]

§ 273. **Phosphuretted Hydrogen.—Phosphine** (PH_3), mol. weight 34, specific gravity 1.178, percentage composition, phosphorus 91.43, hydrogen 8.57 by weight. The absolutely pure gas is not spontaneously inflammable, but that made by the ordinary process is so. It is a colourless, highly poisonous gas, which does not support combustion, but is itself combustible, burning to phosphoric acid ($PH_3 + 2O_2 = PO_4H_3$). Extremely dangerous explosive mixtures may be made by combining phosphine and air or oxygen. Phosphine, when quite dry, burns with a white flame, but if mixed with aqueous vapour, it is green; hence a hydrogen flame containing a mixture of PH_3 possesses a green colour.

If sulphur is heated in a stream of phosphine, hydric sulphide and sulphur phosphide are the products. Oxides of the metals, heated with phosphine, yield phosphides with formation of water. Iodine, warmed in phosphine, gives white crystals of iodine phosphonium, and biniodide of phosphorus, $5I + 4PH_3 = 3PIH_4 + PI_2$. Chlorine inflames the gas, the final result being hydric chloride and chloride of phosphorus, $PH_3 + 8Cl = 3ClH + PCl_5$. One of the most important decompositions for our purpose is the action of phosphine on a solution of nitrate of silver; there is a separation of metallic silver, and nitric and phosphoric acids are found in solution, thus—$8AgNO_3 + PH_3 + 4OH_2 = 8Ag + 8HNO_3 + PO_4H_3$. This is, however, rather the end reaction; for, at first, there is a separation of a black precipitate composed of phosphor-silver. The excess of silver can be separated by hydric chloride, and the

[271] *Zur acuten Phosphor-Vergiftung*, Dorpat, 1866.

[272] Phosphorus is very little soluble in cold acetic acid, and the solubility given is only correct when the boiling acid acts for some time on the phosphorus.

[273] A hound took 200 grms. of red phosphorus in twelve days, and remained healthy.—Sonnenschein.

[274] Schrotter, *Chem. News*, vol. xxxvi. p. 198.

phosphoric acid made evident by the addition of molybdic acid in excess.

§ 274. **The medicinal preparations of phosphorus** are not numerous; it is usually prescribed in the form of pills, made by manufacturers of coated pills on a large scale. The pills are composed of phosphorus, balsam of Tolu, yellow wax, and curd soap, and 3 grains equal 1/30 grain of phosphorus. There is also a *phosphorated oil*, containing about 1 part of phosphorus in 100; that of the French Pharmacopœia is made with 1 part of dried phosphorus dissolved in 50 parts of warm almond oil; that of the German has 1 part in 80; the strength of the former is therefore 2 per cent., of the latter 1.25 per cent. The medicinal dose of phosphorus is from 1/100 to 1/30 grain.

§ 275. **Matches and Vermin Pastes.**—An acquaintance with the percentage of phosphorus in the different pastes and matches of commerce will be found useful. Most of the vermin-destroying pastes contain from 1 to 2 per cent. of phosphorus.

A phosphorus paste that was fatal to a child,[275] and gave rise to serious symptoms in others, was composed as follows:—

	Per cent.
Phosphorus,	1 .4
Flowers of sulphur,	42 .2
Flour,	42 .2
Sugar,	14 .2
	100 .00

Three common receipts give the following proportions:—

	Per cent.
Phosphorus,	1 .5
Lard,	18 .4
Sugar,	18 .4
Flour,	61 .7
	100 .00

	Per cent.
Phosphorus,	1 .2
Warm water,	26 .7
Rye flour,	26 .7
Melted butter,	26 .7
Sugar,	18 .7
	100 .00

	Per cent.
Phosphorus,	1 .6
Nut oil,	15 .7
Warm water,	31 .5
Flour,	31 .5
Sugar,	19 .7
	100 .00

A very common phosphorus paste, to be bought everywhere in England, is sold in little pots; the whole amount of phosphorus contained in these varies from .324 to .388 grm. (5 to 6 grains), the active constituent being a little

[275] Casper's 204th case.

over 4 per cent. Matches differ much in composition. Six matchheads, which had been placed in an apple for criminal purposes, and were submitted to Tardieu, were found to contain 20 mgrms. of phosphorus—*i.e.*, .33 grm. in 100. Mayet found in 100 matches 55 mgrms. of phosphorus. Gonning[276] analysed ten different kinds of phosphorus matches with the following result:—Three English samples contained in 100 matches 34, 33, and 32 mgrms. of phosphorus: a Belgian sample, 38 mgrms.; and 5 others of unknown origin, 12, 17, 28, 32, and 41 mgrms. respectively. Some of the published formularies are as follows:—

(1.)	Glue,	6	parts.	
	Phosphorus,	4	„	or 14.4 per cent.
	Nitre,	10	„	
	Red ochre,	5	„	
	Blue smalts,	2	„	
(2.)	Phosphorus,	9	parts,	or 16.3 per cent.
	Gum,	16	„	
	Nitre,	14	„	
	Smalts,	16	„	
(3.)	Phosphorus,	4	parts,	or 14.4 per cent.
	Glue,	6	„	
	Nitre,	10	„	
	Red lead,	5	„	
	Smalts,	2	„	
(4.)	Phosphorus,	17	parts,	or 17 per cent.
	Glue,	21	„	
	Nitre,	38	„	
	Red lead,	24	„	

Phosphorus poisoning by matches will, however, shortly become very rare, for those containing the ordinary variety of phosphorus are gradually being superseded by matches of excellent quality, which contain no phosphorus whatever.

§ 276. **Statistics.**—The following table gives the deaths for ten years from phosphorus poisoning in England and Wales:—

DEATHS FROM PHOSPHORUS IN ENGLAND AND WALES DURING THE TEN YEARS ENDING 1892.

Accident or Negligence.

Ages,	1-5	5-15	15-25	25-65	65 and above	Total
Males,	11	1	2	8	...	22
Females,	15	2	11	5	...	33
Totals,	26	3	13	13	...	55

Suicide.

[276] *Nederlandsch Tijdschr. voor Geneesk.*, Afl. i., 1866.

Ages,	5-15	15-25	25-65	65 and above	Total
Males,	1	6	20	1	28
Females,	6	33	24	1	64
Totals,	7	39	44	2	92

Phosphorus as a cause of death through accident or negligence occupies the eighth place among poisons, and as a cause of suicide the ninth.

A far greater number of cases of poisoning by phosphorus occur yearly in France and Germany than in England. Phosphorus may be considered as the favourite poison which the common people on the Continent employ for the purpose of self-destruction. It is an agent within the reach of anyone who has 2 sous in his pocket, wherewith to buy a box of matches, but to the educated and those who know the horrible and prolonged torture ensuing from a toxic dose of phosphorus, such a means of exit from life will never be favoured.

Otto Schraube[277] has collected 92 cases from Meischner's work,[278] and added 16 which had come under his own observation, giving in all 108 cases. Seventy-one (or 65 per cent.) of these were suicidal—of the suicides 24 were males, 47 females (12 of the latter being prostitutes); 21 of the cases were those of murder, 11 were accidental, and in 3 the cause was not ascertained. The number of cases in successive years, and the kind of poison used, is given as follows:—

Number of Cases.	In the Years	Phosphorus in Substance, or as Paste.	Phosphorus Matches.
15	1798-1850	13	2
36	1850-1860	15	21
41	1860-1864	6	35
16	1864-1867	5	11

Of the 108 cases, 18 persons recovered and 90 (or 83.3 per cent.) died.

Falck also has collected 76 cases of poisoning from various sources during eleven years; 55 were suicidal, 5 homicidal[279] (murders), and the rest accidental. Of the latter, 2 were caused by the use of phosphorus as a medicine, 13 by accidents due to phosphorus being in the house; in 1 case phosphorus was taken intentionally to try the effects of an antidote.[280] With regard to the form in which the poison was taken, 2 of the 76, as already mentioned, took it as prescribed by physicians, the remaining 74 were divided between poisonings by phosphorus paste (22) and matches (52) = 70 per cent. Of the 76 cases, 6 were children, 43 adult males, 13 adult females, and 14 adults, sex not given. Of the 76 cases, 42, or 55.3 per cent., died—a much smaller rate of mortality than that shown by Schraube's collection.

§ 277. **Fatal Dose.**—The smallest dose on record is that mentioned by Lobenstein Lobel, of Jena, where a lunatic died from taking 7.5 mgrms. (.116 grain). There are other cases clearly indicating that this small quantity may produce dangerous symptoms in a healthy adult.

§ 278. **Effects of Phosphorus.**—Phosphorus is excessively poisonous, and will destroy life, provided only that it enters the body in a fine state of division, but if taken in coarse pieces no symptoms may follow, for it has been proved that single lumps of phosphorus will go the whole length of a dog's intestinal canal without causing appreciable loss of weight, and without destroying life.[281] Magendie injected *oleum phosphoratum* into the veins, and although the animals experimented on exhaled white fumes, and not a few died asphyxiated, yet no symptoms of phosphorus poisoning resulted—an observation confirmed by others—the reason being that the phosphorus

[277] Schmidt's *Jahrbuch der ger. Med.*, 1867, Bd. 186, S. 209-248.

[278] *Die acute Phosphorose und einige Reflexionen über die acute gelbe Leberatrophie, &c., Inaug. Diss.*, Leipzig, 1864.

[279] Dr. Dannenberg has shown by direct experiment that a poisonous dose of phosphorus may be introduced into spirits or coffee, and the mixture have but little odour or taste of phosphorus.—Schuchardt in Maschka's *Handbuch.*

[280] Géry, "*Ueber Terpentinessenz als Gegenmittel gegen Phosphor,*" in *Gaz. Hebd. de Méd.*, 2 sér., x. 2, 1873.

[281] Reveil, *Ann. d'Hygiène Publ.* (3), xii. p. 370.

particles in a comparatively coarse state of division were arrested in the capillaries of the lung, and may be said to have been, as it were, outside the body. On the other hand, A. Brunner,[282] working in L. Hermann's laboratory, having injected into the veins phosphorus in such a fine emulsion that the phosphorus could pass the lung capillaries, found that there were no exhalations of white fumes, but that the ordinary symptoms of phosphorus poisoning soon manifested themselves. Phosphorus paste, by the method of manufacture, is in a state of extreme sub-division, and hence all the phosphorus pastes are extremely poisonous.

§ 279. In a few poisons there is a difference, more or less marked, between the general symptoms produced on man, and those noticeable in the different classes of animals; but with phosphorus, the effects on animals appear to agree fairly with those witnessed most frequently in man. Tardieu (who has written perhaps the best and most complete clinical record of phosphorus poisoning extant) divides the cases under three classes, and to use his own words:—"I think it useful to establish that poisoning by phosphorus in its course, sometimes rapid, sometimes slow, exhibits in its symptoms three distinct forms—a common form, a nervous form, and a hæmorrhagic form. I recognise that, in certain cases, these three forms may succeed each other, and may only constitute periods of poisoning; but it is incontestable that each of them may show itself alone, and occupy the whole course of the illness produced by the poison."[283] Premising that the common form is a blending of irritant, nervous, and hæmorrhagic symptoms, I adopt here in part Tardieu's division. The name of "hæmorrhagic form" may be given to that in which hæmorrhage is the predominant feature, and the "nervous" to that in which the brain and spinal cord are from the first affected. There yet remain, however, a few cases which have an entirely anomalous course, and do not fall under any of the three classes.

From a study of 121 recorded cases of phosphorus poisoning, I believe the relative frequency of the different forms to be as follows:—The common form 83 per cent., hæmorrhagic 10 per cent., nervous 6 per cent., anomalous 1 per cent. The "anomalous" are probably over-estimated, for the reason that cases presenting ordinary features are not necessarily published, but others are nearly always chronicled in detail.

§ 280. **Common Form.**—At the moment of swallowing, a disagreeable taste and smell are generally experienced, and there may be immediate and intense pain in the throat, gullet, and stomach, and almost immediate retching and vomiting. The throat and tongue also may become swollen and painful; but in a considerable number of cases the symptoms are not at once apparent, but are delayed from one to six hours—rarely longer. The person's breath may be phosphorescent before he feels in any way affected, and he may go about his business and perform a number of acts requiring both time and mental integrity. Pain in the stomach (which, in some of the cases, takes the form of violent cramp and vomiting) succeeds; the matters vomited may shine in the dark, and are often tinged with blood. Diarrhœa is sometimes present, sometimes absent; sleeplessness for the first night or two is very common. The pulse is variable, sometimes frequent, sometimes slow; the temperature in the morning is usually from 36.0° to 36.5°, in the evening 37° to 38°.

The next symptom is jaundice. I have notes of the exact occurrence of jaundice in 23 cases, as follows:—In 1 within twenty-four hours, in 3 within thirty-six hours, in 3 within two days, in 11 within three days, in 1 within four days, in 1 within five days, in 1 within nine days, in 1 within eighteen days, and in 1 within twenty-seven days; so that in about 78 per cent. jaundice occurred before the end of the third day. Out of 26 cases, in which the patients lived long enough for the occurrence of jaundice, in 3 (or 11 per cent.) it was entirely absent. In 132 cases recorded by Lewin, Meischner, and Heisler, jaundice occurred in 65, or about 49 per cent., but it must be remembered, that in many of these cases the individual died before it had time to develop. The jaundice having thoroughly pronounced itself, the system may be considered as not only under the influence of the toxic action of phosphorus, but as suffering in addition from all the accidents incidental to the retention of the biliary secretion in the blood; nor is there from this point any special difference between phosphorus poisoning and certain affections of the liver—such, for example, as acute yellow atrophy. There is retention of urine, sleeplessness, headache, frequent vomiting, painful and often involuntary evacuations from the bowels, and occasionally skin affections, such as urticaria or erythema. The case terminates either by acute delirium with fever, followed by fatal coma, or, in a few instances, coma comes on, and the patient passes to death in sleep without delirium. In this common form there is in a few cases, at the end of from twenty-four to thirty hours, a remission of the symptoms, and a non-medical observer might imagine that the patient was about to recover without further discomfort; but then jaundice supervenes, and the course is as described. Infants often do not live long enough for the jaundiced stage to develop, but die within twenty-four hours,

[282] *Arch. f. d. Ges. Physiologie*, iii. p. 1.

[283] *Étude Médico-Légale et Clinique sur l'Empoisonnement*, Paris, 1875, p. 483.

the chief symptoms being vomiting and convulsions.

§ 281. **Hæmorrhagic Form.**—The symptoms set in as just detailed, and jaundice appears, but accompanied by a new and terrible train of events—viz., great effusion of blood. In some cases the blood has been poured out simultaneously from the nose, mouth, bladder, kidneys, and bowels. Among women there is excessive hæmorrhagia. The liver is found to be swollen and painful; the bodily weakness is great. Such cases are usually of long duration, and a person may die months after taking the poison from weakness, anæmia, and general cachexia. In many of its phases the hæmorrhagic form resembles scurvy, and, as in scurvy, there are spots of purpura all over the body.

§ 282. **The nervous form** is less common than the two forms just described. From the beginning, there are strange creeping sensations about the limbs, followed by painful cramps, repeated faintings, and great somnolence. Jaundice, as usual, sets in, erythematous spots appear on the skin, and, about the fifth day, delirium of an acute character breaks out, and lock-jaw and convulsions close the scene.

The following are one or two brief abstracts of anomalous cases in which symptoms are either wanting, or run a course entirely different from any of the three forms described:—

A woman, aged 20, took about 3 grains of phosphorus in the form of rat-paste. She took the poison at six in the evening, behaved according to her wont, and sat down and wrote a letter to the king. During the night she vomited once, and died the next morning at six o'clock, exactly twelve hours after taking the poison. There appear to have been no symptoms whatever, save the single vomiting, to which may be added that in the course of the evening her breath had a phosphorus odour and was luminous.[284]

A girl swallowed a quantity of phosphorus paste, but there were no marked symptoms until the fifth day, on which there was sickness and purging. She died on the seventh day. A remarkable blueness of the finger nails was observed a little before death, and was noticeable afterwards.[285]

§ 283. **Sequelæ.**—In several cases in which the patients have recovered from phosphorus poisoning, there have been observed paralytic affections.[286] O. Bollinger has recorded a case in which paralysis of the foot followed;[287] in another, published by Bettelheim,[288] there were peculiar cerebral and spinal symptoms. Most of these cases are to be explained as disturbance or loss of function from small hæmorrhages in the nervous substance.

§ 284. **Period at which the first Symptoms commence.**—The time when the symptoms commence is occasionally of importance from a forensic point of view. I find that out of 28 cases in which the commencement of evident symptoms—*i.e.*, pain, or vomiting, or illness—is precisely recorded, in 8 the symptoms were described as either immediate or within a few minutes after swallowing the poison; in 6 the symptoms commenced within the hour; in 3 within two hours; in other 3 within four hours; and in 1 within six hours. One was delayed until the lapse of twelve hours, 1 from sixteen to eighteen hours, 1 two, and another five days. We may, therefore, expect that in half the cases which may occur, the symptoms will commence within the hour, and more than 80 per cent. within six hours.

§ 285. **Period of Death.**—In 129 cases death took place as follows:—In 17 within twenty-four hours, in 30 within two days, in 103 within seven days. Three patients lived eight days, 6 nine days, 13 ten days, 1 eleven days, 1 sixteen days, 1 seventeen days, and 1 survived eight months. It hence follows that 79.8 per cent. of the fatal cases die within the week.

§ 286. **Phosphorus Vapour.**—There are one or two cases on record of acute poisoning by phosphorus in the form of vapour. The symptoms are somewhat different from the effects produced by the finely-divided solid, and in general terms it may be said that phosphorus vapour is more apt to produce the rarer "nervous" form of poisoning than the solid phosphorus.

Bouchardat[289] mentions the case of a druggist who, while preparing a large quantity of rat-poison in a close room, inhaled phosphorus vapour. He fainted repeatedly, fell into a complete state of prostration, and died within a week.

The following interesting case came under the observation of Professor Magnus Huss:—A man, thirty-nine years old, married, was admitted into the Seraphin-Lazareth, Stockholm, on the 2nd of February 1842. He had been

[284] Casper's 205th case.
[285] Taylor on *Poisons*, p. 277.
[286] See Gallavardin, *Les Paralyses Phosphoriques*, Paris, 1865.
[287] *Deutsches Archiv f. klin. Med.*, Bd. 6, Hft. 1, S. 94, 1869.
[288] *Wiener Med. Presse*, 1868, No. 41.
[289] *Annuaire de Thérap.*, 1874, p. 109; Schuchardt in Maschka's *Handbuch*; also Schmidt's *Jahrbuch*, 1846, Bd. 51, S. 101.

occupied three years in the manufacture of phosphorus matches, and inhabited the room in which the materials were preserved. He had always been well-conducted in every way, and in good health, until a year previously, when a large quantity of the material for the manufacture of the matches accidentally caught fire and exploded. In his endeavours to extinguish the flames, he breathed a large quantity of the vapour, and he fell for a time unconscious. The spine afterwards became so weak that he could not hold himself up, and he lost, in a great measure, power over his legs and arms. On admission, his condition was as follows:—He could make a few uncertain and staggering steps, his knees trembled, his arms shook, and if he attempted to grasp anything when he lay in bed, there were involuntary twitchings of groups of muscles. There was no pain; the sensibility of the skin was unchanged; he had formication in the left arm; the spine was neither sensitive to pressure, nor unusually sensitive to heat (as, *e.g.*, to the application of a hot sponge); the organs of special sense were not affected, but his speech was somewhat thick. He lived to 1845 in the same condition, but the paralysis became worse. There does not seem to have been any autopsy.

The effects of phosphorus vapour may be still further elucidated by one of Eulenberg's[290] experiments on a rabbit. The vapour of burning phosphorus, mixed with much air, was admitted into a wooden hutch in which a strong rabbit sat. After 5 mgrms. of phosphorus had been in this manner consumed, the only symptoms in half an hour were salivation, and quickened and somewhat laboured respiration. After twenty-four hours had elapsed there was sudden indisposition, the animal fell as if lifeless, with the hind extremities stretched out, and intestinal movements were visible; there was also expulsion of the urine. These epileptiform seizures seem to have continued more or less for twelve days, and then ceased. After fourteen days the experiment was repeated on the same rabbit. The animal remained exposed to the vapour for three-quarters of an hour, when the epilepsy showed itself as before, and, indeed, almost regularly after feeding. Between the attacks the respiration was slowed. Eight weeks afterwards there was an intense icterus, which disappeared at the end of ten weeks.

§ 287. **Chronic phosphorus poisoning** has frequently been noticed in persons engaged either in the manufacture of phosphorus or in its technical application. Some have held that the symptoms are due to an oxidation product of phosphorus rather than to phosphorus itself; but in one of Eulenberg's experiments, in which a dove was killed by breathing phosphorus fumes evolved by phosphorus oil, phosphorus was chemically recognised in the free state in the lungs. The most constant and peculiar effect of breathing small quantities of phosphorus vapour is a necrosis of the lower jaw. There is first inflammation of the periosteum of the jaw, which proceeds to suppuration and necrosis of a greater or smaller portion. The effects may develop with great suddenness, and end fatally. Thus Fournier and Olliver[291] relate the case of a girl, fourteen years old, who, after working four years in a phosphorus manufactory, was suddenly affected with periostitis of the upper jaw, and with intense anæmia. An eruption of purpuric spots ensued, and she died comatose. There is now little doubt, that minute doses of phosphorus have a specific action on the bones generally, and more especially on the bones of the jaw. Wegner[292] administered small daily doses to young animals, both in the state of vapour, and as a finely-divided solid. The condition of the bones was found to be more compact than normal, the medullary canals being smaller than in healthy bone, the ossification was quickened. The formation of callus in fractured limbs was also increased.

§ 288. **Changes in the Urinary Secretion.**—It has been before stated that, at a certain period of the illness, the renal secretion is scantier than in health, the urine diminishing, according to Lebert and Wyss's[293] researches, to one-half on the third, fourth, or fifth day. It frequently contains albumen, blood, and casts. When jaundice is present, the urine has then all the characters noticed in icterus; leucin and tyrosin, always present in acute yellow atrophy of the liver, have been found in small quantity in jaundice through phosphorus; lactic acid is also present. The urea is much diminished, and, according to Schultzen and Riess,[294] may be towards death entirely absent. Lastly, it is said that there is an exhalation of either phosphorus vapour or phosphine from such urine. In some cases the urine is normal, *e.g.*, in a case recorded by E. H. Starling, M.D., and F. G. Hopkins, B.Sc. (*Guy's Hospital Report*, 1890), in which a girl, aged 18, died on the fifth day after taking phosphorus paste, the liver was fatty, and there was jaundice; but the urine contained neither leucin nor tyrosin, and was stated to be generally normal.

§ 289. **Changes in the blood** during life have been several times observed. In a case attended by M. Romellære

[290] *Gewerbe Hygiene*, p. 255.
[291] *Gaz. hebd. de Méd.*, 29, p. 461, 1868.
[292] Virchow's *Arch. f. path. Anat.*, lv. 11.
[293] *Archiv Générale de Méd.*, 6 Sér., Tom. 12, 1868, p. 709.
[294] *Annalen der Charité*, Berlin.

of Brussels,[295] in which a man took the paste from 300 matches, and under treatment by turpentine recovered, the blood was frequently examined, and the leucocytes found much increased in number. There is a curious conflict of evidence as to whether phosphorus prevents coagulation of the blood or not. Nasse asserted that phosphorated oil given to a dog fully prevented coagulation; P. I. Liebreck[296] also, in a series of researches, found the blood dark, fluid, and in perfect solution. These observations were also supported by V. Bibra and Schuchardt.[297] Nevertheless, Lebert and Wyss found the blood, whether in the veins or in extravasations, in a normal condition. Phosphorus increases the fatty contents of the blood. Ritter found that phosphorus mixed with starch, and given to a dog, raised the fatty content from the normal 2 per 1000 up to 3.41 and 3.47 per 1000. Eug. Menard[298] saw in the blood from the jugular and portal veins, as well as in extravasations, microscopic fat globules and fine needle-shaped crystals soluble in ether.

§ 290. **Antidote—Treatment.**—After emptying the stomach by means of emetics or by the stomach-pump, oil of turpentine in full medicinal doses, say 2.5 c.c. (about 40 min.), frequently administered, seems to act as a true antidote, and a large percentage of cases treated early in this way recover.

§ 291. **Poisonous Effects of Phosphine (phosphuretted hydrogen).**—Experiments on pigeons, on rats, and other animals, and a few very rare cases among men, have shown that phosphine has an exciting action on the respiratory mucous membranes, and a secondary action on the nervous system. Eulenberg[299] exposed a pigeon to an atmosphere containing 1.68 per cent. of phosphine. There was immediate unrest; at the end of three minutes, quickened and laboured breathing (100 a minute); after seven minutes, the bird lay prostrate, with shivering of the body and wide open beak; after eight minutes, there was vomiting; after nine minutes, slow breathing (34 per minute); after twelve minutes, convulsive movements of the wings; and after thirteen minutes, general convulsions and death.

The membranes of the brain were found strongly injected, and there were extravasations. In the mucous membrane of the crop there was also an extravasation. The lungs externally and throughout were of a dirty brown-red colour; the entire heart was filled with coagulated blood, which was weakly acid in reaction.

In a second experiment with another pigeon, there was no striking symptom save that of increased frequency of respiration and loss of appetite; at the end of four days it was found dead. There was much congestion of the cerebral veins and vessels, the mucous membrane of the trachea and bronchi were weakly injected, and the first showed a thin, plastic, diphtheritic-like exudation.

Dr. Henderson's[300] researches on rats may also be noticed here. He found that an atmosphere consisting entirely of phosphine killed rats within ten minutes, an atmosphere with 1 per cent. in half an hour. The symptoms observed were almost exactly similar to those noticed in the first experiment on the pigeon quoted above, and the *post-mortem* appearances were not dissimilar. With smaller quantities of the gas, the first symptom was increased frequency of the respiration; then the animals showed signs of suffering intense irritation of the skin, scratching and biting at it incessantly; afterwards they became drowsy, and assumed a very peculiar attitude, sitting down on all-fours, with the back bent forward, and the nose pushed backwards between the forepaws, so as to bring the forehead against the floor of the cage. When in this position, the rat presented the appearance of a curled-up hedgehog. Phosphine, when injected into the rectum, is also fatal; the animals exhale some of the gas from the lungs, and the breath, therefore, reduces solutions of silver nitrate.[301]

Brenner[302] has recorded the case of a man twenty-eight years old, a pharmaceutist, who is supposed to have suffered from illness caused by repeated inhalations of minute quantities of phosphine. He was engaged for two and a half years in the preparation of hypophosphites; his illness commenced with spots before the eyes, and inability to fix the attention. His teeth became very brittle, and healthy as well as carious broke off from very slight causes. Finally, a weakness of the arms and limbs developed in the course of nine months into complete locomotor ataxy.

[295] Tardieu, *op. cit.*, Case 31.

[296] *Diss. de Venefico Phosphoreo Acuto*, Upsal, 1845.

[297] V. Bibra u. Geist, *Die Krankheiten der Arbeiter in den Phosphorzundholz Fabriken*, 1847, S. 59, &c.; Henle u. v. Pfeuffer's *Zeitschr. f. ration. Med.*, N. F., Bd. 7, Hft. 3, 1857.

[298] *Étude Expérimentale sur quelques lésions de l'Empoisonnement aigu par le Phosphore (Thèse)*, Strasbourg, 1869.

[299] *Gewerbe Hygiene*, p. 273.

[300] *Journ. Anat. and Physiol.*, vol. xiii. p. 19.

[301] Dybskowsky, *Med. Chem. Untersuchungen aus Hoppe-Seyler's Labor. in Tübingen*, p. 57.

[302] *St. Petersburg Med. Zeitschr.*, 4 Hft., 1865.

§ 292. Blood takes up far more phosphine than water. Dybskowsky found that putting the coefficient of solubility of phosphine in pure water at .1122 at 15°, the coefficient for venous blood was .13, and for arterial 26.73; hence the richer the blood is in oxygen the more phosphine is absorbed. It seems probable that the poisonous gas reacts on the oxyhæmoglobin of the blood, and phosphorous acid is formed. This is supported by the fact that a watery extract of such blood reduces silver nitrate, and has been also found feebly acid. The dark blood obtained from animals poisoned by phosphine, when examined spectroscopically, has been found to exhibit a band in the violet.

§ 293. **Post-mortem Appearances.**—There are a few perfectly well authenticated cases showing that phosphorus may cause death, and yet no lesion be discovered afterwards. Thus, Tardieu[303] cites a case in which a woman, aged 45, poisoned herself with phosphorus, and died suddenly the seventh day afterwards. Dr. Mascarel examined the viscera with the greatest care, but could discover absolutely no abnormal conditions; the only symptoms during life were vomiting, and afterwards a little indigestion. It may, however, be remarked that the microscope does not seem to have been employed, and that probably a close examination of the heart would have revealed some alteration of its ultimate structure. The case quoted, by Taylor[304] may also be mentioned, in which a child was caught in the act of sucking phosphorus matches, and died ten days afterwards in convulsions. None of the ordinary *post-mortem* signs of poisoning by phosphorus were met with, but the intestines were reddened throughout, and there were no less than ten invaginations; but the case is altogether a doubtful one, and no phosphorus may actually have been taken. It is very difficult to give in a limited space anything like a full picture of the different lesions found after death from phosphorus, for they vary according as to whether the death is speedy or prolonged, whether the phosphorus has been taken as a finely-divided solid, or in the form of vapour, &c. It may, however, be shortly said, that the most common changes are fatty infiltration of the liver and kidneys, fatty degeneration of the heart, enlargement of the liver, ecchymoses in the serous membranes, in the muscular, in the fatty, and in the mucous tissues. When death occurs before jaundice supervenes, there may be little in the aspect of the corpse to raise a suspicion of poison; but if intense jaundice has existed during life, the yellow staining of the skin, and it may be, spots of purpura, will suggest to the experienced pathologist the possibility of phosphorus poisoning. In the mouth and throat there will seldom be anything abnormal. In one or two cases of rapid death among infants, some traces of the matches which had been sucked were found clinging to the gums. The stomach may be healthy, but the most common appearance is a swelling of the mucous membrane and superficial erosions. Virchow,[305] who was the first to call attention to this peculiar grey swelling of the intestinal mucous membrane under the name of *gastritis glandularis* or *gastradenitis*, shows that it is due to a fatty degeneration of the epithelial cells, and that it is by no means peculiar to phosphorus poisoning. The swelling may be seen in properly-prepared sections to have its essential seat in the glands of the mucous membrane; the glands are enlarged, their openings filled with large cells, and each single cell is finely granular. Little centres of hæmorrhage, often microscopically small, are seen, and may be the centres of small inflammations; their usual situation is on the summit of the rugæ. Very similar changes are witnessed after death from septicæmia, pyæmia, diphtheria, and other diseases. The softening of the stomach, gangrene, and deep erosions, recorded by the earlier authors, have not been observed of late years, and probably were due to *post-mortem* changes, and not to processes during life. The same changes are to be seen in the intestines, and there are numerous extravasations in the peritoneum.

The liver shows of all the organs the most characteristic signs; a more or less advanced fatty infiltration of its structure takes place, which was first described as caused by phosphorus by Hauff in 1860.[306] It is the most constant pathological evidence both in man and animal, and seems to occur at a very early period, Munk and Leyden having found a fatty degeneration in the liver far advanced in twenty-four hours[307] after poisoning. In rats and mice poisoned with paste, I have found this evident to the naked eye twelve hours after the fatal dose. The liver is mostly large, but in a case[308] recorded in the *Lancet*, July 14, 1888, the liver was shrunken; it has a pale yellow (or sometimes an

[303] *L'Empoisonnement*, p. 520.

[304] *Poisons*, 3rd ed., p. 276.

[305] Virchow's *Archiv. f. path. Anat.*, Bd. 31, Hft. 3, 399.

[306] Hauff collected 12 cases, and found a fatty liver in 11.—*Würtemb. Med. Corresp. Bl.*, 1860, No. 34.

[307] *Die acute Phosphor-Vergiftung*, Berlin, 1865.

[308] This case, from the similarity of the pathological appearances to those produced by yellow atrophy, deserves fuller notice:—"Frances A. Cowley, aged 20, on her own admission, took some rat paste on Tuesday, June 19th. Death ensued eleven days later. The initial symptoms were not very marked. Nausea and vomiting continued with moderate severity for a few days and then

intense yellow) colour; on section the cut surface presents a mottled appearance; the serous envelopes, especially along the course of the vessels, exhibit extravasations of blood. The liver itself is more deficient in blood than in the normal condition, and the more bloodless it is, the greater the fatty infiltration.

In the Museum of the Royal College of Surgeons there is a preparation (No. 2737) of the section of a liver derived from a case of phosphorus poisoning.

A girl, aged 18, after two days' illness, was admitted into Guy's Hospital. She confessed to having eaten a piece of bread coated with phosphorus paste. She had great abdominal pain, and died on the seventh day after taking the phosphorus. A few hours before her death she was profoundly and suddenly collapsed. The liver weighed 66 ozs. The outlines of the hepatic lobules were very distinct, each central vein being surrounded by an opaque yellowish zone; when fresh the hue was more uniform, and the section was yellowish-white in colour. A microscopical examination of the hepatic cells showed them laden with fat globules, especially in the central parts of the liver.

The microscopic appearances are also characteristic. In a case of suicidal poisoning by phosphorus, in which death took place on the seventh day, the liver was very carefully examined by Dr. G. F. Goodart, who reported as follows:—

"Under a low power the structure of the liver is still readily recognisable, and in this the specimen differs from slides of three cases of acute yellow atrophy that I have in my possession. The hepatic cells are present in large numbers, and have their natural trabecular arrangement. The columns are abnormally separated by dilated blood or lymph-spaces, and the individual cells are cloudy and ill-defined. The portal channels are everywhere characterised by a crowd of small nuclei which stain with logwood deeply. The epithelium of the smaller ducts is cloudy, and blocks the tubes in many cases. Under a high power (one-fifth) it is seen that the hepatic cells are exceedingly ill-defined in outline, and full of granules and even drops of oil. But in many parts, even where the cells themselves are hazy, the nucleus is still fairly visible. It appears to me that, in opposition to what others have described, the nuclei of the cells have in great measure resisted the degenerative process. The change in the cells is uniform throughout each lobule, but some lobules are rather more affected than others. The blood-spaces between the cells are empty, and the liver appears to be very bloodless. The portal canals are uniformly studded with small round nuclei or cells, which are in part, and might be said in great part, due to increase of the connective tissue or to a cirrhotic process. But I am more disposed to favour the view that they are due to migration from the blood-vessels, because they are so uniform in size, and the hepatic cells and connective tissue in their neighbourhood are undergoing no changes in the way of growth whatever. I cannot detect any fatty changes in the vessels, but some of the smaller biliary ducts contain some cloudy albuminous material, and their nucleation is not distinct. No retained biliary pigment is visible."[309]

Oscar Wyss,[310] in the case of a woman twenty-three years old, who died on the fifth day after taking phosphorus, describes, in addition to the fatty appearance of the cells, a new formation of cells lying between the lobules and in part surrounding the gall-ducts and the branches of the portal vein and hepatic artery.

---

ceased. There ensued a feeling of depression. Towards the end insensibility, icterus, and somewhat profuse metrorrhagia supervened. At the necropsy the skin and conjunctivæ were observed of a bright yellow colour. There was no organic disease save of a recent nature, and entirely attributable to the action of the poison ingested. The stomach contained about three-quarters of a pint of dark claret-coloured fluid, consisting largely of blood derived from capillary hæmorrhage from the mucous membrane. There was no solution of continuity of the mucous membrane, which showed traces of recent irritation. The whole surface presented a yellow icteric tint, except the summits of some of the rugæ, which were of a bright pink colour. There was also faint wrinkling of the mucous membrane. The upper part of the small intestine was affected in much the same manner as the stomach. The large intestine contained a quantity of almost colourless fæces. The liver was shrunken, weighing only 26 ozs., and both on its outer and sectional surface exactly resembled the appearances produced by acute yellow atrophy, except that there were greater congestion and interstitial hæmorrhage in patches. The lobules of the liver were in many places unrecognisable; in others they stood in bold relief as brilliant canary-yellow patches, standing in strong contrast to the deep dark-red areas of congestion and extravasation. The gall-bladder contained about 2 drachms of thin greyish fluid, apparently all but devoid of bile. The urinary bladder was empty; the kidneys were enlarged; the cortex was very pale and bile-stained, of greater depth than natural, and of softer consistence. The spleen was not enlarged, nor was it in the least degree softened. In addition to the bleeding from the uterus noticed during life, there was capillary hæmorrhage into the right lung and pleura, into the pericardium, and, as already mentioned, into the stomach. The brain was healthy."

[309] "A Recent Case of Suicide," by Herbert J. Capon, M.D.—*Lancet*, March 18, 1882.

[310] Virchow's *Archiv. f. path. Anat.*, Bd. 33, Hft. 3, S. 432, 1865.

Salkowsky[311] found in animals, which he killed a few hours after administering to them toxic doses of phosphorus, notable hyperæmia of the throat, intestine, liver, and kidneys—both the latter organs being larger than usual. The liver cells were swollen, and the nuclei very evident, but they contained no fat, fatty drops being formed afterwards.

§ 294. **The kidneys** exhibit alterations very similar and analogous to those of the liver. They are mostly enlarged, congested, and flabby, with extravasations under the capsule, and show microscopic changes essentially consisting in a fatty degeneration of the epithelium. In cases attended with hæmorrhage, the tubuli may be here and there filled with blood. The fatty epithelium is especially seen in the contorted tubes, and the walls of the vessels, both of the capsule and of the malpighian bodies, also undergo the same fatty change. In cases in which death has occurred rapidly, the kidneys have been found almost healthy, or a little congested only. The pancreas has also been found with its structure in part replaced by fatty elements.

Of great significance are also the fatty changes in the general muscular system, and more especially in the heart. The muscular fibres of the heart quickly lose their transverse striæ, which are replaced by drops of fat. Probably this change is the cause of the sudden death not unfrequently met with in phosphorus poisoning.

In the lungs, when the phosphorus is taken in substance, there is little "naked-eye" change, but Perls,[312] by manometric researches, has shown that the elasticity is always decreased. According to experiments on animals, when the vapour is breathed, the mucous membrane is red, congested, swollen, and has an acid reaction.

In the nervous system no change has been remarked, save occasionally hæmorrhagic points and extravasations.

§ 295. **Diagnostic Differences between Acute Yellow Atrophy of the Liver and Fatty Liver produced by Phosphorus.**—O. Schultzen and O. L. Riess have collected and compared ten cases of fatty liver from phosphorus poisoning, and four cases of acute yellow atrophy of the liver, and, according to them, the chief points of distinction are as follows:—In phosphorus poisoning the liver is large, doughy, equally yellow, and with the acini well marked; while in acute yellow atrophy the liver is diminished in size, tough, leathery, and of a dirty yellow hue, the acini not being well mapped out. The "phosphorus" liver, again, presents the cells filled with large fat drops, or entirely replaced by them; but in the "atrophy" liver, the cells are replaced by a finely-nucleated detritus and through newly-formed cellular tissue. Yellow atrophy seems to be essentially an inflammation of the intralobular connective tissue, while in phosphorus poisoning the cells become gorged by an infiltration of fat, which presses upon the vessels and lessens the blood supply, and the liver, in consequence, may, after a time, waste.

There is also a clinical distinction during life, not only in the lessening bulk of the liver in yellow atrophy, in opposition to the increase of size in the large phosphorus liver, but also in the composition of the renal secretion. In yellow atrophy the urine contains so much leucine and tyrosin, that the simple addition of acetic acid causes at once a precipitate. Schultzen and Riess also found in the urine, in cases of yellow atrophy, *oxymandelic acid* ($C_8H_8O_4$), but in cases of phosphorus poisoning a nitrogenised acid, fusing at 184° to 185°.

According to Maschka, grey-white, knotty, fæcal masses are found in the intestines in yellow atrophy, but never in cases of phosphorus poisoning. In the latter, it is more common to find a slight intestinal catarrh and fluid excreta.

§ 296. **The Detection of Phosphorus.**—The following are the chief methods in use for the separation and detection of phosphorus:[313]—

1. **Mitscherlich's Process.**—The essential feature of this process is simply distillation of free phosphorus, and observation of its luminous properties as the vapour condenses in the condensing tube. The conditions necessary for success are—(1) that the apparatus should be in total darkness;[314] and (2) that there should be no substance present, such as alcohol or ammonia,[315] which, distilling over with the phosphorus-vapour, could destroy its

[311] *Ibid.*, Bd. 34, Hft. 1 u. 2, S. 73, 1865.

[312] Deutsch. *Archiv f. klin. Med.*, vi. Hft. 1, S. 1, 1869.

[313] It has been recommended to dissolve the phosphorus out from organic matters by carbon disulphide. On evaporation of the latter the phosphorus is recognised by its physical properties. Such a method is of but limited application, although it may sometimes be found useful. I have successfully employed it in the extraction of phosphorus from the crop of a fowl; but on this occasion it happened to be present in large quantity.

[314] Any considerable amount of phosphorescence can, however, be observed in twilight.

[315] Many volatile substances destroy the luminous appearance of phosphorus vapour, *e.g.*, chlorine, hydric sulphide, sulphur dioxide, carbon disulphide, ether, alcohol, petroleum, turpentine, creasote, and most essential oils. On the other hand, bromine, hydrochloric acid, camphor, and carbonate of ammonia do not seem to interfere much with the phosphorescence.

luminosity. A convenient apparatus, and one certain to be in all laboratories, is an ordinary Florence flask, containing the liquid to be tested, fitted to a glass Liebig's condenser, supported on an iron sand-bath (which may, or may not, have a thin layer of sand), and heated by a Fletcher's low temperature burner. The distillate is received into a flask. This apparatus, if in darkness, works well; but should the observer wish to work in daylight, the condenser must be enclosed in a box perfectly impervious to light, and having a hole through which the luminosity of the tube may be seen, the head of the operator and the box being covered with a cloth. If there be a stream of water passing continuously through the condenser, a beautiful luminous ring of light appears in the upper part of the tube, where it remains fixed for some time. Should, however, the refrigeration be imperfect, the luminosity travels slowly down the tube into the receiver. In any case, the delicacy of the test is extraordinary.[316] If the organic liquid is alkaline, or even neutral, there will certainly be some evolution of ammonia, which will distil over before the phosphorus, and retard (or, if in sufficient quantity, destroy) the luminosity. In such a case it is well, as a precaution, to add enough sulphuric acid to fix the ammonia, omitting such addition if the liquid to be operated upon is acid.

2. **The Production of Phosphine** (PH_3).—Any method which produces phosphine (phosphuretted hydrogen), enabling that gas to be passed through nitrate of silver solution, may be used for the detection of phosphorus. Thus, Sonnenschein states that he has found phosphorus in extraordinary small amount, mixed with various substances, by heating with potash in a flask, and passing the phosphine into silver nitrate, separating the excess of silver, and recognising the phosphoric acid by the addition of molybdate of ammonia.[317]

The usual way is, however, to produce phosphine by means of the action on free phosphorus of nascent hydrogen evolved on dissolving metallic zinc in dilute sulphuric acid. Phosphine is formed by the action of nascent hydrogen on solid phosphorus, phosphorous acid, and hypophosphorous acid; but no phosphine can be formed in this way by the action of hydrogen on phosphoric acid.

Since it may happen that no free phosphorus is present, but yet the first product (phosphorous acid) of its oxidation, the production of phosphine becomes a necessary test to make on failure of Mitscherlich's test; if no result follows the proper application of the two processes, the probability is that phosphorus has not been taken.

Blondlot and Dusart evolve hydrogen from zinc and dilute sulphuric acid, and pass the gas into silver nitrate; if the gas is pure, there is of course no reduction; the liquid to be tested is then added to the hydrogen-generating liquid, and if phosphorous or hypophosphorous acids be present, a black precipitate of phosphor-silver will be produced. To prove that this black precipitate is neither that produced by SH_2, nor by antimony nor arsenic, the precipitate is collected and placed in the apparatus to be presently described, and the spectroscopic appearances of the phosphine flame observed.

3. **Tests Dependent on the Combustion of Phosphine** (PH_3).—A hydrogen flame, containing only a minute trace of phosphorus, or of the lower products of its oxidation, acquires a beautiful green tint, and possesses a characteristic *spectrum*. In order to obtain the latter in its best form, the amount of phosphine must not be too large, or the flame will become whitish and livid, and the bands lose their defined character, rendering the spectrum continuous. Again, the orifice of the tube whence the gas escapes must not be too small; and the best result is obtained when the flame is cooled.

M. Salet has proposed two excellent methods for the observation of phosphine by the spectroscope:—

(1) He projects the phosphorus-flame on a plane vertical surface, maintained constantly cold by means of a thin layer of running water; the green colour is especially produced in the neighbourhood of the cool surface.

(2) At the level of the base of the flame, there is an annular space, through which a stream of cold air is continually blown upwards. Thus cooled, the light is very pronounced, and the band δ, which is almost invisible in the ordinary method of examination, is plainly seen.[318]

An apparatus (devised by Blondlot, and improved by Fresenius) for the production of the phosphine flame in medico-legal research, is represented in the following diagram:—

Several of the details of this apparatus may be modified at the convenience of the operator. A is a vessel containing sulphuric acid; B is partly filled with granulated zinc, and hydrogen may be developed at pleasure; *c* contains a solution of nitrate of silver; *d* is a tube at which the gas can be lit; *e*, a flask containing the fluid to be

---

316 Fresenius states that he and Neubauer, with 1 mgrm. of phosphorus in 200,000, recognised the light, which lasted for half an hour.—*Zeitschr. f. anal. Chem.*, i. p. 336.

317 Sonnenschein, *Handbuch der gerichtlichen Chemie*, Berlin, 1869.

318 Consult *Spectres Lumineux*, par M. Lecoq de Boisbaudran, Paris, 1874. See also Christofle and Beilstrom's "Abhandlung," in *Fresenius' Zeitschr. f. anal. Chem.*, B. 2, p. 465, and B. 3, p. 147.

tested, and provided with a tube *f*, at which also the gas issuing can be ignited. The orifice should be provided with a platinum nozzle. When the hydrogen has displaced the air, both tubes are lit, and the two flames, being side by side, can be compared. Should any phosphorus come over from the zinc (a possibility which the interposed silver nitrate ought to guard against), it is detected; the last flask is now gently warmed, and if the flame is green, or, indeed, in any case, it should be examined by the spectroscope.[319]

§ 297. The spectrum, when fully developed, shows one band in the orange and yellow between C and D, but very close to D, and several bands in the green. But the bands δ, γ, α, and β are the most characteristic. The band δ has its centre about the wave-length 599.4; it is easily distinguished when the slit of the spectroscope is a little wide, but may be invisible if the slit is too narrow. It is best seen by M. Salet's second process, and, when cooled by a brisk current of air, it broadens, and may extend closer to D. The band γ has a somewhat decided border towards E, while it is nebulous towards D, and it is, therefore, very difficult to say where it begins or where it ends; its centre may, however, be put at very near 109 of Boisbaudran's scale, corresponding to W. L. 560.5, if the flame is free. This band is more distinct than β, but with a strong current of air the reverse is the case. The middle of the important band α is nearly marked by Fraunhofer's line E. Boisbaudran gives it as coinciding with 122 of his scale W. L. 526.3. In ordinary conditions (that is, with a free uncooled flame) this is the brightest and most marked of all the bands. The approximate middle of the band β is W. L. 510.6 (Boisbaudran's scale 129.00).

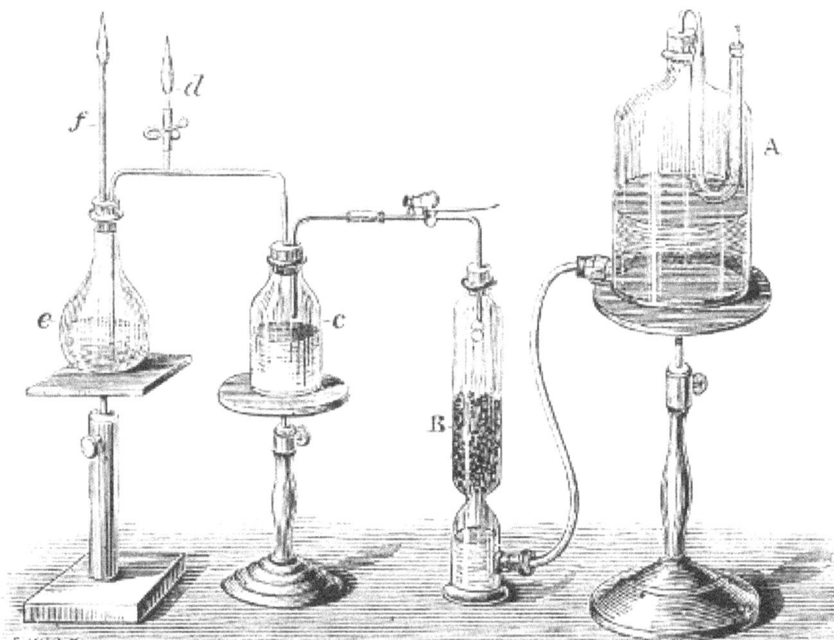

Lipowitz's Sulphur Test.—Sulphur has the peculiar property of condensing phosphorus on its surface, and of this Lipowitz proposed to take advantage. Pieces of sulphur are digested some time with the liquid under research, subsequently removed, and slightly dried. When examined in the dark, should phosphorus be present, they gleam strongly if rubbed with the finger, and develop a phosphorus odour. The test is wanting in delicacy, nor can it well be made quantitative; it has, however, an advantage in certain cases, *e.g.*, the detection of phosphorus in an alcoholic liquid.

Scherer's test, as modified by Hager,[320] is a very delicate and almost decisive test. The substances to be examined are placed in a flask with a little lead acetate (to prevent the possibility of any hydric sulphide being evolved), some ether added, and a strip of filter-paper soaked in a solution of silver nitrate is then suspended in the

[319] F. Selmi has proposed the simple dipping of a platinum loop into a liquid containing phosphoric acid, and then inserting it into the tip of a hydrogen flame.
[320] *Pharm. Central-halle*, 20, 353.

flask; this is conveniently done by making a slit in the bottom of the cork, and in the slit securing the paper. The closed flask is placed in the dark, and if phosphorus is present, in a few minutes there is a black stain. It may be objected that arsine will cause a similar staining, but then arsine could hardly be developed under the circumstances given. It is scarcely necessary to observe that the paper must be wet.

§ 298. **Chemical Examination of the Urine.**—It may be desirable, in any case of suspected phosphorus poisoning, to examine the renal secretion for leucin and tyrosin, &c. Leucin may be found as a deposit in the urine. Its general appearance is that of little oval or round discs, looking like drops of fat. It can be recognised by taking up one or more of these little bodies and placing them in the author's subliming cell. By careful heating it will sublime wholly on to the upper cover. On now adding a little nitric acid to the sublimed leucin, and drying, and then to the dried residue adding a droplet of a solution of sodium hydrate, leucin forms an oily drop. Tyrosin also may occur as a sediment of little heaps of fine needles. The best test for tyrosin is to dissolve in hot water, and then add a drop of a solution of mercuric nitrate and mercurous nitrate, when a rose colour is at once developed, if the tyrosin is in very minute quantity; but if in more than traces, there is a distinct crimson precipitate. To separate leucin and tyrosin from the urine, the best process is as follows:—The urine is filtered from any deposit, evaporated to a thin syrup, and decanted from the second deposit that forms. The two deposits are mixed together and treated with dilute ammonia, which will dissolve out any tyrosin and leave it in needles, if the ammonia is spontaneously evaporated on a watch-glass. The urine is then diluted and treated with neutral and basic acetates of lead, filtered, and the lead thrown out of the filtrate by hydric sulphide. The filtrate is evaporated to a syrup, and it then deposits leucin mixed with some tyrosin. If, however, the syrup refuses to crystallise, it is treated with cold absolute alcohol, and filtered, the residue is then boiled up with spirit of wine, which extracts leucin, and deposits it on cooling in a crystalline form. To obtain oxymandelic acid, the mother liquor, from which leucin and tyrosin have been extracted, is precipitated with absolute alcohol, filtered, and then the alcoholic solution evaporated to a syrup. This syrup is acidified by sulphuric acid, and extracted with ether; the ether is filtered off and evaporated to dryness; the dry residue will be in the form of oily drops and crystals. The crystals are collected, dissolved in water, and the solution precipitated by lead acetate to remove colouring-matters; after filtration it is finally precipitated by basic acetate. On decomposition of the basic acetate, by suspending in water and saturating with hydric sulphide, the ultimate filtrate on evaporation deposits colourless, flexible needles of oxymandelic acid. The nitrogenised acid which Schultzen and Riess obtained from urine in a case of phosphorus poisoning, was found in an alcohol and ether extract—warts of rhombic scales separating out of the syrupy residue. These scales gave no precipitate with basic acetate, but formed a compound with silver nitrate. The silver compound was in the form of shining white needles, and contained 33.9 per cent. of silver; the acid was decomposed by heat, and with lime yielded aniline. Its melting-point is given at from 184° to 185°. The occurrence of some volatile substance in phosphorus urine, which blackens nitrate of silver, and which is probably phosphine, was first noticed by Selmi.[321] Pesci and Stroppa have confirmed Selmi's researches. It is even given off in the cold.

§ 299. **The quantitative estimation of phosphorus** is best carried out by oxidising it into phosphoric acid, and estimating as ammon. magnesian phosphate. To effect this, the substances are distilled in an atmosphere of CO_2 into a flask with water, to which a tube containing silver nitrate is attached; the latter retains all phosphine, the former solid phosphorus. If necessary, the distillate may be again distilled into $AgNO_3$; and in any case the contents of the U-tube and flask are mixed, oxidised with nitromuriatic acid, filtered from silver chloride, and the phosphoric acid determined in the usual way.

In the case of a child poisoned by lucifer matches, Sonnenschein estimated the free phosphorus in the following way:—The contents of the stomach were diluted with water, a measured part filtered, and the phosphoric acid estimated. The other portion was then oxidised by HCl and potassic chlorate, and the phosphoric acid estimated—the difference being calculated as free phosphorus.

§ 300. **How long can Phosphorus be recognised after Death?**—One of the most important matters for consideration is the time after death in which free phosphorus, or free phosphoric acids, can be detected. Any phosphorus changed into ammon. mag. phosphate, or into any other salt, is for medico-legal purposes entirely lost, since the expert can only take cognisance of the substance either in a free state, as phosphine, or as a free acid.

The question, again, may be asked in court—Does the decomposition of animal substances rich in phosphorus develop phosphine? The answer to this is, that no such reaction has been observed.

[321] *Giornale Internaz. della Scienza Med.*, 1879, Nro. 5, p. 645.

A case is related[322] in which phosphorus was recognised, although the body had been buried for several weeks and then exhumed.

The expert of pharmacy of the Provincial Government Board of Breslau has also made some experiments in this direction, which are worthy of note:—Four guinea-pigs were poisoned, each by 0.023 grm. of phosphorus; they died in a few hours, and were buried in sandy-loam soil, 0.5 metre deep. Exhumation of the first took place four weeks after. The putrefying organs—heart, liver, spleen, stomach, and all the intestines—tested by Mitscherlich's method of distillation, showed characteristic phosphorescence for nearly one hour.

The second animal was exhumed after eight weeks in a highly putrescent state. Its entrails, on distillation, showed the phosphorescent appearance for thirty-five minutes.

The third animal was taken from the earth after twelve weeks, but no free phosphorus could be detected, although there was evidence of the lower form of oxidation (PO_3) by Blondlot's method.

The fourth animal was exhumed after fifteen weeks, but neither free phosphorus nor PO_3 could be detected.[323]

A man, as well as a cat, was poisoned by phosphorus. On analysis, twenty-nine days after death, negative results were alone obtained.—*Sonnenschein.*

It will thus be evident that there is no constant rule, and that, even when decomposition is much advanced, an examination *may* be successful.

[322] *Pharm. Zeitsch. f. Russl.*, Jahrg. 2, p. 87.

[323] *Vierteljahrsschrift für gerichtliche Medicin*, Jan. 7, 1876; see also *Zeitschr. f. anal. Chemie*, 1872.

Part VI. Alkaloids And Poisonous Vegetable Principles Separated For The Most Part By Alcoholic Solvents.

DIVISION I.—VEGETABLE ALKALOIDS.

I.—General Methods of Testing and Extracting Alkaloids.

§ 301. **General Tests for Alkaloids.**—In order to ascertain whether an alkaloid is present or not, a method of extraction must be pursued which, while disposing of fatty matters, salts, &c., shall dissolve as little as possible of foreign substances—such a method, *e.g.*, as the original process of Stas, or one of its modern modifications.

If to the acid aqueous solution finally obtained by this method a dilute solution of soda be added, drop by drop, until it is rendered feebly alkaline, *and no precipitate appear*, whatever other poisonous plant-constituents may be present, all ordinary alkaloids[324] are absent.

In addition to this negative test, there are also a number of substances which give well-marked crystalline or amorphous precipitates with alkaloids.

§ 302. These may be called "group reagents." The chief members of the group-reagents are—Iodine dissolved in hydriodic acid, iodine dissolved in potassic iodide solution, bromine dissolved in potassic bromide solution, hydrargo-potassic iodide, bismuth-potassic iodide, cadmic potassic iodide; the chlorides of gold, of platinum, and mercury; picric acid, gallic acid, tannin, chromate of potash, bichromate of potash, phospho-molybdic acid, phospho-tungstic acid, silico-tungstic acid, and Fröhde's reagent. It will be useful to make a few general remarks on some of these reagents.

Iodine in hydriodic acid gives either crystalline or amorphous precipitates with nearly all alkaloids; the compound with morphine, for example, is in very definite needles; with dilute solutions of atropine, the precipitate is in the form of minute dots, but the majority of the precipitates are amorphous, and all are more or less coloured.

Iodine dissolved in a solution of potassic iodide gives with alkaloids a reddish or red-brown precipitate, and this in perhaps a greater dilution than almost any reagent. When added to an aqueous solution, the precipitates are amorphous, but if added to an alcoholic solution, certain alkaloids then form crystalline precipitates; this, for example, is the case with berberine and narceine. By treating the precipitate with aqueous sulphurous acid, a sulphate of the alkaloid is formed and hydriodic acid, so that by suitable operations the alkaloid may readily be recovered from this compound. A solution of bromine in potassic bromide solution also gives similar precipitates to the above, but it forms insoluble compounds with phenol, orcin, and other substances.

Mercuric potassic iodide is prepared by decomposing mercuric chloride with potassic iodide in excess. The proportions are 13.546 grms. of mercuric chloride and 49.8 of potassic iodide, and water sufficient to measure, when dissolved, 1 litre. The precipitates from this reagent are white and flocculent; many of them become, on standing, crystalline.

Bismuthic potassic iodide in solution precipitates alkaloids, and the compounds formed are of great insolubility, but it also forms compounds with the various albuminoid bodies.

Chloride of gold forms with the alkaloids compounds, many of which are crystalline, and most admit of utilisation for quantitative determinations. Chloride of gold does not precipitate amides or ammonium compounds, and on this account its value is great. The precipitates are yellow, and after a while are partly decomposed, when the colour is of a reddish-brown.

Platinic chloride also forms precipitates with most of the alkaloids, but since it also precipitates ammonia and potassic salts, it is inferior to gold chloride in utility.

§ 303. (1.) **Phosphomolybdic Acid as a Reagent for Alkaloids.**—*Preparation*; Molybdate of ammonia is precipitated by phosphate of soda; and the well-washed yellow precipitate is suspended in water and warmed with

---

[324] In the case of morphine tartrate, this test will not answer. See the article on Morphine.

carbonate of soda, until it is entirely dissolved. This solution is evaporated to dryness, and the ammonia fully expelled by heating. If the molybdic acid is fairly reduced by this means, it is to be moistened by nitric acid, and the heating repeated. The now dry residue is warmed with water, nitric acid added to strong acid reaction, and the mixture diluted with water, so that 10 parts of the solution contain 1 of the dry salt. The precipitates of the alkaloids are as follows:—

Aniline,	Bright-yellow, flocculent.
Morphine,	,, ,,
Narcotine,	Brownish-yellow, ,,
Quinine,	Whitish-yellow, ,,
Cinchonine,	,,,,
Codeine,	Brownish-yellow, voluminous.
Strychnine,	White-yellow, ,,
Brucine,	Yelk-yellow, flocculent.
Veratrine,	Bright-yellow, ,,
Jervine,	,, ,,
Aconitine,	,, ,,
Emetine,	,, ,,
Theine,	Bright-yellow, voluminous.
Theobromine,	,,,,
Solanine,	Citron-yellow, pulverulent.
Atropine,	Bright-yellow, flocculent.
Hyoscyamine,	,,,,
Colchicine,	Orange-yellow, ,,
Delphinine,	Grey-yellow, voluminous.
Berberine,	Dirty-yellow, flocculent.
Coniine,	Bright-yellow, voluminous.
Nicotine,	,,,,
Piperine,	Brownish-yellow, flocculent.

(2.) **Silico-Tungstic Acid as a Reagent for Alkaloids.**—Sodium tungstate is boiled with freshly precipitated gelatinous silica. To the solution is added mercurous nitrate, which precipitates the yellow mercurous silico-tungstate. This is filtered, well-washed, and decomposed by an equivalent quantity of hydrochloric acid; silico-tungstic acid then goes into solution, and mercurous chloride (calomel) remains behind. The clear filtrate is evaporated to drive off the excess of hydrochloric acid, and furnishes, on spontaneous evaporation, large, shining, colourless octahedra of silico-tungstic acid, which effloresce in the air, melt at 36°, and are easily soluble in water or alcohol.

This agent produces no insoluble precipitate with any metallic salt. Cæsium and rubidium salts, even in dilute solutions, are precipitated by it; neutral solutions of ammonium chloride give with it a white precipitate, soluble with difficulty in large quantities of water. It precipitates solutions of the salts of quinine, cinchonine, morphine, atropine, &c.; if in extremely dilute solution, an opalescence only is produced: for instance, it has been observed that cinchonine hydrochlorate in $^1/_{200000}$, quinia hydrochlorate in $^1/_{20000}$, morphia hydrochlorate in $^1/_{15285}$ dilution, all gave a distinct opalescence.—*Archiv der Pharm.*, Nov., Dr. Richard Godeffroy.

(3.) **Scheibler's Method for Alkaloids: Phospho-Tungstic Acid.**—Ordinary commercial sodium tungstate is digested with half its weight of phosphoric acid, specific gravity 1.13, and the whole allowed to stand for some days, when the acid separates in crystals. A solution of these crystals will give a distinct precipitate with the most minute quantities of alkaloids, $^1/_{200000}$ of strychnine, and $^1/_{100000}$ of quinine. The alkaloid is liberated by digestion with barium hydrate (or calcium hydrate); and if volatile, may be distilled off, if fixed, dissolved out by chloroform. In complex mixtures, colouring-matter may be removed by plumbic acetate, the lead thrown out by SH_2, and concentrated, so as to remove the excess of SH_2.

§ 304. **Schulze's reagent** is phospho-antimonic acid. It is prepared by dropping a strong solution of antimony trichloride into a saturated solution of sodic phosphate. The precipitation of the alkaloids is effected by this reagent in a sulphuric acid solution.

§ 305. **Dragendorff's reagent** is a solution of potass-bismuth iodide; it is prepared by dissolving bismuth iodide in a hot solution of potassium iodide, and then diluting with an equal volume of iodide of potassium solution. On the addition of an acid solution of an alkaloid, a kermes-red precipitate falls down, which is in many cases crystalline.

Marm's reagent is a solution of potass-cadmium iodide. It is made on similar principles.

Potass-zinc iodide in solution is also made similarly. The precipitates produced in solutions of narceine and codeine are crystalline and very characteristic.

§ 306. **Colour Tests.—Fröhde's reagent** is made by dissolving 1 part of sodic molybdate in 10 parts of strong sulphuric acid; it strikes distinctive colours with many alkaloids.

Mandelin's reagent is a solution of meta-vanadate of ammonia in mono- or dihydrated sulphuric acid. The strength should be 1 part of the salt to 200 of the acid. This reagent strikes a colour with many alkaloids, and aids to their identification. It is specially useful to supplement and correct other tests. The following table gives the chief colour reactions, with the alkaloids. (See earlier for the spectroscopic appearances of certain of the colour tests.)

METHODS OF SEPARATION.

§ 307. **Stas's Process.**—The original method of Stas[325] (afterwards modified by Otto)[326] consisted in extraction of the organic matters by strong alcohol, with the addition of tartaric acid; the filtered solution was then carefully neutralised with soda, and shaken up with ether, the ethereal solution being separated by a pipette. Subsequent chemists proposed chloroform instead of ether,[327] the additional use of amyl-alcohol,[328] and the substitution of acetic, hydrochloric, and sulphuric for tartaric acid.

COLOUR REACTIONS[329] OF CERTAIN ALKALOIDS.

Name of Substance.	Strong Sulphuric Acid.	Fröhde's Reagent.	Mandelin's Reagent.
Strychnine.	...	...	Violet-blue, then lastly cinnabar-red.
Brucine.	Pale red.	Red, then yellow.	Yellow-red to orange, afterwards blood-red.
Curarine.	Fine red.	...	...
Quinine.	...	Greenish.	Weak orange, then blue-green, lastly green-brown.
Atropine.	...	...	Red, then yellow-red, and lastly yellow.
Aconitine.	...	...	...

[325] *Annal d. Chem. u. Pharm.*, 84, 379.

[326] *Ib.*, 100, 44. *Anleitung zur Ausmittel. d. Gifte.*

[327] Rodgers and Girwood, *Pharm. Journ. and Trans.*, xvi. 497; Prollin's *Chem. Centralb.*, 1857, 231; Thomas, *Zeitschr. für analyt. Chem.*, i. 517, &c.

[328] Erdmann and v. Ushlar, *Ann. Chem. Pharm.*, cxx. pp. 121-360.

[329] Caustic potash also gives characteristic colours with certain alkaloids. Out of seventy-two alkaloids (using 0.5 mgrm.), the following alone gave characteristic colours when fused with KHO:—Quinine, grass-green, and peculiar odour; quinidine, becoming yellower and finally brown; cinchonine, at first brownish-red to violet, with green edges, later, bluish-green; cinchonidine, blue passing into grey; cocaine, greenish-yellow, turning to blue, and then dirty red on strong heating.—W. Lenz, *Zeit. f. anal. Chem.*, 25, 29-32.

Veratrine.	Yellow, then orange, blood-red, lastly carmine-red.	Gamboge-yellow, then cherry-red.	Yellow, orange, blood-red, lastly carmine-red.
Morphine.	...	Violet, green, blue-green, and yellow.	Reddish, then blue-violet.
Narcotine.	Yellow, then raspberry colour.	Green, then brown-green, yellow, lastly red.	Cinnabar-red, then carmine-red.
Codeine.	...	Dirty green, then blue, lastly yellow.	Green-blue to blue.
Papaverine.	...	Green, then blue-violet, lastly cherry-red.	Blue-green to blue.
Thebaine.	Blood-red, then yellow-red.	Orange, then colourless.	Red to orange.
Narceine.	Grey-brown, then blood-red.	Brown, green, red, lastly blue.	Violet, then orange.
Nicotine.	...	Yellowish, then red.	Transitory dark colour.
Coniine.	...	Yellow.	...
Colchicine.	Intense yellow.	Yellow to green-yellow.	Blue-green, then brown.
Delphinidine.	Red.	Red-brown.	Red-brown to brown.
Solanine.	Red-yellow, then brown.	Cherry-red, red-brown, yellow, yellow-green.	Yellow-orange, cherry-red, and lastly violet.

§ 308. **Selmi's Process for Separating Alkaloids.**—A method of separating alkaloids from an ethereal solution has been proposed by Selmi.[330] The alcoholic extract of the viscera, acidified and filtered, is evaporated at 65°; the residue taken up with water, filtered, and decolorised by basic acetate of lead. The lead is thrown out by sulphuretted hydrogen; the solution, after concentration, repeatedly extracted with ether; and the ethereal solution saturated with dry CO_2, which generally precipitates some of the alkaloids. The ethereal solution is then poured into clean vessels, and mixed with about half its volume of water, through which a current of CO_2 is passed for twenty minutes; this may cause the precipitation of other alkaloids not thrown down by dry CO_2. If the whole of the alkaloids are not obtained by these means, the solution is dehydrated by agitation with barium oxide, and a solution of tartaric acid in ether is added (care being taken to avoid excess); this throws down any alkaloid still present. The detection of any yet remaining in the viscera is effected by mixing with barium hydrate and a little water, and agitating with *purified* amylic alcohol; from the alcohol the alkaloids may be subsequently extracted by agitation with very dilute sulphuric acid.

Another ingenious method (also the suggestion of Selmi) is to treat the organic substance with alcohol, to which a little sulphuric acid has been added, to filter, digest with alcohol, and refilter. The filtrates are united, evaporated down to a smaller bulk, filtered, concentrated to a syrup, alkalised by barium hydrate, and, after the addition of freshly ignited barium oxide and some powdered glass, exhausted with dry ether; the ether filtered, the filtrate digested with lead hydrate; the ethereal solution filtered, evaporated to dryness, and finally again taken up with

[330] F. Selmi, *Gazett. Chim. Ital.*, vj. 153-166, and *Journ. Chem. Soc.*, i., 1877, 93.

ether, which, this time, should leave on evaporation the alkaloid almost pure.

§ 309. **Dragendorff's Process.**—To Dragendorff we owe an elaborate general method of separation, since it is applicable not only to alkaloids, but to glucosides, and other active principles derived from plants. His process is essentially a combination of those already known, and its distinctive features are the shaking up—(1) of the acid fluid with the solvent, thus removing colouring matters and certain non-alkaloidal principles; and (2) of the same fluid made alkaline. The following is his method in full. It may be advantageously used when the analyst has to search generally for vegetable poison, although it is, of course, far too elaborate for every case; and where, from any circumstance, there is good ground for suspecting the presence of one or two particular alkaloids or poisons, the process may be much shortened and modified.[331]

I. The substance, in as finely-divided form as possible, is digested for a few hours in water acidified with sulphuric acid, at a temperature of 40° to 50°, and this operation is repeated two or three times, with filtering and pressing of the substances; later, the extracts are united. This treatment (if the temperature mentioned is not exceeded) does not decompose the majority of alkaloids or other active substances; but there are a few (*e.g.*, solanine and colchicine) which would be altered by it; and, if such are suspected, maceration at the common temperature is necessary, with substitution of acetic for sulphuric acid.[332]

II. The extract is next evaporated until it begins to be of a syrupy consistence; the residue mixed with three to four times its volume of alcohol, macerated for twenty-four hours at about 34°, allowed to become quite cool, and filtered from the foreign matters which have separated. The residue is washed with alcohol of 70 per cent.

III. The filtrate is freed from alcohol by distillation, the watery residue poured into a capacious flask, diluted (if necessary) with water, and filtered. Acid as it is, it is extracted at the common temperature, with frequent shaking, by freshly-rectified petroleum ether; and, after the fluids have again separated, the petroleum ether is removed, carrying with it certain impurities (colouring matter, &c.), which are in this way advantageously displaced. By this operation ethereal oils, carbolic acid, picric acid, &c., which have not been distilled, besides piperin, may also be separated. The shaking up with petroleum ether is repeated several times (as long as anything remains to be dissolved), and the products are evaporated on several watch-glasses.

RESIDUE OF PETROLEUM ETHER FROM THE ACID SOLUTION.

1. It is Crystalline.	2. It is Amorphous.	3. It is Volatile, with a powerful odour; *ethereal oil, carbolic acid, &c.*
A. *It is yellowish*, and with difficulty volatilised.	A. It is fixed.	
α. The crystals are dissolved by concentrated sulphuric acid, with the production of a clear yellow colour, passing into brown and greenish-brown.	α. Concentrated sulphuric acid dissolves it immediately—violet, and later greenish-blue.	
Piperin.	*Constituents of the black hellebore.*	
β. The solution in sulphuric acid remains yellow; potassic cyanide and caustic potash colour it, on warming, blood-red.	β. It dissolves with a yellow colour, changing into fallow-brown.	
Picric acid.	*Constituents of aconite plant and products of the decomposition of Aconitine.*	
B. It Is Colourless, Liquefies easily, and Smells Strongly.	B. It Is White, Sharp-Tasting, and Reddens the Skin.	
Camphor and similar matters.	*Capsicin.*	

[331] Dragendorff's *Gerichtlich-chemische Ermittelung von Giften*, St. Petersburg, 1876, p. 141.

[332] When blood is to be examined, it is better to dry it, and then powder and extract with water acidified with dilute sulphuric acid. However, if the so-called volatile alkaloids are suspected, this modification is to be omitted.

It may be expected that the substances mentioned under the heads 1, 2, and 3 will be, in general, fully obtained by degrees. This is not the case, however, as regards piperin and picric acid.

IV. The watery fluid is now similarly shaken up with benzene, and the benzene removed and evaporated. Should the evaporated residue show signs of an alkaloid (and especially of theine), the watery fluid is treated several times with a fresh mixture of benzene, till a little of the last-obtained benzene extraction leaves on evaporation no residue. The benzene extracts are now united, and washed by shaking with distilled water; again separated and filtered, the greater part of the benzene distilled from the filtrate, and the remainder of the fluid divided and evaporated on several watch-glasses.

The evaporated residue may contain theine, colchicine, cubebin, digitalin, cantharidin, colocynthin, elaterin, caryophylline, absinthin, cascarillin, populin, santonin, &c., and traces of veratrine, delphinine, physostigmine, and berberine.

A remnant of piperin and picric acid may remain from the previous treatment with petroleum ether.

THE BENZENE RESIDUE FROM THE ACID SOLUTION.

1. It is Crystalline.

A. Well-formed, Colourless Crystals.

α. Sulphuric acid dissolves the hair-like crystals without change of colour; evaporation with chlorine water, and subsequent treatment with ammonia, gives a murexide reaction.

Theine.

β. Sulphuric acid leaves the rhombic crystals uncoloured. The substance, taken up by oil, and applied to the skin, produces a blister.

Cantharidin.

γ. Sulphuric acid leaves the scaly crystals at first uncoloured, then slowly develops a reddening. It does not blister. Warm alcoholic potash-lye colours it a transitory red.

Santonin.

δ. Sulphuric acid colours the crystals almost black, whilst it takes itself a beautiful red colour.

Cubebin.

B. Crystals Pale to Clear Yellow.

α. *Piperin.*

β. *Picric Acid.*

γ. Caustic potash dissolves it purple.

Aloetin.

C. Mostly Undefined Colourless Crystals.

2. It is Amorphous.

A. Colourless or Pale Yellow Residue.

α. Sulphuric acid dissolves it at first yellow; the solution becoming later red. Fröhde's reagent does not colour it violet.

Elaterin.

β. Sulphuric acid dissolves red; Fröhde's reagent violet-red;[333] tannic acid does not precipitate.

Populin.

γ. Sulphuric acid dissolves it with a red colour; Fröhde's reagent[334] a beautiful cherry-red; tannic acid precipitates a yellowish-white.

Colocynthin.

δ. Sulphuric acid colours it gradually a beautiful red, whilst tannin does not precipitate.

Constituents of the Pimento.

B. Pure Yellow Residue.

α. Sulphuric acid dissolves it yellow; on the addition of nitric acid, this solution is green, quickly changing to blue and violet.

Colchicine.

β. Sulphuric acid dissolves with separation of a violet powder; caustic potash colours it red; sulphide of ammonia violet, and, by heating, indigo-blue.

Chrysammic acid.

C. A Greenish Bitter Residue, which dissolves brown in concentrated sulphuric acid; in Fröhde's

[333] Fröhde's reagent is described earlier.

[334] Fröhde's reagent is described earlier.

reagent, likewise, at first brown, then at the edge green, changing into blue-violet, and lastly violet.

Constituents of wormwood, with absynthin, besides quassiin, menyanthin, ericolin, daphnin, cnicin, and others.

α. Sulphuric acid dissolves it green-brown; bromine colours this solution red; dilution with water again green. The substance renders the heart-action of a frog slower.

Digitalin.

β. Sulphuric acid dissolves it orange, then brown, lastly red-violet. Nitric acid dissolves it yellow, and water separates as a jelly out of the latter solution. Sulphuric acid and bromine do not colour it red.

Gratiolin.

γ. Sulphuric acid dissolves it red-brown. Bromine produces in this solution red-violet stripes. It does not act on frogs.

Cascarillin.

D. Generally Undefined Yellow Crystallisation.—Sulphuric acid dissolves it olive-green. The alcoholic solution gives with potassic iodide a colourless and green crystalline precipitate.

Berberin.

V. As a complete exhaustion of the watery solution is not yet attained by the benzene agency, another solvent is tried.

THE WATERY SOLUTION IS NOW EXTRACTED IN THE SAME WAY BY CHLOROFORM.

In chloroform the following substances are especially taken up:—Theobromine, narceine, papaverine, cinchonine, jervine, besides picrotoxin, syringin, digitalin, helleborin, convallamarin, saponin, senegin, smilacin. Lastly, portions of the bodies named in Process IV., which benzene failed to extract entirely, enter into solution, as well as traces of brucine, narcotine, physostigmine, veratrine, delphinine. The evaporation of the chloroform is conducted at the ordinary temperature in four or five watch-glasses.

THE CHLOROFORM RESIDUE FROM THE ACID SOLUTION.[335]

1. The Residue is more or less markedly Crystalline.

A. *It gives in the sulphuric acid solution evidence of an alkaloid by its action towards iodine and iodide of potassium.*

α. Sulphuric acid dissolves it without the production of colour, and chlorine and ammonia give no murexide reaction.

Cinchonine.

β. Sulphuric acid dissolves it without colour, chlorine and ammonia give, as with theine, a murexide reaction.

Theobromine.

2. The Residue is Amorphous.

A. *In acetic acid solution it renders the action of the frog's heart slower, or produces local anæsthesia.*

aa. It does not produce local anæsthesia.

α. Sulphuric acid dissolves it red-brown, bromine produces a beautiful purple colour, water changes it into green, hydrochloric acid dissolves it greenish-brown.

Digitalin.

β. Sulphuric acid dissolves it yellow, then brown-red; on addition of water this solution becomes violet. Hydrochloric acid, on warming, dissolves it red.

Convallamarin.

[335] Chloroform removes small portions of acetate of aconitine from acid solution, Dunstan and Umney, *J. C. S.*, 1892, p. 338.

bb. It produces local anæsthesia.

α. Sulphuric acid dissolves it brown. The solution becomes, by extracting with water, violet, and can even be diluted with two volumes of water without losing its colour.

Saponin.

β. Sulphuric acid dissolves it yellow. On diluting with water the same reaction occurs as in the previous case, but more feebly.

Senegin.

γ. Sulphuric acid does not colour in the cold; on warming, the solution becomes a blue violet.

Papaverine.

γ. Sulphuric acid dissolves brown, and the solution becomes red by the addition of a little water. The action is very weak.

Smilacin.

cc. Sulphuric acid dissolves it with the production of a dirty red, hydrochloric acid, in the cold, with that of a reddish-brown colour, and the last solution becomes brown on boiling.

Constituents of the hellebore, particularly Jervine.

δ. Sulphuric acid dissolves it in the cold with the production of a blue colour.

Unknown impurities, many commercial samples of Papaverine.

ε. Sulphuric acid dissolves it at first grey-brown; the solution becomes in about twenty-four hours blood-red. Iodine water colours it blue.

Narceine.

B. It gives no Alkaloid Reaction.

α. Sulphuric acid dissolves it with a beautiful yellow colour; mixed with nitre, then moistened with sulphuric acid, and lastly treated with concentrated soda-lye, it is coloured a brick-red.

Picrotoxin.

β. Sulphuric acid dissolves it with the production of a splendid red colour. The substance renders the heart-action of a frog slower.

Helleborin.

B. Is inactive, and becomes blue by sulphuric acid; by Fröhde's reagent[336] dark cherry-red. Hydrochloric acid dissolves it red. The solution becomes, by boiling, colourless.

Syringin.

VI. THE WATERY FLUID IS NOW AGAIN SHAKEN UP WITH PETROLEUM ETHER,

in order to take up the rest of the chloroform, and the watery fluid is saturated with ammonia. The watery solution of *aconitine* and *emetine* is liable to undergo, through free ammonia, a partial decomposition; but, on the other hand, it is quite possible to obtain, with very small mixtures of the substances, satisfactory reactions, even out

[336] Described earlier.

of ammoniacal solutions.

VII. THE AMMONIACAL WATERY FLUID WITH PETROLEUM ETHER.

In the earlier stages Dragendorff advises the shaking up with petroleum ether at about 40°, and the removal of the ether as quickly as possible whilst warm. This is with the intention of separating by this fluid strychnine, brucine, emetine, quinine, veratrine, &c. Finding, however, that a full extraction by petroleum ether is either difficult or not practicable, he prefers, as we have seen, to conclude the operation by other agents, coming back again upon the ether for certain special cases. Such are the volatile alkaloids; and here he recommends treatment of the fluid by *cold* petroleum ether, taking care *not* to hasten the removal of the latter. Strychnine and other fixed alkaloids are then only taken up in small quantities, and the greater portion remains for the later treatment of the watery fluid by benzene.

A portion of the petroleum ether, supposed to contain in solution volatile alkaloids, is evaporated in two watch-glasses; to the one, strong hydrochloric acid is added, the other being evaporated without this agent. On the evaporation of the petroleum ether, it is seen whether the first portion is crystalline or amorphous, or whether the second leaves behind a strongly-smelling fluid mass, which denotes a volatile alkaloid. If the residue in both glasses is without odour and fixed, the absence of volatile acids and the presence of fixed alkaloids, strychnine, emetine, veratrine, &c., are indicated.

THE PETROLEUM ETHER RESIDUE FROM AMMONIACAL SOLUTION.

1. It is fixed and Crystalline.	2. It is fixed and Amorphous.	3. It is fixed and Odorous.
A. *The crystals are volatilised with difficulty.*		A. *On adding to the watch-glass a little hydrochloric acid, crystals are left behind.*
aa. Sulphuric acid dissolves it without colour.		*aa.* Its solution is not precipitated by platin chloride.
α. Potassic chromate colours this solution a transitory blue, then red.	α. The purest sulphuric acid dissolves it almost without colour; sulphuric acid containing nitric acid, red quickly becoming orange.	α. The crystals of the hydrochloric compound act on polarised light; and are mostly needle-shaped and columnar.
Strychnine.	*Brucine.*	*Coniine and Methyl-Coniine.*
β. Potassic chromate does not colour it blue; with chlorine water and ammonia it gives a green colour.	β. Sulphuric acid dissolves it yellow, becoming deep red.	β. The crystals are cubical or tetrahedral.
Quinine.	*Veratrine.*	*Alkaloid from Capsicum.*
	γ. Sulphuric acid dissolves it brown-green; Fröhde's reagent red, changing into green.	
	Emetine.	
		bb. The solution of the hydrochlorate of the alkaloid is precipitated by platin chloride.
		Sarracinin.
γ. Sulphuric acid dissolves it		B. The residue of the hydrochlorate of the alkaloid is amorphous, or, by further additions

yellow, and the solution becomes gradually a beautiful deep red.

Sabadilline.

δ. The crystals are easily volatilised.

Coniine.

of HCl, becomes crystalline.

aa. Its diluted aqueous solution is precipitated by platin chloride.

α. The hydrochlorate salt, being quickly treated with Fröhde's reagent, gives after about two minutes a violet solution which gradually fades.

Lobeliin.

β. The hydrochlorate smells like nicotine, and becomes by Fröhde's reagent yellow, and after twenty-four hours pale red.

Nicotine.

γ. The hydrochlorate is without odour, the free base smells faintly like aniline.

Sparteine.

bb. The substance is not precipitated from a diluted solution by platin chloride.

α. Its petroleum ether solution produces no turbidity with a solution of picric acid in petroleum ether; but it leaves behind, when mixed with the above, crystals mostly of three-sided plates.

Trimethylamine.

β. The petroleum ether solution gives, on evaporation, when treated similarly, moss-like crystals. The substance is made blue by chloride of lime, as well as by diluted sulphuric acid and bichromate of potash.

Aniline.

γ. The alkaloid does not smell like methylamine, and is not coloured by chloride of lime, sulphuric acid, or chromate of potash.

Volatile alkaloid of the Pimento.

VIII. THE AMMONIACAL SOLUTION IS SHAKEN UP WITH BENZENE.

In most cases petroleum ether, benzene, and chloroform are more easily separated from acid watery fluids than from ammoniacal, benzene and chloroform causing here a difficulty which has perhaps deterred many from using this method. Dragendorff, however, maintains that he has never examined a fluid in which he could not obtain a complete separation of the benzene and water. If the upper benzene layer is fully gelatinous and emulsive, the under layer of water is to be removed with a pipette as far as possible, and the benzene with a few drops of absolute alcohol and filtration. As a rule, the water goes through first alone, and by the time the greater part has run through, the jelly in the filter, by dint of stirring, has become separated from the benzene, and, finally, the jelly shrinks up to a minimum, and the clear benzene filters off. Dragendorff filters mostly into a burette, from which ultimately the benzene and the water are separated.

The principal alkaloids which are dissolved in benzene are—strychnine, methyl and ethyl strychnine, brucine, emetine, quinine, cinchonine, atropine, hyoscyamine, physostigmine, aconitine, nepalin, the alkaloid of the *Aconitum lycoctonum*, aconellin, napellin, delphinine, veratrine, sabatrin, sabadilline, codeine, thebaine, and narcotine.

THE BENZENE RESIDUE DERIVED FROM THE AMMONIACAL SOLUTION.

1. It is for the most part Crystalline.	2. It is for the most part Amorphous.
a. Sulphuric acid dissolves it without colour, the solution being coloured neither on standing nor on the addition of nitric acid.	*a.* Pure sulphuric acid dissolves it either whitish-red or yellowish.
aa. It dilates the pupil of a cat.	
α. Platin chloride does not precipitate the aqueous solution. The sulphuric acid solution gives, on warming, a peculiar smell.	α. The solution becomes by nitric acid immediately red, then quickly orange.
Atropine.	*Brucine.*
β. Platin chloride applied to the solution precipitates.	β. The solution becomes by little and little brownish-red. The substance is coloured red by chloride of lime solution, and it contracts the pupil.
Hyoscyamine.	*Physostigmine.*
bb. It does not dilate the pupil.	
α. The sulphuric acid solution becomes blue by chromate of potash.	
αα. The substance applied to a frog produces tetanus.	
Strychnine.	
ββ. It lowers the number of respirations in a frog.	
Ethyl and Methyl Strychnine.	
β. Sulphuric acid and bichromate of potash do not colour it blue.	
αα. The sulphuric acid watery solution is fluorescent, and becomes green on the addition of chlorine water and ammonia.	
Quinine and Cinchonine.	
(The last is more difficult to dissolve in petroleum ether than quinine.)	
ββ. The solution is not fluorescent.	
Cinchonine.	
b. Sulphuric acid dissolves it at first colourless; the solution takes on standing a rose or violet-blue; on addition of nitric acid, a blood-red or brown coloration.	*b.* Pure sulphuric acid dissolves it yellow, and the solution becomes later beautiful red (with delphinine, more quickly a darker cherry-red.)
α. A solution in diluted sulphuric acid becomes, on heating, gradually deep blood-red, and, when cooled, violet, with nitric acid. The aqueous solution is precipitated by ammonia.	α. The hydrochloric acid solution becomes red on heating.
Narcotine.	

β. The solution in diluted sulphuric acid becomes, on heating, a beautiful blue. Excess of ammonia does not precipitate in a diluted watery solution.

Codeine.

c. Sulphuric acid dissolves it with the production of a yellow colour.

α. The solution remains yellow on standing.

Acolyctin.

β. It becomes beautifully red.

Sabadilline.

d. Sulphuric acid dissolves it with an immediate deep red-brown colour.

Thebaine.

e. Sulphuric acid dissolves it immediately blue.

Substances accompanying the Papaverins.

αα. The substance acts on a frog, causing, in large doses, tetanus.

Veratrine.

ββ. It is almost without action on frogs.

Sabatrin.

β. The hydrochloric acid solution does not, on heating, become red.

Delphinine.

c. Pure sulphuric acid dissolves it yellow, and the solution becomes later red-brown, and gradually violet-red.

α. The substance even in small doses paralyses frogs, and dilates the pupil of a cat's eye. Ether dissolves it with difficulty.

Nepalin.

β. It is easily soluble in ether, its effects are not so marked, and it does not dilate the pupil.

Aconitine.

γ. Its effects are still feeble; it does not dilate the pupil, and is with difficulty dissolved by ether.

Napellin.

d. Sulphuric acid dissolves it with a dark green colour, and the solution becomes, even after a few seconds, a beautiful blood-red.

Alkaloidal substances out of the Aconitum lycoctonum.

e. Sulphuric acid dissolves it brown-green, and Fröhde's reagent red, becoming beautifully green.

Emetine.

IX. SHAKING OF THE AMMONIACAL WATERY SOLUTION WITH CHLOROFORM.

This extracts the remainder of the cinchonine and papaverine, narceine, and a small portion of morphine, as well as an alkaloid from the celandine.

The Residue from the Chloroform.

aa. The solution, on warming, is only slightly coloured.

α. But, after it is again cooled, it strikes with nitric acid a violet-blue; chloride of iron mixed with the substance gives a blue colour; Fröhde's reagent also dissolves it violet.

Morphine.

β. It is not coloured by nitric acid; it is also indifferent to chloride of iron.

Cinchonine.

bb. The solution becomes by warming violet-blue.

Papaverine.

γ. Sulphuric acid dissolves it greenish-brown, and the solution becomes, on standing, blood-red.

Narceine.

δ. Sulphuric acid dissolves it a violet-blue.

Alkaloidal constituent of the Celandine.

X. SHAKING UP OF THE WATERY FLUID WITH AMYL ALCOHOL.

From this process, besides morphine and solanine, as well as salicin, the remnants of the convallamarin, saponin, senegin, and narceine are also to be expected.

The Amyl Alcohol Residue.

a. Sulphuric acid dissolves it without colour in the cold.

Morphine (see above).

b. Sulphuric acid dissolves it with the production of a clear yellow-red and the solution becomes brownish. Iodine water colours it a deep brown. The alcoholic solution gelatinises.

Solanine.

c. Sulphuric acid dissolves it green-brown, becoming red.

Narceine (see above).

d. Sulphuric acid dissolves it yellow, then brown-red, becoming violet on dilution with water. Hydrochloric acid dissolves it, and it becomes red on warming. It stops the heart-action in the systole.

Convallamarin.

e. Hydrochloric acid dissolves it for the most part without colour.

Saponin.

f. As the foregoing, but acting more feebly.

Senegin.

g. Sulphuric acid dissolves it immediately a pure red. On warming with sulphuric acid and bichromate of potash, a smell of salicylic acid is developed.

Salicin.

XI. DRYING THE WATERY FLUID WITH THE ADDITION OF POWDERED GLASS, AND EXTRACTION OF THE FINELY-DIVIDED RESIDUE BY CHLOROFORM.

The residue of the first chloroform extract lessens the number of respirations of a frog; the residue of the second and third chloroform extract becomes, by sulphuric acid and bichromate of potash, blue, passing into a permanent red.

Another portion of this residue becomes red on warming with diluted sulphuric acid.

Curarine.

Shorter Process for Separating some of the Alkaloids.

§ 310. A shorter process, recommended conditionally by Dragendorff, for brucine, strychnine, quinine, cinchonine, and emetine, is as follows:—

The substance, if necessary, is finely divided, and treated with sulphuric acid (dilute) until it has a marked acid reaction. To every 100 c.c. of the pulp (which has been diluted with distilled water to admit of its being filtered later), at least 5 to 10 c.c. of diluted sulphuric acid (1 : 5) are added. It is digested at 50° for a few hours, filtered, and the residue treated again with 100 c.c. of water at 50°. This extract is, after a few hours, again filtered; both the filtrates are mixed and evaporated in the water-bath to almost the consistency of a thin syrup. The fluid, however, must not be concentrated too much, or fully evaporated to dryness. The residue is now placed in a flask, and treated with three to four times its volume of alcohol of 90 to 95 per cent.; the mixture is macerated for twenty-four hours, and then filtered. The filtrate is distilled alcohol-free, or nearly so, but a small amount of alcohol remaining is not objectionable. The watery fluid is diluted to about 50 c.c., and treated with pure benzene; the mixture is shaken, and after a little time the benzene removed—an operation which is repeated. After the removal the second time of the benzene, the watery fluid is made alkaline with ammonia, warmed to 40° or 50°, and the free alkaloid extracted by twice shaking it up with two different applications of benzene. On evaporation of the latter, if the alkaloid is not left pure, it can be dissolved in acid, precipitated by ammonia, and again extracted by benzene.

§ 311. **Scheibler's Process.**—A method very different from those just described is one practised by Scheibler. This is to precipitate the phosphotungstate of the alkaloid, and then to liberate the latter by digesting the precipitate with either hydrate of barium or hydrate of calcium, dissolving it out by chloroform, or, if volatile, by simple distillation. The convenience of Scheibler's process is great, and it admits of very general application. In complex mixtures, it will usually be found best to precede the addition of phosphotungstic acid[337] by that of acetate of lead, in order to remove colouring matter, &c.; the excess of lead must in its turn be thrown out by SH_2, and the excess of SH_2 be got rid of by evaporation. Phosphotungstic acid is a very delicate test for the alkaloids, giving a distinct precipitate with the most minute quantities ($^1/_{200000}$ of strychnine and $^1/_{100000}$ of quinine). A very similar method is practised by Sonnenschein and others with the aid of phospho-molybdic acid. The details of Scheibler's process are as follows:—

The organic mixture is repeatedly extracted by water strongly acidified with sulphuric acid; the extract is evaporated at 30° to the consistence of a thin syrup; then diluted with water, and, after several hours' standing, filtered in a cool place. To the filtered fluid phosphotungstic acid is added in excess, the precipitate filtered, washed with water to which some phosphotungstic acid solution has been added, and, whilst still moist, rinsed into a flask. Caustic baryta or carbonate of potash is added to alkaline reaction, and after the flask has been connected with bulbs containing HCl, it is heated at first slowly, then more strongly. Ammonia and any volatile alkaloids are driven over into the acid, and are there fixed, and can be examined later by suitable methods. The residue in the flask is carefully evaporated to dryness (the excess of baryta having been precipitated by CO_2), and then extracted by strong alcohol. On evaporation of the alcohol, the alkaloid is generally sufficiently pure to be examined, or, if not so, it may be obtained pure by re-solution, &c.

The author has had considerable experience of Scheibler's process, and has used it in precipitating various animal fluids, but has generally found the precipitate bulky and difficult to manage.

§ 312. **Grandval and Lajoux's Method.**[338]—The alkaloids are precipitated from a solution slightly acidified by hydrochloric or sulphuric acid by a solution of hydrarg-potassium iodide. The precipitate is collected on a filter, washed and then transferred to a flask; drop by drop, a solution of sodium sulphide is added; after each addition the suspended precipitate is shaken and allowed to stand for a few minutes, and a drop of the liquid taken out and tested with lead acetate; directly a slight brown colour appears, sufficient sodic sulphide has been added. The liquid is now left for half-an-hour, with occasional shaking. Then sulphuric acid is added until it is just acid, and the liquid is filtered and the mercury sulphide well washed. In the filtrate will be the sulphate of any alkaloid in solution; this liquid is now made alkaline with soda carbonate and shaken up, as in Dragendorff's process, with appropriate solvents; such, for example, as ether, or chloroform, or acetone, or amylic alcohol, according to the particular alkaloid the analyst is searching for, and the solvent finally separated and allowed to evaporate, when the alkaloid is found in the residue.

§ 313. **Identification of the Alkaloids.**—Having obtained, in one way or other, a crystalline or amorphous substance, supposed to be an alkaloid, or, at all events, an active vegetable principle, the next step is to identify it. If the tests given in Dragendorff's process have been applied, the observer will have already gone a good way towards the identification of the substance; but it is, of course, dangerous to trust to one reaction.

In medico-legal researches there is seldom any considerable quantity of the material to work upon. Hence the greatest care must be taken from the commencement not to waste the substance in useless tests, but to study well at the outset what—by the method of extraction used, the microscopic appearance, the reaction to litmus paper, and the solubility in different menstrua—it is likely to be. However minute the quantity may be, it is essential to divide it into different parts, in order to apply a variety of tests; but as any attempt to do this on the solid substance will probably entail loss, the best way is to dissolve it in a watch-glass in half a c.c. of alcohol, ether, or other suitable solvent. Droplets of this solution are then placed on watch-glasses or slips of microscopic glass, and to these drops, by the aid of a glass rod, different reagents can be applied, and the changes watched under the microscope as the drops slowly evaporate.

§ 314. **Sublimation of the Alkaloids.**—A very beautiful and elegant aid to the identification of alkaloids, and vegetable principles generally, is their behaviour towards heat.

Alkaloids, glucosides, the organic acids, &c., when carefully heated, either—(1) sublime wholly without decomposition (like theine, cytisin, and others); or (2) partially sublime with decomposition; or (3) are changed into new bodies (as, for example, gallic acid); or (4) melt and then char; or (5) simply char and burn away.

Many of these phenomena are striking and characteristic, taking place at different temperatures, subliming in

[337] The method of preparing this reagent is as follows:—Ordinary commercial sodium tungstate is treated with half its weight of phosphoric acid, specific gravity, 1.13, and then allowed to stand for some days. Phosphotungstic acid separates in crystals.

[338] "Dosage des alcaloides à l'aide de l'iodure double de mercure et de potassium," par MM. A. Grandval et Henri Lajoux, *Journ. de Pharmacie*, 5 sér. t. xxviii. 152-156.

characteristic forms, or leaving characteristic residues.

One of the first to employ sublimation systematically, as a means of recognition of the alkaloids, &c., was Helwig.[339] His method was to place a small quantity (from ½ to $\frac{1}{4000}$ of a mgrm.) in a depression on platinum foil, cover it with a slip of glass, and then carefully heat by a small flame. After Helwig, Dr. Guy[340] greatly improved the process by using porcelain discs, and more especially by the adoption of a convenient apparatus, which may be termed "the subliming cell." It is essentially composed of a ring of glass from ⅛ to ⅔ of an inch in thickness, such as may be obtained by sections of tubing, the cut surfaces being ground perfectly smooth. This circle is converted into a closed cell by resting it on one of the ordinary thin discs of glass used as a covering for microscopic purposes, and supporting a similar disc. The cell was placed on a brass plate, provided with a nipple, which carried a thermometer, and was heated by a small flame applied midway between the thermometer and the cell; the heat was raised very gradually, and the temperature at which any change took place was noted. In this way Dr. Guy made determinations of the subliming points of a large number of substances, and the microscopic appearances of the sublimates were described with the greatest fidelity and accuracy. On repeating with care Dr. Guy's determinations, however, I could in no single instance agree with his subliming points, nor with the apparatus he figures and describes could two consecutive observations exactly coincide. Further, on examining the various subliming temperatures of substances, as stated by different authors, the widest discrepancies were found—differences of 2 or even 3 degrees might be referred to errors of observation, a want of exact coincidence in the thermometers employed, and the like; but to what, for example, can we ascribe the irreconcilable statements which have been made with regard to theine? According to Strauch, this substance sublimes at 177°; according to Mulder, at 184.7°. But that both of these observations deviate more than 70° from the truth may be proved by any one who cares to place a few mgrms. of theine, enclosed between two watch-glasses, over the water-bath; in a few minutes a distinct sublimate will condense on the upper glass, and, in point of fact, theine will be found to sublime several degrees below 100°.

Since this great divergency of opinion is not found either in the specific gravity, or the boiling-points, or any of the like determinations of the physical properties of a substance, it is self-evident that the processes hitherto used for the determination of subliming points are faulty. The sources of error are chiefly—

(1.) Defects in the apparatus employed—the temperature read being rather that of the metallic surface in the immediate vicinity of the thermometer than of the substance itself.

(2.) The want of agreement among observers as to what should be called a sublimate—one considering a sublimate only that which is evident to the naked eye, another taking cognisance of the earliest microscopic film.

(3.) No two persons employing the same process.

With regard to the apparatus employed, I adopt Dr. Guy's subliming cell; but the cell, instead of resting on a metallic solid, floats on a metallic fluid. For any temperature a little above 100° this fluid is mercury, but for higher temperatures fusible metal is preferable.

The exact procedure is as follows:—A porcelain crucible (*a* in fig.), about 3 inches in diameter, is nearly filled with mercury or fusible metal, as the case may be; a minute speck (or two or three crystals of the substance to be examined) is placed on a thin disc of microscopic covering glass, floated on the liquid, and the cell is completed by the glass ring and upper disc. The porcelain crucible is supported on a brass plate (*b*), fixed to a retort-stand in the usual way, and protected from the unequal cooling effects of currents of air by being covered by a flask (*c*), from which the bottom has been removed. The neck of the flask conveniently supports a thermometer, which passes through a cork, and the bulb of the thermometer is immersed in the bath of liquid metal. In the first examination of a substance the temperature is raised somewhat rapidly, taking off the upper disc with a forceps at every 10° and exchanging it for a fresh disc, until the substance is destroyed. The second examination is conducted much more slowly, and the discs exchanged at every 4° or 5°, whilst the final determination is effected by raising the temperature with great caution, and exchanging the discs at about the points of change (already partially determined) at every half degree. All the discs are examined microscopically. The most convenient definition of a sublimate is this—the most minute films, dots, or crystals, which can be observed by ¼-inch power, and which are obtained by keeping the subliming cell at a definite temperature for 60 seconds. The commencement of many sublimates assumes the shape of dots of extraordinary minuteness, quite invisible to the unaided eye; and, on the other hand, since the practical value of sublimation is mainly as an aid to other methods for the recognition of substances, if we go beyond

339 *Das Mikroskop in der Toxicologie.*

340 *Pharm. Journ. Trans.* (2), viij. 719; ix. 10, 58. *Forensic Medicine*, London, 1875.

short intervals of time, the operation, otherwise simple and speedy, becomes cumbersome, and loses its general applicability.

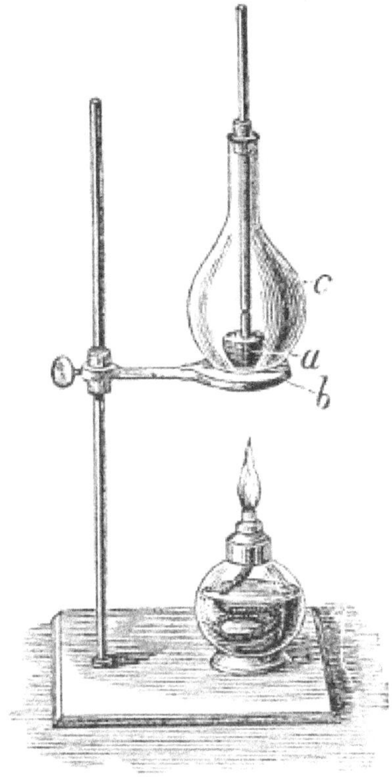

Subliming Cell.

There is also considerable discrepancy of statement with regard to the melting-point of alkaloidal bodies; in many instances a viscous state intervenes before the final complete resolution into fluid, and one observer will consider the viscous state, the other complete fluidity, as the melting-point.

In the melting-points given below, the same apparatus was used, but the substance was simply placed on a thin disc of glass floating on the metallic bath before described (the cell not being completed), and examined from time to time microscopically, for by this means alone can the first drops formed by the most minute and closely-adherent crystals to the glass be discovered.

Cocaine melts at 93°, and gives a faint sublimate at 98°; if put between two watch-glasses on the water-bath, in fifteen minutes there is a good cloud on the upper glass.

Aconitine turns brown, and melts at 179° C.; it gives no characteristic sublimate up to 190°.

Morphine, at 150°, clouds the upper disc with nebulæ; the nebulæ are resolved by high magnifying powers into minute dots; these dots gradually become coarser, and are generally converted into crystals at 188°; the alkaloid browns at or about 200°.

Thebaine sublimes in theine-like crystals at 135°; at higher temperatures (160° to 200°), needles, cubes, and prisms are observed. The residue on the lower disc, if examined before carbonisation, is fawn-coloured with non-characteristic spots.

Narcotine gives no sublimate; it melts at 155° into a yellow liquid, which, on raising the temperature, ever becomes browner to final blackness. On examining the residue before carbonisation, it is a rich brown amorphous substance; but if narcotine be heated two or three degrees above its melting-point, and then cooled slowly, the residue is crystalline—long, fine needles radiating from centres being common.

Narceine gives no sublimate; it melts at 134° into a colourless liquid, which undergoes at higher temperatures the usual transition of brown colours. The substance, heated a few degrees above its melting-point, and then allowed to cool slowly, shows a straw-coloured residue, divided into lobes or drops containing feathery crystals.

Papaverine gives no sublimate; it melts at 130°. The residue, heated a little above its melting-point, and then slowly cooled, is amorphous, of a light-brown colour, and in no way characteristic.

Hyoscyamine gives no crystalline sublimate; it melts at 89°, and appears to volatilise in great part without decomposition. It melts into an almost colourless fluid, which, when solid, may exhibit a network not unlike vegetable parenchyma; on moistening the network with water, interlacing crystals immediately appear. If, however, hyoscyamine be kept at 94° to 95° for a few minutes, and then slowly cooled, the edges of the spots are arborescent, and the spots themselves crystalline.

Atropine (daturine) melts at 97°; at 123° a faint mist appears on the upper disc. Crystals cannot be obtained; the residue is not characteristic.

Solanine.—The upper disc is dimmed with nebulæ at 190°, which are coarser and more distinct at higher temperatures; at 200° it begins to brown, and then melts; the residue consists of amber-brown, non-characteristic drops.

Strychnine gives a minute sublimate of fine needles, often disposed in lines, at 169°; about 221° it melts, the residue (at that temperature) is resinous.

Brucine melts at 151° into a pale yellow liquid, at higher temperatures becoming deep-brown. If the lower disc, after melting, be examined, no crystals are observed, the residue being quite transparent, with branching lines like the twigs of a leafless tree; light mists, produced rather by decomposition than by true sublimation, condense on the upper disc at 185°, and above.

Saponin neither melts nor sublimes; it begins to brown about 145°, is almost black at 185°, and quite so at 190°.

Delphinine begins to brown about 102°; it becomes amber at 119°, and melts, and bubbles appear. There is no crystalline sublimate; residue not characteristic.

Pilocarpine gives a distinct crystalline sublimate at 153°; but thin mists, consisting of fine dots, may be observed as low as 140°. Pilocarpine melts at 159°; the sublimates at 160° to 170° are in light yellow drops. If these drops are treated with water, and the water evaporated, feathery crystals are obtained; the residue is resinous.

Theine wholly sublimes; the first sublimate is minute dots, at 79°; at half a degree above that very small crystals may be obtained; and at such a temperature as 120°, the crystals are often long and silky.

Theobromine likewise wholly sublimes; nebulæ at 134°, crystals at 170°, and above.

Salicin melts at 170°; it gives no crystalline sublimate. The melted mass remains up to 180° almost perfectly colourless; above that temperature browning is evident. The residue is not characteristic.

Picrotoxin gives no crystalline sublimate. The lowest temperature at which it sublimes is 128°; the usual nebulæ then make their appearance; between 165° and 170° there is slight browning; at 170° it melts. The residue, slowly cooled, is not characteristic.

Cantharidin sublimes very scantily between 82° and 83°; at 85° the sublimate is copious.

The active principles of plants may, in regard to their behaviour to heat, be classed for practical purposes into—

- 1. Those which give a decided crystalline sublimate:
  - (*a.*) Below 100°, *e.g.*, cocaine, theine, thebaine, cantharidin.
  - (*b.*) Between 100° and 150°, *e.g.*, quinetum.
  - (*c.*) Between 150° and 200°, *e.g.*, strychnine, morphine, pilocarpine.
- 2. Those which melt, but give no crystalline sublimate:
  - (*a.*) Below 100°, *e.g.*, hyoscyamine, atropine.
  - (*b.*) Between 100° and 150°, *e.g.*, papaverine.
  - (*c.*) Between 150° and 200°, *e.g.*, salicin.
  - (*d.*) Above 200°, *e.g.*, solanine.
- 3. Those which neither melt nor give a crystalline sublimate, *e.g.*, saponin.

§ 315. **Melting-point.**—The method of sublimation just given also determines the melting-point; such a determination will, however, seldom compare with the melting-points of the various alkaloids as given in text-books, because the latter melting-points are not determined in the same way. The usual method of determining melting-points is to place a very small quantity in a glass tube closed at one end; the tube should be almost capillary. The tube is fastened to a thermometer by means of platinum wire, and then the bulb of the thermometer, with its attached tube, is immersed in strong sulphuric acid or paraffin, contained in a flask. The thermometer should be suspended midway in the liquid and heat carefully applied, so as to raise the temperature gradually and equably. It will be found that rapidly raising the heat gives a different melting-point to that which is obtained by slowly raising the heat. During the process careful watching is necessary: most substances change in hue before they actually melt.

A constant melting-point, however often a substance is purified by recrystallisation, is a sign of purity.

§ 316. **Identification by Organic Analysis.**—In a few cases (and in a few only) the analyst may have sufficient material at hand to make an organic analysis, either as a means of identification or to confirm other tests. By the vacuum process described in "Foods," in which carbon and nitrogen are determined by measuring the gases evolved by burning the organic substance in as complete a vacuum as can be obtained, very minute quantities of a substance can be dealt with, and the carbon and nitrogen determined with fair accuracy. It is found in practice that the carbon determinations appear more reliable than those of the nitrogen, and there are obvious reasons why this should be so.

Theoretically, with the improved gas-measuring appliances, it is possible to measure a c.c. of gas; but few chemists would care to create a formula on less than 10 c.c. of CO_2. Now, since 10 c.c. of CO_2 is equal to 6.33 mgrms. of carbon, and alkaloids average at least half their weight of carbon, it follows that 12 mgrms. of alkaloid represent about the smallest quantity with which a reliable single combustion can be made.

The following table gives a considerable number of the alkaloids and alkaloidal bodies, arranged according to their content in carbon:—

TABLE SHOWING THE CONTENT OF CARBON AND NITROGEN IN VARIOUS ALKALOIDAL BODIES.

	Carbon.		Nitrogen.	
Asparagin,	36	.36	21	.21
Methylamine,	38	.71	45	.17
Betaine,	44	.44	10	.37
Theobromine,	46	.67	31	.11
Theine,	49	.48	28	.86
Indican,	49	.60	2	.22
Muscarine,	50	.42	11	.77
Lauro-cerasin,	52	.47	1	.53
Amanitine,	57	.69	13	.46
Narceine,	59	.63	3	.02
Colchicine,	60	.53	4	.15
Oxyacanthine,	60	.57	4	.42
Solanine,	60	.66	1	.68
Trimethylamine,	61	.02	23	.73
Jervine,	61	.03	5	.14
Sabadilline,	61	.29	3	.46
Aconitine,	61	.21	2	.16
Nepaline,	63	.09	2	.12
Colchicein,	63	.44	4	.38
Veratroidine,	63	.8	3	.1
Narcotine,	63	.92	3	.39
Veratrine,	64	.42	2	.91
Delphinine,	64	.55	3	.42
Physostigmine,	65	.49	15	.27
Rhœadine,	65	.79	3	.65
Cocaine,	66	.44	4	.84
Gelsemine,	67	.00	7	.10
Conhydrine,	67	.12	9	.79
Staphisagrine,	67	.5	3	.6
Chelidonine,	68	.06	12	.34
Atropine, Hyoscyamine,	70	.58	4	.84

Sanguinarine,	70	.59	4	.33
Papaverine,	70	.79	4	.13
Delphinoidine,	70	.9	3	.9
Morphine and Piperine,	71	.58	4	.91
Berberine,	71	.64	4	.18
Codeine,	72	.24	4	.68
Thebaine,	73	.31	4	.50
Cytisine,	73	.85	12	.92
Nicotine,	74	.08	17	.28
Quinine,	75	.02	8	.64
Coniine,	76	.81	11	.20
Strychnine,	77	.24	8	.92
Curarine,	81	.51	5	.28

§ 317. **Quantitative Estimation of the Alkaloids.**—For medico-legal purposes the alkaloid obtained is usually weighed directly, but for technical purposes other processes are used. One of the most convenient of these is titration with normal or decinormal sulphuric acid, a method applicable to a few alkaloids of marked basic powers—*e.g.*, quinine is readily and with accuracy estimated in this way, the alkaloid being dissolved in a known volume of the acid, and then titrated back with soda. If a large number of observations are to be made, an acid may be prepared so that each c.c. equals 1 mgrm. of quinine. A reagent of general application is found in the so-called *Mayer's reagent*, which consists of 13.546 grms. of mercuric chloride, and 49.8 grms. of iodide of potassium in a litre of water. Each c.c. of such solution precipitates—

Of	Strychnine,	.0167	grm.
„	Brucine,	.0233	„
„	Quinine,	.0108	„
„	Cinchonine,	.0102	„
„	Quinidine,	.0120	„
„	Atropine,	.0145	„
„	Aconitine,	.0268	„
„	Veratrine,	.0269	„
„	Morphine,	.0200	„
„	Narcotine,	.0213	„
„	Nicotine,	.00405	„
„	Coniine,	.00416	„

The final reaction is found by filtering, from time to time, a drop on to a glass plate, resting on a blackened surface, and adding the test until no precipitate appears. The results are only accurate when the strength of the solution of the alkaloid is about 1 : 200; so that it is absolutely necessary first to ascertain approximatively the amount present, and then to dilute or concentrate, as the case may be, until the proportion mentioned is obtained.

A convenient method of obtaining the sulphate of an alkaloid for quantitative purposes, and especially from organic fluids, is that recommended by Wagner. The fluid is acidulated with sulphuric acid, and the alkaloid precipitated by a solution of iodine in iodide of potassium. The precipitate is collected and dissolved in an aqueous solution of hyposulphite of soda. The filtered solution is again precipitated with the iodine reagent, and the precipitate dissolved in sulphurous acid, which, on evaporation, leaves behind the pure sulphate of the base.

It is also very useful for quantitative purposes to combine an alkaloid with gold or platinum, by treating the solution with the chlorides of either of those metals—the rule as to selection being to give that metal the preference which yields the most insoluble and the most crystallisable compound.

The following table gives the percentage of gold or platinum left on ignition of the double salt:—

	Gold.		Platinum.	
Atropine,	31	.57	...	
Aconitine	20	.0	...	
Amanitine,	44	.23	...	
Berberine,	29	.16	18	.11
Brucine,	...		16	.52
Cinchonine,	...		27	.36
Cinchonidine,	...		27	.87
Codeine,	...		19	.11
Coniine,	...		29	.38
Curarine,	...		32	.65
Delphinine,	26	.7	...	
Delphinoidine,	29	.0	15	.8
Emetine,	...		29	.7
Hyoscyamine,	34	.6	...	
Morphine,	...		19	.52
Muscarine,	43	.01	...	
Narcotine,	15	.7	15	.9
Narceine,	...		14	.52
Nicotine,	...		34	.25
Papaverine,	...		17	.82
Pilocarpine,	35	.5	23	.6 to 25.2.
Piperine,	...		12	.7
Quinine,	40	.0	26	.26
Strychnine,	29	.15	18	.16
Thebaine,	...		18	.71
Theine,	37	.02	24	.58
Theobromine,	...		25	.55
Veratrine,	21	.01	...	

II.—Liquid Volatile Alkaloids.

THE ALKALOIDS OF HEMLOCK—NICOTINE—PITURIE—SPARTEINE.

1. THE ALKALOIDS OF HEMLOCK (CONIUM).

§ 318. The *Conium maculatum*, or spotted hemlock, is a rather common umbelliferous plant, growing in waste places, and flowering from about the beginning of June to August. The stem is from three to five feet high, smooth, branched, and spotted with purple; the leaflets of the partial involucres are unilateral, ovate, lanceolate, with an attenuate point shorter than the umbels; the seeds are destitute of vittæ, and have five prominent crenate wavy ridges. The whole plant is fœtid and poisonous. Conium owes its active properties to a volatile liquid alkaloid, *Coniine*, united with a crystalline alkaloid, *Conhydrine*.

§ 319. **Coniine (conia, conicine)**, ($C_8H_{17}N$)—specific gravity 0.862 at 0°; melting-point, -2.5°; boiling-point, 166.6°. Pure coniine has been prepared synthetically by Ladenburg, and found to be propyl-piperidine $C_5H_{10}NC_3H_7$, but the synthetically-prepared piperidine has no action on polarised light. By uniting it with dextro-tartaric acid, and evaporating, it is possible to separate the substance into dextro-propyl-piperidine and lævo-propyl-piperidine. The former is in every respect identical with coniine from hemlock; it is a clear, oily fluid, possessing a peculiarly unpleasant, mousey odour. One part is soluble in 150 parts of water,[341] in 6 parts of ether, and in almost all

[341] The saturated watery solution of coniine at 15°, becomes cloudy if gently warmed, and clears again on cooling.

proportions of amyl alcohol, chloroform, and benzene. It readily volatilises, and, provided air is excluded, may be distilled unchanged. It ignites easily, and burns with a smoky flame. It acts as a strong base, precipitating the oxides of metals and alkaline earths from their solutions, and it coagulates albumen. Coniine forms salts with hydrochloric acid ($C_8H_{15}N.HCl$), phosphoric acid, iodic acid, and oxalic acid, which are in well-marked crystals. The sulphate, nitrate, acetate, and tartrate are, on the other hand, non-crystalline.

If coniine is oxidised with nitric acid, or bichromate of potash, and diluted sulphuric acid, butyric acid is formed; and since the latter has an unmistakable odour, and other characteristic properties, it has been proposed as a test for coniine. This may be conveniently performed thus:—A crystal of potassic bichromate is put at the bottom of a test-tube, and some diluted sulphuric acid with a drop of the supposed coniine added. On heating, the butyric acid reveals itself by its odour, and can be distilled into baryta water, the butyrate of baryta being subsequently separated in the usual way, and decomposed by sulphuric acid, &c.

Another test for coniine is the following:—If dropped into a solution of alloxan, the latter is coloured after a few minutes an intense purple-red, and white needle-shaped crystals are separated, which dissolve in cold potash-lye into a beautiful purple-blue, and emit an odour of the base.[342] Dry hydrochloric acid gives a purple-red, then an indigo-blue colour, with coniine; but if the acid is not dry, there is formed a bluish-green crystalline mass. This test, however, is of little value to the toxicologist, the pure substance alone responding with any definite result.

The ordinary precipitating agents, according to Dragendorff, act as follows:—

Potass bismuth iodide.

- 1 : 2000, a strong orange precipitate.
- 1 : 3000. The drop of the reagent is surrounded with a muddy border.
- 1 : 4000. The drop of the reagent is surrounded with a muddy border.
- 1 : 5000, still perceptible.
- 1 : 6000. The last limit of the reaction.

Phosphomolybdic acid gives a strong yellow precipitate; limit, 1 : 5000.

Potass. mercuric iodide gives a cheesy precipitate; limit, 1 : 1000 in neutral, 1 : 800 in acid, solutions.

Potass. cadmic iodide gives an amorphous precipitate, 1 : 300. The precipitate is soluble in excess of the precipitant. (Nicotine, under similar circumstances, gives a crystalline precipitate.)

Flückiger recommends the following reaction:[343]—"Add to 10 drops of ether in a shallow glass crystallising dish 2 drops of coniine, and cover with filter paper. Set upon the paper a common-sized watch-glass containing bromine water, and invert a beaker over the whole arrangement. Needle-shaped crystals of coniine hydro-bromine soon form in the dish as well as in the watch-glass." Hydrochloric acid, used in the same way, instead of bromine water, forms with coniine microscopic needles of coniine hydrochlorate; both the hydro-bromide and the hydrochlorate doubly refract light. Nicotine does not respond to this reaction.

Coniine forms with carbon disulphide a thiosulphate and a sulphite. If carbon disulphide, therefore, be shaken with an aqueous solution of coniine, the watery solution gives a brown precipitate with copper sulphate, colours ferric chloride solution dark brown red, and gives a milky opalescence with dilute acids. If coniine itself is added to carbon disulphide, there is evolution of heat, separation of sulphur, and formation of thiosulphate. Nicotine does not respond to this reaction.

§ 320. **Other Coniine Bases.**—Methyl- and ethyl-coniine have been prepared synthetically, and are both similar in action to coniine, but somewhat more like curarine. By the reduction of coniine with zinc dust conyrine ($C_8H_{11}N$) is formed; between coniine and conyrine stands coniceine ($C_8H_{15}NO$). De Coninck has made synthetically by the addition of 6 atoms of hydrogen to β collidine, a new fluid alkaloid ($C_8H_{11}N + 6H = C_8H_{17}N$), which he has called *isocicutine*: it has the same formula as coniine. Paraconiine Schiff prepared synthetically from ammonia and normal butyl aldehyde; it has the formula $C_8H_{15}N$, and therefore differs from coniine in containing two atoms less of hydrogen. All the above have a similar physiological action to coniine. α-stillbazoline ($C_{11}H_{19}N$), prepared by Baurath from benzaldehyde and picoline, is analogous to coniine, and according to Falck has similar action, but is more powerful.

§ 321. **Pharmaceutical Preparations.**—The percentage of coniine in the plant itself, and in pharmaceutical

[342] Schwarzenbach, *Vierteljahrsschr. f. prakt. Pharm.*, viij. 170.

[343] *Reactions*, by F. A. Flückiger, Detroit, 1893.

preparations, can be approximately determined by distilling the coniine over, in a partial vacuum,[344] and titrating the distillate with Mayer's reagent, each c.c. = about .00416 grm. of coniine. It appears to be necessary to add powdered potassic chloride and a small quantity of diluted sulphuric acid before titrating, or the precipitate does not separate. In any case, the end of the reaction is difficult to observe.[345]

The fresh plant is said to contain from about .04 to .09 per cent., and the fruit about 0.7 per cent. of coniine.

The officinal preparations are—the leaves, the fruit, a tincture of the fruit, an extract of the leaves, the juice of the leaves (*Succus conii*), a compound hemlock pill (composed of extract of hemlock, ipecacuanha, and treacle), an inhalation of coniine (*Vapor conii*), and a poultice (*Cataplasma conii*) made with the leaves.

§ 322. **Statistics of Coniine Poisoning.**—F. A. Falck[346] has been able to collect 17 cases of death recorded in medical literature, up to the year 1880, from either coniine or hemlock. Two of these cases were criminal (murders), 1 suicidal, 2 cases in which coniine had been used medicinally (in one instance the extract had been applied to a cancerous breast; in the other, death was produced from the injection of an infusion of hemlock leaves). The remaining 12 were cases in which the root, leaves, or other portions of the plant had been ignorantly or accidentally eaten.

§ 323. **Effects on Animals.**—It destroys all forms of animal life. The author made some years ago an investigation as to its action on the common blow-fly. Droplets of coniine were applied to various parts of blow-flies, which were then placed under glass shades. The symptoms began within a minute by signs of external irritation, there were rapid motions of the wings, and quick and aimless movements of the legs. Torpor set in speedily, the buzz soon ceased, and the insects lay on their sides, motionless, but for occasional twitching of the legs. The wings, as a rule, became completely paralysed before the legs, and death occurred at a rather variable time, from ten minutes to two hours. If placed in a current of air in the sun, a fly completely under the influence of coniine may recover. Coniine causes in frogs, similar to curarine, peripheral paralysis of the motor nerves, combined with a transitory stimulation, and afterwards a paralysis of the motor centres; in frogs the paralysis is not preceded by convulsions. Dragendorff experimented on the action of coniine when given to five cats, the quantities used being .05 to .5 grm. The symptoms came on almost immediately, but with the smaller dose given to a large cat, no effect was witnessed until twenty-five minutes afterwards; this was the longest interval. One of the earliest phenomena was dilatation of the pupil, followed by weakness of the limbs passing into paralysis, the hinder legs being affected prior to the fore. The respiration became troubled, and the frequency of the breathing diminished; the heart in each case acted irregularly, and the sensation generally was blunted; death was preceded by convulsions. In the cases in which the larger dose of .4 to .5 grm. was administered, death took place within the hour, one animal dying in eight minutes, a second in eighteen minutes, a third in twenty minutes, and a fourth in fifty-eight minutes. With the smaller dose of .051 grm. given to a large cat, death did not take place until eight hours and forty-seven minutes after administration.

§ 324. **Effects on Man.**—In a case recorded by Bennet,[347] and quoted in most works on forensic medicine, the symptoms were those of general muscular weakness deepening into paralysis. The patient had eaten hemlock in mistake for parsley; in about twenty minutes he experienced weakness in the lower extremities, and staggered in walking like a drunken man; within two hours there was perfect paralysis of both upper and lower extremities, and he died in three and a quarter hours. In another case, related by Taylor, the symptoms were also mainly those of paralysis, and in other instances stupor, coma, and slight convulsions have been noted.

§ 325. **Physiological Action.**—It is generally agreed that coniine paralyses, first the ends of the motor nerves, afterwards their trunks, and lastly, the motor centre itself. At a later period the sensory nerves participate. In the earlier stage the respiration is quickened, the pupils contracted, and the blood-pressure increased; but on the development of paralysis the breathing becomes slowed, the capillaries relaxed, and the blood-pressure sinks. Death takes place from cessation of the respiration, and not primarily from the heart, the heart beating after the breathing has stopped. Coniine is eliminated by the urine, and is also in part separated by the lungs, while a portion is, perhaps, decomposed in the body.

---

[344] This is easily effected by uniting a flask containing the alkaloidal fluid, air-tight, with a Liebig's condenser and a receiver, the latter being connected with Bunsen's water-pump, or one of the numerous exhausting apparatuses now in use in every laboratory.

[345] Dragendorff, *Die Chemische Werthbestimmung einiger starkwirkender Droguen*, St. Petersb., 1874.

[346] *Prakt. Toxicologie*, p. 273.

[347] *Edin. Med. and Surg. Journ.*, July 1845, p. 169.

§ 326. **Post-mortem Appearances.**—There is nothing characteristic in the appearances after death.

Fatal Dose.—The fatal dose of coniine is not accurately known; it is about 150 mgrms. (2.3 grains). In the case of Louise Berger, 10 to 15 drops appear to have caused death in a few minutes. The auto-experiments of Dworzak, Heinrich, and Dillaberger would indicate that one drop may cause unpleasant symptoms. Albers, in the treatment of a woman suffering from cancer of the breast, witnessed convulsions and loss of consciousness from a third dose of 4 mgrms. (.06 grain); and Eulenberg, its full narcotic effects on a child after subcutaneous injection of 1 mgrm. (.015 grain).

§ 327. **Separation of Coniine from Organic Matters or Tissues.**—The substances are digested with water, acidulated with H_2SO_4, at a temperature not exceeding 40°, and then filtered. If the filtrate should be excessive, it must be concentrated; alcohol is then added, the liquid refiltered, and from the filtrate the alcohol separated by distillation.

On cooling, the acid fluid is agitated with benzene, and the latter separated in the usual way. The fluid is now alkalised with ammonia, and shaken up once or twice with its own volume of petroleum ether; the latter is separated and washed with distilled water, and the alkaloid is obtained almost pure. If the petroleum ether leaves no residue, it is certain that the alkaloid was not present in the contents of the stomach or intestine.

The affinity of coniine with ether or chloroform is such, that its solution in either of these fluids, passed through a *dry* filter, scarcely retains a drop of water. In this way it may be conveniently purified, the impurities dissolved by water remaining behind.

In searching for coniine, the stomach, intestines, blood, urine, liver, and lungs are the parts which should be examined. According to Dragendorff, it has been discovered in the body of a cat six weeks after death.

Great care must be exercised in identifying any volatile alkaloid as coniine, for the sources of error seem to be numerous. In one case[348] a volatile coniine-like ptomaine, was separated from a corpse, and thought to be coniine; but Otto found that in its behaviour to platinic chloride, it differed from coniine; it was very poisonous—.07 was fatal to a frog, .44 to a pigeon, in a few minutes. In the seeds of *Lupinus luteus* there is a series of coniine-like substances,[349] but they do not give the characteristic crystals with hydrochloric acid.

2. TOBACCO—NICOTINE.

§ 328. The different forms of tobacco are furnished by three species of the tobacco plant, viz., *Nicotianum tabacum*, *N. rustica*, and *N. persica*.

Havanna, French, Dutch, and the American tobaccos are in the main derived from *N. tabacum*; Turkish, Syrian, and the Latakia tobaccos are the produce of *N. rustica*. There seems at present to be little of *N. persica* in commerce.

All the species of tobacco contain a liquid, volatile, poisonous alkaloid (*Nicotine*), probably united in the plant with citric and malic acids. There is also present in tobacco an unimportant camphor (*nicotianin*). The general composition of the plant may be gathered from the following table:—

TABLE SHOWING THE COMPOSITION OF FRESH LEAVES OF TOBACCO (POSSELT AND RIENMANN).

Nicotine,	0.060
Concrete volatile oil,	0.010
Bitter extractive,	2.870
Gum with malate of lime,	1.740
Chlorophyl,	0.267
Albumen and gluten,	1.308
Malic acid,	0.510
Lignine and a trace of starch,	4.969
Salts (sulphate, nitrate, and malate of potash, chloride of potassium, phosphate and malate of lime, and malate of ammonia,)	- 0.734
Silica,	0.088
Water,	88.280

[348] Otto, *Anleitung z. Ausmittlung d. Gifte*, 1875.

[349] Sievert, *Zeitschrift für Naturwissenschaften*.

100.836

§ 329. **Quantitative Estimation of Nicotine in Tobacco.**—The best process (although not a perfectly accurate one) is the following:—25 grms. of the tobacco are mixed with milk of lime, and allowed to stand until there is no odour of ammonia; the mixture is then exhausted by petroleum ether, the ether shaken up with a slight excess of normal sulphuric acid, and titrated back by baryta water; the sulphate of baryta may be collected and weighed, so as to control the results. With regard to the percentage of nicotine in commercial tobacco, Kosutany found from 1.686 to 3.738 per cent. in dry tobacco; Letheby, in six samples, from 1.5 to 3.2 per cent.; whilst Schlössing gives for Havanna 2 per cent., Maryland 2.29 per cent., Kentucky 6.09 per cent., Virginian 6.87 per cent., and for French tobacco, quantities varying from 3.22 to 7.96 per cent. Again, Lenoble found in Paraguay tobacco from 1.8 to 6 per cent.; and Wittstein, in six sorts of tobacco in Germany, 1.54 to 2.72 per cent.

Mr. Cox[350] has recently determined the amount of nicotine in a number of tobaccos. The results are tabulated in the following table as follows:—

TABLE OF RESULTS, ARRANGED ACCORDING TO PER CENT. OF NICOTINE.

	Variety examined.	Nicotine per cent.
1.	Syrian leaves (*a*),	.612
2.	American chewing,	.935
3.	Syrian leaves (*b*),	1 .093
4.	Chinese leaves,	1 .902
5.	Turkish (coarse cut),	2 .500
6.	Golden Virginia (whole strips),	2 .501
7.	Gold Flake (Virginia),	2 .501
8.	"Navy-cut" (light coloured),	2 .530
9.	Light returns (Kentucky),	2 .733
10.	"Navy-cut" (dark "all tobacco"),	3 .640
11.	Best "Birds-eye,"	3 .931
12.	Cut Cavendish (*a*),	4 .212
13.	"Best Shag" (*a*),	4 .907
14.	"Cut Cavendish" (*b*),	4 .970
15.	"Best Shag" (*b*),	5 .000
16.	French tobacco,	8 .711
17.	Algerian tobacco (*a*),	8 .813
18.	Algerian tobacco (*b*),	8 .900

It is therefore obvious that the strength of tobacco in nicotine varies between wide limits.

Twenty-five grammes (or more or less, according to the amount of the sample at disposal) of the dried and powdered tobacco were intimately mixed with slaked lime, and distilled in a current of steam until the condensed steam was no longer alkaline; the distillate was slightly acidulated with dilute H_2SO_4, and evaporated to a conveniently small bulk. This was made alkaline with soda, and agitated repeatedly with successive portions of ether. The separated batches of ethereal solution of nicotine were then mixed and exposed to the air in a cool place. This exposure to the air carries away ammonia, if any be present, as well as ether.

Water was added to the ethereal residue, and the amount of nicotine present determined by decinormal H_2SO_4, using methyl-orange as an indicator. One c.c. of decinormal H_2SO_4 represents 0.0162 gramme of nicotine ($C_{10}H_{14}N_2$).

§ 330. **Nicotine** ($C_{10}H_{14}N_2$).—Hexahydro dipyridyl $(C_5H_4N)_2H_6$, when pure, is an oily, colourless fluid, of

[350] *Pharm. Journ.*, Jan. 20, 1894.

1.0111, specific gravity at 15°.[351] It evaporates under 100° in white clouds, and boils at about 240°, at which temperature it partly distils over unchanged, and is partly decomposed—a brown resinous product remaining. It volatilises with aqueous and amyl alcohol vapour notably, and is not even fixed at -10°. It has a strong alkaline reaction, and rotates a ray of polarised light to the right. Its odour, especially on warming, is strong and unpleasantly like tobacco, and it has a sharp caustic taste. It absorbs water exposed to the air, and dissolves in water in all proportions, partly separating from such solution on the addition of a caustic alkali. The aqueous solution acts in many respects like ammonia, saturating acids fully, and may therefore be in certain cases estimated with accuracy by titration, 49 parts of H_2SO_4 corresponding to 162 of nicotine. It gives on oxidation nicotinic acid = m(β) pyridincarbo acid $C_5H_4N(COOH)$, and by oxidation with elimination of water dipyridyl $(C_5H_4N)_2$, and through reduction dipiperydil $(C_5H_{10}N)_2$.

Alcohol and ether dissolve nicotine in every proportion; if such solutions are distilled, nicotine goes over first. The salts which it forms with hydrochloric, nitric, and phosphoric acids crystallise with difficulty; tartaric and oxalic acid form white crystalline salts, and the latter, oxalate of nicotine, is soluble in alcohol, a property which distinguishes it from the oxalate of ammonia. The best salts are the oxalate and the acid tartrate of nicotine, from which to regenerate nicotine in a pure state.

Hydrochloride of nicotine is more easily volatilised than the pure base. Nicotine is precipitated by alkalies, &c., also by many oxyhydrates, lead, copper, &c. By the action of light, it is soon coloured yellow and brown, and becomes thick, in which state it leaves, on evaporation, a brown resinous substance, only partly soluble in petroleum ether.

A very excellent test for nicotine, as confirmatory of others, is the beautiful, long, needle-like crystals obtained by adding to an ethereal solution of nicotine a solution of iodine in ether. The crystals require a few hours to form.

Chlorine gas colours nicotine blood-red or brown; the product is soluble in alcohol, and separates on evaporation in crystals.

Cyanogen also colours nicotine brown; the product out of alcohol is not crystalline. Platin chloride throws down a reddish crystalline precipitate, soluble on warming; and gallic acid gives a flocculent precipitate. A drop of nicotine poured on dry chromic acid blazes up, and gives out an odour of tobacco camphor; if the ignition does not occur in the cold, it is produced by a gentle heat. It is scarcely possible to confound nicotine with ammonia, by reason of its odour; and, moreover, ammonia may always be excluded by converting the base into the oxalate, and dissolving in absolute alcohol.

On the other hand, a confusion between coniine and nicotine is apt to occur when small quantities only are dealt with. It may, however, be guarded against by the following tests:—

(1.) If coniine be converted into oxalate, the oxalate dissolved in alcohol, and coniine regenerated by distillation (best in *vacuo*) with caustic lye, and then hydrochloric acid added, a crystalline hydrochlorate of coniine is formed, which doubly refracts light, and is in needle-shaped or columnar crystals, or dendritic, moss-like forms. The columns afterwards become torn, and little rows of cubical, octahedral, and tetrahedral crystals (often cross or dagger-shaped) grow out of yellow amorphous masses. Crystalline forms of this kind are rare, save in the case of dilute solutions of chloride of ammonium (the presence of the latter is, of course, rendered by the treatment impossible); and nicotine does not give anything similar to this reaction.

(2.) Coniine coagulates albumen; nicotine does not.

(3.) Nicotine yields a characteristic crystalline precipitate with an aqueous solution of mercuric chloride; the similar precipitate of coniine is amorphous.

(4.) Nicotine does not react with CS_2 to form thiosulphate.

§ 331. **Effects on Animals.**—Nicotine is rapidly fatal to all animal life—from the lowest to the highest forms. That tobacco-smoke is inimical to insect-life is known to everybody; very minute quantities in water kill infusoria. Fish of 30 grms. weight die in a few minutes from a milligram of nicotine; the symptoms observed are rapid movements, then shivering and speedy paralysis, with decreased motion of the gills, and death. With frogs, if doses not too large are employed, there is first great restlessness, then strong tetanic convulsions, and a very peculiar position of the limbs; the respiration after fatal doses soon ceases, but the heart beats even after death. Birds also show tetanic convulsions followed by paralysis and speedy death. The symptoms witnessed in mammals poisoned by nicotine are not essentially dissimilar. With large doses the effect is similar to that of prussic acid—viz., a cry, one or two shuddering convulsions, and death. If the dose is not too large, there is trembling of the limbs, excretion

[351] J. Skalweit, *Ber. der. deutsch. Chem. Gesell.*, 14, 1809.

of fæces and urine, a peculiar condition of stupor, a staggering gait, and then the animal falls on its side. The respiration, at first quickened, is afterwards slowed, and becomes deeper than natural; the pulse, also, with moderate doses, is first slowed, then rises in frequency, and finally, again falls. Tetanic convulsions soon develop, during the tetanus the pupils have been noticed to be contracted, but afterwards dilated, the tongue and mouth are livid, and the vessels of the ear dilated. Very characteristic of nicotine poisoning as witnessed in the cat, the rabbit, and the dog, is its peculiarly violent action, for after the administration of from one to two drops, the whole course from the commencement of symptoms to the death may take place in five minutes. F. Vas has drawn the smoke of tobacco from an immense pipe, and condensed the products; he finds the well-washed tarry products without physiological action, but the soluble liquid affected the health of rabbits,—they lost weight, the number of the blood corpuscles was decreased, and the hæmoglobin of the blood diminished.[352]

The larger animals, such as the horse, are affected similarly to the smaller domestic animals. A veterinary surgeon, Mr. John Howard, of Woolwich,[353] has recorded a case in which a horse suffered from the most violent symptoms of nicotine-poisoning, after an application to his skin of a strong decoction of tobacco. The symptoms were trembling, particularly at the posterior part of the shoulders, as well as at the flanks, and both fore and hind extremities; the superficial muscles were generally relaxed and felt flabby; and the pupils were widely dilated. There was also violent dyspnœa, the respirations being quick and short, pulse 32 per minute, and extremely feeble, fluttering, and indistinct. When made to walk, the animal appeared to have partly lost the use of his hind limbs, the posterior quarter rolling from side to side in an unsteady manner, the legs crossing each other, knuckling over, and appearing to be seriously threatened with paralysis. The anus was very prominent, the bowels extremely irritable, and tenesmus was present. He passed much flatus, and at intervals of three or four minutes, small quantities of fæces in balls, partly in the liquid state, and coated with slimy mucus. There was a staring, giddy, intoxicated appearance about the head and eyes, the visible mucous membrane being of a dark-red colour. A great tendency to collapse was evident, but by treatment with cold douches and exposure to the open air, the horse recovered.

In a case occurring in 1863, in which six horses ate oats which had been kept in a granary with tobacco, the symptoms were mainly those of narcosis, and the animals died.[354]

§ 332. **Effects on Man.**—Poisoning by the pure alkaloid nicotine is so rare that, up to the present, only three cases are on record. The first of these is ever memorable in the history of toxicology, being the first instance in which a pure alkaloid had been criminally used. The detection of the poison exercised the attention of the celebrated chemist Stas. I allude, of course, to the poisoning of M. Fougnies by Count Bocarmé and his wife. For the unabridged narrative of this interesting case the reader may consult Tardieu's *Étude Médico-Légale sur L'Empoisonnement.*

Bocarmé actually studied chemistry in order to prepare the alkaloid himself, and, after having succeeded in enticing his victim to the chateau of Bitremont, administered the poison forcibly. It acted immediately, and death took place in five minutes. Bocarmé now attempted to hide all traces of the nicotine by pouring strong acetic acid into the mouth and over the body of the deceased. The wickedness and cruelty of the crime were only equalled by the clumsy and unskilful manner of its perpetration. The quantity of nicotine actually used in this case must have been enormous, for Stas separated no less than .4 grm. from the stomach of the victim.

The second known case of nicotine-poisoning was that of a man who took it for the purpose of suicide. The case is related by Taylor. It occurred in June 1863. The gentleman drank an unknown quantity from a bottle; he stared wildly, fell to the floor, heaving a deep sigh, and died quietly without convulsion. The third case happened at Cherbourg,[355] where an officer committed suicide by taking nicotine, but how much had been swallowed, and what were the symptoms, are equally unknown, for no one saw him during life.

Poisoning by nicotine, pure and simple, then is rare. Tobacco-poisoning is very common, and has probably been experienced in a mild degree by every smoker in first acquiring the habit. Nearly all the fatal cases are to be ascribed to accident; but criminal cases are not unknown. Christison relates an instance in which tobacco in the form of snuff was put into whisky for the purpose of robbery. In 1854, a man was accused of attempting to poison his wife by putting snuff into her ale, but acquitted. In another case, the father of a child, ten weeks old, killed the infant by putting tobacco into its mouth. He defended himself by saying that it was applied to make the child sleep.

[352] *Archiv. f. Exper. Pathol. u. Pharm.*, Bd. 33.
[353] *Veter. Journal*, vol. iii.
[354] *Annales Vétérinaires*, Bruxelles, 1868.
[355] *Ann. d'Hygiène*, 1861, x. p. 404.

In October 1855,[356] a drunken sailor swallowed (perhaps for the purpose of suicide) his quid of tobacco, containing from about half an ounce to an ounce. He had it some time in his mouth, and in half an hour suffered from frightful tetanic convulsions. There was also diarrhœa; the pupils were dilated widely; the heart's action became irregular; and towards the end the pupils again contracted. He died in a sort of syncope, seven hours after swallowing the tobacco.

§ 333. In 1829 a curious instance of poisoning occurred in the case of two girls, eighteen years of age, who suffered from severe symptoms of tobacco-poisoning after drinking some coffee. They recovered; and it was found that tobacco had been mixed with the coffee-berries, and both ground up together.[357]

Accidents have occurred from children playing with old pipes. In 1877[358] a child, aged three, used for an hour an old tobacco-pipe, and blew soap bubbles with it. Symptoms of poisoning soon showed themselves, and the child died in three days.

Tobacco-juice, as expressed or distilled by the heat developed in the usual method of smoking, is very poisonous. Sonnenschein relates the case of a drunken student, who was given a dram to drink, into which his fellows had poured the juice from their pipes. The result was fatal. Death from smoking is not unknown.[359] Helwig saw death follow in the case of two brothers, who smoked seventeen and eighteen German pipefuls of tobacco. Marshall Hall[360] records the case of a young man, nineteen years of age, who, after learning to smoke for two days, attempted two consecutive pipes. He suffered from very serious symptoms, and did not completely recover for several days. Gordon has also recorded severe poisoning from the consecutive smoking of nine cigars. The external application of the leaf may, as already shown in the case of the horse, produce all the effects of the internal administration of nicotine. The old instance, related by Hildebrand, of the illness of a whole squadron of hussars who attempted to smuggle tobacco by concealing the leaf next to their skin, is well known, and is supported by several recent and similar cases. The common practice of the peasantry, in many parts of England, of applying tobacco to stop the bleeding of wounds, and also as a sort of poultice to local swellings, has certainly its dangers. The symptoms—whether nicotine has been taken by absorption through the broken or unbroken skin, by the bowel, by absorption through smoking, or by the expressed juice, or the consumption of the leaf itself—show no very great difference, save in the question of time. Pure nicotine acts with as great a rapidity as prussic acid; while if, so to

[356] *Edin. Med. Journ.*, 1855.

[357] Barkhausen, *Pr. Ver. Ztg.*, v. 17, p. 83, 1838.

[358] *Pharm. Journ.* [3], 377, 1877.

[359] The question as to whether there is much nicotine in tobacco-smoke cannot be considered settled; but it is probable that most of the poisonous symptoms produced are referable to the pyridene bases of the general formula ($C_nH_{2n-5}N$). Vohl and Eulenberg (*Arch. Pharmac.*, 2, cxlvi. p. 130) made some very careful experiments on the smoke of strong tobacco, burnt both in pipes and also in cigars. The method adopted was to draw the smoke first through potash, and then through dilute sulphuric acid. The potash absorbed prussic acid, hydric sulphide, formic, acetic, propionic, butyric, valeric, and carbolic acids; while in the acid the bases were fixed, and these were found to consist of the whole series of pyridene bases, from pyridene (C_5H_5N), boil. point 117°, picoline (C_6H_7N), boil. point 133°, lutidine (C_7H_9N), boil. point 154°, upwards. When smoked in pipes, the chief yield was pyridene; when in cigars, collidine ($C_8H_{11}N$); and in general, pipe-smoking was found to produce a greater number of volatile bases. The action of these bases has been investigated by several observers. They all have a special action on the organism, and all show an increase in physiological activity as the series is ascended. The lowest produce merely excitement from irritation of the encephalic nervous centres, and the highest, paralysis of those centres. Death proceeds from gradual failure of the respiratory movements, leading to asphyxia—(Kendrick and Dewar, *Proc. Roy. Soc.*, xxii. 442; xxiii. 290). The most recent experimental work is that of A. Gautier; he found that tobacco smoked in a pipe produced basic compounds, a large quantity of nicotine, and a higher homologue of nicotine, $C_{11}H_{16}N_2$, which pre-exists in tobacco leaves, and a base C_6H_9NO, which seems to be a hydrate of picoline—(*Compt. Rend.*, t. cxv. p. 992, 993). The derivatives of the pyridene series are also active. The methiodides strongly excite the brain and paralyse the extremities. A similar but more energetic action is exerted by the ethyl and allyl derivatives; the iodyallyl derivatives are strong poisons. Methylic pyridene carboxylate is almost inactive, but the corresponding ammonium salt gives rise to symptoms resembling epilepsy—(Ramsay, *Phil. Mag.*, v. 4, 241). One member of the pyridene series β-lutidine has been elaborately investigated by C. Greville Williams and W. H. Waters—(*Proc. Roy. Soc.*, vol. xxxii. p. 162, 1881). They conclude that it affects the heart profoundly, causing an increase in its tonicity, but the action is almost confined to the ventricles. The auricles are but little affected, and continue to beat after the ventricles have stopped. The rate of the heart's beat is slowed, and the inhibitory power of the vagus arrested. By its action on the nervous cells of the spinal cord, it in the first place lengthens the time of reflex action, and then arrests that function. Finally, they point out that it is antagonistic to strychnine, and may be successfully employed to arrest the action of strychnine on the spinal cord.

[360] *Edin. Med. and Surg. Jour.*, xii., 1816.

speak, it is entangled in tobacco, it takes more time to be separated and absorbed; besides which, nicotine, taken in the concentrated condition, is a strong enough base to have slight caustic effects, and thus leaves some local evidences of its presence. In order to investigate the effects of pure nicotine, Dworzak and Heinrich made auto-experiments, beginning with 1 mgrm. This small dose produced unpleasant sensations in the mouth and throat, salivation, and a peculiar feeling spreading from the region of the stomach to the fingers and toes. With 2 mgrms. there was headache, giddiness, numbness, disturbances of vision, torpor, dulness of hearing, and quickened respirations. With 3 to 4 mgrms., in about forty minutes there was a great feeling of faintness, intense depression, weakness, with pallid face and cold extremities, sickness, and purging. One experimenter had shivering of the extremities and cramps of the muscles of the back, with difficult breathing. The second suffered from muscular weakness, fainting, fits of shivering, and creeping sensations about the arms. In two or three hours the severer effects passed away, but recovery was not complete for two or three days. It is therefore evident, from these experiments and from other cases, that excessive muscular prostration, difficult breathing, tetanic cramps, diarrhœa, and vomiting, with irregular pulse, represent both tobacco and nicotine poisoning. The rapidly-fatal result of pure nicotine has been already mentioned; but with tobacco-poisoning the case may terminate lethally in eighteen minutes. This rapid termination is unusual, with children it is commonly about an hour and a half, although in the case previously mentioned, death did not take place for two days.

§ 334. **Physiological Action.**—Nicotine is absorbed into the blood and excreted unchanged, in part by the kidneys and in part by the saliva (*Dragendorff*). According to the researches of Rosenthal and Krocker,[361] nicotine acts energetically on the brain, at first exciting it, and then lessening its activity; the spinal marrow is similarly affected. The convulsions appear to have a cerebral origin; paralysis of the peripheral nerves follows later than that of the nerve centres, whilst muscular irritability is unaffected. The convulsions are not influenced by artificial respiration, and are therefore to be considered as due to the direct influence of the alkaloid on the nervous system. Nicotine has a striking influence on the respiration, first quickening, then slowing, and lastly arresting the respiratory movements: section of the vagus is without influence on this action. The cause of death is evidently due to the rapid benumbing and paralysis of the respiratory centre. Death never follows from heart-paralysis, although nicotine powerfully influences the heart's action, small doses exciting the terminations of the vagus in the heart, and causing a slowing of the beats. Large doses paralyse both the controlling and exciting nerve-centres of the heart; the heart then beats fast, irregularly, and weakly. The blood-vessels are first narrowed, then dilated, and, as a consequence, the blood-pressure first rises, then falls. Nicotine has a special action on the intestines. As O. Nasse[362] has shown, there is a strong contraction of the whole tract, especially of the small intestine, the lumen of which may be, through a continuous tetanus, rendered very small. This is ascribed to the peripheral excitation of the intestinal nerves and the ganglia. The uterus is also excited to strong contraction by nicotine; the secretions of the bile and saliva are increased.

§ 335. **Fatal Dose.**—The fatal dose for dogs is from ½ to 2 drops; for rabbits, a quarter of a drop; for an adult not accustomed to tobacco the lethal dose is probably 6 mgrms.

§ 336. **Post-mortem Appearances.**—There seem to be no appearances so distinctive as to be justly ascribed to nicotine or tobacco-poisoning and no other.

A more or less fluid condition of the blood, and, generally, the signs of death by the lungs, are those most frequently found. In tobacco-poisoning, when the leaves themselves have been swallowed, there may be some inflammatory redness of the stomach and intestine.

§ 337. **Separation of Nicotine from Organic Matters, &c.**—The process for the isolation of nicotine is precisely that used for coniine. It appears that it is unaltered by putrefaction, and may be separated and recognised by appropriate means a long time after death. Orfila detected it in an animal two or three months after death; Melsens discovered the alkaloid unmistakably in the tongues of two dogs, which had been buried in a vessel filled with earth for seven years; and it has been found, by several experiments, in animals buried for shorter periods. Nicotine should always be looked for in the tongue and mucous membrane of the mouth, as well as in the usual viscera. The case may be much complicated if the person supposed to be poisoned should have been a smoker; for the defence would naturally be that there had been either excessive smoking or chewing, or even swallowing accidentally a quid of

[361] *Ueber die Wirkung des Nicotines auf den thierischen Organismus*, Berlin, 1868.

[362] *Beiträge zur Physiologie der Darmbewegung, Leipsic*, 1866.

tobacco.[363] A ptomaine has been discovered similar to nicotine. Wolckenhaar separated also an alkaloid not unlike nicotine from the corpse of a woman addicted to intemperate habits; but this base was not poisonous, nor did it give any crystals when an ethereal solution was added to an ether solution of iodine. It will be well always to support the chemical evidence by tests on animal life, since the intensely poisonous action of nicotine seems not to be shared by the nicotine-like ptomaines.

3. PITURIE.[364]

§ 338. Piturie (C_6H_8N) is a liquid, nicotine-like alkaloid, obtained from the *Duboisia hopwoodii*, a small shrub or tree belonging to the natural order *Solanaceæ*, indigenous in Australia. The natives mix piturie leaves with ashes from some other plant, and chew them. Piturie is obtained by extracting the plant with boiling water acidified with sulphuric acid, concentrating the liquid by evaporation, and then alkalising and distilling with caustic soda, and receiving the distillate in hydrochloric acid. The solution of the hydrochlorate is afterwards alkalised and shaken up with ether, which readily dissolves out the piturie. The ether solution of piturie is evaporated to dryness in a current of hydrogen, and the crude piturie purified by distillation in hydrogen, or by changing it into its salts, and again recovering, &c. It is clear and colourless when pure and fresh, but becomes yellow or brown when exposed to air and light. It boils and distils at 243° to 244°. It is soluble in all proportions in alcohol, water, and ether; its taste is acrid and pungent; it is volatile at ordinary temperatures, causing white fumes with hydrochloric acid; it is very irritating to the mucous membranes, having a smell like nicotine at first, and then, when it becomes browner, like pyridine. It forms salts with acids, but the acetate, sulphate, and hydrochlorate are varnish-like films having no trace of crystallisation; the oxalate is a crystalline salt. Piturie gives precipitates with mercuric chloride, cupric sulphate, gold chloride, mercur-potassic iodide, tannin, and an alcoholic solution of iodine. If an ethereal solution of iodine is added to an ethereal solution of piturie, a precipitate of yellowish-red needles, readily soluble in alcohol, is deposited. The iodine compound melts at 110°, while the iodine compound of nicotine melts at 100°. Piturie is distinguished from coniine by its aqueous solution not becoming turbid either on heating or on the addition of chlorine water; it differs from picoline in specific gravity, picoline being .9613 specific gravity at 0°, and piturie sinking in water; it differs from aniline by not being coloured by chlorinated lime. From nicotine it has several distinguishing marks, one of the best being that it does not change colour on warming with hydrochloric acid and the addition to the mixture afterwards of a little nitric acid. The physiological action seems to be but little different from that of nicotine. It is, of course, poisonous, but as yet has no forensic importance.

4. SPARTEINE.

§ 339. In 1851 Stenhouse[365] separated a poisonous volatile alkaloid from *Spartium scoparium*, the common broom, to which he gave the name of sparteine. At the same time a crystalline non-poisonous substance, *scoparin*, was discovered.

Sparteine is separated from the plant by extraction with sulphuric acid holding water, and then alkalising the acid solution and distilling: it has the formula ($C_{15}H_{26}N_2$), and belongs to the class of tertiary diamines. It is a clear, thick, oily substance, scarcely soluble in water, to which it imparts a strong, alkaline reaction; it is soluble in alcohol, in ether, and chloroform; insoluble in benzene and in petroleum; it boils at 288°. Sparteine neutralises acids fully, but the oxalate is the only one which can be readily obtained in crystals. It forms crystalline salts with platinic chloride, with gold chloride, with mercuric chloride, and with zinc chloride. The picrate is an especially beautiful salt, crystallising in long needles, which, when dried and heated, explode. On sealing sparteine up in a tube with ethyl iodide and alcohol, and heating to 100° for an hour, ethyl sparteine iodide separates in long, needle-like crystals, which are somewhat insoluble in cold alcohol.

Effect on Animals.—A single drop kills a rabbit; the symptoms are similar to those produced by nicotine, but the pupils are dilated.[366]

5. ANILINE.

§ 340. **Properties.**—Aniline or amido-benzol ($C_6H_5NH_2$) is made by the reduction of nitro-benzol. It is an oily fluid, colourless when quite pure, but gradually assuming a yellow tinge on exposure to the air. It has a peculiar and

---

363 In an experiment of Dragendorff's, nicotine is said to have been detected in 35 grms. of the saliva of a person who had half an hour previously smoked a cigar.

364 See "The Alkaloid from Piturie," by Prof. Leversidge, *Chem. News*, March 18 and 25, 1881.

365 *Phil. Trans.*, 1851.

366 To the nicotine group, gelsemine ($C_{24}H_{28}N_2O_4$) and oxalathylin ($C_6H_{10}N_2$) also belong, in a physiological sense, but gelsemine, like sparteine, dilates the pupil.

distinctive smell. It boils at 182.5°, and can be congealed by a cold of 8°. It is slightly soluble in water, 100 parts of water at 16° retaining about 3 of aniline, and easily soluble in alcohol, ether, and chloroform. It does not blue red-litmus paper, but nevertheless acts as a weak alkali, for it precipitates iron from its salts. It forms a large number of crystalline salts. The hydrochloride crystallises in white plates, and has a melting-point of 192°. The platinum compound has the formula of $(C_6H_5NH_2HCl)_2PtCl_4$, and crystallises in yellow needles.

§ 341. **Symptoms and Effects.**—Aniline, like picric acid, coagulates albumin. Aniline is a blood poison; it produces, even during life, in some obscure way, methæmoglobin, and it disintegrates the red blood corpuscles; both these effects lessen the power of the blood corpuscles to convey oxygen to the tissues, hence the cyanosis observed so frequently in aniline poisoning is explained. Engelhardt[367] has found that aniline black is produced; in every drop of blood there are fine black granules, the total effect of which produce a pale blue or grey-blue colour of the skin. Aniline has also an action on the central nervous system, at first stimulating, and then paralysing. Schmiedeberg finds that para-amido-phenol-ether-sulphuric acid is produced, and appears in the urine as an alkali salt; a small quantity of fuchsine is also produced, and has been found in the urine. Some aniline may be excreted unchanged.

The symptoms are giddiness, weakness, cyanosis, blueness of the skin, sinking of the temperature, and dilatation of the pupil. The pulse is small and frequent, the skin moist and cold. The patient smells of aniline. Towards the end coma and convulsions set in. The urine may be brown to brown-black, and may contain hyaline cylinders. The blood shows the spectrum of methæmoglobin, and has the peculiarities already mentioned. Should the patient recover, jaundice often follows. The outward application of aniline produces eczema.

Chronic poisoning by aniline is occasionally seen among workers in the manufacture of aniline. Headache, loss of muscular power, diminished sensibility of the skin, vomiting, loss of appetite, pallor, eruptions on the skin, and general malaise are the chief symptoms. The perspiration has been noticed to have a reddish colour.

Cases of aniline poisoning are not common; Dr. Fred. J. Smith has recorded one in the *Lancet* of January 13, 1894.[368] The patient, a woman, 42 years of age, of alcoholic tendencies, swallowed, 13th December 1893, at 1.40 P.M., about 3 ounces of marking ink, the greatest part of which consisted of aniline; in a very little while she became unconscious, and remained so until death. At 3 P.M. her lips were of a dark purple, the general surface of the skin was deadly white, with a slight bluish tinge; the pupils were small and sluggish, the breathing stertorous, and the pulse full and slow—60 per minute. The stomach was washed out, ether injected, and oxygen administered, but the patient died comatose almost exactly twelve hours after the poison had been taken.

The *post-mortem* examination showed slight congestion of the lungs; the heart was relaxed in all its chambers, and empty of blood; it had a peculiar green-blue appearance. All the organs were healthy. The blood was not spectroscopically examined.

§ 342. **Fatal Dose.**—This is not known, but an adult would probably be killed by a single dose of anything over 6 grms. Recovery under treatment has been known after 10 grms.; the fatal dose for rabbits is 1-1.5 grms., for dogs 3-5 grms.

§ 343. **Detection of Aniline.**—Aniline is easily separated and detected. Organic fluids are alkalised by a solution of potash, and distilled. The organs, finely divided, are extracted with water acidulated with sulphuric acid, the fluid filtered, and then alkalised and distilled. The distillate is shaken up with ether, the ether separated and allowed to evaporate spontaneously. Any aniline will be in the residue left after evaporation of the ether, and may be identified by the following tests:—An aqueous solution of aniline or its salts is coloured blue by a little chloride of lime or hypochlorite of soda; later on the mixture becomes red. The blue colour has an absorption band, when examined spectroscopically, extending from W.L. 656 to 560, and therefore in the red and yellow from Fraunhofer's line C, and overlapping D. Another test for aniline is the addition of kairine, hydrochloric acid, and sodium nitrite, which strikes a blue colour.

III.—The Opium Group of Alkaloids.

§ 344. **General Composition.**—Opium contains a larger number of basic substances than any plant known. The list reaches at present to 18 or 19 nitrogenised bases, and almost each year there have been additions. Some of these alkaloids exist in very small proportion, and have been little studied. Morphine and narcotine are those which,

[367] *Beiträge zur Tox. des Anilins. Inaug.-Diss.*, Dorpat, 1888.

[368] See also a case reported by K. Dehio, in which a person drank 10 grms. and recovered, *Ber. klinis. Wochen.*, 1888, Nr. 1.

alone, are toxicologically important. Opium is a gummy mass, consisting of the juice of the incised unripe fruit of the *Papaver somniferum* hardened in the air. The following is a nearly complete list of the constituents which have been found in opium:—

Morphine, $C_{17}H_{19}NO_3$.
Narcotine, $C_{22}H_{23}NO_7$.
Narceine, $C_{23}H_{29}NO_9$.
Apomorphine, $C_{17}H_{10}NO_2$ } By dehydration of morphine and codeine respectively.
Apocodeine, $C_{18}H_{19}NO_2$ }
Pseudomorphine, $C_{17}H_{19}NO_4$.
Codamine, $C_{20}H_{25}NO_4$.
Ladanine, $C_{20}H_{25}NO_4$.
Ladanosine, $C_{21}H_{27}NO_4$.
Protapine, $C_{20}H_{19}NO_5$.
Cryptopine, $C_{21}H_{23}NO_5$.
Lanthopine, $C_{23}H_{25}NO_4$.
Hydrocotarnine, $C_{12}H_{15}NO_3$.
Opianine, $C_{21}H_{21}NO_7$.
Cnoscopine, $C_{34}H_{36}N_2O_{11}$.
Rhœadine, $C_{20}H_{21}NO_7$.
Codeine, $C_{18}H_{21}NO_3$.
Thebaine, $C_{19}H_{21}NO_3$.
Papaverine, $C_{20}H_{21}NO_4$.
Meconidine, $C_{21}H_{23}NO_4$.
Meconin, $C_{10}H_{10}O_4$.
Meconic acid, $C_7H_4O_7$.
Thebolactic acid.
Fat.
Resin.
Caoutchouc.
Gummy matters—Vegetable mucus.
Ash, containing the usual constituents.

The various opiums differ, the one from the other, in the percentages of alkaloids, so that only a very general statement of the mean composition of opium can be made. The following statement may, however, be accepted as fairly representative of these differences:—

	Per cent.
Morphine,	6 to 15
Narcotine,	4 to 8
Other alkaloids,	5 to 2
Meconin,	Under 1
Meconic acid,	3 to 8
Peculiar resin and caoutchouc,	5 to 10
Fat,	1 to 4
Gum and soluble humoid acid matters,	40 to 50
Insoluble matters and mucus,	18 to 20
Ash,	4 to 8

Water, 8 to 30

The general results of the analysis of 12 samples of Turkey opium, purchased by Mr. Bott,[369] from leading druggists in London, Dublin, and Edinburgh, are as follows:—

Water.—Highest, 31.2; lowest, 18.4; mean, 22.4 per cent.

Insoluble Residue.—Highest, 47.9; lowest, 25.45; mean, 32.48 per cent.

Aqueous Extract.—Highest, 56.15; lowest, 20.90; mean, 45.90 per cent.

Crude Morphine (containing about 7/10 of pure morphine).—Highest, 12.30; lowest, 6.76; mean, 9.92 per cent., which equals 12.3 per cent. of the dried drug.

Persian Opium, examined in the same way, varied in crude morphine from 2.1 to 8.5 per cent.; Malwa, from 5.88 to 7.30. In 18 samples of different kinds of opium, the mean percentage of crude morphine was 8.88 per cent. (11 per cent. of the dried opium). According to Guibourt, Smyrna opium, dried at 100°, yields 11.7 to 21.46 per cent., the mean being 12 to 14 per cent.; Egyptian, from 5.8 to 12 per cent.; Persian, 11.37 per cent. In East Indian Patna opium, for medical use, he found 7.72; in a sample used for smoking, 5.27 per cent.; in Algerian opium, 12.1 per cent.; in French opium, 14.8 to 22.9 per cent.

§ 345. **Action of Solvents on Opium.**—The action of various solvents on opium has been more especially studied by several scientists who are engaged in the extraction of the alkaloids.

Water dissolves nearly everything except resin, caoutchouc, and woody fibre. Free morphine would be left insoluble; but it seems always to be combined with meconic and acetic acids. The solubility of free narcotine in water is extremely small.

Alcohol dissolves resin and caoutchouc, and all the alkaloids and their combinations, with meconic acid, &c.

Amylic Alcohol dissolves all the alkaloids, if they are in a free state, and it also takes up a little of the resin.

Ether, Benzene, and Carbon Sulphide do not dissolve the resin, and only slightly morphine, if free; but they dissolve the other free alkaloids as well as caoutchouc.

Acids dissolve all the alkaloids and the resin.

Fixed Alkalies, in excess, dissolve in part resin; they also dissolve morphine freely; narcotine remains insoluble.

Lime Water dissolves morphine, but is a solvent for narcotine only in presence of morphine.

Ammonia dissolves only traces of morphine; but narceine and codeine readily. It does not dissolve the other alkaloids, nor does it dissolve the resin.

§ 346. **Assay of Opium.**—The following processes may be described:—

Process of Teschemacher and Smith.—This process, with a few modifications, is as follows:—10 grms. of opium are as completely exhausted with proof spirit at a boiling temperature as possible. The resulting alcoholic extract is treated with a few drops of ammonium oxalate solution, and the solution is almost neutralised with ammonia. The solution is concentrated to one-third, cooled, and filtered. The filtrate is farther concentrated to 5 c.c., and transferred to a small flask, it is washed into this flask by 4 c.c. of water, and 3 c.c. of 90 per cent. alcohol; next 2 c.c. solution of ammonia (sp. gr. 0.960) and 25 c.c. of dry ether are added. The flask is corked, shaken, and then allowed to rest over-night.

The ether is decanted as completely as possible. Two filter papers are taken and counterpoised—that is to say, they are made precisely the same weight. The filters are placed one inside the other, and the precipitate collected on the inner one; the precipitate is washed with morphinated water—that is to say, water in which morphine has been digested for some days. The filter papers with their contents are washed with benzene and dried, the outer paper put on the pan of the balance carrying the weights, and the inner filter with the precipitate weighed. The precipitate is now digested with a known volume of decinormal acid, and then the excess of acid ascertained by titration with decinormal alkali, using either litmus or methyl orange; each c.c. of decinormal acid is equal to 30.3 mgrms. of morphine.[370]

Dott's Process.—Dott has recently proposed a new process, which he states has given good results. The process is as follows:—10 grammes of powdered opium are digested with 25 c.c. water; 1.8 gramme barium chloride dissolved in about 12 c.c. water is then added, the solution made up to 50 c.c., well mixed, and after a short time filtered. 22 c.c. (representing 5 grammes opium) are mixed with dilute sulphuric acid in quantity just sufficient to precipitate the barium. About 1 c.c. is required, and the solution should be warmed to cause the precipitate to

[369] *Year Book of Pharmacy*, 1876.

[370] *Pharm. Journal*, xix. 45, 82; xxii. 746. Wright and Farr, *Chemist and Druggist*, 1893, i. 78.

subside, and the solution to filter clear. To this filtered solution a little dilute ammonia, about 0.5 c.c. is added to neutralise the free acid, and the solution concentrated to 6 or 7 c.c., and allowed to cool. 1 c.c. spirit and 1 c.c. ether are then added, and next ammonia in slight excess. The ammonia should be added gradually until there is no further precipitation, and a perceptible odour of ammonia remains after well stirring and breaking down any lumps with the stirring rod. After three hours the precipitate is collected on counterpoised filters and washed. Before filtering, it should be noted that the solution has a faint odour of ammonia: if not, one or two drops of ammonia solution should be added. The dried precipitate is washed with benzene or chloroform, dried, and weighed. It is then titrated with $^{n}/_{10}$ acid, until the morphine is neutralised, as indicated by the solution reddening litmus paper.[371]

§ 347. **Medicinal and other Preparations of Opium.**—The chief mixtures, pills, and other forms, officinal and non-officinal, in which opium may be met with, are as follows:—

(1.) Officinal.

Compound Tincture of Camphor, P. B. (Paregoric).—Opium, camphor, benzoic acid, oil of anise, and proof spirit: the opium is in the proportion of about 0.4 per cent., or 1 grain of opium in 240 minims.

Ammoniated Tincture of Opium (Scotch paregoric).—Strong solution of ammonia, rectified spirit, opium, oil of anise, saffron, and benzoic acid. Nearly 1 per cent. or 1 grain of opium in every 96 minims.

The Compound Powder of Kino, P. B.

Opium,	5	per cent.
Cinnamon,	20	„
Kino,	75	„

The Compound Powder of Opium, P. B.

Opium,	10.00	per cent.
Black Pepper,	13.33	„
Ginger,	33.33	„
Caraway Fruit,	40.00	„
Tragacanth,	3.33	„

[371] Other methods of opium assay have been published: see Mr. A. B. Prescott's method (*Proceedings of Amer. Pharm. Assoc.*, 1878); Allen (*Commercial Org. Analysis*, vol. ii. p. 473); E. R. Squibb's modification of Flückiger's method (*Pharm. Journ.* (3), xii. p. 724); a rapid mode of opium assay, MM. Portes and Lanjlois (*Journ. de Pharm. et de Chim.*, Nov. 1881); *Year Book of Pharmacy*, 1882.

To the above may be added—(1.) *Schacht's Method.*—5 to 10 grms. of dry, finely-powdered opium are digested with sufficient distilled water to make a thin pulp. After twenty-four hours the whole is thrown on a weighed filter, and washed until the washings are almost colourless and tasteless. The portion insoluble in water is dried at 100° and weighed; in good opium this should not exceed 40 per cent. The filtrate is evaporated until it is about one-fifth of the weight of the opium taken originally; cooled, filtered, and treated with pure animal charcoal, until the dark brown colour is changed into a brownish-yellow. The liquid is then refiltered, precipitated with a slight excess of ammonia, allowed to stand in an open vessel until all odour of ammonia disappears, and at the same time frequently stirred, in order that the precipitate may not become crystalline—a form which is always more difficult to purify. The precipitate is now collected on a tared filter, washed, dried, and weighed. With an opium containing 10 per cent. of morphine, its weight is usually 14 per cent. A portion of the precipitate is then detached from the filter, weighed, and exhausted, first with ether, and afterwards with boiling alcohol (0.81 specific gravity). Being thus purified from narcotine, and containing a little colouring-matter only, it may now be dried and weighed, and the amount of morphine calculated, on the whole, from the data obtained.

(2.) *Fleury* has proposed a titration by oxalic acid as follows:—2 grms. of the powdered opium are macerated a few hours with 8 c.c. of aqueous oxalate of ammonia, brought on a filter, and washed with 5 c.c. of water. To the filtrate an equal volume of 80 per cent. alcohol and ammonia to alkaline reaction is added; and, after standing twenty-four hours in a closed flask, it is filtered, and the flask rinsed out with some c.c. of 40 per cent. alcohol. The filter, with its contents, after drying, is placed in the same flask (which should not be cleansed), a few drops of alcoholic logwood solution are added, with an excess of oxalic acid solution of known strength, the whole being made up to 100 c.c. This is divided into two parts, and the excess of acid titrated back with diluted soda-lye. If the oxalic acid solution is of the strength of 4.42 grms. to the litre, every c.c. of the oxalic acid solution which has become bound up with morphine, corresponds to 0.02 grm. of morphine.

Pill of Lead and Opium, P. B.

Acetate of Lead,	75.0	per cent.
Opium,	12.5	„
Confection of Roses,	12.5	„

Tincture of Opium (Laudanum).—Opium and proof spirit. One grain of opium in 14.8 min.—that is, about 6.7 parts by weight in 100 by measure.

The amount of opium actually contained in laudanum has been investigated by Mr. Woodland,[372] from fourteen samples purchased from London and provincial chemists. The highest percentage of extract was 5.01, the lowest 3.21, the mean being 4.24; the highest percentage of morphine was .70 per cent., the lowest .32, the mean being .51 per cent. It is, therefore, clear that laudanum is a liquid of very uncertain strength.

Aromatic Powder of Chalk and Opium.—Opium 2.5 per cent., the rest of the constituents being cinnamon, nutmeg, saffron, cloves, cardamoms, and sugar.

Compound Powder of Ipecacuanha (Dover's Powder).

Opium,	10 per cent.
Ipecacuanha,	10 „
Sulphate of Potash,	80 „

Confection of Opium (Confectio opii) is composed of syrup and compound powder of opium; according to its formula, it contains 2.4 per cent. of opium by weight.

Extract of Opium contains the solid constituents capable of extraction by water; it should contain 20 per cent. of morphine, and is therefore about double the strength of dry powdered opium.

Liquid Extract of Opium has been also examined by Mr. Woodland:[373] ten samples yielded as a mean 3.95 per cent. of dry extract, the highest number being 4.92 per cent., the lowest 3.02. The mean percentage of morphine was .28 per cent., the highest amount being .37, and the lowest .19 per cent.

Liniment of Opium is composed of equal parts of laudanum and soap liniment; it should contain about 0.0375 per cent. morphine.

The Compound Soap-pill is made of soap and opium, one part of opium in every 5.5 of the mass—*i.e.*, about 18 per cent.

Ipecacuanha and Morphine Lozenges, as the last, with the addition of ipecacuanha; each lozenge contains 1⁄36 grain (1.8 mgrms.) morphine hydrochlorate, 1⁄12 grain (5.4 mgrms.) ipecacuanha.

Morphia Suppositories are made with hydrochlorate of morphine, benzoated lard, white wax, and oil of theobroma; each suppository contains ½ grain (32.4 mgrms.) of morphine salt.

Opium Lozenges are composed of opium extract, tincture of tolu, sugar, gum, extract of liquorice, and water. Each lozenge contains 1⁄10 grain (6.4 mgrms.) of extract of opium, or about 1⁄50 grain (1.3 mgrm.) morphine.

The Ointment of Galls and Opium contains one part of opium in 14.75 parts of the ointment—*i.e.*, opium 6.7 per cent.

Opium Wine, P. B.—Sherry, opium extract, cinnamon, and cloves. About 5 of opium extract by weight in 100 parts by measure (22 grains to the ounce).

Solutions of Morphine, both of the acetate and hydrochlorate, P. B., are made with a little free acid, and with rectified spirit. The strength of each is half a grain in each fluid drachm (.0324 grm. in 3.549), or .91 part by weight in 100 by measure.

Solution of Bimeconate of Morphine.—One fluid oz. contains 5½ grains of bimeconate of morphine.

Morphia Lozenges are made with the same accessories as opium lozenges, substituting morphine for opium; each lozenge contains 1⁄36 grain of hydrochlorate of morphia (1.8 mgrm.).

Syrup of Poppies.—The ordinary syrup of poppies is sweetened laudanum. It should, however, be what it is described—viz., a syrup of poppy-heads. As such, it is said to contain one grain of extract of opium to the ounce.

(2.) Patent and other Non-Officinal Preparations of Opium.

Godfrey's Cordial is made on rather a large scale, and is variable in strength and composition. It usually

[372] *Year Book of Pharmacy*, 1882.

[373] *Op. cit.*

contains about 1½ grains of opium in each fluid ounce,[374] and, as other constituents: sassafras, molasses or treacle, rectified spirit, and various flavouring ingredients, especially ginger, cloves, and coriander; aniseed and caraways may also be detected.

Grinrod's Remedy for Spasms consists of hydrochlorate of morphine, spirit of sal-volatile, ether, and camphor julep; strength, 1 grain of the hydrochlorate in every 6 ounces.

Lemaurier's Odontalgic Essence is acetate of morphine dissolved in cherry-laurel water; strength, 1 grain to the ounce.

Nepenthe is a preparation very similar to *Liq. Opii sedativ.*, and is of about the same strength as laudanum.[375]

Black Drop (known also by various names, such as Armstrong's Black Drop) is essentially an acetic acid solution of the constituents of opium. It is usually considered to be of four times the strength of laudanum. The wholesale receipt for it is: Laudanum, 1 oz., and distilled vinegar 1 quart, digested for a fortnight. The original formula proposed by the Quaker doctor of Durham, Edward Tunstall, is—Opium, sliced, ½ lb.; good verjuice,[376] 3 pints; and nutmeg, 1½ oz.; boiled down to a syrup thickness; ¼ lb. of sugar and 2 teaspoonfuls of yeast are then added. The whole is set in a warm place for six or eight weeks, after which it is evaporated in the open air until it becomes of the consistence of a syrup. It is lastly decanted and filtered, a little sugar is added, and the liquid made up to 2 pints.

"Nurse's Drops" seem to be composed of oil of caraway and laudanum.

Powell's Balsam of Aniseed, according to evidence in the case of *Pharmaceutical Society v. Armson* (*Pharm. Journ.*, 1894), contains in every oz. 1/10 grain of morphine.

Dalby's Carminative—

Carbonate of magnesia,	40	grains.
Tincture of castor, and compound tincture of cardamoms, of each	15	drops.
Laudanum,	5	"
Oil of aniseed,	3	"
Oil of nutmeg,	2	"
Oil of peppermint,	1	"
Peppermint water,	2	fl. ounces

Dose, from a half to one teaspoonful. Another recipe has no laudanum, but instead syrup of poppies.

Chlorodyne—Brown's Chlorodyne is composed of—

Chloroform,	6	drachms.
Chloric ether,	1	"
Tincture of capsicum,	½	"
Hydrochlorate of morphine,	8	grains.
Scheele's prussic acid,	12	drops
Tincture of Indian hemp,	1	drachm.
Treacle,	1	"

Atkinson's Infant Preserver—

Carbonate of magnesia,	6	drachms.
White sugar,	2	ounces
Oil of aniseed,	20	drops.
Spirit of sal-volatile,	2 ½	drachms.
Laudanum,	1	"
Syrup of saffron,	1	ounce.
Caraway water, to make up,	1	pint.

[374] If made according to Dr. Paris' formula, 1⅙ grains in an ounce.

[375] It may be regarded as a purified alcoholic solution of meconate of morphia, with a little excess of acid, and of about the same strength as laudanum.—*Taylor.*

[376] Verjuice is the juice of the wild crab.

Boerhave's Odontalgic Essence—

Opium,	½ drachm.
Oil of cloves,	2 „
Powdered camphor,	5 „
Rectified spirit,	1 ½ fl. ounce.

§ 348. **Statistics.**—During the ten years 1883-1892 no less than 1424 deaths in England and Wales were attributed to some form or other of opium or its active constituents; 45 of these deaths were ascribed to various forms of soothing syrup or to patent medicines containing opium or morphine; 876 were due to accident or negligence; 497 were suicidal and 6 were homicidal deaths. The age and sex distribution of the deaths ascribed to accident and those ascribed to suicide are detailed in the following tabular statement:—

DEATHS IN ENGLAND AND WALES DURING THE TEN YEARS 1883-1892 FROM OPIUM, LAUDANUM, MORPHINE, &c.

Accident.

Ages,	0-1	1-5	5-15	15-25	25-65	65 and above	Total
Males,	72	27	1	16	302	85	503
Females,	50	23	4	21	189	86	373
Total,	122	50	5	37	491	171	876

Suicide.

Ages,	5-15	15-25	25-65	65 and above	Total
Males,	1	26	269	34	330
Females,	...	24	126	17	167
Total,	1	50	395	51	497

Of European countries, England has the greatest proportional number of opium poisonings. In France, opium or morphine poisoning accounts for about 1 per cent. of the whole; and Denmark, Sweden, Switzerland, Germany, all give very small proportional numbers; arsenic, phosphorus, and the acids taking the place of opiates. The more considerable mortality arises, in great measure, from the pernicious practice—both of the hard-working English mother and of the baby-farmer—of giving infants various forms of opium sold under the name of "*soothing syrups*," "*infants' friends*," "*infants' preservatives*," "*nurses' drops*" and the like, to allay restlessness, and to keep them during the greater part of their existence asleep. Another fertile cause of accidental poisoning is mistakes in dispensing; but these mistakes seem to happen more frequently on the Continent than in England. This is in some degree due to the decimal system, which has its dangers as well as its advantages, *e.g.*:—A physician ordered .5 decigrm. of morphine acetate in a mixture for a child, but omitted the decimal point, and the apothecary, therefore, gave ten times the dose desired, with fatal effect. Again, morphine hydrochlorate, acetate, and similar soluble salts are liable to be mistaken for other white powders, and in this way unfortunate accidents have occurred—accidents that, with proper dispensing arrangements, should be impossible.

§ 349. **Poisoning of Children by Opium.**—The drugging of children by opium—sometimes with a view to destroy life, sometimes merely for the sake of the continual narcotism of the infant—is especially rife in India.[377] A little solid opium is applied to the roof of the mouth, or smeared on the tongue, and some Indian mothers have been known to plaster the nipples with opium, so that the child imbibes it with the milk. Europeans, again and again,

[377] See Dr. Chevers's *Jurisprudence*, 3rd ed., 232 *et seq.*

have discovered the native nurses administering opiates to the infants under their care, and it is feared that in many cases detection is avoided.

The ignorant use of poppy-tea has frequently caused the death of young children; thus in 1875 an inquest was held at Chelsea on the body of a little boy two years and a half old. He had been suffering from whooping-cough and enlargement of the bowels, and poppy-tea was by the advice of a neighbour given to him. Two poppy-heads were used in making a quart of tea, and the boy, after drinking a great portion of it, fell into a deep sleep, and died with all the symptoms of narcotic poisoning.

§ 350. **Doses of Opium and Morphia.**—Opium in the solid state is prescribed for adults in quantities not exceeding 3 grains, the usual dose being from 16.2 mgrms. to 64.8 mgrms. ($^1/_4$ to 1 grain). The extract of opium is given in exactly the same proportions (special circumstances, such as the habitual use of opium, excepted); the dose of all the compounds of opium is mainly regulated by the proportion of opium contained in them.

The dose for children (who bear opium ill) is usually very small; single drops of laudanum are given to infants at the breast, and the dose cautiously increased according to age. Most practitioners would consider half a grain a very full dose, and, in cases requiring it, would seldom prescribe at first more than $^1/_{16}$ to $^1/_4$ grain.

The dose of solid opium for a horse is from 1.77 grm. to 7.08 grms. ($^1/_2$ drachm to 2 drachms); in extreme cases, however, 4 drachms (14.16 grms.) have been given.

The dose for large cattle is from .648 grm. to 3.88 grms. (10 to 60 grains); for calves, .648 grm. (10 grains); for dogs it is greatly regulated by the size of the animal, 16.2 to 129.6 mgrms. ($^1/_4$ grain to 2 grains).

Fatal Dose.—Cases are recorded of infants dying from extremely small doses of opium, *e.g.*, .7, 4.3, and 8.1 mgrms. ($^1/_{90}$, $^1/_{15}$, and $^1/_8$ of a grain); but in such instances one cannot help suspecting some mistake. It may, however, be freely conceded that a very small quantity might be fatal to infants, and that 3 mgrms. given to a child under one year would probably develop serious symptoms.

The smallest dose of solid opium known to have proved fatal to adults was equal to 259 mgrms. (4 grains) of crude opium (*Taylor*), and the smallest dose of the tincture (laudanum), 7.0 c.c. (2 drachms), (*Taylor*); the latter is, however, as already shown, uncertain in its composition.

A dangerous dose (save under special circumstances) is:—For a horse, 14.17 grms. (4 drachms); for cattle, 7.04 grms. (2 drachms); for a dog of the size and strength of a foxhound, 204 mgrms. (3 grains).

Enormous and otherwise fatal doses may be taken under certain conditions by persons who are not opium-eaters. I have seen 13 cgrms. (2 grains) of morphine acetate injected hypodermically in a strong man suffering from rabies with but little effect. Tetanus, strychnine, convulsions, and excessive pain all decrease the sensibility of the nervous system to opium.

§ 351. **General Method for the Detection of Opium.**—It is usually laid down in forensic works that, where poisoning by opium is suspected, it is sufficient to detect the presence of meconic acid in order to establish that of opium. In a case of adult poisoning there is generally substance enough available to obtain one or more alkaloids, and the presence of opium may, without a reasonable doubt, be proved, if meconic acid (as well as either morphine, narcotine, thebaine, or other opium alkaloid) has been detected. Pills containing either solid opium or the tincture usually betray the presence of the drug by the odour, and in such a case there can be no possible difficulty in isolating morphine and meconic acid, with probably one or two other alkaloids. The method of extraction from organic fluids is the same as before described, but it may, of course, be modified for any special purpose. If opium, or a preparation of opium, be submitted to Dragendorff's process, the following is a sketch of the chief points to be noticed.

If the solution is *acid*—

(1.) **Benzene** mainly extracts *meconin,* which dissolves in sulphuric acid very gradually (in twenty-four to forty-eight hours), with a green colour passing into red. Meconin has no alkaloidal reaction.

(2.) **Amyl alcohol** dissolves small quantities of *meconic acid,* identified by striking a blood-red colour with ferric chloride.

If now the amyl alcohol is removed with the aid of petroleum ether, and the fluid made alkaline by ammonia—

(1.) **Benzene** extracts *narcotine*, *codeine*, and *thebaine*. On evaporation of the benzene the alkaloidal residue may be dissolved in water, acidified with sulphuric acid, and after filtration, on adding ammonia *in excess*, *thebaine and narcotine* are precipitated, *codeine* remaining in solution. The dried precipitate, if it contain thebaine, becomes blood-red when treated with cold concentrated sulphuric acid, while narcotine is shown by a violet colour developing gradually when the substance is dissolved in dilute sulphuric acid 1 : 5, and gently warmed. The codeine in the ammoniacal solution can be recovered by shaking up with benzene, and recognised by the red colour which the solid substance gives when treated with a little sugar and sulphuric acid.

(2.) **Chloroform** especially dissolves the *narceine*, which, on evaporation of the chloroform, may be identified by its general characters, and by its solution in Fröhde's reagent becoming a beautiful blue colour. Small quantities of morphine may be extracted with codeine.

(3.) **Amyl alcohol** extracts from the alkaline solution morphine, identified by its physical characters, by its forming a crystalline precipitate with iodine and hydriodic acid, and the reaction with iodic acid to be described.

§ 352. **Morphine** ($C_{17}H_{17}NO(OH)_2 + H_2O$).—Morphine occurs in commerce as a white powder, sp. gr. 1.205, usually in the form of more or less perfect six-sided prisms, but sometimes in that of white silky needles. When heated in the subliming cell, faint nebulæ, resolved by high microscopic powers into minute dots, appear on the upper disc at 150°. As the temperature is raised the spots become coarser, and at 188° distinct crystals may be obtained, the best being formed at nearly 200°, at which temperature morphine begins distinctly to brown, melt, and carbonise. At temperatures below 188°, instead of minute dots, the sublimate may consist of white circular spots or foliated patterns. One part of morphine, according to P. Chastaing, is soluble at a temperature of 3° in 33,333 parts of water; at 22°, in 4545 parts; at 42°, 4280; and at 100°, 4562. It is scarcely soluble in ether or benzene. Absolute alcohol, according to Pettenkofer, dissolves in the cold one-fortieth of its weight; boiling, one-thirtieth. Amyl alcohol, in the cold, dissolves one-fourth per cent., and still more if the alkaloid be thrown out of an aqueous acid solution by ammonia in the presence of amyl alcohol; for under such circumstances the morphine has no time to become crystalline. According to Schlimpert, 1 part of morphine requires 60 of chloroform for solution; according to Pettenkofer, 175.

Morphine is easily soluble in dilute acids, as well as in solutions of the caustic alkalies and alkaline earths; carbonated alkalies and chloride of ammonium also dissolve small quantities. The acid watery, and the alcoholic solutions, turn the plane of polarisation to the left; for sulphuric, nitric, and hydrochloric acids $[\alpha]r$ = 89.8°; in alkaline solution the polarisation is less, $[\alpha]r$ = 45.22°. It is alkaline in reaction, neutralising acids fully; and, in fact, a convenient method of titrating morphine is by the use of a centinormal sulphuric acid—each c.c. equals 2.85 mgrms. of anhydrous morphine.

§ 353. The salts of morphine are for the most part crystalline, and are all bitter, neutral, and poisonous. They are insoluble in amylic alcohol, ether, chloroform, benzene, or petroleum ether.

Morphine meconate is one of the most soluble of the morphine salts; it is freely soluble in water. Of all salts this is most suitable for subcutaneous injection; it is the form in which the alkaloid exists in opium.

Morphine hydrochlorate ($C_{17}H_{19}NO_3HCl$) crystallises in silky fibres; it is readily soluble in alcohol, and is soluble in cold, more freely in boiling water. The purest morphine hydrochlorate is colourless, but that which is most frequently met with in commerce is fawn or buff-coloured.

Morphine acetate is a crystallisable salt, soluble in water or alcohol; it is in part decomposed by boiling the aqueous solution, some of the acetic acid escaping.

Morphine Tartrates.—These are readily soluble salts, and it is important to note that the morphine might escape detection, if the expert trusted alone to the usual test of an alkaloidal salt giving a precipitate when the solution is alkalised by the fixed or volatile alkalies; for the tartrates of morphine do not give this reaction, nor do they give any precipitate with calcic chloride. By adding a solution of potassium acetate in spirit, and also alcohol and a little acetic acid to the concentrated solution, the tartrate is decomposed, and acid tartrate of potassium is precipitated in the insoluble form; the morphine in the form of acetate remains in solution, and then gives the usual reactions.

The solubility of morphine salts in water and alcohol has been investigated by Mr. J. U. Lloyd. His results are as follows:—

Morphine Acetate.

11 .70 parts of water by weight at 15.0° dissolve 1 part of morphine acetate.

61 .5 parts of water by weight at 100° dissolve 1 part of morphine acetate.

68 .30 parts of alcohol by weight (.820 specific gravity) at 15.0° dissolve 1 part of morphine acetate.

13 .30 parts of alcohol by weight (.820 specific gravity) at 100° dissolve 1 part of morphine acetate.

Morphine Hydrochlorate.

23 .40 parts of water dissolve at 15° 1 morphine hydrochlorate.

.51 part of water dissolves at 100° 1 morphine hydrochlorate.
62 .70 parts of alcohol (.820 specific gravity) dissolve at 15° 1 morphine hydrochlorate.
30 .80 parts of alcohol (.820 specific gravity) dissolve at 100° 1 morphine hydrochlorate.

Morphine Sulphate.

21 .60 parts of water at 15° dissolve 1 morphine sulphate.
.75 part of water at 100° dissolves 1 morphine sulphate.
701.5 parts of alcohol (.820) at 15° dissolve 1 morphine sulphate.
144.00 parts of alcohol (.820) at 100° dissolve 1 morphine sulphate.

§ 354. **Constitution of Morphine.**—The chief facts bearing on the constitution of morphine are as follows:—

It certainly contains two hydroxyl groups, because by the action of acetic anhydride, acetyl morphine and diacetyl morphine, $C_{17}H_{18}(CH_3CO)NO_3$ and $C_{17}H_{17}(CH_3CO)_2NO_3$ are produced. The formation of the monomethyl ether of morphine (codeine), $C_{17}H_{17}(OH)(OCH_3)NO$, is also a testimony to the existence of hydroxyl groups. One of the hydroxyl groups has phenolic functions, the other alcoholic functions. By suitable oxidation morphine yields trinitrophenol (picric acid), and by fusion with an alkali, protocatechuic acid; both of these reactions suggest a benzene ring. On distilling with zinc dust phenanthrene, pyridine, pyrrol, trimethylamine, and ammonia are formed; evidence of a pyridine nucleus. If morphine is mixed with 10 to 15 times its weight of a 20 per cent. solution of potash, and heated at 180° for from four to six hours, air being excluded, a phenol-like compound is formed, and a volatile amine, ethylmethylamine (the amine boils at 34° to 35°, and its hydrochloride melts at 133°). This reaction is interpreted by Z. H. Skrauk[378] and L. Wiegmann to indicate that the nitrogen is directly connected with two alkyl groups—that is, ethyl and methyl.

G. N. Vis,[379] after a careful review of the whole of the reactions of morphine, has proposed the following constitutional formula as the one that agrees best with the facts:—

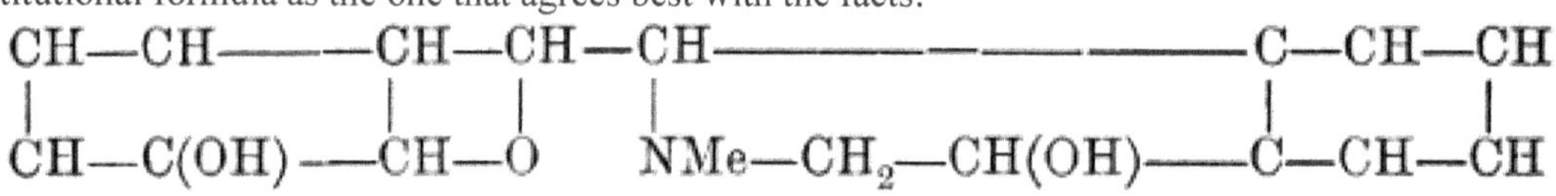

§ 355. **Tests for Morphine.**—(1.) One hundredth of a milligrm. of pure morphine gives a blue colour to a paste of ammonium molybdate in sulphuric acid; 20 mgrms. of ammonium molybdate are rubbed with a glass rod in a porcelain dish, and well mixed with 5 drops of pure strong sulphuric acid and the morphine in a solid form applied; titanic acid and tungstates give similar reactions.

(2.) Morphine possesses strong reducing properties; a little solid morphine dissolved in a solution of ferric chloride gives a Prussian blue precipitate when ferridcyanide solution is added. A number of ptomaines and other substances also respond to this test, so that in itself it is not conclusive.

(3.) **Iodic Acid Test.**—The substance supposed to be morphine is converted into a soluble salt by adding to acid reaction a few drops of hydrochloric acid, and then evaporating to dryness. The salt thus obtained is dissolved in as little water as possible—this, as in toxicological researches only small quantities are recovered, will probably be but a few drops. A little of the solution is now mixed with a very small quantity of starch paste, and evaporated to dryness at a gentle heat in a porcelain dish. After cooling, a drop of a solution of 1 part of iodic acid in 15 of water is added to the dry residue; and if even the $^1/_{20000}$ of a grain of morphine be present, a blue colour will be developed.

Another way of working the iodic acid test is to add the iodic acid solution to the liquid in which morphine is supposed to be dissolved, and then shake the liquid up with a few drops of carbon disulphide. If morphine be present,

---

378 *Monatsb.*, x. 110-114.

379 *J. pr. Chemie* (2), xlvii. 584. Knorr's formula is—

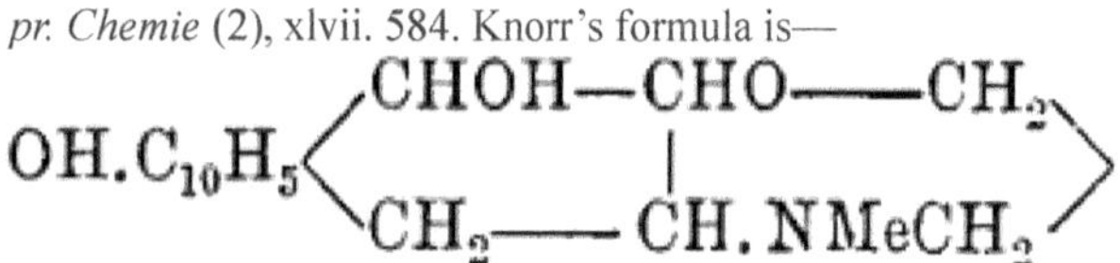

Ber., xxii. 1113-1119.

the carbon disulphide floats to the top distinctly coloured pink. Other substances, however, also set free iodine from iodic acid, and it has, therefore, been proposed to distinguish morphine from these by the after addition of ammonia. If ammonia is added to the solution, which has been shaken up with carbon disulphide, the pink or red colour of the carbon disulphide is deepened, if morphine was present; on the contrary, if morphine was *not* present, it is either discharged or much weakened.

Other Reactions.—There are some very interesting reactions besides the two characteristic tests just mentioned. If a saturated solution of chloride of zinc be added to a little solid morphine, and heated over the water-bath for from fifteen minutes to half-an-hour, the liquid develops a beautiful and persistent green colour. This would be an excellent test for morphine were it not for the fact that the colour is produced with only pure morphine. For example, I was unable to get the reaction from morphine in very well-formed crystals precipitated from ordinary laudanum by ammonia, the least trace of resinous or colouring-matter seriously interfering. By the action of nitric acid on morphine, the liquid becomes orange-red, and an acid product of the formula $C_{10}H_9NO_9$ is produced, which, when heated in a closed tube with water at 100°, yields trinitrophenol or picric acid. This interesting reaction points very decidedly to the phenolic character of morphine. On adding a drop of sulphuric acid to solid morphine in the cold, the morphine solution becomes of a faint pink; on gently warming and continuing the heat until the acid begins to volatilise, the colour changes through a series of brownish and indefinite hues up to black. On cooling and treating the black spot with water, a green solution is obtained, agreeing in hue with the same green produced by chloride of zinc. Vidali[380] has proposed the following test:—Morphine is dissolved in strong sulphuric acid, and a little arsenate of sodium is added; on gently warming, a passing blue colour develops; on raising the temperature higher, the liquid changes into green, then into blue, and finally again into green. Codeine acts very similarly. The following test originated with Siebold (*American Journal of Pharmacy*, 1873, p. 544):—The supposed morphine is heated gently with a few drops of concentrated sulphuric acid and a little pure potassic perchlorate. If morphine be present the liquid immediately takes a pronounced brown colour—a reaction said to be peculiar to morphine, and to succeed with $\frac{1}{10}$ of a mgrm. In order to obtain absolutely pure perchlorate, potassic perchlorate is heated with hydrochloric acid so long as it disengages chlorine; it is then washed with distilled water, dried, and preserved for use. There is also a test known as "Pellagri's"; it depends on the production of apomorphine. The suspected alkaloid is dissolved in a little strong hydrochloric acid, and then a drop of concentrated sulphuric acid is added, and the mixture heated for a little time from 100° to 120°, until it assumes a purple-black colour. It is now cooled, some hydrochloric acid again added, and the mixture neutralised with sodic carbonate. If morphine be present, on the addition of iodine in hydriodic acid, a cherry-red colour is produced, passing into green. Morphine and codeine are believed alone to give this reaction.

The acetate of morphine, and morphine itself, when added to ferric chloride solution, develop a blue colour. When 1 molecule of morphine is dissolved in alcohol, containing 1 molecule of sodium hydroxide, and 2 vols. of methyl iodide are added, and the mixture gently heated, a violent reaction sets in and the main product is codeine methiodide ($C_{17}H_{18}NO_2OCH,MeI$). If only half the quantity of methyl iodide is added, then free codeine is in small quantity produced; if ethyl iodide be substituted for methyl, a new base is formed homologous with codeine—codeine is therefore the methyl ether of morphine. If morphine is heated with iodide of methyl and absolute alcohol in a closed tube for half an hour at 100°, methyl iodide of morphine is obtained in colourless, glittering, quadratic crystals, easily soluble in water ($C_{17}H_{19}NO_3MeI + H_2O$); similarly the ethyl iodide compound can be produced.

If morphine is heated for from two to three hours in a closed tube with dilute hydrochloric acid, water is eliminated—

$$(C_{17}H_{19}NO_3 = C_{17}H_{17}NO_2 + H_2O),$$

and the hydrochlorate of apomorphine is produced. This succeeds when even $\frac{1}{2}$ mgrm. is heated with $\frac{1}{10}$ c.c. of strong HCl, and the tests for apomorphine applied.

If concentrated sulphuric acid be digested on morphine for twelve to fifteen hours (or heated for half an hour at 100°), on adding to the cooled violet-coloured solution either a crystal of nitrate of potash or of chlorate of potash, or a drop of dilute nitric acid, a beautiful violet-blue colour is produced, which passes gradually into a dark blood-red. $\frac{1}{100}$ of a mgrm. will respond distinctly to this test. Fröhde's reagent strikes with morphine a beautiful violet colour, passing from blue into dirty green, and finally almost vanishing. $\frac{1}{200}$ of a mgrm. will respond to the test, but it is not itself conclusive, since papaverine and certain glucosides give an identical reaction.

§ 356. **Symptoms of Opium and Morphine Poisoning.**—The symptoms of opium and morphine poisoning

[380] D. Vidali, *Bull. Farmaceut.*, Milano, 1881, p. 197; D. E. Dott, *Year Book of Pharmacy*, 1882.

are so much alike, that clinically it is impossible to distinguish them; therefore they may be considered together.

Action on Animals—Frogs.—The action of morphine or opium on frogs is peculiar: the animal at first springs restlessly about, and then falls into a condition extremely analogous to that seen in strychnine poisoning, every motion or external irritation producing a tetanic convulsion. This condition is, however, sometimes not observed. The tetanic stage is followed by paralysis of reflex movements and cessation of breathing, the heart continuing to beat.

Dogs.—0.2 to 0.5 grm. of morphine meconate, or acetate, injected directly into the circulation of a dog, shows its effects almost immediately. The dog becomes uneasy, and moves its jaws and tongue as if some peculiar taste were experienced; it may bark or utter a whine, and then in a minute or two falls into a profound sleep, which is often so deep that while it lasts—usually several hours—an operation may be performed. In whatever attitude the limbs are placed, they remain. The respiration is rapid and stertorous, and most reflex actions are extinguished. Towards the end of the sleep, any sudden noise may startle the animal, and when he wakes his faculties are evidently confused. A partial paralysis of the hind legs has often been noticed, and then the dog, with his tail and pelvis low, has something the attitude of the hyena. Hence this condition (first, I believe, noticed by Bernard) has been called the "hyenoid" state. If the dose is larger than 2 to 3 grms. (31 to 46 grains), the symptoms are not dissimilar, save that they terminate in death, which is generally preceded by convulsions.[381]

Goats.—According to Guinard, goats are proof against the narcotic influence of morphine. Large doses kill goats, but death is caused by interference with the respiratory function. A young goat weighing 30 kilos, showed little effect beyond a slightly increased cerebral excitability after two doses of 8 and 8.5 grms. respectively of morphine hydrochlorate had been administered by intravenous injection, the second being given an hour and a half after the first. To the same animal two days afterwards 195 grms. were administered in the same way, yet the goat recovered. The lethal dose for a goat seems to be no less than 1000 times that which will produce narcotism in man, and lies somewhere between 0.25 to 0.30 per kilo. of the body weight.[382]

Cats and the Felidæ.—According to Guinard,[383] morphine injected subcutaneously or intravenously into cats, in doses varying from 0.4 mgrm. to 90 mgrms. per kilo., never produces sleep or narcotic prostration. On the contrary, it causes a remarkable degree of excitement, increasing in intensity with the dose given. This excitement is evidently accompanied by disorder in the functions of the brain, and if the dose is large convulsions set in, ending in death. According to Milne-Edwards, the same symptoms are produced in lions and tigers.

Birds, especially pigeons, are able to eat almost incredible quantities of opium. A pigeon is said[384] to have consumed 801 grains of opium, mixed with its food, in fourteen days. The explanation of this is that the poison is

---

[381] MM. Grasset and Amblard have studied the action of morphine in causing convulsions in the mammalia. They found that if small doses of hydrochlorate of morphine (from 1 to 15 centigrammes) are administered to dogs, the brief sleep which is produced may be accompanied by partial muscular contractions (in one paw, for instance), which are renewed at variable intervals. Then occur true convulsive shocks in the whole body or in the hind limbs. After an interval, the phenomena recur in more intense degree, and are followed by true convulsions. Regularly, ten or sixteen times a minute, at each inspiration, the hind limbs present a series of convulsive movements, which may become general. Sometimes they are excited by external stimulation, but they are usually spontaneous. The sleep may continue profound during this convulsive period, or it may become distinctly lighter. These convulsive phenomena may continue, with intervals, for an hour. Differences are observed with different animals; but the chief characters of the phenomena are as described. In certain animals, and with small doses, there may be a brief convulsive phase at the commencement of the sleep, but it is much less constant than the later period of spasm. These convulsions, the authors believe, have not previously been described, except as a consequence of very large doses, amounting to grammes. The period of cerebral excitement, described by Claude Bernard as occurring at the commencement of the sleep from morphine, is a phenomenon of a different order. The conclusions drawn from the experiments are—(1) That morphia is not diametrically opposed to thebaine, as is often stated, since it has, to a certain degree, the convulsive properties of the latter alkaloid. (2) That the excitomotor action of opium cannot be exclusively attributed to the convulsive alkaloids, but is, in fact, due to those which are soporific. According to the ordinary composition of opium, 5 centigrammes of morphine represent about a milligramme of thebaine. But these experiments show that the quantity of morphine has a much more powerful convulsive action than a milligramme of thebaine. (3) There is not the supposed antagonism between the action of morphine on the frog and on the mammalia. (4) The researches hitherto undertaken on the antagonism between morphine and other agents need to be repeated, and a separate study made of the substances which antagonise the convulsive and soporific action.

[382] *Compt. Rend.*, t. cxvi. pp. 520-522.

[383] *Compt. Rend.*, t. cxi. pp. 981-983. The *bovine* animals also get excited, and no narcotic effect is produced by dosing them with morphine.—*Compt. Rend. Soc. de Biologie*, t. iv., v.

[384] Hermann's *Lehrbuch der exper. Toxicologie*, p. 374.

not absorbed; for subcutaneous injections of salts of morphine act rapidly on all birds hitherto experimented upon.

§ 357. **Physiological Action.**—From experiments on animals, the essential action of morphine on the nervous and arterial systems has in some measure been examined. There is no very considerable action on the heart. The beats are first accelerated, then diminished in frequency; but very large doses introduced directly into the circulation at once diminish the pulsations, and no acceleration is noticed. The slowing may go on to heart-paralysis. The slowing is central in its origin, for on the vagi being cut, morphine always quickens. With regard to the peripheric ends of the vagi, small doses excite, large paralyse. If all the nerves going to the heart are divided, there is first a considerable acceleration, and then a slowing and weakening of the pulsations. The arterial blood-pressure, at first increased, is afterwards diminished. This increase of blood-pressure is noticed during the acceleration of the pulse, and also during some portion of the time during which the pulse is slowed. Stockman and D. B. Dott,[385] experimenting on rabbits and frogs, consider that a medium dose of morphine first of all depresses the spinal cord and then excites it, for tetanus follows. If morphine is in sufficient quantity thrown into the circulation then tetanus at once occurs. It would thus appear that depression and stimulation is entirely a matter of dosage. Gescheidlen, in his researches on the frog, found the motor nerves at first excited, and then depressed. When the doses were large, there was scarcely any excitement, but the reverse effect, in the neighbourhood of the place of application. According to other observers, the function of the motor nerves may be annihilated.[386] According to Meihuizen, reflex action, at first much diminished, is later, after several hours, normal, and later still again increased. The intestinal movements are transitorily increased. In the dog there has been noticed a greater flow of saliva than usual, and the flow of bile from the gall-bladder is diminished. The pupils in animals are mostly contracted, but, if convulsions occur towards death, they are dilated.

§ 358. **Physiological Effect of Morphine Derivatives.**—By introducing methyl, or amyl, or ethyl, into the morphine molecule, the narcotic action is diminished, while the tetanic effects are increased. Acetyl, diacetyl, benzoyl, and dibenzoyl morphine, morphine sulphuric ether, and nitrosomorphine are all weaker narcotics than morphine, but, on the other hand, they depress the functions of the spinal cord and bring on, in large doses, tetanus.

The introduction of two methyl groups into morphine, as in metho-codeine, $C_{17}H_{17}MeNO(OH)\text{-}Me$, entirely alters the physiological effect. This compound has an action on voluntary muscle causing gradual paralysis.

The chlorine derivatives, trichlormorphine and chlorcodeine, have the characteristic action of the morphine group on the central nervous system and, in addition, act energetically as muscle poisons, soon destroying the contractile power of the voluntary muscles with which they first come into contact at the place of injection, and more gradually affecting the other muscles of the body.[387]

§ 359. **Action on Man.**—There are at least three forms of opium poisoning:—(1) *The common form*, as seen in about 99 per cent. of cases; (2) A very *sudden form*, in which death takes place with fearful rapidity (the *foudroyante* variety of the French);[388] and (3) a very rare entirely *abnormal form*, in which there is no coma, but convulsions.

In the *common form* there are three stages, viz.:—(1) Excitement; (2) Narcosis; (3) Coma. In from half an hour to an hour[389] the first symptoms commence, the pulse is quickened, the pupils are contracted, the face flushes, and the hands and feet reddened,—in other words, the capillary circulation is active. This stage has some analogy to the action of alcohol; the ideas mostly flow with great rapidity, and instead of a feeling of sleepiness, the reverse is the case. It, however, insensibly, and more or less rapidly, passes into the next stage of heaviness and stupor. There is an irresistible tendency to sleep; the pulse and the respiration become slower; the conjunctivæ are reddened; the face and head often flushed. In some cases there is great irritability of the skin, and an eruption of nettle-rash. If the poison has been taken by the mouth, vomiting may be present. The bowels are usually—in fact almost invariably—constipated. There is also some loss of power over the bladder.

In the next stage, the narcosis deepens into dangerous coma; the patient can no longer be roused by noises, shaking, or external stimuli; the breathing is loud and stertorous; the face often pale; the body covered with a clammy sweat. The pupils are still contracted, but they may in the last hours of life dilate: and it is generally agreed that, if

[385] *Brit. Med. Journ.* (2), 1890, 189-192.

[386] *Arch. f. d. Ges. Physiol.*, vii. p. 201.

[387] R. Stockman and Dott, *Brit. Med. Journ.* (2), 1890, 189-192.

[388] Tardieu, *Étude Méd. Légale sur l'Empoisonnement.*

[389] In a remarkable case related by Taylor, a lady took a large dose (supposed to be 1½ oz.) of laudanum, and there were no symptoms for four and a half hours. She died in twenty-two hours.

a corpse is found with the pupils dilated, this circumstance, taken in itself, does not contra-indicate opium or morphine poisoning. Death occasionally terminates by convulsion.

The *sudden form* is that in which the individual sinks into a deep sleep almost immediately—that is, within five or ten minutes—and dies in a few hours. In these rapid cases the pupils are said to be constantly dilated.

Examples of the *convulsive form* are to be sought among opium-eaters, or persons under otherwise abnormal conditions.

A man, forty years old, who had taken opiates daily since his twenty-second year—his dose being 6 grms. (92.4 grains) of solid opium—when out hunting, of which sport he was passionately fond, took cold, and, as a remedy, administered to himself three times his accustomed dose. Very shortly there was contraction of the left arm, disturbance of vision, pain in the stomach, faintness, inability to speak, and unconsciousness which lasted half an hour. Intermittent convulsions now set in, and pains in the limbs. There was neither somnolence nor delirium, but great agitation; repeated vomiting and diarrhœa followed. After five hours these symptoms ceased; but he was excessively prostrate.[390] There was complete recovery.

One may hazard a surmise that, in such a case, tolerance has been established for morphine, but not for other morphine alkaloids in the same degree, and that the marked nervous symptoms were in no small degree the effect of some of the homologous alkaloids, which, in such an enormous dose, would be taken in sufficient quantity to have a physiological action.

There are several instances of a relapsing or remittent form of poisoning—a form in which the patient more or less completely recovers consciousness, and then sinks back into a fatal slumber. One of the best known is the case of the Hon. Mrs Anson (January 1859), who swallowed an ounce and a half of laudanum by mistake. After remaining in a comatose condition for more than nine hours, she revived. The face became natural, the pulse steady. She was able to recognise her daughter, and in a thick voice to give an account of the mistake. But this lasted only ten minutes, when she again became comatose, and died in fourteen hours.[391]

In a Swedish case quoted by Maschka,[392] a girl, nine years old, in weak health and suffering from slight bronchitis, had been given a non-officinal acetate of morphia lozenge, which was supposed to contain 5 mgrms. (.075 grain) of morphine acetate. She took the lozenge at eight in the evening; soon slept, woke at ten, got out of bed, laughed, talked, and joked with the nurse, again got into bed, and very quickly fell asleep. At four A.M. the nurse came and found her breathing with a rattling sound, and the physician, who arrived an hour later, found the girl in a state of coma, with contracted pupils, breathing stertorously, and the pulse scarcely to be felt. Despite all attempts to rouse the patient, she died at eight in the morning, twelve hours after taking the lozenge.

The *post-mortem* examination showed some hyperæmia of the brain and serous effusion in the ventricles, and there was also tubercle in the pleura. Three lozenges similar to the one taken by the patient were chemically investigated by Hamberg, who found that the amount of acetate was very small, and that the lozenges, instead of morphine acetate, might be considered as prepared with almost pure morphine; the content in the three of morphine being respectively 35, 37, and 42 mgrms. (that is, from half a grain to three-fifths of a grain). There was a difference of opinion among the experts as to whether in this case the child died from morphine poisoning or not—a difference solely to be attributed to the waking up of the child two hours after taking the poison. Now, considering the great probability that a large dose for a weakly child of that age had been taken, and that this is not the only case in which a relapse has occurred, it seems just to infer that it was really a case of poisoning.

As unusual symptoms (or rather sequelæ) may be noted in a few cases, hemiplegia, which soon passes off; a weakness of the lower extremities may also be left, and inability to empty the bladder thoroughly; but usually on recovery from a large dose of opium, there is simply heaviness of the head, a dry tongue, constipation, and loss of appetite. All these symptoms in healthy people vanish in a day or two. There have also been noticed slight albuminuria, eruptions on the skin, loss of taste, and numbness of parts of the body.

Opium, whether taken in substance, or still more by subcutaneous injection, in some individuals constantly causes faintness. In my own case, I have several times taken a single grain of opium to relieve either pain or a catarrh; almost invariably within an hour afterwards there has been great coldness of the hands and feet, lividity of

---

[390] Demontporcellet, *De l'Usage Quotidien de l'Opium*, Paris, 1874.

[391] Taylor, *op. cit.*

[392] Maschka's *Handbuch*, Band ii. p. 438; also Svenska, *Läk-Sällsk. Förhandl.*, Apr. 1, p. 90; Apr. 8, p. 160, 1873. For other cases see Nasmyth, *Edin. Med. Journ.*, Dec. 1878; Kirby, *Dub. Med. Press*, Dec. 24, 1845; W. Boyd Muschet, *Med. Times and Gaz.*, March 20, 1858.

the face, a feeling of deadly faintness followed by vomiting; this stage (which has seldom lasted more than half an hour) passed, the usual narcotic effects have been produced.

Some years ago I injected one-sixth of a grain of morphine hydrochlorate subcutaneously into an old gentleman, who was suffering from acute lumbago, but was otherwise healthy, and had no heart disease which could be detected; the malady was instantly relieved, and he called out, "I am well; it is most extraordinary." He went out of the front door, and walked some fifty yards, and then was observed to reel about like a drunken man. He was supported back and laid in the horizontal posture; the face was livid, the pulse could scarcely be felt, and there was complete loss of consciousness. This state lasted about an hour, and without a doubt the man nearly died. Medical men in practice, who have been in the habit of using hypodermic injections of morphine, have had experiences very similar to this and other cases, and although I know of no actual death, yet it is evident that morphine, when injected hypodermically even in a moderate dose, may kill by syncope, and within a few minutes.[393] Absorption by hypodermic administration is so rapid that by the time, or even before the needle of the syringe is withdrawn, a contraction of the pupil may be observed.

Opium or morphine is poisonous by whatever channel it gains access to the system, the intestinal mucous membrane absorbs it readily, and narcotic effects may be produced by external applications, whether a wound is present or not. A case of absorption of opium by a wound is related in Chevers's *Jurisprudence*.[394] A Burman boy, about nine or ten years of age, was struck on the forehead by a brick-bat, causing a gaping wound about an inch long; his parents stuffed the wound with opium. On the third day after the accident, and the opium still remaining in the wound, he became semi-comatose, and, in short, had all the symptoms of opium narcosis; with treatment he recovered. The unbroken skin also readily absorbs the drug. Tardieu states that he had seen 30 grms. of laudanum, applied on a poultice to the abdomen, produce death. Christison has also cited a case in which a soldier suffered from erysipelas, and died in a narcotic state, apparently produced from the too free application of laudanum to the inflamed part.

To these cases may be added the one cited by Taylor, in which a druggist applied 30 grains of morphine to the surface of an ulcerated breast, and the woman died with all the symptoms of narcotic poisoning ten hours after the application—an event scarcely surprising. It is a curious question whether sufficient of the poison enters into the secretions—*e.g.*, the milk—to render it poisonous. An inquest was held in Manchester, Nov. 1875, on the body of a male child two days old, in which it seemed probable that death had occurred through the mother's milk. She was a confirmed opium-eater, taking a solid ounce per week.

§ 360. **Diagnosis of Opium Poisoning.**—The diagnosis is at times between poisoning by opium or other narcotic substances, at others, between opium and disease. Insensibility from chloral, from alcohol, from belladonna or atropine, and from carbon oxide gas, are all more or less like opium poisoning. With regard to chloral, it may be that only chemical analysis and surrounding circumstances can clear up the matter. In alcohol poisoning, the breath commonly smells very strongly of alcohol, and there is no difficulty in separating it from the contents of the stomach, &c., besides which the stomach is usually red and inflamed. Atropine and belladonna invariably dilate the pupil, and although just before death opium has the same effect, yet we must hold that mostly opium contracts, and that a widely-dilated pupil during life would, *per se*, lead us to suspect that opium had not been used, although, as before mentioned, too much stress must not be laid upon the state of the pupils. In carbon oxide, the peculiar rose-red condition of the body affords a striking contrast to the pallor which, for the most part, accompanies opium poisoning. In the rare cases in which convulsions are a prominent symptom, it may be doubtful whether opium or strychnine has been taken, but the convulsions hitherto noticed in opium poisoning seem to me to have been rather of an epileptiform character, and very different from the effects of strychnine. No rules can be laid down for cases which do not run a normal course; in medicine such are being constantly met with, and require all the care and acumen of the trained observer. Cases of disease render a diagnosis often extremely difficult, and the more so in those instances in which a dose of laudanum or other opiate has been administered. In a case under my own observation, a woman, suffering from emphysema and bronchitis, sent to a chemist for a sleeping draught, which she took directly it arrived. A short time afterwards she fell into a profound slumber, and died within six hours. The draught had been contained in an ounce-and-a-half bottle; the bottle was empty, and the druggist stated in evidence that it only contained 20 minims of laudanum, 10 grains of potassic bromide, and water. On, however, diluting the

[393] See a case of morphia poisoning by hypodermic injection, and recovery, by Philip E. Hill, M.R.C.S., *Lancet*, Sept. 30, 1882. In this instance a third of a grain introduced subcutaneously caused most dangerous symptoms in a gardener, aged 48.
[394] Third ed., p. 228.

single drop remaining in the bottle, and imitating its colour with several samples of laudanum diluted in the same way, I came to the conclusion that the quantity of laudanum which the bottle originally contained was far in excess of that which had been stated, and that it was over 1 drachm and under 2 drachms. The body was pallid, the pupils strongly contracted, the vessels of the brain membranes were filled with fluid blood, and there was about an ounce of serous fluid in each ventricle. The lungs were excessively emphysematous, and there was much secretion in the bronchi; the liver was slightly cirrhotic. The blood, the liver, and the contents of the stomach were exhaustively analysed with the greatest care, but no trace of morphine, narcotine, or meconic acid could be separated, although the woman did not live more than six hours after taking the draught. I gave the opinion that it was, in the woman's state, improper to prescribe a sedative of that kind, and that probably death had been accelerated, if not directly caused, by opium.

Deaths by apoplexy will only simulate opium-poisoning during life; a *post-mortem* examination will at once reveal the true nature of the malady. In epilepsy, however, it is different, and more than once an epileptic fit has occurred and been followed by coma—a coma which certainly cannot be distinguished from that produced by a narcotic poison. Death in this stage may follow, and on examining the body no lesion may be found.

§ 361. **Opium-eating.**—The consumption of opium is a very ancient practice among Eastern nations, and the picture, drawn by novelist and traveller, of poor, dried-up, yellow mortals addicted to this vice, with their faculties torpid, their skin hanging in wrinkles on their wasted bodies, the conjunctivæ tinged with bile, the bowels so inactive that there is scarcely an excretion in the course of a week, the mental faculties verging on idiocy and imbecility, is only true of a percentage of those who are addicted to the habit. In the *British Medical Journal* for 1894, Jan. 13 and 20, will be found a careful digest of the evidence collated from 100 Indian medical officers, from which it appears that opium is taken habitually by a very large number of the population throughout India, those who are accustomed to the drug taking it in quantities of from 10 to 20 grains in the twenty-four hours; so long as this amount is not exceeded they do not appear to suffer ill-health or any injurious effect. The native wrestlers even use it whilst training. The habitual consumption of opium by individuals has a direct medico-legal bearing. Thus in India, among the Rajpoots, from time immemorial, infused opium has been the drink both of reconciliation and of ordinary greeting, and it is no evidence of death by poison if even a considerable quantity of opium be found in the stomach after death, for this circumstance taken alone would, unless the history of the case was further known, be considered insufficient proof. So, again, in all climates, and among all races, it is entirely unknown what quantity of an opiate should be considered a poisonous dose for an opium-eater. Almost incredible quantities have, indeed, been consumed by such persons, and the commonly-received explanation, that the drug, in these cases, passes out unabsorbed, can scarcely be correct, for Hermann mentions the case of a lady of Zurich who daily injected subcutaneously 1 to 2 grms. (15-31 grains) of a morphine salt. In a case of uterine cancer, recorded by Dr. W. C. Cass,[395] 20 grains of morphine in the twelve hours were frequently used subcutaneously; during thirteen months the hypodermic syringe was used 1350 times, the dose each time being 5 grains. It is not credible that an alkaloid introduced into the body hypodermically should not be absorbed.

Opium-smoking is another form in which the drug is used, but it is an open question as to what poisonous alkaloids are in opium smoke. It is scarcely probable that morphine should be a constituent, for its subliming point is high, and it will rather be deposited in the cooler portion of the pipe. Opium, specially prepared for smoking, is called "Chandoo"; it is dried at a temperature not exceeding 240°. H. Moissan[396] has investigated the products of smoking chandoo, but only found a small quantity of morphine. N. Gréhant and E. Martin[397] have also experimented with opium smoke; they found it to have no appreciable effect on a dog; one of the writers smoked twenty pipes in succession, containing altogether 4 grms. of chandoo. After the fourth pipe there was some headache, at the tenth pipe and onwards giddiness. Half an hour after the last pipe the giddiness and headache rapidly went off. In any case, opium-smoking seems to injure the health of Asiatics but little. Mr. Vice-Consul King, of Kew-Kiang, in a tour through Upper Yangtse and Stechnan, was thrown much into the company of junk sailors and others, "almost every adult of whom smoked more or less." He says:—"Their work was of the hardest and rudest, rising at four and working with hardly any intermission till dark, having constantly to strip and plunge into the stream in all seasons, and this often in the most dangerous parts. The quantity of food they eat was simply prodigious, and from this and their work it seems fairly to be inferred that their constitution was robust. The two most addicted to the habit were

[395] *Lancet*, March 25, 1882. See also Dr. Boulton's case, *Lancet*, March 18, 1882.
[396] *Compt. Rend.*, cxv. 988-992.
[397] *Compt. Rend.*, 1012-1014.

the pilot and the ship's cook. On the incessant watchfulness and steady nerve of the former the safety of the junk and all on board depended, while the second worked so hard from 3 A.M. to 10 P.M., and often longer, and seemed so independent of sleep or rest, that to catch him seated or idle was sufficient cause for good-humoured banter. This latter had a conserve of opium and sugar which he chewed during the day, as he was only able to smoke at night."

§ 362. **Treatment of Opium or Morphine Poisoning.**—The first thing to be done is doubtless to empty the stomach by means of the flexible stomach tube; the end of a sufficiently long piece of indiarubber tubing is passed down into the pharynx and allowed to be carried into the stomach by means of the natural involuntary movements of the muscles of the pharynx and gullet; suction is then applied to the free end and the contents syphoned out; the stomach is, by means of a funnel attached to the tube, washed out with warm water, and then some coffee administered in the same way.

Should morphine have been taken, and permanganate of potash be at hand, it has been shown that under such circumstances potassic permanganate is a perfect antidote, decomposing at once any morphine remaining in the stomach, but it, of course, will have no effect upon any morphine which has already been absorbed. In a case of opium poisoning, reported in the *Lancet* of June 2, 1894, by W. J. C. Merry, M.B., inhalations of oxygen, preceded by emptying the stomach and other means, appeared to save a man, who, three hours before the treatment, had drank 2 ozs. of chlorodyne. It is also the received treatment to ward off the fatal sleep by stimulation; the patient is walked about, flicked with a towel, made to smell strong ammonia, and so forth. This stimulation must, however, be an addition, but must never replace the measures first detailed.

§ 363. **Post-mortem Appearances.**—There are no characteristic appearances after death save hyperæmia of the brain and blood-vessels of the membranes, with generally serous effusion into the ventricles. The pupils are sometimes contracted, sometimes dilated, the dilatation occurring, as before mentioned, in the act of dying. The external surface of the body is either livid or pale. The lungs are commonly hyperæmic, the bladder full of urine; still, in not a few cases, there is nothing abnormal, and in no single case could a pathologist, from the appearance of the organs only, declare the cause of death with confidence.

§ 364. **Separation of Morphine from Animal Tissues and Fluids.**—Formerly a large proportion of the opium and morphine cases submitted to chemical experts led to no results; but owing to the improved processes now adopted, failure, though still common, is less frequent. The constituents of opium taken into the blood undergo partial destruction in the animal body, but a portion may be found in the secretions, more especially in the urine and fæces. First Bouchardat[398] and then Lefort[399] ascertained the excretion of morphine by the urine after medicinal doses; Dragendorff and Kauzmann showed that the appearance of morphine in the urine was constant, and that it could be easily ascertained and separated from the urine of men and animals; and Levinstein[400] has also shown that the elimination from a single dose may extend over five or six days. The method used by Dragendorff to extract morphine from either urine or blood is to shake the liquid (acidified with a mineral acid) several times with amyl alcohol, which, on removal, separates urea and any bile acids. The liquid thus purified is then alkalised, and shaken up with amyl alcohol, and this amyl alcohol should contain any morphine that was present. On evaporation it may be pure enough to admit of identification, but if not, it may be redissolved and purified on the usual principles. Considerable variety of results seems to be obtained by different experimenters. Landsberg[401] injected hypodermically doses of .2 to .4 grm. of morphine hydrochlorate into dogs, making four experiments in all, but failed to detect morphine in the urine. A large dose with 2.4 mgrms. of the salt gave the same result. On the other hand, .8 grm. of morphine hydrochlorate injected direct into the jugular vein, was partly excreted by the kidneys, for 90 c.c. of the urine yielded a small quantity of morphine. Voit, again, examined the urine and fæces of a man who had taken morphine for years; he could detect none in the urine, but separated morphine from the fæces.[402] Morphine may occasionally be recognised in the blood. Dragendorff[403] found it in the blood of a cat twenty-five minutes after a subcutaneous dose, and he also separated it from the blood of a man who died of morphine poisoning

[398] *Bull. Gén. de Thérap.*, Dec. 1861.

[399] *Journ. de Chim.*, xi. 93, 1861.

[400] *Berl. klin. Wochenschr.*, 1876, 27.

[401] *Pflüger's Archiv.*, 23, 433, 413-433. *Chem. Soc. Journ.*, May 1882, 543.

[402] *Arch. Pharm.*, pp. [3], vii. pp. 23-26.

[403] Kauzmann, *Beiträge für den gerichtlich-chemischen Nachweis des Morphia u. Narcotins*, Dissert., Dorpat, 1868. Dragendorff, *Pharm. Zeitschr. f. Russland*, 1868, Hft. 4.

in six hours. Haidlen[404] recognised morphine in the blood of a suicide who had taken opium extract.

On the other hand, in a case recorded earlier, where a woman died in six hours from a moderate dose, probably of laudanum, although the quantity of blood operated upon was over a pound in weight, and every care was taken, the results were entirely negative. In poisoning by laudanum there may be some remaining in the stomach, and also if large doses of morphine have been taken by the mouth; but when morphine has been administered hypodermically, and in all cases in which several hours have elapsed, one may almost say that the organ in which there is the least probability of finding the poison is the stomach. It may, in some cases, be necessary to operate on a very large scale;—to examine the fæces, mince up the whole liver, the kidney, spleen, and lungs, and treat them with acid alcohol. The urine will also have to be examined, and as much blood as can be obtained. In cases where all the evidence points to a minute quantity (under a grain) of morphine, it is decidedly best to add these various extracts together, to distil off the alcohol at a very gentle heat, to dry the residue in a vacuum, to dissolve again in absolute alcohol, filter, evaporate again to dryness, dissolve in water, and then use the following process:—

§ 365. **Extraction of Morphine.**—To specially search for morphine in such a fluid as the urine, it is, according to the author's experience, best to proceed strictly as follows:—The urine is precipitated with acetate of lead, the powdered lead salt being added to the warm urine contained in a beaker on the water-bath, until a further addition no longer produces a precipitate; the urine is then filtered, the lead precipitate washed, and the excess of lead thrown down by SH_2; the lead having been filtered off, and the precipitate washed, the urine is concentrated down to a syrup in a vacuum. The syrup is now placed in a separating tube (if not acid, it is acidified with hydrochloric acid), and shaken up successively with petroleum ether, chloroform, ether, and, lastly, with amylic alcohol (the latter should be warm); finally, the small amount of amylic alcohol left dissolved in the liquid is got rid of by shaking it up with petroleum ether. To get rid of the last traces of petroleum ether, it may be necessary to turn the liquid into an evaporating dish, and gently heat for a little time over the water-bath. The acid liquid is now again transferred to the separating tube, and shaken up with ether, after being made alkaline with ammonia; this will remove nearly all alkaloids save morphine,—under the circumstances, a very small quantity of morphine may indeed be taken up by the ether, but not the main bulk. After separating the ether, the liquid is again made slightly acid, so as to be able to precipitate morphine in the presence of the solvent; the tube is warmed on the water-bath, at least its own bulk of hot amylic alcohol added and the liquid made alkaline, and the whole well shaken. The amylic alcohol is removed in the usual way, and shaken with a small quantity of decinormal sulphuric acid; this washes out the alkaloid from the amyl alcohol, and the same amyl alcohol can be used again and again. It is best to extract the liquid for morphine at least thrice, and to operate with both the solution and the amyl hot. The decinormal acid liquid is made slightly alkaline with ammonia, and allowed to stand for at least twelve hours; any precipitate is collected and washed with ether, and then with water; the alkaline liquid from which the morphine has been separated is concentrated to the bulk of 5 c.c. on the water bath, and again allowed to stand for twelve hours; a little more morphine may often in this way be obtained.

The author in some test experiments, in which weighed small quantities of morphine (60-80 mgrms.) were dissolved in a little decinormal sulphuric acid, and added to large quantities of urine, found the process given to yield from 80 to 85 per cent. of the alkaloid added, and it was always recovered in fine crystals of a slight brown tint, which responded well to tests.

Various other methods were tried, but the best was the one given; the method not only separates the alkaloid with but little loss, but also in a sufficiently pure state to admit of identification.

From the tissues the alkaloid may be dissolved out by the general method given earlier, and the ultimate aqueous solution, reduced to a bulk of not more than 25 c.c., treated by the ethereal solvents in the way just described.

§ 366. **Narcotine** ($C_{22}H_{23}NO_7$) crystallises out of alcohol or ether in colourless, transparent, glittering needles, or groups of needles, belonging to the orthorhombic system.

It is only slightly soluble in boiling, and almost insoluble in cold water. One part requires 100 parts of cold, and 20 of boiling 84 per cent. alcohol; 126 parts of cold, 48 of boiling ether (specific gravity 0.735); 2.69 parts of chloroform; 400 of olive oil; 60 of acetic ether; 300 of amyl alcohol; and 22 parts of benzene, for solution. The neutral solution of narcotine turns the plane of polarisation to the left $[\alpha]r = 130.6$; the acid solution to the right. Narcotine has no effect on red litmus paper.

Narcotine gives no crystalline sublimate; its behaviour in the subliming cell is described earlier. Its melting-point, taken in a tube, is about 176°.

404 *Würtbg. Correspondenzbl.*, xxxiv. 16, 1863.

Behaviour of Narcotine with Reagents.—Narcotine, dissolved in dilute hydrochloric acid, and then treated with a little bromine, gives a yellow precipitate, which on boiling is dissolved; by gradually adding solution of bromine and boiling, a fine rose colour is produced, readily destroyed by excess of bromine. This is perhaps the best test for the presence of narcotine. Concentrated sulphuric acid dissolves narcotine; the solution in the cold is at first colourless, after a few minutes yellow, and in the course of a day or longer the tints gradually deepen. If the solution is warmed, it first becomes orange-red, then at the margin violet-blue; and if heated until hydric sulphate begins to volatilise, the colour is an intense red-violet. If the heating is not carried so far, but the solution allowed to cool, a delicate cherry-red hue slowly develops. If the sulphuric acid solution contains 1 : 2000 of the alkaloid, this test is very evident; with 1 : 40,000, the colour is only a faint carmine.—*A. Husemann.*

A solution of narcotine in pure sulphuric acid, to which a drop of nitric acid has been added, becomes of a red colour; if the solution is warmed to 150°, hypochlorite of soda develops a carmine-red; and chloride of iron, first a violet, then a cherry-red. The precipitants of narcotine are—phosphomolybdic acid, picric acid, sulphocyanide of potash, potassio cadmic iodide, mercuric chloride, platinic chloride, auric chloride, and several other reagents.

From the brown mass left after heating narcotine above 200°, hydrochloric acid extracts a small portion of a base but little studied. The residue consists of humopic acid ($C_{40}H_{19}O_{14}$), which can be obtained by dissolving in caustic potash, precipitating with HCl, dissolving the precipitate in boiling alcohol, and finally throwing it down by water.

§ 367. **Effects.**—Narcotine in itself has toxic action only in rather large doses; from 1 to 2 grms. have been given to man, and slight hypnotic effects have followed. It is poisonous in very large doses; an ordinary-sized cat is killed by 3 grms. The symptoms are mainly convulsions.

§ 368. **Codeine (Codomethylene)**, $C_{17}H_{17}OCH_3(OH)NO + H_2O$, is the methyl of morphine; it is an alkaloid contained in opium in small quantity only. Mulder, indeed, quotes .66 to .77 per cent. as present in Smyrna opium, but Merck and Schindler give .25 per cent. Schindler found in Constantinople, .5 per cent.; and Merck, in Bengal, .5 per cent. also.

Codeine crystallises out of dry ether in small, colourless, anhydrous, crystals; but crystallised slowly from an aqueous solution, the crystals are either in well-defined octahedra, or in prisms, containing one atom of water, and melting in boiling-water to an oily fluid. The anhydrous crystals have a melting-point of 150°, and solidify again on cooling. Its watery solution is alkaline to litmus paper.

It requires 80 parts of cold, 17 of boiling water, 10 parts of benzole, and 7 parts of amyl alcohol respectively, for solution. Alcohol, benzene, ether, carbon disulphide, and chloroform freely dissolve it, but in petroleum ether it is almost insoluble. Further, it is also soluble in aqueous ammonia, and in dilute acids, but insoluble in excess of caustic potash or soda, and may thus be thrown out of an aqueous solution. A solution of codeine turns the plane of polarisation to the left, $[\alpha]r = 118.2°$.

Concentrated sulphuric acid dissolves codeine without colour, but after eight days the solution becomes blue; this reaction is quicker if the acid contains a trace of nitric acid. If the sulphuric acid solution be warmed to 150°, and a drop of nitric acid be added after cooling, a blood-red colour is produced. Fröhde's reagent produces a dirty green colour, soon becoming Prussian blue, and terminating after twenty-four hours in a pale yellow.

Cyanogen gas, led into an alcoholic solution of codeine, gives first a yellow and then a brown colour; lastly, a crystalline precipitate falls. On warming with a little sulphuric acid and ferric chloride, a blue colour is produced. This blue colour is apparently common to all ethers of the codeine class.

Of the group reagents, the following precipitate solutions of codeine:—Mercuric potassium iodide, mercuric chloride, mercuric bromide, picric acid, and tannin solutions. The following do not precipitate:—Mercuric cyanide and potassium ferrocyanide solutions. Potassium dichromate gives no immediate precipitate, but crystals form on long standing. It does not give the reaction with iodic acid like morphine; it is distinguished from narceine by dropping a small particle of iodine into the aqueous solution, the iodine particle does not become surrounded with fine crystals.

§ 369. **Effects.**—The physiological action of codeine on animals has been investigated by Claude Bernard, Magendie, Crum Brown and Fraser, Falck, and a large number of others.[405] It has also been administered to man, and has taken in some degree the place of morphine. Claude Bernard showed that, when given to dogs in sufficient quantity to produce sleep, the sleep was different in some respects to that of morphine sleep, especially in its after-effects. Thus, in his usual graphic way, he describes the following experiment:—"Two young dogs, accustomed to

[405] *Ann. Chem. Phys.* [5], 27, pp. 273-288; also, *Journ. Chem. Soc.*, No. ccxliv., 1883, p. 358.

play together, and both a little beyond the average size, received in the cellular tissue of the axillæ, by the aid of a subcutaneous syringe, the one 5 centigrammes of morphine hydrochloride, the other 5 centigrammes of codeine hydrochloride. At the end of a quarter of an hour both dogs showed signs of narcosis. They were placed on their backs in the experimental trough, and slept tranquilly for three or four hours. When the animals woke, they presented the most striking contrast. The morphine dog ran with a hyena-like gait (*démarche hyénoid*), the eye wild, recognising no one, not even his codeine comrade, who vainly bit him playfully, and jumped sportively on his back. It was not until the next day that the morphine dog regained his spirits and usual humour. A couple of days after, the two dogs being in good health, I repeated the same experiment, but in an inverse order—that is to say, I gave the codeine to that which previously had the morphine, and *vice versâ*. Both dogs slept about as long as the first time; but on waking the attitudes were completely reversed, just as the administration of the two substances had been. The dog which, two days before, after having been codeinised, woke lively and gay, was now bewildered and half paralysed at the end of his morphine sleep; whilst the other was wide awake and in the best spirits."

Subsequent experimenters found what Bernard does not mention—viz., that codeine produced epileptiform convulsions. Falck made some very careful experiments on pigeons, frogs, and rabbits. To all these in high enough doses it was fatal. Falk puts the minimum lethal dose for a rabbit at 51.2 mgrms. per kilo. Given to man, it produces a sleep very similar to that described by Claude Bernard—that is, a sleep which is very natural, and does not leave any after-effect. Therefore it is declared to be the best alkaloid of a narcotic nature to give when lengthened slumber is desired, more especially since it does not confine the bowels, nor has it been found to produce any eruption on the skin. Before it has a full narcotic effect, vomiting has often been excited, and in a few cases purging. The maximum dose for an adult is about .1 grm. (1.5 grain); three times this quantity, .3 grms. (4-5 grains), would probably produce unpleasant, if not dangerous, symptoms.[406]

§ 370. **Narceine,** $C_{23}H_{27}NO_8 + 3H_2O$.—Two of the three molecules of water are expelled at 100°, the other molecule requires a higher temperature; anhydrous narceine is hygroscopic, and melts in a tube at about 140°; when exposed to air it unites with one molecule of water, and then melts at about 160°.

The constitution of narceine is probably that of a substituted phenylbenzylketone, and the following structural formula has been attributed to it:[407]—

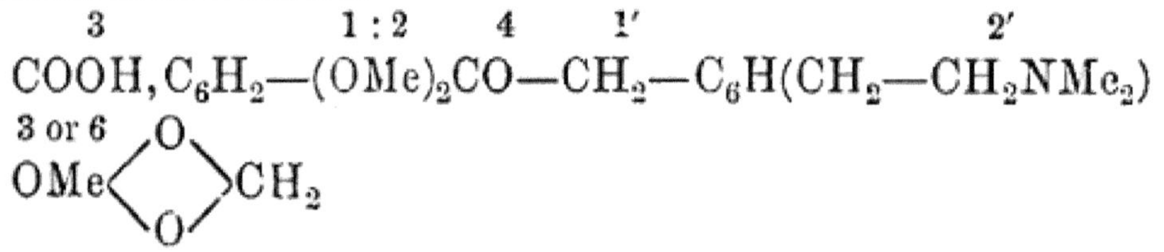

It therefore contains three methoxyl groups.

Narceine forms good crystals, the form being that of long, four-sided rhombic prisms or fine bushy united needles.

Narceine hydrochloride crystallises with $5\frac{1}{2}H_2O$ and with $3H_2O$; the anhydrous salt melts at 190°-192°. The platinochloride is a definite salt, m.p. 190°-191°; it decomposes at 195°-196°. The nitrate forms good crystals, which decompose at 97°. Narceine also forms crystalline salts with potassium and sodium; these may be obtained by heating the base at 60°-70° with a 33 per cent. of NaHO or KHO.

The potassium compound melts at 90°, the sodium at 159°-160°. The alkaloid is regenerated when the alkali salts are treated with acids or with CO_2. Crude narceine may be purified by means of the sodium salt; the latter is dissolved in alcohol and precipitated with ether.

It is soluble in alcohol, but almost insoluble in alcohol and ether, or benzene and ether; it is slightly soluble in ether, carbon disulphide, and chloroform. It has no reaction on moist litmus paper.

Benzole and petroleum ether extract narceine neither from acid nor alkaline solutions; chloroform extracts narceine both from acid and from alkaline solutions, the latter in small proportion only. Narceine turns the plane of polarisation to the left, $[\alpha]r = 66.7°$. Narceine may be separated from narcotine by the addition of ammonia to the acid aqueous solution; narcotine is fully precipitated by ammonia, but narceine is left in solution.

[406] For further details as to the action of codeine, the reader is referred to L. O. Wach's monograph, *Das Codein* (1868), which contains reference to the earlier literature. See also Harley, *The Old Vegetable Neurotics*, London.
[407] M. Freund and G. B. Frankforter, *Annalen*, 277, pp. 20-58.

In the subliming cell it melts at 134°, but gives no crystalline sublimate. The tube melting-point of the trihydrate is 170°. The melted substance is at first colourless; but on raising the temperature, the usual transitions of colour through different shades of brown to black are observed. If melted, and kept a few degrees above its melting-point, and then cooled slowly, the residue is straw-coloured, divided into lobes, most of which contain feathery crystals.

At high temperatures narceine develops a herring-like odour; the residue becomes darkish blue with iron chloride. Concentrated nitric acid dissolves it with a yellow colour; on heating, red vapours are produced; the fluid contains crystals of oxalic acid, and develops with potash a volatile base. Concentrated sulphuric acid colours pure narceine brown; but if impure, a blood-red or blue colour may be produced. It does not reduce iron salts.

Fröhde's reagent colours it first brown-green, then red, passing into blue. Narceine forms precipitates with bichromate of potash, chloride of gold, bichloride of platinum, and several other reagents. The one formed by the addition of potassio zinc iodide is in hair-like crystals, which after twenty-four hours become blue.

Weak iodine solution colours narceine crystals a black-blue; they dissolve in water at 100° without colour, but on cooling again separate with a violet or blue colour. If on a saturated solution of narceine a particle of iodine is strewn, fine needle-like grey crystals form around the iodine. A drop of "Nessler" solution, added to solid narceine, at once strikes a brown colour; on diluting the drop with a little water, beautiful little bundles of crystals appear.—*Flückiger.*

The following group reagents precipitate narceine:—picric acid, tannin solution, and potassium dichromate on long standing. The following give no precipitate:—mercuric cyanide, mercuric potas. iodide, mercuric chloride, mercuric bromide, and potas. ferrocyanide solutions.

§ 371. **Effects.**—The physiological action of narceine has been variously interpreted by different observers. Claude Bernard[408] thought it the most somniferous of the opium alkaloids. He said that "the narceinic sleep was characterised by a profound calm and absence of the excitability of morphine, the animals narcotised by narceine on awaking returning to their natural state without enfeeblement of the hind limbs or other sequelæ." It has been amply confirmed that narceine possesses somniferous properties, but certainly not to the extent that Bernard's observations led physiologists to expect. In large doses there is some irritation of the stomach and intestines, and vomiting occurs, and even diarrhœa; moderate doses induce constipation. The maximum medicinal dose may be put at .14 grm. (or 2.26 grains), and a probably dangerous dose would be three times that quantity.[409]

§ 372. **Papaverine** ($C_{21}H_{21}NO_4$) crystallises from alcohol in white needles or scales. It possesses scarcely any alkaline reaction, but its salts have an acid reaction; it has but little effect on a ray of polarised light. It is almost insoluble in water; it is easily soluble in acetone, amyl alcohol, alcohol, and chloroform. One part of the alkaloid is dissolved in 36.6 of benzene, and in 76 parts of amyl alcohol. Petroleum ether dissolves it by the aid of heat, but the alkaloid separates in crystals on cooling. Chloroform extracts it from either acid or alkaline solutions. Papaverine gives no crystalline sublimate. The melting-point of pure samples in a tube is 147°, with scarcely any colour; it solidifies again to crystals on cooling; in the subliming cell it melts at 130°, and decomposes about 149°; the vapours are alkaline; the residue is amorphous, light brown, and is not characteristic. Concentrated sulphuric acid colours it a deep violet-blue, and dissolves it to a violet, slowly fading. This solution, by permanganate of potash, is first green and then grey. Fröhde's reagent gives a beautiful violet colour, which becomes blue, and vanishes after twenty-four hours. Diluted solutions of salts of papaverine are not precipitated by phosphomolybdic acid. It is precipitated by ammonia, by the caustic and carbonated alkalies, by potassic-cadmic iodide, iodine in hydriodic acid, and by alkaloidal reagents generally—save by the important exception mentioned above. A solution in amyl alcohol is also precipitated by bromine; the precipitate is crystalline. An alcoholic solution of platinic chloride also separates papaverine platin chloride in crystals. An alcoholic solution of iodine, added to an alcoholic solution of papaverine, separates in a little time crystals of the composition $C_{21}H_{21}NO_4I_3$. From the mother-liquor, by concentration, can be obtained needles of another iodine combination, $C_{21}H_{21}NO_4I_5$; the latter heated above 100° parts with free iodine. These compounds with iodine are decomposed by ammonia and potash, papaverine separating. The decomposition may be watched under the microscope. Nitric acid precipitates from a solution of the sulphate a white nitrate soluble in excess; the precipitate does not appear at once, but forms in the course of an hour; it is at first amorphous, but subsequently crystalline; this, with its physical properties, is a great assistance to identification.

[408] *Compt. Rend.*, lix. p. 406, 1864.

[409] See J. Bouchardat, *La Narcéine*, Thèse, Paris, 1865; Harley, *The Old Vegetable Neurotics*, Lond.; Ch. Liné, *Études sur la Narcéine et son Emploi Thérapeutique*, Thèse, Paris, 1865; also, Husemann's *Planzenstoffe*, in which these and other researches are summarised.

§ 373. **Effects.**—Claude Bernard ranked papaverine with the convulsants; probably the papaverine he had was impure. In any case, subsequent observations have shown that it is to be classed rather with the hypnotic principles of opium. Leidesdorf[410] administered it to the insane, and noted slowness of the pulse, muscular weakness, and drowsiness to follow. The doses were given subcutaneously (.42 grm. of the hydrochloride). Baxt,[411] experimenting with the frog, found that a milligramme caused deep sleep and slowing of the heart's action. This action on the heart is witnessed also on the recently-removed frog's heart. Guinea-pigs, and other small animals poisoned by strychnine or thebaine, and then given papaverine, did not seem to be so soon affected with tetanus as when no such remedy was administered. The fatal dose of papaverine for a man is unknown. I should conjecture that the least quantity that would cause dangerous symptoms would be 1 grm. (15.4 grains).

§ 374. **Thebaine**, $C_{17}H_{15}NO(OCH_3)_2$.—Opium seldom contains much more than 1 per cent. of this alkaloid. It usually forms needles or short crystals. It is alkaline, and by rubbing becomes negatively electric. It is almost insoluble in water, aqueous ammonia, and solutions of the alkalies. It requires 10 parts of cold alcohol for solution, and dissolves readily in hot. Ether, hot or cold, is also a good solvent. 100 parts of benzene are required for 5.27 parts of thebaine, and 100 of amyl alcohol for 1.67 parts. Chloroform dissolves thebaine with difficulty out of both acid and alkaline solutions; petroleum ether extracts it from neither. Thebaine melts in a tube at 193°, sublimes at 135°. The sublimate is in minute crystals, similar to theine; at higher temperatures (160° to 200°) needles, cubes, and prisms are obtained. The residue is fawn coloured. Fröhde's reagent (as well as concentrated sulphuric acid) dissolves it, with the production of a blood-red colour, passing gradually into yellow. The precipitate with picric acid is yellow and amorphous; with tannic acid yellow; with gold chloride, red-yellow; and with platinic chloride, citron-yellow, gradually becoming crystalline. A concentrated alcoholic solution of thebaine, just neutralised with HCl, deposits well-formed rhombic crystals of the composition $C_{19}H_{21}NO_3HCl + H_2O$.

If 200 mgrms. of thebaine are heated to boiling with 1.4 c.c. of HCl and 2.8 c.c. of water, and the solution diluted, after boiling, with 4 c.c. of water, crystals of thebaine hydrochloride form in the yellow fluid in the course of a few hours.—*Flückiger.*

§ 375. **Effects.**—There is no disagreement of opinion as to the action of thebaine. By the united testimony of all who have experimented with it, the alkaloid belongs to those poisons which produce tetanus, and the symptoms can scarcely be differentiated from strychnia. In Baxt's experiments on frogs he showed that there was some considerable difference in details in the general course of the symptoms, according to the dose of the poison. A small dose (such, for example, as .75 mgrm.) injected into a frog subcutaneously produces immediate excitement, the animal jumping about, and this stage lasting for about a minute; it then becomes quieter, and has from three to six minutes' sleep; in a little time this comatose state is followed by reflex tetanic spasms and then spontaneous tetanic spasms. With three times the dose, the tetanic convulsions commence early, and death takes place in from two to six hours. Baxt[412] found 6 to 7 mgrms. kill rabbits with tetanic convulsions in from fifteen to twenty-five minutes. Crum Brown and Fraser also found that 12 mgrms. injected into rabbits were fatal; it may then be presumed that the lethal dose for a rabbit is about 5 mgrms. per kilo. A frog's heart under the action of thebaine, and removed from the body, beats quicker and ceases earlier than one in distilled water. Thebaine has been administered to the insane subcutaneously in doses of from 12 to 40 mgrms., when a rise of temperature and an increase in the respiratory movements and in the circulation were noticed.[413]

The fatal dose for a man is not known; .5 grm., or about 8 grains, would probably be a poisonous quantity.

§ 376. **Cryptopine** ($C_{21}H_{23}NO_5$) was discovered by T. & H. Smith in 1867.[414] It is only contained in very minute traces in opium—something like .003 per cent. It is a crystalline substance, the crystals being colourless, six-sided prisms, without odour, but with a bitter taste, causing an after-sensation like peppermint. The crystals melt at 217°, and congeal in a crystalline form again at 171°; at high temperatures they are decomposed with evolution of ammoniacal vapour. Cryptopine is insoluble, or almost so, in ether, water, and oil of turpentine; it is soluble in acetone, benzene, and chloroform; the latter is the best solvent, or hot alcohol; it is insoluble in aqueous ammonia and in solutions of the caustic alkaloids. Cryptopine is strongly basic, neutralising fully mineral acids. Concentrated sulphuric acid colours cryptopine pure blue, the tint gradually fading from absorption of water from the atmosphere.

---

[410] *Ztschr. d. Wien. Aerzte*, pp. 13, 115, 1868.

[411] *Arch. Anat. Phys.*, p. 70, 1869.

[412] *Sitzungsber. d. Wien. Akadem.*, lvi. pp. 2, 89, 1867; *Arch. f. Anat. u. Physiol.*, Hft. 1, p. 112, 1869.

[413] F. W. Müller, *Das Thebaine, eine Monographie*, Diss., Marburg 1868.

[414] *Pharm. Journ. Trans.* [2], viii. pp. 495 and 716.

On a crystal of potassic nitrate being added, the colour changes into a permanent green. With ferric chloride cryptopine gives no colour—thus distinguishing it from morphine. The physiological properties of cryptopine have been investigated by Dr. Harley;[415] it has a narcotic action, about double as strong as narceine, and four times weaker than morphine. Munk and Sippell[416] found that it gave rise in animals to paralysis of the limbs, and occasionally asphyxic convulsions before death.

§ 377. **Rhœadine** ($C_{21}H_{21}NO_6$).—Rhœadine was separated from *Papaver rhœas* by Hesse, and has also been found in *Papaver somniferum* and in opium. Rhœadine is in the form of small anhydrous tasteless prisms, melting at 230° and partly subliming. In a vacuum sublimation is almost complete, and at a much lower temperature. It is a very insoluble substance, and is scarcely dissolved, when crystalline, by water, alcohol, ether, chloroform, benzene, and solutions of the fixed or volatile alkalies. When in an amorphous state it is rather soluble in ether, and may be dissolved out of any substance by treating with dilute acetic acid, and neutralising by ammonia, and shaking up with ether before the precipitate becomes crystalline. Rhœadine is easily recognised by its striking a red colour with hydrochloric acid. Either spontaneously or on gentle warming, the colour is produced—one part of rhœadine will colour in this way 10,000 parts of acid water blue or purple-red, 200,000 rose-red, and 800,000 pale red. The reaction depends on a splitting up of the rhœadine into a colourless substance, *rhœadin*, and a red colouring-matter. Rhœadine is not poisonous.

§ 378. **Pseudomorphine** ($C_{17}H_{19}NO_4$).—Pseudomorphine was discovered by Pelletier and Thiboumery in 1835. As precipitated by ammonia out of the hot solution, pseudomorphine falls as a white crystalline precipitate; but if the solution is cold, the precipitate is gelatinous. It possesses no taste, and has no action on vegetable colours. On heating, it decomposes and then melts. It dissolves easily in caustic alkalies and in milk of lime, but is insoluble in all the ordinary alcoholic and ethereal solvents, as well as in diluted sulphuric acid. The most soluble salt is the hydrochlorate ($C_{17}H_{19}NO_4HCl + H_2O$), and that requires 70 parts of water at 20° for solution. Various salts, such as the sulphate, oxalate, &c., may be prepared from the hydrochlorate by double decomposition. Concentrated sulphuric acid dissolves pseudomorphine gradually, with the production of an olive-green colour.

§ 379. **Opianine** ($C_{66}H_{72}N_4O_{21}$).—Opianine crystallises in colourless, glittering ortho-rhombic needles. Ammonia precipitates it from its solution in hydrochloric acid as a fine white powder. It is without odour, and has a bitter taste. It is a strong base, and is soluble in cold, but slightly soluble in boiling water. It is also but little soluble in boiling alcohol.

An alcoholic solution of the alkaloid gives a voluminous precipitate with mercuric chloride; after standing a little time, the precipitate becomes crystalline, the crystals being in the shape of fine needles. They have the following composition—$C_{66}H_{72}N_4O_{21}$, 2HCl, 2HgCl—and are with difficulty soluble in water or alcohol.

Opianine, administered to cats in doses of .145 grm., produces complex symptoms—*e.g.*, dilated pupils, foaming at the mouth, uncertain gait, paralysis of the hinder extremities, and stupor—but the alkaloid is rare, and few experiments have been made with it.

§ 380. **Apomorphine** ($C_{17}H_{19}NO_3$).—Apomorphine is a derivative of morphine, and is readily prepared by saponifying morphine by heating it with dilute hydrochloric acid in sealed tubes. The result is apomorphine hydrochloride, the morphine losing one molecule of water, according to the equation $C_{17}H_{19}NO_3 = C_{17}H_{17}NO_2 + H_2O$.

To extract apomorphine, the bases are precipitated by sodic bicarbonate, and the precipitate extracted by ether or chloroform, either of which solvents leaves morphine undissolved. The apomorphine is again converted into hydrochloride, and once more precipitated by sodic bicarbonate, and is lastly obtained as a snow-white substance, rapidly becoming green on exposure to the air. The mass dissolves with a beautiful green colour in water, and also in alcohol, whilst it colours ether purple-red, and chloroform violet.

A test for apomorphine is the following:—The chloride is dissolved in a little acetic acid and shaken with a crystal of potassic iodate (KIO_3); this immediately turns red from liberated iodine on shaking it up with a little chloroform; on standing, the chloroform sinks to the bottom, and is coloured by the alkaloid a beautiful blue colour; on now carefully pouring a little CS_2 on the surface of the liquid at the point of junction it is coloured amethyst owing to dissolved iodine, and apocodeine gives a similar reaction.

Apomorphine is the purest and most active emetic known: whether injected beneath the skin or taken by the

[415] *The Old Vegetable Neurotics.*

[416] Munk, *Versuche über die Wirkung des Cryptopins*, Berlin, 1873. Sippell, *Beiträge zur Kentniss des Cryptopins*, Marburg, 1874.

mouth, the effect is the same—there is considerable depression, faintness, and then vomiting. The dose for an adult is about 6 mgrms. (.092 grain) subcutaneously administered.

§ 381. The reactions of some of the rarer alkaloids of opium with sulphuric acid and ferric chloride are as follows: none of them have at present any toxicological importance:—

TABLE SHOWING SOME OF THE REACTIONS OF THE RARER ALKALOIDS OF OPIUM.

Alkaloid.	Formula.	Reaction with Warm Sulphuric Acid.	Reaction with Ferric Chloride.
Codamine, Landamine,	$C_{20}H_{25}NO_4$ $C_{20}H_{25}NO_4$	Dirty red-violet colour, turning dark violet on the addition of HNO_3.	Dark green.
Landanosine, Protapine,	$C_{20}H_{27}NO_4$ $C_{20}H_{19}NO_5$	Dirty green to brownish-green.	No colour.
Lanthopine,	$C_{23}H_{25}NO_4$	Dark brown or black.	No colour.
Hydrocotarnine,	$C_{12}H_{15}NO_3$	Dirty red-violet; not changed by trace of HNO_3.	No colour.

§ 382. **Tritopine** ($C_{42}H_{54}N_2O_7$).—This is a rare alkaloid that has been found in small quantities in opium. It is crystalline, separating in transparent prisms. Melting-point 182°. It is soluble in alcohol and chloroform, and slightly soluble in ether.[417]

§ 383. **Meconin (Opianyl)** ($C_{10}H_{10}O_4$) is in the form of white glittering needles, which melt under water at 77° and in air at 90°, again coagulating at 75°. It may be sublimed in beautiful crystals. It is soluble in 22 parts of boiling, and 700 of cold water; dissolves easily in alcohol, ether, acetic acid, and ethereal oil, and is not precipitated by acetate of lead. Its solution in concentrated sulphuric acid becomes, on warming, purple, and gives, on the addition of water, a brown precipitate. Meconin may be prepared by treating narcotine with nitric acid. Meconin, in large doses, is a feeble narcotic; 1.25 grm. (20 grains) has been given to man without result.

§ 384. **Meconic Acid** ($C_7H_4O_7$) crystallises in white shining scales or small rhombic prisms, with three atoms of water ($C_7H_4O_7 + 3H_2O$), but at 100° this is lost, and it becomes an opaque white mass. It reddens litmus, and has a sourish taste. It is soluble in 115 parts of cold, but dissolves in 4 parts of boiling water; it dissolves easily in alcohol, less so in ether. It forms well-marked salts; the barium and calcium salt crystallise with one atom of water, the former having the composition $BaH_4(C_7HO_7)_2$; the latter, if ammonium meconate is precipitated by calcium chloride, $CaH_4(C_7HO_7)_2$; but if calcium chloride is added to the acid itself, the salt has the composition $C_7H_2CaO_7 + H_2O$. If meconic acid is gently heated, it decomposes into carbon dioxide and comenic acid ($C_6H_4O_5$). If the heat is stronger, pyromeconic acid ($C_5H_4O_3$)—carbon dioxide, water, acetic acid, and benzole are formed. Pyromeconic acid is readily sublimed in large transparent tables. Chloride of iron, and soluble iron salts generally, give with meconic acid (even in great dilution) a lively red colour, which is not altered by heat, nor by the addition of HCl nor by that of gold chloride. Sugar of lead and nitrate of silver each give a white precipitate; and mercurous and mercuric nitrates white and yellow precipitates. In any case where the analyst has found only meconic acid, the question may be raised in court as to whether it is a poison or not. The early experiments of Sertürner,[418] Langer, Vogel, Sömmering, and Grape[419] showed that, in comparatively speaking large doses, it had but little, if any, action on dogs or men. Albers[420] has, however, experimented on frogs, and found that in doses of .1 to .2 grm. there is, first, a narcotic action, and later, convulsions and death. According to Schroff,[421] there is a slight narcotic action on

[417] E. Kander, *Arch. Pharm.*, 228, pp. 419-431.

[418] *Ann. Phys.*, xxv. 56; xxvii. 183.

[419] *De opio et de illis quibus constat partibus*, Berol., 1822.

[420] *Arch. Path. Anat.*, xxvi. 248.

[421] *Med. Jahresb.*, 1869.

man.

The most generally accepted view at the present time is that the physiological action of meconic acid is similar to that of lactic acid—viz., large doses cause some depression and feeble narcosis.

In a special research amongst organic fluids for meconic acid, the substances are extracted by alcohol *feebly* acidulated with nitric acid; on filtration the alcohol, after the addition of a little water, is distilled off, and to the remaining fluid a solution of acetate of lead is added, and the whole filtered. The filtrate will contain any alkaloids, whilst meconic acid, if present, is bound up with the lead on the filter. The meconate of lead may be either washed or digested in strong acetic acid to purify it, suspended in water, and freed from lead by SH_2; the filtrate from the lead sulphide may be tested by ferric chloride, or preferably, at once evaporated to dryness, and weighed. After this operation it is identified. If the quantity is so small that it cannot be conveniently weighed, it may be estimated colorimetrically, by having a standard solution of meconic acid, containing 1 mgrm. in every c.c. A few drops of neutral ferric chloride are added in a Nessler cylinder to the liquid under examination; and the tint thus obtained is imitated in the usual way, in another cylinder, by means of ferric chloride, the standard solution, and water. It is also obvious that the weight of the meconic acid may be increased by converting it into the barium salt—100 parts of anhydrous baric meconate, ($Ba_2C_7H_2O_7$), being equivalent to 42.3 of meconic acid ($C_7H_4O_7$).

IV.—The Strychnine or Tetanus-Producing[422] Group of Alkaloids.

1. NUX VOMICA GROUP—STRYCHNINE—BRUCINE—IGASURINE.

§ 385. Nux vomica is found in commerce both in the entire state and as a powder. It is the seed of the *Strychnos nux vomica*, or Koochla tree. The seed is about the size of a shilling, round, flattened, concavo-convex, of a yellowish-grey or light-brown colour, covered with a velvety down of fine, radiating, silky hairs, which are coloured by a solution of iodine beautiful gold-yellow; the texture is tough, leathery, and not easily pulverised; the taste is intensely bitter. The powder is not unlike that of liquorice, and, if met with in the pure state, gives a dark orange-red colour with nitric acid, which is destroyed by chloride of tin; the aqueous infusion gives a precipitate with tincture of galls, is reddened by nitric acid, and gives an olive-green tint with persulphate of iron. The best method, however, of recognising quickly and with certainty that the substance under examination is nux vomica powder, is to extract strychnine from it by the following simple process:—The powder is completely exhausted by boiling alcohol (90 per cent.), the alcoholic extract evaporated to dryness, and then treated with water; the aqueous solution is passed through a wet filter, and concentrated by evaporation to a small bulk. To this liquid a drop or so of a concentrated solution of picric acid is added, and the yellow precipitate of picrates thus obtained is separated, treated with nitric acid, the picric acid removed by ether, and the pure alkaloid precipitated by soda, and shaken out by chloroform.

§ 386. **Chemical Composition.**—Nux vomica contains at least four distinct principles:—

- (1.) Strychnine.
- (2.) Brucine.
- (3.) Igasurine.
- (4.) Strychnic or igasuric acid.

§ 387. **Strychnine** ($C_{21}H_{22}N_2O_2$) is contained in the bean of S. *ignatius*, in the bark (*false angustura bark*) and seeds of the *Strychnos nux vomica*, in the *Strychnos colubrina*, L., in the *Strychnos tieuté*, Lesch, and probably in various other plants of the same genus.

Commercial strychnine is met with either in colourless crystals or as a white powder, the most usual form being that of the alkaloid itself; but the nitrate, sulphate, and acetate are also sold to a small extent.

The *microscopical appearance* of strychnine, as thrown down by the solution of vapour of ammonia, may be referred to three leading forms—the long rectangular prism, the short hexagonal prism, or the regular octahedron. If obtained from the slow evaporation of an alcoholic solution, it is usually in the form of four-sided pyramids or long prisms; but if obtained by speedy evaporation or rapid cooling, it appears as a white granular powder. If obtained from a benzene solution, the deposit is usually crystalline, but without a constant form, though at times the crystals are extremely distinct, the short six-sided prism prevailing; but triangular plates, dodecahedral, rhomboidal, and pentagonal, may also be met with. An ethereal solution on evaporation assumes dendritic forms, but may contain

[422] To this group also belong some of the opium alkaloids. See "Thebaine," "Landamine," "Codeine," "Hydrocotarnine."

octahedra and four-sided prisms. A chloroform solution deposits rosettes, veined leaves, stellate dotted needles, circles with broken radii, and branched and reticulated forms of great delicacy and beauty.—*Guy.*

Strychnine is very insoluble in water, although readily dissolved by acidulated water. According to Wormley's repeated experiments, one part of strychnine dissolves in 8333 parts of cold water; and, according to Pelletier and Cahours, it dissolves in 6667 parts of cold, and 2500 parts of boiling water. It may be convenient, then, to remember that a gallon of cold water would hardly dissolve more than 10 grains (.142 grm. per litre); the same amount, if boiling, about 30 grains (.426 grm. per litre) of strychnine. The solubility of one part of strychnine in other menstrua is as follows:—Cold alcohol, 0.833 specific gravity, 120, boiling, 10 parts (*Wittstein*); cold alcohol, 0.936 specific gravity, 240 parts (*Merck*); cold alcohol, 0.815 specific gravity, 107 parts (*Dragendorff*); amyl alcohol, 181 parts; benzene, 164; chloroform, 6.9 (*Schlimpert*), 5 (*Pettenkofer*); ether, 1250 parts; carbon disulphide, 485 parts; glycerin, 300 parts. Creosote and essential and fixed oils also dissolve strychnine.

Of all the above solvents, it is evident that chloroform is the best for purposes of separation, and next to chloroform, benzene.

If a speck of strychnine be placed in the subliming cell, it will be found to sublime usually in a crystalline form at 169°. A common form at this temperature, according to the writer's own observations, is minute needles, disposed in lines; but, as Dr. Guy has remarked, the sublimate may consist of drops, of waving patterns, and various other forms; and, further, while the sublimates of morphia are made up of curved lines, those of strychnine consist of lines either straight or slightly curved, with parallel feathery lines at right angles. On continuing the heat, strychnine melts at about 221°, and the lower disc, if removed and examined, is found to have a resinous residue; but it still continues to yield sublimates until reduced to a spot of carbon. The melting-point taken in a tube is 268°.

Strychnine is so powerfully bitter, that one part dissolved in 70,000 of water is distinctly perceptible; it is a strong base, with a marked alkaline reaction, neutralising the strongest acids fully, and precipitating many metallic oxides from their combinations, often with the formation of double salts. Most of the salts of strychnine are crystalline, and all extremely bitter. Strychnine, in the presence of oxygen, combines with SH_2 to form a beautiful crystalline compound:—

$2C_{21}H_{22}N_2O_2 + 6H_2S + O_3 = 2C_{21}H_{22}N_2O_23H_2S_2 + 3H_2O$.

On treatment with an acid this compound yields H_2S_2.—Schmidt, *Ber. Deutsch. Chem. Ges.*, 8, 1267.

An alcoholic solution of strychnine turns the plane of polarisation to the left, $[\alpha]r$ = -132.08° to 136.78° (*Bouchardat*); but acid solutions show a much smaller rotatory power.

The salts used in medicine are—the *sulphate*, officinal only in the French pharmacopœia; the *nitrate*, officinal in the German, Austrian, Swiss, Norse, and Dutch pharmacopœias; and the *acetate*, well known in commerce, but not officinal.

The commercial **Sulphate** ($C_{21}H_{22}N_2O_2H_2SO_4 + 2H_2O$) is an acid salt crystallising in needles which lose water at 150°, the neutral sulphate ($2C_{21}H_{22}N_2O_2,H_2SO_4 + 7H_2O$) crystallises in four-sided, orthorhombic prisms, and is soluble in about 50 parts of cold water.

The **Nitrate** ($C_{21}H_{22}N_2O_2,HNO_3$) crystallises on evaporation from a warm solution of the alkaloid in dilute nitric acid, in silky needles, mostly collected in groups. The solubility of this salt is considerable, one part dissolving in 50 of cold, in 2 of boiling water; its solubility in boiling and cold alcohol is almost the same, taking 60 of the former and 2 of the latter.

The **Acetate** crystallises in tufts of needles; as stated, it is not officinal in any of the European pharmacopœias.

The chief precipitates or sparingly soluble crystalline compounds of strychnine are—

(1.) **The Chromate of Strychnine** ($C_{21}H_{22}N_2O_2CrHO_2$), formed by adding a neutral solution of chromate of potash to a solution of a strychnine salt, crystallises out of hot water in beautiful, very insoluble, orange-yellow needles, mixed with plates of various size and thickness. The salt is of great practical use to the analyst; for by its aid strychnine may be separated from a variety of substances, and in part from brucine—the colour tests being either applied direct to the strychnine chromate, or the chromate decomposed by ammonia, and the strychnine recovered from the alkaline liquid by chloroform.

(2.) **Sulphocyanide of Strychnine** ($C_{21}H_{22}N_2O_2CNHS$) is a thick, white precipitate, produced by the addition of a solution of potassic sulphocyanide to that of a strychnine salt; on warming it dissolves, but on cooling reappears in the form of long silky needles.

(3.) **Double Salts.**—The platinum compound obtained by adding a solution of platinic chloride to one of strychnine chloride has the composition $C_{21}H_{22}N_2O_2HClPtCl_2$, and crystallises out of weak boiling alcohol (in which it is somewhat soluble) in gold-like scales. The similar palladium compound ($C_{21}H_{22}N_2O_2HCl,PdCl$) is in dark brown needles, and the gold compound ($C_{21}H_{22}N_2O_2HClAuCl_3$) in orange-coloured needles.

(4.) **Strychnine Trichloride.**—The action of chlorine on strychnine—by which chlorine is substituted for a portion of the hydrogen—has been proposed as a test. The alkaloid is dissolved in very dilute HCl, so as to be only just acid; on now passing through chlorine gas, a white insoluble precipitate is formed, which may be recrystallised from ether; it has probably the composition $C_{21}H_{19}Cl_3N_2O_2$, and is extremely insoluble in water.

(5.) **The Iodide of Strychnine** ($C_{21}H_{22}N_2O_2HI_3$) is obtained by the action of iodine solution on strychnine sulphate; on solution of the precipitate in alcohol, and evaporation, it forms violet-coloured crystals, very similar to those of potassic permanganate.

§ 388. **Pharmaceutical and other Preparations of Nux Vomica and Strychnine, with Suggestions for their Valuation.**

An aqueous extract of nux vomica, officinal in the German pharmacopœia, appears to contain principally brucine, with a small percentage of strychnine; the proportion of brucine to strychnine being about four-fifths to one-fifth. Blossfield found in a sample 4.3 per cent. of total alkaloid, and two samples examined by Grundmann consisted (No. 1) of strychnine, 0.6 per cent.; brucine, 2.58 per cent.—total, 3.18 per cent.; (No. 2) strychnine, 0.68 per cent.; brucine, 2.62 per cent.—total, 3.3 per cent. A sample examined by Dragendorff yielded—strychnine, 0.8 per cent.; brucine, 3.2 per cent.—total, 4 per cent. The maximum medicinal dose is put at .6 grm. ($9\frac{1}{14}$ grains).

The spirituous extract of nux vomica, officinal in the British and all the Continental pharmacopœias, differs from the aqueous in containing a much larger proportion of alkaloids, viz., about 15 per cent., and about half the total quantity being strychnine. The medicinal dose is 21.6-64.8 mgrms. ($\frac{1}{3}$ grain to a grain).

There is also an **extract of St. Ignatius bean** which is used in the United States; nearly the whole of its alkaloid may be referred to strychnine.

The tincture of nux vomica, made according to the British Pharmacopœia, contains in 1 fl. oz. 1 grain of alkaloids, or 0.21 part by weight in 100 by volume, but the strength of commercial samples often varies. Lieth found in one sample 0.122 per cent. of strychnine and 0.09 per cent. brucine; and two samples examined by Wissel consisted respectively of 0.353 per cent. and 0.346 per cent. of total alkaloids. Dragendorff found in two samples .2624 per cent. and .244 per cent. of total alkaloids, about half of which was strychnine.

Analysis.—Either of the extracts may be treated for a few hours on the water-bath, with water acidulated by sulphuric acid, filtered, the residue well washed, the acid liquid shaken up with benzene to separate impurities, and, on removal of the benzene, alkalised with ammonia, and shaken up two or three times with chloroform; the chloroform is then evaporated in a tared vessel, and the total alkaloids weighed. The alkaloids can then be either (*a*) treated with 11 per cent. of nitric acid on the water-bath until all the brucine is destroyed, and then (the liquid being neutralised) precipitated by potassic chromate; or (*b*) the alkaloids may be converted into picrates. Picrate of strychnine is very insoluble in water, 1 part requiring no less than 10,000 of water.[423] The tincture is analysed on precisely similar principles, the spirit being got rid of by distillation, and the residue treated by acidified water, &c.

The nux vomica powder itself may be valued as follows:—15 to 20 grms., pulverised as finely as possible, are treated three times with 150 to 300 c.c. of water, acidified with sulphuric acid, well boiled, and, after each boiling, filtered and thoroughly pressed. The last exhaustion must be destitute of all bitter taste. The united filtrates are then evaporated to the consistence of a thick syrup, which is treated with sufficient burnt magnesia to neutralise the acid. The extract is now thoroughly exhausted with boiling alcohol of 90 per cent.; the alcoholic extract, in its turn, is evaporated nearly to dryness, and treated with acidulated water; this acid solution is freed from impurities by shaking up with benzene, and lastly alkalised with ammonia, and the alkaloids extracted by shaking up with successive portions of chloroform. The chloroformic extract equals the total alkaloids, which may be separated in the usual way.

In four samples of nux vomica examined by Dragendorff, the total alkaloids ranged from 2.33 to 2.42 per cent. Grate found in two samples 2.88 per cent. and 2.86 per cent. respectively; while Karing from one sample separated only 1.65 per cent. The strychnine and brucine are in about equal proportions, Dragendorff[424] finding 1.187 per cent. strychnine and 1.145 per cent. brucine.[425]

---

[423] Dolzler, *Arch. Pharm.* [3], xxiv. 105-109.

[424] Dragendorff, *Die chemische Werthbestimmung einiger starkwirkenden Droguen*, St. Petersburg, 1874.

[425] These details are very necessary, as bearing on the question of the fatal dose of nux vomica, which Taylor tells us (*Med. Jurisprud.*, i. 409) was of some importance in *Reg.* v. *Wren*, in which 47 grains were attempted to be given in milk. The fatal dose of nux vomica must be ruled by its alkaloidal content, which may be so low as 1 per cent., and as high as nearly 3 per cent.

The **vermin-killers** in use in this country are those of Miller, Battle, Butler, Clift, Craven, Floyd, Gibson, Hunter, Stenier, and Thurston. Ten samples from these various makers were examined recently by Mr. Allen (*Pharm. Journal*, vol. xii., 1889), and the results of the analyses are embodied in the following table:—

Name or Mark.	Weight of Powder in Grains.	Price.	Strychnine. Weight in Grains.	Strychnine. Per-centage.	Nature of Starch.	Colouring Matter.
1	5.6	3*d.*	0.61	10.9	Wheat	?
2	11.8	3*d.*	0.80	6.7	Wheat	Ultramarine.
3	13.1	3*d.*	1.12	8.7	Rice	Ultramarine.
4	11.6	3*d.*	1.28	11.1	Rice	Ultramarine.
5	13.1	3*d.*	1.70	13.0	Rice	Ultramarine.
6	21.5	6*d.*	2.42	11.2	Wheat	Prussian blue.
7	49.2	3*d.*	2.85	5.8	Wheat	Soot.
8	30.5	3*d.*	3.45	11.3	Wheat	Prussian blue.
9	16.6	3*d.*	3.81	19.4	Rice	Carmine.
10	10.0	3*d.*	4.18	41.8	Rice	Ultramarine.

§ 389. **Statistics.**—In England, during the ten years 1883-92, out of 6666 total deaths from poison, strychnine, nux vomica, and vermin-killer account for 325. Out of these deaths, 118 were ascribed to "vermin-killer." "Vermin-killer" may be presumed to include not only strychnine mixtures, but also phosphorus and arsenic pastes and powders, so that there are no means of ascertaining the number of strychnine cases comprised under this heading. Taking the deaths actually registered as due to strychnine or nux vomica, they are about 4.7 per cent. of the deaths from all sorts of poison. Of these deaths, 268, or 82.4 per cent., were suicidal, 8 were homicidal, and 49 only were accidental.

Schauenstein has collected from literature 130 cases of poisoning by strychnine, but most of these occurred during the last twenty-five years; 62 of the 130, or about one-half, were fatal, and 15 were homicidal. It has been stated that strychnine is so very unsuitable for the purpose of criminal poisoning as to render it unlikely to be often used. Facts, however, do not bear out this view; for, allowing its intensely bitter taste, yet it must be remembered that bitter liquids, such as bitter ale, are in daily use, and a person accustomed to drink any liquid rapidly might readily imbibe sufficient of a toxic liquid to produce death before he was warned by its bitterness. It is, indeed, capable of demonstration, that taste is more vivid *after* a substance has been taken than just in the act of swallowing, for the function of taste is not a rapid process, and requires a very appreciable interval of time.

The series of murders by Thomas Neill, or, more correctly, Thomas Neill Cream, is an example of the use of strychnine for the purposes of murder. Thomas Neill Cream was convicted, October 21, 1892, for the murder of Matilda Clover on October 20, 1891; there was also good evidence that the same criminal had murdered Ellen Dunworth, October 13, 1891; Alice Marsh, April 12, 1892; Emma Shrivell, April 12, 1892, and had attempted the life of Louie Harvey. The agent in all these cases was strychnine. There was no evidence as to what form of the poison was administered in the case of Clover, but Ellen Dunworth, who was found dying in the streets at 7.45 P.M., and died less than two hours afterwards, stated that a gentleman gave her "two drops" of white stuff to drink.

In the cases of Marsh and Shrivell, Neill Cream had tea with them on the night of April 11, and gave them both "three long pills;" half an hour after Neill Cream left them they were found to be dying, and died within six hours. From Marsh 7 grains, from Shrivell nearly 2 grains of strychnine were separated; the probability is that each pill contained at least 3 grains of strychnine. The criminal met Louie Harvey on the Embankment, and gave her "some pills" to take; she pretended to do so, but threw them away. Hence it seems probable that Neill Cream took advantage of the weakness that a large number of the population have for taking pills, and mostly poisoned his victims in this manner. Clover's case was not diagnosed during life, but strychnine was found six or seven months after burial in

30 grains have proved fatal (*Taylor*); if the powder in this instance was of the ordinary strength, the person died from less than a grain (.0648 grm.) of the united alkaloids.

the body. It may be mentioned incidentally that the accused himself furnished the clue which led to his arrest, by writing letters charging certain members of the medical profession with poisoning these poor young prostitutes with strychnine.

§ 390. **Fatal Dose.**—In a research, which may, from its painstaking accuracy, be called classical, F. A. Falck has thrown much light upon the minimum lethal dose of strychnine for various animals. It would seem that, in relation to its size, the frog is by no means so sensible to strychnine as was believed, and that animals such as cats and rabbits take a smaller dose in proportion to their body-weight. The method used by Falck was to inject subcutaneously a solution of known strength of strychnine nitrate, and, beginning at first with a known lethal dose, a second experiment was then made with a smaller dose, and if that proved fatal, with a still smaller, and so on, until such a quantity was arrived at, that the chances as determined by direct observation were as great of recovery as of death. Operating in this way, and making no less than 20 experiments on the rabbit, he found that the least fatal dose for that animal was .6 mgrm. of strychnine nitrate per kilogramme. Cats were a little less susceptible, taking .75 mgrm. Operating on fowls, he found that strychnine taken into the crop in the usual way was very uncertain; 50 mgrms. per kilo, taken with the food had no effect, but results always followed if the poison was introduced into the circulation by the subcutaneous needle—the lethal dose for fowls being, under those circumstances, 1 to 2 mgrms. per kilo. He made 35 experiments on frogs, and found that to kill a frog by strychnine nitrate, at least 2 mgrms. per kilo, must be injected. Mice take a little more, from 2.3 to 2.4 mgrms. per kilo. In 2 experiments on the ring adder, in one 62.5 mgrms. per kilo. of strychnine nitrate, injected subcutaneously, caused death in seven hours; in the second, 23.1 mgrms. per kilo. caused death in five days; hence the last quantity is probably about the least fatal dose for this particular snake.

These observations may be conveniently thrown into the following table, placing the animals in order according to their relative sensitiveness.[426]

Now, the important question arises, as to the place in this series occupied by man—a question difficult to solve, because so few cases are recorded in which strychnine has been administered by subcutaneous injection with fatal result. Eulenberg has observed poisonous symptoms, but not death, produced by 6 mgrms. (1/11 grain) and by 10 mgrms. (about 1/6 grain). Bois observed poisonous symptoms from the similar subcutaneous administrations of 8 mgrms. to a child six years old, and 4 mgrms. to another child four years old—the latter dose, in a case recorded by Christison, actually killing a child of three years of age. On the other hand, the smallest lethal dose taken by an adult was swallowed in solution. Dr. Warner took 32 mgrms. (1/2 grain) of strychnine sulphate, mistaking it for morphine sulphate, and died in twenty minutes. In other cases 48 mgrms. (7/10 grain) have been fatal. It will be safe to conclude that these doses by the stomach would have acted still more surely and energetically if injected subcutaneously. The case of Warner is exceptional, for he was in weak health; and, if calculated out according to body-weight, presuming that Dr. Warner weighed 68 kilos., the relative dose as strychnine nitrate would be .24 per kilo.—a smaller dose than for any animal hitherto experimented upon. There is, however, far more reason for believing that the degree of sensitiveness in man is about the same as that of cats or dogs, and that the least fatal dose for man is .70 per kilo., the facts on record fairly bearing out this view. It is, therefore, probable that death would follow if 38 mgrms. (7/10 grain) were injected subcutaneously into a man of the average weight of 68 kilos. (150 lbs.). Taylor estimates the fatal dose of strychnine for adults as from 32.4 to 129.6 mgrms. (.5 to 2 grains); Guy puts the minimum at 16.2 mgrms. (.25 grain).

TABLE SHOWING THE ACTION OF STRYCHNINE ON ANIMALS.

Animal.	Manner of Application.	Reckoned on 1 Kilo. of Body-weight.	
		Lowest Experimental Lethal Dose.	Highest Experimental Lethal Dose.

[426] According to Christison's researches, 0.2 grm. (about 1/3 grain) is fatal to swine; .03 grm. (1/2 grain) to bears, if injected into the pleura. 1 to 3 grains (.0648 to .1944 grm.) is given to horses in cases of paralysis, although 3 grains cannot but be considered a dangerous dose, unless smaller doses have been previously administered without effect; 10 grains would probably kill a horse, and 15 grains (.972 grm.) have certainly done so.

		Dose of Strychnine Nitrate in Mgrms.	
Rabbit,	Subcutaneous.	0 .50	0 .60
Cat,	„	...	0 .75
Dog,	„	...	0 .75
„	Taken by the Stomach.	2 .0	3 .90
„	„Rectum.	...	2 .00
„	„Bladder.	5 .50	...
Fox,	Subcutaneous.	...	1 .00
Hedgehog,	„	1 .00	2 .00
Fowl,	„	...	2 .00
Frog,	„	2 .00	2 .10
Mouse,	„	2 .36	2 .36
Ring Adder,	„	...	23 .10

Large doses of strychnine may be recovered from if correct medical treatment is sufficiently prompt. Witness the remarkable instances on record of duplex poisonings, in which the would-be-suicide has unwittingly defeated his object by taking strychnine simultaneously with some narcotic, such as opium or chloral. In a case related by Schauenstein,[427] a suicidal pharmacist took .48 grm. or .6 grm. (7.4 to 9.25 grains) of strychnine nitrate dissolved in about 30 c.c. of bitter-almond water, and then, after half an hour, since no symptoms were experienced, .6 grm. (9.25 grains) of morphine acetate, which he likewise dissolved in bitter-almond water and swallowed. After about ten minutes, he still could walk with uncertain steps, and poured some chloroform on the pillow-case of his bed, and lay on his face in order to breathe it. In a short time he lost consciousness, but again awoke, and lay in a half-dreamy state, incapable of motion, until some one entered the room, and hearing him murmur, came to his bedside. At that moment—two and a quarter hours after first taking the strychnine—the pharmacist had a fearful convulsion, the breathing was suspended, and he lost consciousness. Again coming to himself, he had several convulsions, and a physician who was summoned found him in general tetanus. There were first clonic, then tonic convulsions, and finally opisthotonus was fully developed. The treatment consisted of emetics, and afterwards tannin and codeine were given separately. The patient slept at short intervals; in ten hours after the taking of the poison the seizures were fewer in number and weaker in character, and by the third day recovery was complete. Dr. Macredy[428] has also placed on record an interesting case, in which the symptoms, from a not very large dose of strychnine, were delayed by laudanum for eight hours. A young woman, twenty-three years of age, pregnant, took at 10 A.M. a quantity of strychnine estimated at 1.5 grain, in the form of Battle's vermin-killer, and immediately afterwards 2 ounces of laudanum. She was seen by Dr. Macredy in four hours, and was then suffering from pronounced narcotic symptoms. A sulphate of zinc emetic was administered. In eight hours after taking the strychnine, there were first observed some clonic convulsive movements of the hands, and, in a less degree, the legs. These convulsions continued, at times severe, for several hours, and were treated with chloral. Recovery was speedy and complete.

In a similar case related by Dr. Harrison,[429] a man, aged 54, took a packet of Battle's vermin-killer, mixed with about a drachm and a half of laudanum and some rum. At the time he had eaten no food for days, and had been drinking freely; yet fifty minutes elapsed before the usual symptoms set in, and no medical treatment was obtained until four hours after taking the dose. He was then given chloral and other remedies, and made a rapid recovery.

§ 391. **Action on Animals.**—The action of strychnine has been experimentally studied on all classes of animals, from the infusoria upwards. The effects produced on animal forms which possess a nervous system are strikingly alike, and even in the cephalopoda, tetanic muscular spasm may be readily observed. Of all animals the frog shows the action of strychnine in its purest form, especially if a dose be given of just sufficient magnitude to produce toxic effects. The frog sits perfectly still and quiet, unless acted upon by some external stimuli, such as a breath of air, a

[427] Maschka's *Handbuch*, from Tschepke, *Deutsche Klinik*, 1861.
[428] *Lancet*, November 28, 1882.
[429] *Lancet*, May 13, 1882.

loud noise, or the shaking of the vessel which contains it, then an immediate tetanic convulsion of all the muscles is witnessed, lasting a few seconds only, when the animal again resumes its former posture. This heightened state of reflex action has its analogue in hydrophobia as well as in idiopathic tetanus. If the frog thus poisoned by a weak dose is put under a glass shade, kept moist, and sheltered from sound, or from other sources of irritation, no convulsions occur, and after some days it is in its usual health. If, on the other hand, by frequent stimuli, convulsions are excited, the animal dies. M. Richet[430] has contributed a valuable memoir to the Academy of Sciences on the toxic action of strychnine. He has confirmed the statement of previous observers that, with artificial respiration, much larger doses of strychnine may be taken without fatal result than under normal conditions, and has also recorded some peculiar phenomena. Operating on dogs and rabbits, after first securing a canula in the trachea, and then injecting beneath the skin or into the saphena vein 10 mgrms. of strychnine hydrochlorate, the animal is immediately, or within a few seconds, seized with tetanic convulsions, and this attack would be mortal, were it not for artificial respiration. Directly this is practised the attack ceases, and the heart, after a period of hurried and spasmodic beats, takes again its regular rhythm. Stronger and stronger doses may then be injected without causing death. As the dose is thus augmented, the symptoms differ. M. Richet distinguishes the following periods:—(1.) A period of tetanus. (2.) A period of convulsion, characterised by spasmodic and incessant contraction of all the muscles. (3.) A little later, when the quantity exceeds 10 mgrms. per kilo., a choreic period, which is characterised by violent rhythmic shocks, very sudden and short, repeated at intervals of about three to four seconds; during these intervals there is almost complete relaxation. (4.) A period of relaxation; this period is attained when the dose exceeds 40 mgrms. per kilo. Reflex action is annihilated, the spontaneous respiratory movements cease, the heart beats tumultuously and regularly in the severe tetanic convulsions at first, and then contracts with frequency but with regularity. The pupils, widely dilated at first, become much contracted. The arterial pressure, enormously raised at the commencement, diminishes gradually, in one case from 0.34 mm. to 0.05 mm. The temperature undergoes analogous changes, and during the convulsions is extraordinarily elevated; it may even attain 41° or 42°, to sink in the period of relaxation to 36°. Dogs and rabbits which have thus received enormous quantities of strychnine (*e.g.*, 50 mgrms. per kilo.), may, in this way, live for several hours, but the slightest interruption to the artificial respiration, in the relaxed state, is followed by syncope and death.

§ 392. **Effects on Man: Symptoms.**—The commencement of symptoms may be extremely rapid, the rapidity being mainly dependent on the form of the poison and the manner of application. A soluble salt of strychnine injected subcutaneously will act within a few seconds;[431] in a case of amaurosis, related by Schuler,[432] 5.4 mgrms. of a soluble strychnine salt were introduced into the punctum lachrymale;—in less than four minutes there were violent tetanic convulsions. In a case related by Barker, the symptoms commenced in three minutes from a dose of .37 grm. (5.71 grains).[433] Here the poison was not administered subcutaneously. Such short periods, to a witness whose mind

[430] *De l'Action de la Strychnine à très forte dose sur les Mammifères. Comptes Rend.*, t. xcl. p. 131.

[431] In one of M. Richet's experiments, a soluble strychnine salt injected into a dog subcutaneously acted in fourteen seconds.

[432] Quoted by Taylor from *Med. Times and Gazette*, July, 1861.

[433] A non-fatal dose may show its effects rapidly, *e.g.*, there is a curious case of symptoms of poisoning caused by the *last* dose of a mixture which is recorded in *Pharm. Journ.*, 1893, 799. A medical practitioner prescribed the following mixture:—

℞.	Tr. strophanthi,		ʒi.
	Liq. strychni hydrochlorici,		ʒiiss.
	Sol. bismuthi et pepsin. (Richardson's),		℥iss.
	Sp. ammon. aromat.,		...
	Sp. chloroformi,	aa.	℥iss.
	Aquam ad,		℥vi.
	ft. mist.		

Shake the bottle.

Two teaspoonfuls when the attack threatens, and repeat in an hour if necessary.

Richardson's liquor bismuth contains ⅟₂₀ grain of strychnine in each drachm. The mixture was alkaline; it contained 1.7 grain of strychnine and 38.25 minims of chloroform.

The patient, a woman, 54 years of age, had taken the previous doses with considerable relief; but ten minutes after the last dose, which she described as far more bitter than those she had taken previously, she was seized with the usual symptoms of strychnine poisoning, but recovered after five hours.

The explanation is pretty obvious; the mixture was alkaline, so that the strychnine was not in the form of a salt, but in the

was occupied during the time, might seem immediate. On the other hand, when nux vomica powder has been taken, and when strychnine has been given in the form of pill, no such rapid course has been observed, or is likely to occur, the usual course being for the symptoms to commence within half an hour. It is, however, also possible for them to be delayed from one to two hours, and under certain circumstances (as in the case related by Macredy) for eight hours. In a few cases, there is first a feeling of uneasiness and heightened sensibility to external stimuli, a strange feeling in the muscles of the jaw, and a catching of the respiration; but generally the onset of the symptoms is as sudden as epilepsy, and previous to their appearance the person may be pursuing his ordinary vocation, when, without preliminary warning, there is a shuddering of the whole frame, and a convulsive seizure. The convulsions take the form of violent general tetanus; the limbs are stretched out involuntarily, the hands are clenched, the soles of the feet incurved, and, in the height of the paroxysm, the back may be arched and rigid as a board, the sufferer resting on head and heels, and the abdomen tense. In the grasp of the thoracic muscles the walls of the chest are set immovable, and from the impending suffocation the face becomes congested, the eyes prominent and staring. The muscles of the lower jaw—in "disease tetanus" the first to be affected—are in "strychnos tetanus," as a rule, the last; a distinction, if it were more constant, of great clinical value. The convulsions and remissions recur until death or recovery, and, as a rule, within two hours from the commencement of the symptoms the case in some way or other terminates. The number of the tetanic seizures noted has varied—in a few cases the third spasm has passed into death, in others there have been a great number. The duration of the spasm is also very different, and varies from thirty seconds to five or even eight minutes, the interval between lasting from forty-five seconds[434] to one or even one and a half hours.[435]

§ 393. **Diagnosis of Strychnine Poisoning.**—However striking and well defined the picture of strychnine tetanus may be, mistakes in diagnosis are rather frequent, especially when a medical man is hastily summoned, has never seen a case of similar poisoning, and has no suspicion of the possible nature of the seizure. If a young woman, for instance, is the subject, he may put it down to hysteria, and certainly hysteria not unfrequently affects somewhat similar convulsions. In a painful case in which the author was engaged, a young woman either took or was given (for the mystery was never cleared up fully) a fatal dose of strychnine, and though the symptoms were well marked, the medical attendant was so possessed with the view that the case was due to hysteria, that, even after making the *post-mortem* examination, and finding no adequate lesion, he theorised as to the possibility of some fatal hysteric spasm of the glottis, while there was ample chemical evidence of strychnine, and a weighable quantity of the alkaloid was actually separated from the contents of the stomach. The medical attendant of Matilda Clover, one of Neill's victims, certified that the girl died from *delirium tremens* and syncope, although the symptoms were typically those produced by strychnine. Such cases are particularly sad, for we now know that, with judicious treatment, a rather large dose may be recovered from.

If the case is a male, a confusion with epilepsy is possible, though hardly to be explained or excused; while in both sexes idiopathic tetanus is so extremely similar as to give rise to the idea that all cases of idiopathic tetanus are produced by poison, perhaps secreted by the body itself. As for the distinction between idiopathic and strychnic tetanus, it is usually laid down (1) that the intervals in the former are characterised by no relaxation of the muscles, but that they continue contracted and hard; and (2) that there is a notable rise of temperature in disease tetanus proper, and not in strychnine tetanus. Both statements are misleading, and the latter is not true, for in strychnic poisoning the relaxation is not constant, and very high temperatures in animals have been observed.

§ 394. **Physiological Action.**—The tetanic convulsions are essentially reflex, and to be ascribed to a central origin; the normal reflex sensibility is exaggerated and unnaturally extended. If the ischiatic plexus supplying the one leg of an animal is cut through, that leg takes no part in the general convulsions, but if the artery of the leg alone is tied, then the leg suffers from the muscular spasm, as well as the limbs in which the circulation is unrestrained. In an experiment by Sir B. W. Richardson, a healthy dog was killed, and, as soon as practicable, a solution of strychnine was injected through the systemic vessels by the aorta—the whole body became at once stiff and rigid as a board. These facts point unmistakably to the spinal marrow as the seat of the toxic influence. Strychnine is, *par*

---

free state, and was therefore dissolved by the chloroform; the amount of strychnine taken in each dose wholly depended on whether or not the mixture was shaken violently and poured out into the teaspoon immediately after shaking; if allowed to repose the globules of chloroform saturated with strychnine would settle at the bottom, and there form a stratum rich in strychnine; so that the last dose would certainly contain an excess.

[434] White, *Brit. Med. Journ.*, 1867.

[435] Folkes, *Med. Times*, 1869.

excellence, a spinal poison. On physiological grounds the grey substance of the cord is considered to have an inhibitory action upon reflex sensibility, and this inhibitory power is paralysed by strychnine. The spinal cord, it would appear, has the power of collecting strychnine from the circulation and storing it up in its structure.[436]

Much light has been thrown upon the cause of death by Richet's experiments.[437] It would seem that, in some cases, death takes place by a suffocation as complete as in drowning, the chest and diaphragm being immovable, and the nervous respiratory centres exhausted. In such a case, immediate death would be averted by a tracheal tube, by the aid of which artificial respiration might be carried on; but there is another asphyxia due to the enormous interstitial combustion carried on by muscles violently tetanised. "If," says Richet, "after having injected into a dog a mortal dose of strychnine, and employed artificial respiration according to the classic method twenty or thirty times a minute, the animal dies (sometimes at the end of ten minutes, and in every case at the end of an hour or two), and during life the arterial blood is examined, it will be ascertained that it is black, absolutely like venous blood."

This view is also supported by the considerable rise of temperature noticed: the blood is excessively poor in oxygen, and loaded with carbon dioxide. That this state of the blood is produced by tetanus, is proved by the fact that an animal poisoned by strychnine, and then injected subcutaneously with curare in quantity just sufficient to paralyse the muscular system, does not exhibit these phenomena. By the aid of artificial respiration, together with the administration of curare, an animal may live after a prodigious dose of strychnine.

Meyer[438] has investigated carefully the action of strychnine on the blood-pressure—through a strong excitement of the vaso-motor centre, the arteries are narrowed in calibre, and the blood-pressure much increased; the action of the heart in frogs is slowed, but in the warm-blooded animals quickened.

§ 395. **Post-mortem Appearances.**—There is but little characteristic in the *post-mortem* appearances from strychnine poisoning. The body becomes very stiff a short time after death, and this rigidity remains generally a long time. In the notorious Palmer case, the body was rigid two months after death, but, on the other hand, the *rigor mortis* has been known to disappear within twenty-four hours. If the convulsions have been violent, there may be minute hæmorrhages in the brain and other parts. I have seen considerable hæmorrhage in the trachea from this cause. When death occurs from asphyxia, the ordinary signs of asphyxia will be found in the lungs, &c. The heart mostly has its right side gorged with blood, but in a few cases it is empty and contracted.

In a case which Schauenstein has recorded[439] he found strychnine still undissolved, coating the stomach as a white powder; but this is very unusual, and I believe unique. The bladder often contains urine, which, it need scarcely be said, should be preserved for chemical investigation.

§ 396. **Treatment.**—From the cases detailed, and from the experiments on animals, the direction which treatment should take is very clear. As a matter of course, if there is the slightest probability of any of the poison remaining in the stomach, it should be removed. It is doubtful whether the stomach pump can be ever applied with benefit in strychnine poisoning, the introduction of the tube is likely to aggravate the tetanus, but apomorphine can be injected subcutaneously. Large and frequent doses of chloral should be administered in order to lessen the frequency of convulsions, or prevent their occurrence, and it may be necessary in a few cases, where death threatens by suffocation, to perform tracheotomy, and to use artificial respiration. Where chloral or chloroform is not at hand, and in cases of emergency, where this may easily happen, the medical man must administer in full doses the nearest narcotic at hand.[440]

§ 397. **Separation of Strychnine from Organic Matters.**—The separation of strychnine from organic matters, &c., is undertaken strictly on the general principles already detailed. It may happen, however, that in cases of poisoning there is the strongest evidence from symptoms in the person or animal that strychnine alone is to be sought for. In an instance of the kind, if a complex organic liquid (such as the contents of the stomach) is under examination, it is best to remove the solid substances by filtration through glass, wool, or linen, and evaporate nearly to dryness over the water-bath, acidifying with acetic acid, and then exhausting the residue repeatedly with boiling

[436] R. W. Lovett, *Journ. Physiol.*, ix. 99-111.

[437] *Op. cit.*

[438] *Wiener Akad. Sitzungsber.*, 1871.

[439] *Op. cit.*

[440] It is certain that lutidine would be a valuable antidote for strychnine. C. G. Williams found that lutidine injected into frogs already under the influence of strychnine, arrested the convulsions, or if given first, and then followed by a fatal dose of strychnine, it prevented the appearance of the tetanus. (See *ante*, footnote.)

alcohol of 80 per cent. The alcoholic extract is in its turn evaporated to dryness, and taken up with water; the aqueous solution is passed through a wet filter, and then shaken up with the usual succession of fluids, viz., petroleum ether, benzene, chloroform, and amyl alcohol, which will remove a great number of impurities, but will not dissolve the strychnine from the acid solution. The amyl alcohol may lastly be removed by petroleum ether; and on removal of the final extractive (which should be done as thoroughly as possible) chloroform is added, and the fluid is alkalised by ammonia, which precipitates the alkaloid in the presence of the solvent. Should the reverse process be employed—that is, ammonia added first, and then chloroform—the strychnine is not so perfectly dissolved, since it has time to assume a crystalline condition. On separation and evaporation of the chloroform, the residue (if much discoloured, or evidently impure) may be dissolved in alcohol or benzene, and recrystallised several times. Cushman has published an improved method of separating strychnine, which, according to test experiments, appears to give good results. He describes the method as follows:[441]—

"The stomach contents or viscera properly comminuted are weighed, and an aliquot part taken for analysis. The mass is digested in a beaker over night, at a warm temperature, with water acidulated with acetic acid. The contents of the beaker are filtered by pressing through muslin, and then passing through paper. The clear filtrate is evaporated on the water-bath to soft dryness, an excess of ordinary 80 per cent. alcohol added, and boiled ten minutes with stirring, and allowed to stand one half hour at a warm temperature. This extraction is repeated, the alcohol extracts united, filtered, evaporated to soft dryness, and the residue taken up with a little water acidulated with acetic acid, and shaken out with pure acetic ether in a separating funnel. Successive fresh portions of acetic ether are used until the solvent shows by its colour, and by the evaporation of a few drops, that it does not contain extractive matter. As many as twelve extractions are sometimes necessary to accomplish this. Care should be taken in each case to allow time for as complete separation as possible between the two layers. The purified acid aqueous liquid, which need not exceed in bulk 50 c.c., is now returned to the separator, an equal quantity of fresh acetic ether added, and enough sodic carbonate in solution to render the mixture slightly alkaline, and the separator is then thoroughly shaken for several minutes. All the alkaloid should now be in solution in the acetic ether, but a second shaking of the alkaline liquid, with acetic ether, is always made, the two extracts united, and evaporated in a glass dish over hot water to dryness. It will now be found that the residue shows the alkaloid fairly pure, but not pure enough for quantitative results. The residue is dissolved in a few drops of dilute acetic acid, warmed to complete solution, filtered if necessary, diluted to about 30 c.c., and the solution transferred to a small separating funnel; 30 c.c. of ether-chloroform (1-1) are now added, and the separator shaken. After separation the heavier ether-chloroform is allowed to run off, another lot of 30 c.c. of ether-chloroform is added, the separator shaken, and immediately enough ammonia-water added to render the mixture alkaline, and the whole vigorously agitated for several minutes. After separation is complete, the ether-chloroform layer is run out into a clean 50 c.c. glass-stoppered burette. The alkaline water solution is agitated with 20 c.c. more of the ether-chloroform, separated, and this extract added to that in the burette. The burette is now supported over a small weighed glass dish, which is kept warm on a water-bath, and the liquid allowed to evaporate gently, drop by drop, until a sufficient quantity of the pure alkaloid has collected in the centre of the dish to render an accurate weighing possible, or else all of the alkaloid may be collected and weighed at once. After all possible tests have been made upon the weighed alkaloid, the remainder is re-dissolved in a drop or two of acetic acid, a little water added, and the dish exposed under a bell-glass to the fumes of ammonia. After standing some time all the strychnine is found crystallised out in the beautiful characteristic needle-formed crystals. The mother-liquor is drawn off with a small fine-pointed tube and rubber bulb, the crystals carefully washed with a little water and dried over sulphuric acid. The glass dish containing these crystals is kept as the final exhibit, and is shown in evidence. Another convenient exhibit may be prepared by moistening a small filter-paper with a solution of the alkaloid in dilute acetic acid, then moistening with a solution of potassium dichromate: this paper, on being dried, may be kept indefinitely. On moistening it, and touching it at any time with a drop of strong sulphuric acid, a violet film, changing to cherry-red, is formed at the place of contact."

Should search be made for minute portions of strychnine in the tissues, considering the small amount of the poison which may produce death, it is absolutely necessary to operate on a very large quantity of material. It would be advisable to take the whole of the liver, the brain, spinal cord, spleen, stomach, duodenum, kidneys, all the blood that can be obtained, and a considerable quantity of muscular tissue, so as to make in all about one-eighth to one-tenth of the whole body; this may be cut up into small pieces, and boiled in capacious flasks with alcohol, acidified with acetic acid. Evaporation must be controlled by adapting to the cork an upright condenser.

[441] "The *post-mortem* Detection and Estimation of Strychnine," by Allerton S. Cushman—*Chem. News*, vol. lxx. 28.

Should the analyst not have apparatus of a size to undertake this at one operation, it may be done in separate portions—the filtrate from any single operation being collected in a flask, and the spirit distilled off in order to be used for the next. In this way, a large quantity of the organs and tissues can be exhausted by half a gallon of alcohol. Finally, most of the alcohol is distilled off, and the remainder evaporated at a gentle heat in a capacious dish, the final extract being treated, evaporating to a syrup, and using Cushman's process (*ante*) as just described. It is only by working on this large scale that there is any probability of detecting absorbed strychnine in those cases where only one or two grains have destroyed life, and even then it is possible to miss the poison.

Strychnine is separated by the kidneys rapidly. In a suicidal case recorded by Schauenstein,[442] death took place in an hour and a half after taking strychnine, yet from 200 c.c. of the urine, Schauenstein was able to separate nitrate of strychnine in well-formed crystals. Dr. Kratter[443] has made some special researches on the times within which strychnine is excreted by the kidneys. In two patients, who were being treated by subcutaneous injection, half an hour after the injection of 7.5 mgrms. of strychnine nitrate the alkaloid was recognised in the urine. The strychnine treatment was continued for eight to ten days, and then stopped; two days after the cessation, strychnine was found in the urine, but none on the third day, and the inference drawn is that the elimination was complete within forty-eight hours.

Strychnine has been detected in the blood of dogs and cats in researches specially undertaken for that purpose, but sometimes a negative result has been obtained, without apparent cause. Dragendorff[444] gave dogs the largest possible dose of strychnine daily. On the first few days no strychnine was found in the urine, but later it was detected, especially if food was withheld. M'Adam was the first who detected the absorbed poison, recognising it in the muscles and urine of a poisoned horse, and also in the urine of a hound. Dragendorff has found it in traces in the kidneys, spleen, and pancreas; Gay, in different parts of the central nervous system, and in the saliva. So far as the evidence goes, the liver is the best organ to examine for strychnine; but all parts supplied with blood, and most secretions, may contain small quantities of the alkaloid. At one time it was believed that strychnine might be destroyed by putrefaction, but the question of the decomposition of the poison in putrid bodies may be said to be settled. So far as all evidence goes, strychnine is an extremely stable substance, and no amount of putrescence will destroy it. M'Adam found it in a horse a month after death, and in a duck eight weeks after; Nunneley in 15 animals forty-three days after death, when the bodies were much decomposed; Roger in a body after five weeks' interment; Richter in putrid tissues exposed for eleven years to decomposition in open vessels; and, lastly, W. A. Noyes[445] in an exhumed body after it had been buried 308 days.

It would appear from Ibsen's[446] experiments that strychnine gets dissolved in the fluids of the dead body—so that whether strychnine remains or not, greatly depends as to whether the fluids are retained or are allowed to soak away; it is, therefore, most important in exhumations to save as much of the fluid as possible.

§ 398. **Identification of the Alkaloid.**—A residue containing strychnine, or strychnine mixed with brucine, is identified—

(1.) By its alkaline reaction and its bitter taste. No substance can possibly be strychnine unless it tastes remarkably bitter.

(2.) By the extremely insoluble chromate of strychnine, already described.[447] A fluid containing 1 : 1000 of strychnine gives with chromate of potash (if allowed to stand over-night) a marked precipitate, dissimilar to all others, except those of lead and baryta chromates, neither of which can possibly occur if any of the processes described are followed.

(3.) If the chromate just described is treated on a porcelain plate with a drop of pure strong sulphuric acid, a deep rich blue colour, passing through purple into red, rapidly makes its appearance. This colour possesses an absorption spectrum (figured earlier). Dr. Guy, neglecting intermediate colours, aptly compares the succession—(1) to the rich blue of the Orleans plum; (2) to the darker purple of the mulberry; and (3) to the bright clear red of the

[442] Maschka's *Handbuch*, Band 2, p. 620.

[443] *Ibid.*

[444] In an animal rapidly killed by a subcutaneous injection of acetate of strychnine, no strychnine was detected either in the blood or liver.—*Dragendorff.*

[445] *Journ. Americ. Chem. Soc.*, xvi. 2.

[446] *Viertel. f. gericht. Med.*, Bd. viii.

[447] 1 grm. of strychnine gave 1.280 grms. of the chromate, = 78.1 per cent. of strychnine; 3 gave 3.811 of the chromate, = 78.77 per cent. of strychnine.—*Mohr.*

sweet orange. These characters—viz., alkalinity, bitterness, and the property of precipitation by potassic chromate in a definite crystalline form, the crystals giving the colours detailed—belong to no other substance known save strychnine, and for all purposes sufficiently identify the alkaloid. The same colour is obtained by mixing a drop of sulphuric acid with strychnine and a crystal, or speck, of any one of the following substances:—Ferridcyanide of potash, permanganate of potash, peroxide of lead, peroxide of manganese, and cerous hydroxide.

Potassic permanganate and sulphuric acid is the most delicate, and will detect 0.001 mgrm. of strychnine; cerous hydroxide is, on the other hand, most convenient, for cerous hydroxide is white; all the others have colours of their own. Cerous hydroxide is prepared strychnine; 3 gave 3.811 of the chromate, = 78.77 per cent. of strychnine.—*Mohr.* by dissolving cerium oxalate in dilute sulphuric acid and precipitating with ammonia, filtering and well washing the precipitate; and the latter may be used while moist, and responds well to $^1/_{100}$ mgrm. of strychnine.

The influence of mixtures on the colour reactions of strychnine have been studied by Flückiger, who states:—

"No strychnine reaction appears with sulphuric acid containing chromic acid (made by dissolving 0.02 grm. of pot. bichromate in 10 c.c. of water, and then adding 30 grms. strong sulphuric acid) when brucine and strychnine mixed in equal parts are submitted to the test; it succeeds, however, in this proportion with sulphuric acid containing potassium permanganate (.02 grm. pot. permanganate in 10 c.c. of water, and 30 grms. of strong sulphuric acid).

"If the brucine is only one-tenth of the mixture, the blue-violet colour is obtained. A large excess of atropine does not prevent or obscure the strychnine reaction. A solution of 1 milligrm. atropine sulphate evaporated to dryness, together with 5 c.c. of a solution of strychnine (1 : 100,000) has no influence on the reaction, neither in the proportion of 1 mgrm. to 1 c.c. of the same solution; neither has cinchonine nor quinine any effect.

"Morphine obscures the reaction in the following proportions:—

"A solution of 0.01 mgrm. strychnine evaporated with a solution of 1 mgrm. of morphine sulphate on a water-bath, yields a blurred strychnine reaction when the residue is dissolved in sulphuric acid, and a crystal of potassic permanganate added. But still there is evidence whereby to *suspect* the presence of strychnine.

"A solution of 2 mgrms. of morphine sulphate treated in like manner with 0.01 mgrm. of strychnine yields like results.

"A solution of 3 mgrms. of morphine sulphate evaporated to dryness, with a solution of 0.01 mgrm. strychnine yielded results with the potassic permanganate test the same as if no strychnine was present.

"A solution of 1 mgrm. of morphine sulphate, treated as above, with a solution of 0.1 mgrm. strychnine, offered positive proof of the presence of the latter."[448]

Dragendorff was able to render evident .025 mgrm. mixed with twenty times its weight of quin. sulphate; the same observer likewise recognised .04 mgrm. of strychnine in thirty-three times its weight of caffeine. Veratrine is likewise not injurious.

The physiological test consists in administering the substance to some small animal (preferably to a frog), and inducing the ordinary tetanic symptoms. It may be at once observed that if definite chemical evidence of strychnine has been obtained, the physiological test is quite unnecessary; and, on the other hand, should the application of a liquid or substance to a frog induce tetanus, while chemical evidence of the presence of strychnine was wanting, it would be hazardous to assert that strychnine was present, seeing that caffeine, carbolic acid, picrotoxin, certain of the opium alkaloids, hypaphorine, some of the ptomaines, and many other substances induce similar symptoms. The best method (if the test is used at all) is to take two frogs,[449] and insert under the skin of the one the needle of a subcutaneous syringe, previously charged with a solution of the substance, injecting a moderate quantity. The other frog is treated similarly with a very dilute solution of strychnine, and the two are then placed under small glass shades, and the symptoms observed and compared. It is not absolutely necessary to inject the solution under the skin, for if applied to the surface the same effects are produced; but, if accustomed to manipulation, the operator will find the subcutaneous application more certain, especially in dealing with minute quantities of the alkaloid.[450]

§ 399. **Hypaphorine.**—One substance is known which neither physiological test nor the colour reactions

[448] Flückiger's *Reactions*, translated by Nagelvoort, Detroit, 1893.

[449] A very practical disadvantage of the physiological test is the great difficulty of obtaining frogs exactly when wanted.

[450] Methyl strychnine, as well as methyl brucine, has been shown by Brown and Fraser to have an effect exactly the opposite to that of strychnine, paralysing the muscles like curare. In the case, therefore, of the methyl compounds, a physiological test would be very valuable, since these compounds do not respond to the ordinary tests.

suffice to distinguish from strychnine, viz., hypaphorine,[451] the active matter of a papilionaceous tree growing in Java—the *Hypaphorus subumbrans*; a small quantity of the alkaloid is in the bark, a larger quantity is in the seed.

Hypaphorine forms colourless crystals which brown, without melting, above 220°, and exhale a vapour smelling like napththylamine. The free alkaloid is soluble in water, but has no action on litmus. The salts are less soluble than the free alkaloid, so that acids, such as nitric or hydrochloric, produce in a short time precipitates on standing. Solutions of the salts are not precipitated by alkalies; chloroform, ether, benzene, all fail to extract it from either alkaline or acid solutions. It gives no precipitate with potassic chromate, but most general alkaloidal reagents precipitate.

It gives a precipitate with iodine trichloride, and has therefore probably a pyridine nucleus, it may be an acid anilide.[452] It gives the same colours as strychnine with sulphuric acid and potassic permanganate or potassic chromate; it causes in frogs tetanus, but the dose has to be much larger than that of strychnine. The duration of life in doses of 15 mgrms. may extend to five days, and frogs may even recover after 50 mgrms.

The distinction between strychnine and hypaphorine is therefore easy; besides it will not occur in a chloroform extract, and it will not give a precipitate with potassic chromate.

§ 400. **Quantitative Estimation of Strychnine.**—The best process of estimating the proportion of each alkaloid in a mixture of strychnine and brucine, is to precipitate them as picrates, and to destroy the brucine picrate by nitric acid after obtaining the combined weight of the mixed picrates; then to weigh the undestroyed strychnine picrate.

To carry out the process, the solution of the mixed alkaloids must be as neutral as possible. A saturated solution of picric acid is added drop by drop to complete precipitation. A filter paper is dried and weighed, and the precipitate collected on to this filter paper; the precipitate is washed with cold water, dried at 105°, and weighed. This weight gives the combined weight of both strychnine and brucine picrates.

The precipitate is now detached from the filter, washed into a small flask, and heated on the water-bath for some time with nitric acid diluted to 1.056 gravity (about 11 per cent. HNO_3). This process destroys the brucine picrate, but leaves the strychnine picrate untouched. The acid liquid is now neutralised with ammonia or soda, and a trace of acetic acid added; the precipitate of strychnine picrate is now collected and weighed. The weight of this subtracted from the first weight, of course, gives that of the brucine picrate.

One part of strychnine picrate is equal to 0.5932 strychnine; and one part of brucine picrate is equal to 0.6324 brucine.

From the strychnine picrate the picric acid may be recovered and weighed by dissolving the picrate in a mineral acid and shaking out with ether; from the acid liquid thus deprived of picric acid the alkaloid may be separated by alkalising with ammonia and shaking out with chloroform.

§ 401. **Brucine** ($C_{23}H_{26}N_2O_4 + 4H_2O$)[453] occurs associated with strychnine in the plants already mentioned; its best source is the so-called *false angustura* bark, which contains but little strychnine. Its action is similar to that of strychnine. If crystallised out of dilute alcohol it contains 4 atoms of water, easily expelled either in a vacuum over sulphuric acid or by heat. Crystallised thus, it forms transparent four-sided prisms, or arborescent forms, like boric acid. If thrown down by ammonia from a solution of the acetate, it presents itself in needles or in tufts.

The recently-crystallised alkaloid has a solubility different from that which has effloresced, the former dissolving in 320 parts of cold, and 150 parts of boiling water; whilst the latter (according to Pelletier and Caventou) requires 500 of boiling, and 850 parts of cold water for solution. Brucine is easily soluble in absolute, as well as in ordinary alcohol; 1 part dissolves in 1.7 of chloroform, in 60.2 of benzene. Petroleum ether, the volatile and fatty oils and glycerine, dissolve the alkaloid slightly, amyl alcohol freely; it is insoluble in *anhydrous* ether. The behaviour of brucine in the subliming cell is described earlier. Anhydrous brucine melts in a tube at 178°. The alcoholic solution of brucine turns the plane of polarisation to the left $[\alpha]r = -11.27°$. The taste is bitter and acrid. Soubeiran maintains that it can be recognised if 1 part is dissolved in 500,000 parts of water. If nitric trioxide be passed into an alcoholic solution of brucine, first brucine nitrate is formed; but this passes again into solution, from which, after a time, a heavy, granular, blood-red precipitate separates: it consists of dinitro-brucine

[451] Dr. C. Plugge, *Arch. f. exp. Path. u. Ph.*, Bd. xxxii. 313.

[452] Julius Tafel (*Ber.*, 1890, 412) has shown that the colour reactions with H_2SO_4 and oxidising agents are the characteristic tests of an acid anilide.

[453] Sonnenschein has asserted that brucine may be changed into strychnine by the action of NO_3. This statement has been investigated by A. J. Cownley, but not confirmed.—*Pharm. Journ.* (3), vi. p. 841.

($C_{23}H_{24}(NO_2)_2N_2O_4$). Brucine fully neutralises acids, and forms salts, which are for the most part crystalline. The neutral sulphate ($C_{23}H_{25}N_2O_4SH_2O_4 + 3\frac{1}{2}H_2O$) is in long needles, easily soluble in water. The acetate is not crystalline, that of strychnine is so.

Brucine is precipitated by ammonia, by the caustic and carbonated alkalies, and by most of the group reagents. Ammonia does not precipitate brucine, if in excess; on the other hand, strychnine comes down if excess of ammonia is added immediately. This has been proposed as a method of separation; if the two alkaloids are present in acid solution, ammonia in excess is added, and the solution is immediately filtered; the quantitative results are, however, not good, the strychnine precipitate being invariably contaminated by brucine.

Chromate and dichromate of potassium give no precipitate with neutral salts of brucine; on the other hand, strychnine chromate is at once formed if present. It might, therefore, be used to separate strychnine from brucine. The author has attempted this method, but the results were not satisfactory.

§ 402. **Physiological Action.**—The difference between the action of strychnine and that of brucine on man or animals is not great. Mays states that strychnine affects more the anterior, brucine the posterior extremities. In strychnine poisoning, convulsions occur early, and invariably take place before death; but death may occur from brucine without any convulsions, and in any case they develop late. Brucine diminishes local sensibility when applied to the skin; strychnine does not.[454] In a physiological sense, brucine may be considered a diluted strychnine. The lethality of brucine, especially as compared with strychnine, has been investigated by F. A. Falck.[455] He experimented on 11 rabbits, injecting subcutaneously brucine nitrate, in doses of varying magnitude, from 100 mgrms. down to 20 mgrms. per kilogram of body-weight. He found that brucine presented three stages of symptoms. In the first, the respiration is quickened; in 3 of the 11 cases a strange injection of the ear was noticed; during this period the pupils may be dilated. In the second stage, there are tetanic convulsions, trismus, opisthotonus, oppressed respiration, and dilated pupils. In the third stage, the animal is moribund. Falck puts the minimum lethal dose for rabbits at 23 mgrms. per kilo. Strychnine kills 3.06 times more quickly than brucine, the intensity of the action of strychnine relative to that of brucine being as 1 : 117.4. Falck has also compared the minimum lethal dose of strychnine and brucine with the tetanising opium alkaloids, as shown in the following table:—

TABLE SHOWING THE LETHAL DOSES OF VARIOUS TETANISING POISONS.

	Minimum Lethal Dose for every Kilogram Weight of Rabbit. Mgrms.	Proportional Strength.
Strychnine nitrate,	0.6	...
Thebaine nitrate,	14.4	24 .0
Brucine nitrate,	23.0	38 .33
Landanine nitrate,	29.6	49 .33
Codeine nitrate,	51.2	85 .33
Hydrocotarnine nitrate,	203.8	339 .66

If these views are correct, it follows that the least fatal dose for an adult man would be 1.64 grm. (about 24.6 grains) of brucine nitrate.

§ 403. Tests.—If to a solution of brucine in strong alcohol a little methyl iodide is added, at the end of a few minutes circular rosettes of crystal groups appear (see fig.): they are composed of methyl brucine iodide ($C_{23}H_{25}(CH_3)N_2O_4HI$). Crystals identical in shape are also obtained if an alcoholic solution of iodine, or hydriodic acid with iodine, is added to an alcoholic solution of brucine. A solution of strychnine gives with methyl iodide no similar reaction. Strychnine in alcoholic solution, mixed with, brucine in no way interferes with the test. The methyl iodide test may be confirmed by the action of nitric acid. With that reagent it produces a scarlet colour, passing into blood-red, into yellow-red, and finally ending in yellow. This can be made something more than a mere colour test, for it is possible to obtain a crystalline body from the action of nitric acid on brucine. If a little of the latter be put

[454] *Journ. Physiol.*, viii. 391-403.

[455] *Brucin u. Strychnin; eine toxikologische Parallele*, von Dr. F. A. Falck. *Vierteljahrsschr. f. gerichtl. Med.*, Band xxiii. p. 78.

in a test-tube, and treated with nitric acid of 1.4 specific gravity (immersing the test-tube in cold water to moderate the action), the red colour is produced. On spectroscopic examination of the blood-red liquid a broad, well-marked absorption band is seen, the centre of which is between E. & F. [W. L. about 500]. There is also a development of nitric oxide and carbon dioxide, and the formation of methyl nitrite, oxalic acid, and kakotelin ($C_{23}H_{26}N_2O_4$ + $5NHO_3$ = $C_{20}H_{22}N_4O_9$ + $N(CH_3)O_2$ + $C_2H_2O_4$ + $2NO$ + $2H_2O$). On diluting abundantly with water, the kakotelin separates in yellow flocks, and may be crystallised out of dilute hydrochloric or dilute nitric acid in the form of yellow or orange-red crystals, very insoluble in water, but dissolving readily in dilute acid. On removal by dilution of the product just named, neutralisation with ammonia, and addition of a solution of chloride of calcium, the oxalate of lime is thrown down. The nitric acid test is, therefore, a combined test, consisting of—the production by the action of nitric acid (1) of a red colour; (2) of yellow scales or crystals insoluble in water; (3) of oxalic acid. No alkaloid save brucine is known to give this reaction.

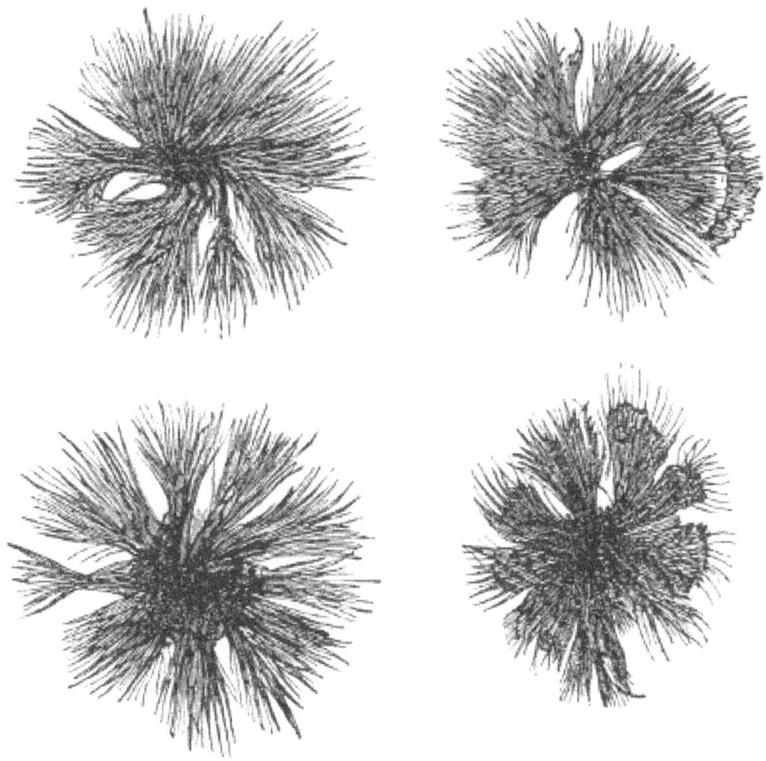

Brucine Crystals. (*From a Photograph.*)

There are other methods of producing the colour test. If a few drops of nitric acid are mixed with the substance in a test-tube, and then sulphuric acid cautiously added, so as to form a layer at the bottom, at the junction of the liquids a red zone, passing into yellow, is seen.

A solution of brucine is also coloured red by chlorine gas, ammonia changing the colour into yellow.

Flückiger[456] has proposed as a test mercurous nitrate, in aqueous solution with a little free nitric acid. On adding this reagent to a solution of brucine salt, and gently warming, a fine carmine colour is developed.

In regard to the separation of brucine from organic fluids or tissues, the process already detailed for strychnine suffices. It is of very great importance to ascertain whether both strychnine and brucine are present or not—the presence of both pointing to nux vomica or one of its preparations. The presence of brucine may, of course, be owing to impure strychnine; but if found in the tissues, that solution of the question is improbable, the commercial strychnine of the present day being usually pure, or at the most containing so small a quantity of brucine as would

[456] *Archiv f. Pharm.* (3), vi. 404.

hardly be separated from the tissues.

§ 404. **Igasurine** is an alkaloid as yet but little studied; it appears that it can be obtained from the boiling-hot watery extract of nux vomica seeds, through precipitating the strychnine and brucine by lime, and evaporation of the filtrate. According to Desnoix,[457] it forms white crystals containing 10 per cent. of water of crystallisation.

It is said to be poisonous, its action being similar to that of strychnine and brucine, and in activity standing midway between the two.

§ 405. *Strychnic Acid.*—Pelletier and Caventou obtained by boiling with spirit small, hard, warty crystals of an organic acid, from *S. ignatius*, as well as from nux vomica seeds. The seeds were first exhausted by ether, the alcohol solution was filtered and evaporated, and the extract treated with water and magnesia, filtered, and the residue first washed with cold water, then with hot spirit, and boiled lastly with a considerable quantity of water. The solution thus obtained was precipitated with acetate of lead, the lead thrown out by SH_2, and the solution evaporated, the acid crystallising out. It is a substance as yet imperfectly studied, and probably identical with malic acid.

2. THE QUEBRACHO GROUP OF ALKALOIDS.

§ 406. The bark of the *Quebracho Blanco*[458] (*Aspidosperma quebracho*) contains, according to Hesse's researches, no fewer than six alkaloids—Quebrachine, Aspidospermine, Aspidospermatine, Aspidosamine, and Hypoquebrachine. The more important of these are *Aspidospermine* and *Quebrachine.*

Aspidospermine ($C_{22}H_{30}N_2O_2$) forms colourless needles which melt at 206°. They dissolve in about 6000 parts of water at 14°—48 parts of 90 per cent. alcohol, and 106 parts of pure ether. The alkaloid gives a fine magenta colour with perchloric acid.

Quebrachine ($C_{21}H_{26}N_2O_3$) crystallises in colourless needles, melting-point (with partial decomposition) 215°. The crystals are soluble in chloroform, with difficulty soluble in cold alcohol, but easily in hot. The alkaloid, treated with sulphuric acid, and peroxide of lead, strikes a beautiful blue colour. It also gives with sulphuric acid and potassic chromate the strychnine colours. Quebrachine, dissolved in sulphuric acid containing iron, becomes violet-blue, passing into brown. The alkaloid, treated with strong sulphuric acid, becomes brown; on adding a crystal of potassic nitrate, a blue colour is developed; on now neutralising with caustic soda no red coloration is perceived. Dragendorff has recently studied the best method of extracting these alkaloids for toxicological purposes. He recommends extraction of the substances with sulphuric acid holding water, and shaking up with solvents. Aspidospermine is not extracted by petroleum ether or benzene from an acid watery extract, but readily by chloroform or by amyl alcohol. It is also separated from the same solution, alkalised by ammonia, by either amyl alcohol or chloroform; with difficulty by petroleum ether; some is dissolved by benzene. Quebrachine may be extracted from an acid solution by chloroform, but not by petroleum ether. Alkalised by ammonia, it dissolves freely in chloroform and in amyl alcohol. Traces are taken up by petroleum, somewhat more by benzene. Aspidospermine is gradually decomposed in the body, but Quebrachine is more resistant, and has been found in the stomach, intestines, blood, and urine. The toxicological action of the bark ranks it with the tetanic class of poisons. In this country it does not seem likely to attain any importance as a poison.

3. PEREIRINE.

§ 407. **Pereirine**—an alkaloid from pereira bark—gives a play of colours with sulphuric acid and potassic bichromate similar to but not identical with that of strychnine. Fröhde's reagent strikes with it a blue colour. On dissolving pereirine in dilute sulphuric acid, and precipitating by gold chloride, the precipitate is a beautiful red, which, on standing and warming, is deepened. Pereirine may be extracted from an acid solution, after alkalising with ammonia, by ether or benzene.

4. GELSEMINE.

§ 408. Gelsemine ($C_{22}H_{28}N_2O_4$) is an alkaloid[459] which has been separated from *Gelsemium sempervirens*, the Carolina jessamine, a plant having affinities with several natural orders, and placed by De Candolle among the *Loganiaceæ*, by Chapman among the *Rubiaceæ* and by Decaisne among the *Apocynaceæ*. It grows wild in Virginia

[457] *Journ. Pharm.* (3), xxv. 202.

[458] See Liebig's *Annal.*, 211, 249-282; *Ber. der deutsch. Chem. Gesellsch.*, 11, 2189; 12, 1560.

[459] Dr. T. G. Wormley separated, in 1870, a non-nitrogenised remarkably fluorescent body, which he named gelsemic acid (*Amer. Journ. of Pharm.*, 1870), but Sonnenschein and C. Robbins afterwards found gelsemic acid to be identical with æsculin (*Ber. der deutsch. Chem. Ges.*, 1876, 1182). Dr. Wormley has, however, contested this, stating that there are differences. (*Amer. Journ. of Pharm.*, 1882, p. 337. *Yearbook of Pharmacy*, 1882, p. 169.)

and Florida.[460] Gelsemine is a strong base; it is yellowish when impure, but a white amorphous powder when pure. It fuses below 100° into a transparent vitreous mass, at higher temperatures it condenses on glass in minute drops; its taste is extremely bitter; it is soluble in 25 parts of ether, in chloroform, bisulphide of carbon, benzene, and in turpentine; it is not very soluble in alcohol, and still less soluble in water, but it freely dissolves in acidulated water. The caustic alkalies precipitate it, the precipitate being insoluble in excess; it is first white, but afterwards brick-red. Tannin, picric acid, iodised potassic iodide, platinic chloride, potassio-mercuric iodide, and mercuric chloride all give precipitates. Fröhde's reagent gives with gelsemine a brown changing to green.

Sulphuric acid dissolves gelsemine with a reddish or brownish colour; after a time it assumes a pinkish hue, and if warmed on the water-bath, a more or less purple colour; if a small crystal of potassic bichromate be slowly stirred in the sulphuric acid solution, reddish purple streaks are produced along the path of the crystal; ceric oxide exhibits this better and more promptly, so small a quantity as .001 grain showing the reaction. This reaction is something like that of strychnine, but nitric acid causes gelsemine to assume a brownish-green, quickly changing to a deep green—a reaction which readily distinguishes gelsemine from strychnine and other alkaloids.

§ 409. **Fatal Dose.**—10 mgrms. killed a frog within four hours, and 8 mgrms. a cat within fifteen minutes. A healthy woman took an amount of concentrated tincture, which was equivalent to 11 mgrms. (⅙ grain), and died in seven and a half hours.

§ 410. **Effects on Animals—Physiological Action.**—Gelsemine acts powerfully on the respiration; for example, Drs. Sydney Ringer and Murrell[461] found, on operating on the frog, that in two minutes the breathing had become distinctly slower; in three and a half minutes, it had been reduced by one-third; and in six minutes, by one-half; at the expiration of a quarter of an hour, it was only one-third of its original frequency; and in twenty minutes, it was so shallow and irregular that it could no longer be counted with accuracy. In all their experiments they found that the respiratory function was abolished before reflex and voluntary motion had become extinct. In several instances the animals could withdraw their legs when their toes were pinched, days after the most careful observations had failed to detect the existence of any respiratory movement. The heart was seen beating through the chest wall long after the complete abolition of respiration.

In their experiments on warm-blooded animals (cats), they noticed that in a few minutes the respirations were slowed down to 12 and even to 8, and there was loss of power of the posterior extremities, while at short intervals the upper half of the body was convulsed. In about half an hour paralysis of the hind limbs was almost complete, and the respiratory movements so shallow that they could not be counted. In the case of a dog, after all respiration had ceased tracheotomy was performed, and air pumped in: the animal recovered.

Ringer and Murrell consider that gelsemine produces no primary quickening of the respiration, that it has no direct action on either the diaphragm or intercostal muscles, that it paralyses neither the phrenic nor the intercostal nerves, and that it diminishes the rate of respiration after both vagi have been divided. They do not consider that gelsemine acts on the cord through Setschenow's inhibitory centre, but that it destroys reflex power by its direct action on the cord, and that probably it has no influence on the motor nerves. Dr. Burdon Sanderson has also investigated the action of gelsemine on the respiration, more especially in relation to the movements of the diaphragm. He operated upon rabbits; the animal being narcotised by chloral, a small spatula, shaped like a teaspoon, was introduced into the peritoneal cavity through an opening in the linea alba, and passed upwards in front of the liver until its convex surface rested against the under side of the centrum tendineum. The stem of the spatula was brought into connection with a lever, by means of which its to-and-fro movements (and consequently that of the diaphragm) were inscribed. The first effect is to augment the depth but not the frequency of the respiratory movements; the next is to diminish the action of the diaphragm both in extent and frequency. This happens in accordance with the general principle applicable to most cases of toxic action—viz., that paresis of a central organ is preceded by over-action. The diminution of movement upon the whole is progressive, but this progression is

[460] The following are its botanical characters:—Calyx five-parted, corolla funnel-shaped, five-lobed, somewhat oblique, the lobes almost equal, the posterior being innermost in bud; stamens five; anthers oblong sagittate, style long and slender; stigmas two, each two-parted, the divisions being linear; fruit elliptical, flattened contrary to the narrow partition, two-celled, septicidally two-valved, the valves keeled; seeds five to six in each cell, large, flat, and winged; embryo straight in fleshy albumen; the ovate flat, cotyledons much shorter than the slender radicle; stem smooth, twining and shrubby; leaves opposite, entire, ovate, or lanceolate, shining on short petioles, nearly persistent; flowers large, showy, very fragrant, yellow, one to five in the axil of the leaves.

[461] *Lancet*, vol. i., 1876, p. 415.

interrupted, because the blood is becoming more and more venous, and, therefore, the phenomena of asphyxia are mixed up with the toxical effects. Dr. Sanderson concludes that the drug acts by paralysing the automatic respiratory centre; the process of extinction, which might be otherwise expected to be gradual and progressive, is prevented from being so by the intervention of disturbances of which the explanation is to be found in the imperfect arterialisation of the circulating blood. Ringer and Murrell have also experimented upon the action of gelsemine on the frog's heart. In all cases it decreased the number of beats; a small fatal dose produced a white contracted heart, a large fatal dose, a dark dilated heart; in either case arrest of the circulation of course followed.

§ 411. **Effects on Man.**—The preparations used in medicine are the fluid extract and the tincture of gelsemine; the latter appears to contain the resin of the root as well as the active principle. There are several cases on record of gelsemine, or the plant itself, having been taken with fatal effect.[462] Besides a marked effect on the respiration, there is an effect upon the eye, better seen in man than in the lower animals; the motor nerves of the eye are attacked first, objects cannot be fixed, apparently dodging their position, the eyelids become paralysed, droop, and cannot be raised by an effort of the will; the pupils are largely dilated, and at the same time a feeling of lightness has been complained of in the tongue; it ascends gradually to the roof of the mouth, and the pronunciation is slurred. There is some paresis of the extremities, and they refuse to support the body; the respiration becomes laboured, and the pulse rises in frequency to 120 or 130 beats per minute, but the mind remains clear. The symptoms occur in about an hour and a half after taking an overdose of the drug, and, if not excessive, soon disappear, leaving no unpleasantness behind. If, on the other hand, the case proceeds to a fatal end, the respiratory trouble increases, and there may be convulsions, and a course very similar to that seen in experimenting on animals. Large doses are especially likely to produce tetanus, which presents some clinical differences distinguishing it from strychnine tetanus. Gelsemine tetanus is always preceded by a loss of voluntary reflex power, respiration ceases before the onset of convulsions, the posterior extremities are most affected, and irritation fails to excite another paroxysm till the lapse of some seconds, as if the exhausted cord required time to renew its energy; finally, the convulsions only last a short time.

§ 412. *Extraction from Organic Matters, or the Tissues of the Body.*—Dragendorff states that, from as little as half a grain of the root, both gelsemine and gelsemic acid may be extracted with acid water, and identified. On extracting with water acidified with sulphuric acid, and shaking up the acid liquid with chloroform, the gelsemic acid (æsculin?) is dissolved, and the gelsemine left in the liquid. The chloroform on evaporation leaves gelsemic acid in little micro-crystals; it may be identified by (1) its crystallising in little tufts of crystals; (2) its strong fluorescent properties, one part dissolved in 15,000,000 parts of water showing a marked fluorescence, which is increased by the addition of an alkali; and (3) by splitting up into sugar and another body on boiling with a mineral acid. After separation of gelsemic acid, the gelsemine is obtained by alkalising the liquid, and shaking up with fresh chloroform; on separation of the chloroform, gelsemine may be identified by means of the reaction with nitric acid, and also the reaction with potassic bichromate and sulphuric acid.

5. COCAINE.

§ 413. **Cocaine** ($C_{17}H_{21}NO_4$).—There are two cocaines—the one rotating a ray of polarised light to the left, the other to the right. The left cocaine is contained in the leaves of *Erythroxylon coca* with other alkaloids, and is in commerce.

Cocaine has been used most extensively in medicine since the year 1884—its chief use being as a local anæsthetic. Chemically cocaine is a derivative of ecgonin, being ecgonin-methyl-ester. It has a pyridine nucleus, and may be written $C_5H_4N(CH_3)—H_3CHO—(COC_6H_5)—CH_2COOCH_3$, or expressed graphically as follows:—

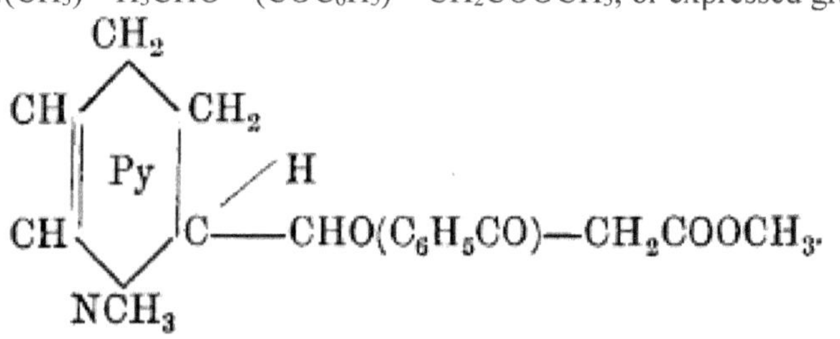

[462] See *Lancet*, 1873, vol. ii. p. 475; *Brit. Med. and Surg. Journ.*, April 1869; *Phil. Med. and Surg. Reporter*, 1861.

Properties.—Cocaine is in the form of four- to six-sided prisms of the monoclinic system. It is one of the few alkaloids which melt under the temperature of boiling water, the melting-point being as low as 85° in water. It readily furnishes a sublimate at 100°, partially decomposing. On boiling with hydrochloric acid cocaine is decomposed into methyl alcohol, ecgonin, and benzoic acid, according to the following reaction:—

Cocaine.				Benzoic acid.		Ecgonin.		Alcohol.
$C_{17}H_{21}NO_4$	+	$2H_2O$	=	C_6H_5COOH	+	$C_9H_{15}NO_3$	+	CH_3OH.

Cocaine is but little soluble in water, but easily dissolves in ether, alcohol, benzene, chloroform, and carbon disulphide; an aqueous solution is alkaline to methyl-orange, but not to phenol-phthalein. It can be made synthetically by the reaction of ecgonin-methyl-ester with benzoyl chloride.

§ 414. **Cocaine Hydrochlorate** ($C_{17}H_{21}NO_4HCl$).—Crystallised from alcohol, cocaine hydrochlorate appears in prismatic crystals; these crystals, according to Hesse,[463] when perfectly pure, should melt at 186°, although the melting-point is generally given as 200° or even 202°. Cocaine hydrochlorate is soluble in half its weight of water, insoluble in dry ether, but readily soluble in alcohol, amyl alcohol, or chloroform.

§ 415. **Pharmaceutical Preparations.**—Cocaine hydrochlorate is officinal. Gelatine discs, weighing 1.31 mgrms. ($^1/_{50}$ grain), and each containing 0.33 mgrm. ($^1/_{200}$ grain) of the salt are officinal, and used by ophthalmic surgeons. A solution of the hydrochlorate, containing 10 per cent. of cocaine hydrochlorate and (for the purposes of preserving the solution) 0.15 per cent. of salicylic acid is also officinal. Stronger solutions may also be met with; for instance, a 20 per cent. solution in oil of cloves for external application in cases of neuralgia.

§ 416. **Separation of Cocaine and Tests.**—Cocaine may be shaken out of solutions made slightly alkaline by ammonia by treatment with benzene; it also passes into petroleum ether under the same circumstances. The best method is to extract a solution, made feebly alkaline, thoroughly by ether, and then shake it out by benzene and evaporate the separated benzene at the ordinary air temperature. The property of the alkaloid to melt at or below the temperature of boiling water, and the ready decomposition into benzoic acid and other products, render cocaine easy of identification. If, for instance, a small particle of cocaine is put in a tube, a drop of strong sulphuric acid added and warmed by the water-bath, colourless crystals of benzoic acid sublime along the tube, and an aromatic odour is produced.

Flückiger has recommended the production of benzoate of iron as a useful test both for cocaine and for cocaine hydrochlorate.

One drop of a dilute solution of ferric chloride added to a solution of 20 mgrms. of cocaine hydrochlorate in 2 c.c. of water, gives a yellow fluid, which becomes red on boiling from the production of iron benzoate. This reaction is of little use unless a solution of the same strength of ferric chloride, but to which the substance to be tested has not been added, is boiled at the same time for comparison, because all solutions of ferric chloride deepen in colour on heating.

A solution of the alkaloid evaporated to dryness on the water-bath, after being acidulated with nitric acid, and then a few drops of alcoholic solution of potash or soda added, develops an odour of benzoic ethyl-ester. Cocaine hydrochlorate, when triturated with calomel, blackens by the slightest humidity or by moistening it with alcohol. Cocaine in solution is precipitated by most of the group reagents, but is not affected by mercuric chloride, picric acid, nor potassic bichromate.

Added to the tests above mentioned, there is the physiological action; cocaine dilates the pupil, tastes bitter, and, for the time, arrests sensation; hence the after-effect on the tongue is a sensation of numbness.

§ 417. **Symptoms.**—A large number of accidents occur each year from the external application of cocaine; few, however, end fatally. Cocaine has thus produced poisonous symptoms when applied to the eye, to the rectum, to the gums, to the urethra, and to various other parts. There have been a few fatal cases, both from its external and internal administration; Mannheim, for example, has collected eleven of such instances.

The action of cocaine is twofold; there is an action on the central and the peripheral nervous system. In small doses cocaine excites the spinal cord and the brain; in large it may produce convulsions and then paralysis. The peripheral action is seen in the numbing of sensation. There is always interference with the accommodation of

[463] O. Hesse, *Annalen*, 276, 342-344.

vision, and dilatation of the pupil. The eyelids are wider apart than normal, and there may be some protrusion of the eyeball.

The usual course of an acute case of poisoning is a feeling of dryness in the nose and throat, difficulty of swallowing, faintness, and there is often vomiting; the pulse is quickened; there is first cerebral excitement, followed usually by great mental depression. Occasionally there is an eruption on the skin. Hyperæsthesia of the skin is followed by great diminution of sensation, the pupils, as before stated, are dilated, the eyes protruding, the eyelids wide open, the face is pale, and the perspiration profuse. Convulsions and paralysis may terminate the scene. Death takes place from paralysis of the breathing centre; therefore the heart beats after the cessation of respiration. As an antidote, nitrite of amyl has apparently been used with success.

There is a form of chronic poisoning produced from the taking of small doses of cocaine daily. The symptoms are very various, and are referable to disturbance of the digestive organs, and to the effect on the nervous system. The patients become extremely emaciated, and it seems to produce a special form of mania.

§ 418. **Post-mortem Appearances.**—The appearances found in acute cases of poisoning have been hyperæmia of the liver, spleen, and kidneys, as well as of the brain and spinal cord.

In the experimental poisoning of mice with cocaine Ehrlich[464] found a considerable enlargement of the liver.

§ 419. **Fatal Dose.**—The fatal dose, according to Mannheim,[465] must be considered as about 1 grm. (15.4 grains); the smallest dose known to have been fatal is 0.08 grm. (1.2 grain) for an adult, and 0.05 grm. (0.7 grain) for a child.

6. CORYDALINE.

§ 420. **Corydaline** ($C_{22}H_{28}NO_4$) is an alkaloid discovered by Wackenroder (1826) in the tubers of *Corydalis tuberosa*; crystallised in the cold and away from light, out of a mixture of absolute alcohol and ether, corydaline forms colourless, flat, prismatic crystals, which quickly turn yellow on exposure to light or heat. Pure corydaline changes colour at about 125°, softens at about 133°, and melts finally at 134° to 135°. It dissolves in ether, chloroform, carbon disulphide, and benzene, but not so readily in alcohol. It is almost insoluble in cold water, and but slightly soluble in boiling water. Water precipitates it from a solution in alcohol. It is also soluble in dilute hydrochloric and sulphuric acids. It gives a precipitate with potassium iodide if a solution of the hydrochloride be used. The precipitate crystallises out of hot water in clusters of short lemon-yellow prismatic crystals, and has the formula of $C_{22}H_{28}NO_4HI$. Corydaline platinochloride has the composition of $(C_{22}H_{28}NO_4)_2H_2PtCl_6$, containing Pt 16.94 per cent., and 2.44 per cent. of N.—Dobbie & Lauder, *Journ. Chem. Soc.*, March 1892, 244.

Corydaline in large doses causes epileptiform convulsions. Death takes place from respiratory paralysis.

V.—The Aconite Group of Alkaloids.

§ 421. The officinal aconite is the *Aconitum napellus*—monkshood or wolfsbane—a very common garden plant in this country, and one cultivated for medicinal purposes. Many varieties of aconite exist in other regions, which either are, or could be, imported. Of these the most important is the *Aconitum ferox*, a native of the Himalayan mountains, imported from India.

All the aconites, so far as known, are extremely poisonous, and it appears probable that different species contain different alkaloids. The root of *A. napellus* is from 2 to 4 inches long, conical in shape, brown externally, and white internally. The leaves are completely divided at the base into five wedge-shaped lobes, each of the five lobes being again divided into three linear segments. The numerous seeds are three-sided, irregularly twisted, wrinkled, of a dark-brown colour, in length one-sixth of an inch, and weighing 25 to the grain (*Guy*). The whole plant is one of great beauty, from 2 to 6 feet high, and having a terminal spike of conspicuous blue flowers. The root has been fatally mistaken for horse-radish, an error not easily accounted for, since no similarity exists between them.

§ 422. **Pharmaceutical Preparations of Aconite.**—The preparations of aconite used in medicine are—

Aconitine, officinal in all the pharmacopœias.

Aconite liniment (linimentum aconiti), made from the root with spirit, and flavoured with camphor; officinal in the British Pharmacopœia. It may contain about 2.0 per cent. of aconitine.

Aconite tincture, officinal in all the pharmacopœias.

Aconite ointment, 8 grains of aconitine to the oz. (*i.e.*, 1.66 per cent.); officinal in the British Pharmacopœia.

---

464 *Deutsche med. Wochens.*, 1890, No. 32.

465 *Deutsch. Arch. f. klin. Med.*, Bd. viii., 1891, 380.

Aconite extract, the juice of the leaves evaporated; officinal in most of the pharmacopœias. The strength in alkaloid of the extract varies; in six samples examined by F. Casson, the least quantity was 0.16 per cent., the maximum 0.28 per cent.[466]

Fleming's tincture of aconite is not officinal, but is sold largely in commerce. It is from three to four times stronger than the B.P. tincture.

§ 423. **The Alkaloids of Aconite.**—The researches of Dr. Alder Wright and Luff, and especially those of Professor Dunstan,[467] have established that in the root of the true aconite there exist four alkaloids, one only of which has been as yet crystallised.

Three of the alkaloids have been fairly well worked out; the fourth homo-napelline has not yet been satisfactorily investigated.

The three alkaloids are aconitine, aconine and benzoyl-aconine; besides which pyraconitine and pyraconine can be obtained by suitable treatment from aconitine and aconine.

The formulæ of the alkaloids and their derivatives are as follows:—

Aconitine (acetyl-benzoyl-aconine),	m.p., 188.60°,	$C_{33}H_{45}NO_{12}$
Benzoyl-aconine,	m.p., 268.0°,	$C_{31}H_{43}NO_{11}$
Pyraconitine (anhydro-benzoyl-aconine),	m.p., 188-190°,	$C_{31}H_{41}NO_{10}$
Aconine,	m.p., 132°,	$C_{24}H_{39}NO_{10}$
Pyraconine (anhydro-aconine),		$C_{24}H_{37}NO_9$

§ 424. **Aconitine**, $C_{33}H_{45}NO_{12}$.—This base has been shown by Dunstan to be acetyl-benzoyl-aconine; one molecule of the base breaking up, on complete hydrolysis, into one molecule of aconine, one of acetic acid, and one of benzoic acid—

$$C_{33}H_{45}NO_{12} + 2H_2O = \underset{\text{Acetic Acid.}}{C_2H_4O_2} + \underset{\text{Benzoic Acid.}}{C_7H_6O_2} + \underset{\text{Aconine.}}{C_{24}H_{39}NO_{10}}.$$

That is to say that 100 parts of aconitine, according to theory, should yield:—

Acetic acid, 9.37 per cent.; benzoic acid, 18.85 per cent.; and aconine, 77.52 per cent.

Pure aconitine has a tube melting-point of 188.6°. The behaviour of a sample of Merck's aconitine in the subliming cell, which had a melting-point of 184°, was as described earlier.

Aconitine dissolves in water at 22° in the proportion of 1 in 4431 (*Dunstan*); it is soluble in 37 of absolute alcohol, 64 of anhydrous ether, 5.5 parts of chloroform and benzene (*A. Jurgens*); it has basic properties, and a cold watery solution has an alkaline reaction to cochineal, but not to litmus nor to phenol-phthalein. Aconitine is not precipitated by mercuric potassium iodide, but gives a voluminous precipitate with an aqueous solution of iodine in potassium iodide.

It gives a crystalline yellow gold compound with gold chloride, which has a melting-point of 135.5°, and according to its composition, $C_{33}H_{45}NO_{12}HAuCl_4$, should give 19.9 per cent. of gold.

Aconitine is best extracted from the plant, or from organic matters generally, by a 1 per cent. sulphuric acid; this strength is stated not to hydrolyse aconitine if acting in the cold; after purifying the acid liquid by shaking it with amyl alcohol, and then with chloroform, *always operating in the cold*, the liquid is precipitated by ammonia in very slight excess, and the liquid shaken with ether; the ether is removed, dehydrated by standing over calcium chloride, and then evaporated spontaneously; should the aconitine be mixed with the other alkaloids, advantage can be taken of the method of separating aconitine by converting it into hydrobromide, as described under "Benzoyl-aconine."

§ 425. **Tests for Aconitine.**—The most satisfactory and the most delicate is the physiological test; the minutest trace of an aconite-holding liquid, applied to the tongue or lips, causes a peculiar numbing, tingling sensation which, once felt, can readily be remembered.

466 *Pharm. Journ.*, 1894, 901.

467 Various papers in *Journ. Chem. Soc.*, 1892-1894.

An alkaloidal substance which, heated in a tube, melts approximately near the melting-point of aconitine, and gives off an acid vapour, would render one suspicious of aconitine, for most alkaloids give off alkaline vapours. Aconitine also may, by heating with dilute acids, be made to readily yield benzoic acid, an acid easy of identification. Aconitine dissolved in nitric acid, evaporated to dryness, and then treated with alcoholic potash, gives off an unmistakable odour of benzoic ester.

Should there be sufficient aconitine recovered to convert it into the gold salt, the properties of the gold salt (that is, its melting-point, and the percentage of gold left after burning) assist materially in the identification.

A minute quantity of aconitine dissolved in water, acidified with acetic acid, and a particle of KI added and the solution allowed to evaporate, gives crystals of aconitine hydriodide, from which water will dissolve out the KI. Iodine water gives a precipitate of a reddish-brown colour in a solution of 1 : 2000.[468]

The chemical tests are supplementary to the physiological; if the alkaloidal extract does not give the tingling, numbing sensation, aconitine cannot be present.

§ 426. **Benzoyl-aconine ("isaconitine")**, $C_{31}H_{43}NO_{11}$, is obtained from aconitine by heating an aqueous solution of the sulphate or hydrochloride in a closed tube at 120°-130° for two or three hours, a molecule of acetic acid (9.27 per cent.) being split off, and benzoyl-aconine left.

It may be separated from the mixed alkaloids of the *Aconitum napellus* by dissolving in a 5 per cent. solution of hydrobromic acid (excess of acid being avoided), precipitating with a slight excess of ammonia, and shaking out with ether. The residue left after the ether is evaporated chiefly consists of aconitine; it is dissolved in just sufficient hydrobromic acid and the exactly neutral hydrobromate solution allowed to evaporate spontaneously in a desiccator; crystals of aconitine hydrobromide separate out, the mother liquor containing some benzoyl-aconine and "homonapelline." The aqueous solution which has been exhausted with ether is now shaken out with chloroform. This chloroform solution contains most of the benzoyl-aconine, and on separation the residue is dissolved in just sufficient hydrochloric acid to form a neutral solution; this solution is concentrated on the water-bath with constant stirring, crystals of the hydrochloride form, and are filtered off from time to time and washed with a little cold water, the washings being added to the original liquid; the different fractions are mixed together, and the process repeated until they have a melting-point of 268°. Benzoyl-aconine is obtained from the hydrochloride by precipitating the aqueous solution by the addition of dilute ammonia, and extracting the solution with ether; the solution in ether is washed with water, dried by means of calcium chloride, and then distilled off. Benzoyl-aconine is left as a transparent colourless non-crystalline varnish of a melting-point near 125°.

The solution in water is alkaline to litmus. The base is readily soluble in alcohol, in chloroform, and in ether. The alcoholic solution is dextrorotatory. The solutions are bitter, but do not give the tingling sensation characteristic of aconitine. The hydrochloride, the hydrobromide, the hydriodide, and the nitrate have been obtained in a crystalline state. The most characteristic salt is, however, the aurochlor derivative. When aqueous solutions of benzoyl-aconine chloride and auric chloride are mixed, a yellow precipitate is thrown down, which (dissolved in alcohol, after being dried over calcium chloride, and slowly evaporated in a desiccator) deposits colourless crystals entirely different from the yellow crystals of aconitine gold chloride. These crystals have the composition $C_{31}H_{42}(AuCl_2)NO_{11}$, and therefore, by theory, should yield 22.6 per cent. of gold, and 8.2 per cent. of chlorine.

By hydrolysis benzoyl-aconine yields benzoic acid, which can be shaken out of an acid solution by ether and identified; one molecule of benzoic acid is formed from one molecule of benzoyl-aconine. Twenty per cent. of benzoic acid should, according to the formula, be obtained; Professor Dunstan found only 18.85 per cent.[469]

Benzoic acid in the subliming cell begins to give a cloud at about 77°-80°, and at or near 100° sublimes most rapidly.

Benzoic acid, recovered from an acid solution by shaking out with ether, may be recognised as follows:—To the film left on evaporating off the ether add a drop of H_2SO_4, and a few crystals of sodic nitrate, and heat gently for a short time; pour the clear liquid into ammonia water, and add a drop of ammonium sulphide. A red-brown colour indicates benzoic acid. The *rationale* of the test is as follows:—Dinitro-benzoic acid is first formed, and next, by the action of ammonium sulphide, this is converted into the red-brown ammonium diamidobenzoate.—E. Mohler, *Bull. Soc. Chem.* (3), iii. 414-416.

§ 427. **Pyraconitine**, $C_{31}H_{41}NO_{10}$, is anhydro-benzoyl-aconine; it differs from benzoyl-aconine by a molecule

---

[468] A. Jurgens, *Arch. Pharm.* (3), xxiv. 127, 128.

[469] Professor Dunstan found, as a means of two determinations, 21.6 per cent. of gold, and 7.8 per cent. of chlorine, which comes nearer his old formula of $C_{33}H_{44}(AuCl_2)NO_{12}$.—*Journ. Chem. Soc.*, April 1893.

of water; picraconitine is obtained by keeping aconitine at its melting-point (188°-190°) for some time, when acetic acid distils over and pyraconitine is left. Pyraconitine is an amorphous varnish, sparingly soluble in water, but readily dissolving in alcohol, chloroform, and ether; it gives a pale yellow precipitate with gold chloride, and forms crystalline salts with hydriodic, hydrobromic, and hydrochloric acids. Pyraconitine readily undergoes hydrolysis by the action of dilute acids, or by potash or soda, or with water in a closed tube; the products are benzoic acid and an alkaloid, to which the name of pyraconine has been given.

§ 428. **Pyraconine**, $C_{24}H_{37}NO_9$.—This base is anhydro-aconine, the formula differing from aconine by one atom of water. It is amorphous, closely resembling aconine; it is soluble in water and ether; the aqueous solution has a somewhat sweet taste, and is lævorotatory; it combines with acids to form crystalline salts, which are very soluble in water.

§ 429. **Aconine**, $C_{24}H_{39}NO_{10}$, m.p. 132°.—Aconine does not crystallise. Its aqueous solution is decidedly alkaline, and, like aconitine, it is lævorotatory, although to a less degree. Its taste is bitter, but causes no tingling sensation. Aconine is very soluble in water or alcohol, and slightly in chloroform, but insoluble in ether or in petroleum ether. It does, however, dissolve, in the presence of aconitine, slightly in ether. The aqueous solutions reduce the salts of gold and silver, and also Fehling's solution. A solution of aconine gives precipitates with the general alkaloidal reagents; with mercuric chloride it gives a copious yellow precipitate, which darkens on standing.

Aconine hydrochloride, the hydriodide, the hydrobromide, and the sulphate, have all been crystallised; solutions of these salts are lævorotatory.

§ 430. **Commercial Aconitine and the Lethal Dose of Aconitine.**—Commercial aconitine has in the past varied in appearance from that of a gummy amorphous mass up to a purer kind in white crystals.

Professor Dunstan[470] has recently examined fourteen samples, some of them of considerable age, and only found two samples (one of English, another of German make) which approached in melting-point and crystalline appearance pure aconitine; the one, the English, melted at 186°-187°, and contained about 3 per cent. of benzoyl-aconine; the other, a German specimen, was almost pure; the melting-point was 187.5°. At the present time it is, however, not difficult to obtain fairly pure crystalline aconitine, and to assay it accurately by determining the proportion of acetic and benzoic acids. The physiological action of commercial aconitine is, however, in all cases the same, the difference being in quantitative not qualitative action; in the small doses usually administered, the physiological action depends wholly upon the true aconitine present, the other bases being practically without toxic action. Professor Plugge[471] has made some researches on the fatal dose (for the lower animals) of Petit's, Merck's, and Friedländer's aconitine nitrate, which in 1882 were the purest in commerce. He administered the following doses to the animals mentioned:—

TABLE SHOWING FATAL DOSES (FOR ANIMALS) OF ACONITINE.
PETIT'S CRYSTALLINE ACONITINE NITRATE.

Animals Experimented upon.	Dose Given.	Dose per Kilogrm.	Result.
A Frog,	.4 mgrm.	16 .0	Death in 60 Minutes.
A Rabbit,	.8 ,,	.5- .6	,,30 ,,
A Dog,	1 .6 ,,	.21	,,20 ,,
,,	.45 ,,	.10	,,140 ,,
,,	.50 ,,	.054	Recovered.
,,	.60 ,,	.075	Recovered.
A Pigeon	.07 ,,	.22	Death in 21 Minutes.

MERCK'S ACONITINE NITRATE.

[470] *Journ. Chem. Soc. Trans.*, 1893, 491.
[471] *Archiv de Pharm.*, Jan. 7, 1882.

Animals Experimented upon.	Dose Given.	Dose per Kilogrm.	Result.
A Frog,	.4 mgrm.	16	Recovered.
„	1 .0 „	40	Died in 110-360 Min.
„	2 .0 „	80	„75-130 „
„	4 .0 „	160	„50„
A Rabbit,	3 .5 „	2	„75„
„	10 „	6 .50	„15„
A Dog,	10 „	1 .65	„15„
A Pigeon,	...	1 .65	Recovered.

FRIEDLÄNDER'S ACONITINE NITRATE.

Animals Experimented upon.	Dose Given.	Dose per Kilogrm.	Result.
A Frog,	4 mgrms.	160	Recovered.
„	10 „	400	Death in more than 60 minutes.
„	20 „	800	
„	40 „	1600	
A Rabbit,	6 „	4 .11	Recovered.
„	24 „	18 .00	„
„	50 „	85 .50	„
A Dog,	28 „	6 .00	„
A Pigeon,	10 „	33 .4	„

The conclusions Plugge draws from his researches are that Petit's aconitine was at least eight times stronger than that of Merck, and seventy times more toxic than that of Friedländer, while Merck's "aconitine again was twenty to thirty times stronger than Friedländer's." He was inclined to put seven commercial samples which he has examined in the following diminishing order of toxicity:—(1) Petit's crystalline aconitine nitrate; (2) Morson's aconitine nitrate; (3) Hottot's aconitine nitrate; (4) Hopkins & Williams' pseudaconitine; (5) Merck's aconitine nitrate; (6) Schuchart's aconitine sulphate; and (7) Friedländer's aconitine nitrate.

From a study of Dr. Harley's experiments,[472] however, made a few years ago, there would appear to have been but little difference between the activity of Petit's and Morson's aconitine. Dr. Harley experimented on a young cat, 3 lbs. in weight, and nearly killed it with a $\frac{1}{1000}$ of a grain of Morson's aconitine; two other cats, also weighing 3 lbs. each, died in seven and a half hours and three-quarters of an hour respectively, killed from a subcutaneous dose of of a grain. Reducing these values to the ordinary equivalents, the dose, after which the cat recovered with difficulty, is equal to about .048 mgrm. per kilo., while a certainly fatal dose is .092 mgrm. per kilo.; therefore, it seems likely that the least fatal dose for Morson's, as for Petit's, is some number between .075 and .09 mgrm. per kilo.

Man is evidently more sensitive to aconitine than any of the dogs or cats experimented upon, since, in the German cases to be recorded, 1.6 mgrm. of Petit's aconitine nitrate, taken by the mouth, gave rise to symptoms so violent that it was evidently a dangerous dose, while 4 mgrms. were rapidly fatal; but if man took the same amount per kilo. as dogs or cats, he would require a little over 6 mgrms. to be certainly fatal. It seems, then, from the evidence obtainable, that .03 grain (2 mgrms.) is about the least fatal dose for an adult man of standard weight. This dose is equal to .028 mgrm. per kilo., and, of course, refers either to Morson's aconitine or French aconitine, the alkaloid being taken by the mouth. If given by subcutaneous injection, probably 1.5 mgrm. would kill, for the whole

[472] "On the Action and Use of Aconitine," *St. Thos. Hosp. Report*, 1874.

of the poison is then thrown on the circulation at one time, and there is no chance of its elimination by vomiting.

The lethal dose of the pure alkaloid being even approximately settled, it is possible to get a more exact idea as to the suitable medicinal dose of the tincture and extract, and also to study more profitably the "quantitative toxicity." The English officinal tincture, although variable in strength, may for our purposes be regarded as averaging 1 per cent. of alkaloid—that is, in every 100 parts by volume there will be 1 part of the alkaloid by weight, and Fleming's tincture may be considered as one-third stronger, containing in every 100 parts 1.3 part of alkaloid. The medicinal dose of the P.B. tincture is laid down as from 5 to 15 min.—equal to from .005 to .015 grain of aconitine. The German pharmacopœia gives the maximum single dose as 1 c.c. (say 15 mins.), and the maximum quantity to be taken in the twenty-four hours as four times that quantity. As before stated, 2 mgrms. (.030 grain) of aconitine being considered a fatal dose, this is equivalent to about 2 c.c. (30 mins.) of the P.B. tincture, or to 1.2 c.c. (20 mins.) of Fleming's tincture in a single dose; and on these theoretical grounds I should consider this dose dangerous, and in the absence of prompt treatment likely to be fatal to an adult man. The usual least fatal dose laid down in medical toxicological works, however, is greater than this—viz., 3.75 c.c. (a drachm).

In 1863 a woman took 70 minims of Fleming's tincture, and a grain of acetate of morphine, and died in about four hours; but as this was a complex case of poisoning, it is not of much value. Fifteen minims of the tincture caused very serious symptoms in the case of a woman under the care of Dr. Topham,[473] the effects lasting many hours. Probably the smallest quantity of the tincture recorded as having destroyed life is in the case of Dr. Male, of Birmingham.[474] He died from the effects of 80 drops taken in ten doses, extending over a period of four days—the largest dose at any one time being 10 drops, the total quantity would perhaps equal .08 grain of aconitine.

The P.B. extract is not a very satisfactory preparation, varying much in strength. It may be taken to average about .6 per cent., and if so, applying the same reasoning as before, from .26 to .32 grm. (4 to 5 grains) would be a fatal dose.[475] On the other hand, there is an alcoholic extract which is very powerful, and averages 5 per cent. of aconitine: 40 mgrms. (.6 grain) of this extract would be likely to be fatal. With regard to the root itself, 3.8 grms. (60 grains) have been known to produce death, and from the average alkaloidal contents it is probable that .648 grm. (10 grains) would be a highly dangerous dose. Dunstan's researches will now alter probably the whole of the pharmacy of aconite, and the tendency will be to make the preparations of greater activity, and, consequently, to make the dangerous doses smaller than formerly.

§ 431. **Effects of Aconitine on Animal Life.**—There are few substances which have been experimented upon in such a variety of ways and upon so many classes of animals as aconitine in different forms; but there does not seem to be any essential difference in the symptoms produced in different animals save that which is explained by the organisation of the life-form under experiment.

Insects.—The author has made experiments with the active principles of aconite upon blow-flies. An extract was made by allowing the ordinary tincture to evaporate spontaneously at the temperature of the atmosphere. If a minute dot of this is placed upon the head of a blow-fly, absorption of the active principle takes place in from fifteen to thirty minutes, and marked symptoms result. The symptoms consist essentially of muscular weakness, inability to fly, and to walk up perpendicular surfaces; there is also, in all cases, a curious entanglement of the legs, and very often extrusion of the proboscis; trembling of the legs and muscular twitchings are frequent. A progressive paralysis terminates in from four to five hours in death; the death is generally so gradual that it is difficult to know when the event occurs, but in one case there were violent movements of the body, and sudden death.[476]

Fish.—The action on fish has been studied by Schulz and Praag. There is rapid loss of power and diminished

[473] *Lancet*, July 19, 1851, p. 56.

[474] *Med. Gaz.*, vol. xxxvi. p. 861, quoted by Taylor, *Prin. of Med. Juris.*, vol. i. p. 426.

[475] But there is a case reported by Dr. Vachell, of Cardiff, in which 2 grains of extract of aconite taken in pills proved fatal. Now 2 grains is the medicinal dose, laid down as a maximum in the pharmacopœia; a complete revolution is, therefore, necessary in the use of these active remedies. No extract or tincture should be used until its approximate strength in active principles is determined.

[476] It may be well to quote in full a typical experiment. Six P.M., a little extract smeared on the head of a blow-fly. Forty-five minutes after—makes no attempt to fly, great muscular weakness, no trembling or convulsive movements. Fifty minutes after—partial paralysis of right half of body, so that the fly, on moving, goes in a circular direction, the second pair of legs are curiously bent forward and useless; the wings seem fairly strong. Seventy-five minutes—fly very dull, always in one spot, without movement; when placed on a horizontal glass surface, and the glass then very slowly inclined, until it is at last quite perpendicular, the fly falls. There is now a strange entanglement of the legs. 125 minutes—perfectly paralysed; 145 minutes—dead.

breathing; the respiration seems difficult, and the fish rapidly die.

Reptiles—Frogs.—The most recent experiments on frogs are those of Plugge, and although his interpretation of the phenomena in some points is different from that of previous observers, the symptoms themselves are, as might have been expected, not different from those described by Achscharumow, L. v. Praag, and others. Plugge found no qualitative difference in the action of any of the commercial samples of aconitine. This fact gives the necessary value to all the old experiments, for we now know that, although they were performed with impure or weak preparations, yet there is no reason to believe that the symptoms described were due to any other but the alkaloid aconitine in varying degrees of purity or dilution. Frogs show very quickly signs of weakness in the muscular power; the respiration invariably becomes laboured, and ceases after a few minutes; the heart's action becomes slowed, irregular, and then stops in diastole. The poisoned heart, while still pulsating, cannot be arrested either by electrical stimulation of the vagus or by irritation of the sinus, nor when once arrested can any further contraction be excited in it. Opening of the mouth and apparent efforts to vomit, Plugge observed both with *Rana esculenta* and *Rana temporaria*. He considers them almost invariable signs of aconitine poisoning. A separation of mucus from the surface of the body of the frog is also very constantly observed. Dilatation of the pupils is frequent, but not constant; there may be convulsions, both of a clonic and tonic character, before death, but fibrillar twitchings are seldom. (With regard to the dose required to affect frogs, see *ante*.)

Birds.—There is a discrepancy in the descriptions of the action of aconitine on birds. L. v. Praag thought the respiration and circulation but little affected at first; while Achscharumow witnessed in pigeons dyspnœa, dilatation of the pupils, vomiting, shivering, and paresis. It may be taken that the usual symptoms observed are some difficulty in breathing, a diminution of temperature, a loss of muscular power generally (but not constantly), dilatation of the pupils, and convulsions before death.

Mammals.—The effects vary somewhat, according to the dose. Very large doses kill rabbits rapidly. They fall on their sides, are violently convulsed, and die in an asphyxiated condition; but with smaller doses the phenomena first observed are generally to be referred to the respiration. Thus, in an experiment on the horse, Dr. Harley found that the subcutaneous administration of .6 mgrm. (.01 grain) caused in a weakly colt some acceleration of the pulse and a partial paralysis of the dilator narium. Double the quantity given to the same animal some time after, caused, in six hours and a half, some muscular weakness, and an evident respiratory trouble. The horse recovered in eighteen hours. 2.7 mgrms. ($\frac{1}{24}$ grain) given in the same way, after a long interval of time, caused, at the end of an hour, more pronounced symptoms; the pulse, at the commencement 50, rose in an hour and a half to 68, then the respiration became audible and difficult. In an hour and three-quarters there were great restlessness and diminution of muscular power. Two hours after the injection the muscular weakness increased so much that the horse fell down; he was also convulsed. After eight hours he began to improve. In another experiment, 32.4 mgrms. ($\frac{1}{2}$ grain) killed a sturdy entire horse in two hours and twenty minutes, the symptoms commencing within the hour, and consisting of difficulty of breathing, irregularity of the heart's action, and convulsions.

The general picture of the effects of fatal, but not excessive, doses given to dogs, cats, rabbits, &c., resembles closely that already described. The heart's action is at first slowed, then becomes quick and irregular, there is dyspnœa, progressive paralysis of the muscular power, convulsions, and death in asphyxia. Vomiting is frequently observed, sometimes salivation, and very often dilatation of the pupil. Sometimes the latter is abnormally active, dilating and contracting alternately. Diarrhœa also occurs in a few cases. Vomiting is more frequent when the poison is taken by the mouth than when administered subcutaneously.[477]

[477] The more important physiological researches on the action of aconite are contained in the following works and papers:—

Fleming, A.—*An Inquiry into the Physiological and Medicinal Properties of the Aconitum napellus*, to which are added observations on several other species of aconite, 8vo, Lond., 1845.

Schulz, F. W.—*De Aconitini Effectu in Organismum Animalium.*

V. Praag.—*Arch. f. Path. Anat.*, vii. p. 438, 1854.

Hottot, E.—*De l'Aconitine et de ses Effets Physiologiques*, 4to, Paris, 1863.

Achscharumow.—*Arch. f. Anatom. u. Physiol.*, 1866.

Böhn.—*Herzgifte*, 1871.

Ewers, C.—*Ueber die physiologischen Wirkungen des aus Aconitum ferox dargestellten Aconitins* (*Pseudoaconitin, Aconitinum anglicum, Nepalin*), 8vo, Dorpat, 1873.

Guilaud.—*De l'Aconite et de l'Aconitine*, 4to, Montpellier, 1874.

Francheschini, M. A.—*Contribution a l'Étude de l'Action Physiologique et Thérapeutique de l'Aconitine*, 4to, Paris, 1875.

Lewin.—*Exp. Untersuch. über die Wirkung d. Aconitins auf's Herz. Diss.*, Berlin, 1875.

§ 432. **Statistics.**—During the ten years, 1883-92, there were recorded in England and Wales, 40 accidental deaths from the various forms of aconite (19 males, 21 females); and 19 suicidal deaths (9 males, 10 females) from the same cause, which makes a total of 59.

§ 433. **Effects on Man.**—I have collected from European medical literature, 87 cases of poisoning by aconite in some form or other. These comprise only 2 cases of murder, 7 of suicide, and 77 which were more or less accidental. Six of the cases were from the use of the alkaloid itself; 10 were from the root; in two cases children eat the flowers; in 1, the leaves of the plant were cooked and eaten by mistake; in 7, the tincture was mistaken for brandy, sherry, or liqueur; the remainder were caused by the tincture, the liniment, or the extract.

§ 434. **Poisoning by the Root.**—A case of murder which occurred some years ago in America, and also the Irish case which took place in 1841 (*Reg.* v. *M'Conkey*), were, until the recent trial of Lamson, the only instances among English-speaking people of the use of aconite for criminal purposes; but if we turn to the Indian records, we find that it has been largely used from the earliest times as a destroyer of human life. In 1842 a tank of water destined for the use of the British army in pursuit of the retreating Burmese, was poisoned by intentional contamination with the bruised root of *Aconitum ferox*; it was fortunately discovered before any harm resulted. A preparation of the root is used in all the hill districts of India to poison arrows for the destruction of wild beasts. A Lepcha described the root to a British officer as being "useful to sportsmen for destroying elephants and tigers, useful to the rich for putting troublesome relations out of the way, and useful to jealous husbands for the purpose of destroying faithless wives." From the recorded cases, the powdered root, mixed with food, or the same substance steeped in spirituous liquor, is usually the part chosen for administration. In M'Conkey's case, the man's wife purchased powdered aconite root, mixed it with pepper, and strewed it over some greens, which she cooked and gave to him. The man complained of the sharp taste of the greens, and soon after the meal vomited, and suffered from purging, became delirious with lock-jaw, and clenching of the hands; he died in about three hours. The chief noticeable *post-mortem* appearance was a bright red colour of the mucous membrane of the stomach.

The symptoms in this case were, in some respects, different from those met with in other cases of poisoning by the root. A typical case is given by Dr. Chevers (*op. cit.*), in which a man had taken by mistake a small portion of aconite root. Immediately after chewing it he felt a sweetish taste, followed immediately by tingling of the lips and tongue, numbness of the face, and severe vomiting. On admission to hospital he was extremely restless, tossing his limbs about in all directions and constantly changing his position. He complained of a burning sensation in the stomach, and a tingling and numbness in every part of the body, excepting his legs. The tingling was specially marked in the face and tongue—so much so that he was constantly moving the latter to and fro in order to scratch it against the teeth. Retching and vomiting occurred almost incessantly, and he constantly placed his hand over the cardiac region. His face was anxious, the eyes suffused, the lips pale and exsanguine, the eyelids swollen, moderately dilated, and insensible to the stimulus of light; the respiration was laboured, 64 in a minute; the pulse 66, small and feeble. There was inability to walk from loss of muscular power, but the man was perfectly conscious. The stomach-pump was used, and albumen and milk administered. Three and three-quarter hours after taking the root the symptoms were increased in severity. The tongue was red and swollen, the pulse intermittent, feeble, and slower. The tingling and numbness had extended to the legs. On examining the condition of the external sensibility with a pair of scissors, it was found that, on fully separating the blades and bringing the points in contact with the skin over the arms and forearms, he felt them as one, although they were 4 inches apart. But the sensibility of the thighs and legs was less obtuse, for he could feel the two points distinctly when they were 4 inches apart, and continued to do so until the distance between the points fell short of $2\frac{3}{4}$ inches. He began to improve about the ninth hour, and gradually recovered, although he suffered for one or two days from a slight diarrhœa. As in the case detailed, no water was passed for a long time, as if the bladder early lost its power.

§ 435. **Poisoning by the Alkaloid Aconitine.**—Probably the earliest instance on record is the case related by Dr. Golding Bird in 1848.[478] What kind of aconitine was then in commerce I know not, and since apparently a person

---

Giulini, P.—*Experimentelle Untersuchungen ueber die Wirkung des Aconitins auf das Nervensystem, das Herz, u. die Athmung*, 8vo, Erlangen, 1876.

Harley, Dr. John.—"On the Action and Uses of Aconitia," *St. Thos. Hosp. Reports*, 1874.

V. Schroff, C. Jr.—*Beitrag zur Kenntniss des Aconit.*, 8vo, Wien, 1876.

Plugge, P. C.—"Untersuchungen ueber die physiologische Wirkung verschiedener Handelssorten von Aconitin, u. Pseudoaconitin auf Muskeln u. Nerven," *Virch. Archiv*, Bd. 87, 1882, S. 410.

[478] *Lancet*, vol. i. p. 14.

of considerable social rank was the subject of the poisoning, the case has been imperfectly reported. It seems, however, that, whether for purposes of suicide, or experiment, or as a medicine, two grains and a half of aconitine were swallowed. The symptoms were very violent, consisting of vomiting, collapse, and attacks of muscular spasm; the narrator describes the vomiting as peculiar. "It, perhaps, hardly deserved that title; the patient was seized with a kind of general spasm, during which he convulsively turned upon his abdomen, and with an intense contraction of the abdominal muscles, he jerked out, as it were, with a loud shout the contents of his stomach, dependent apparently on the sudden contraction of the diaphragm." On attempting to make him swallow any fluid, a fearful spasm of the throat was produced; it reminded his medical attendants of hydrophobia. The patient recovered completely within twenty-four hours.

One of three cases reported by Dr. Albert Busscher,[479] of poisoning by aconitine nitrate, possesses all the exact details of an intentional experiment, and is of permanent value to toxicological literature.

A labourer of Beerta, sixty-one years of age, thin, and of somewhat weak constitution, suffered from neuralgia and a slight intermittent fever; Dr. Carl Meyer prescribed for his ailment:—

℞. Aconiti Nitrici, 2 grm.
Tr. Chenopodii Ambrosioid., 100 grms. M.D.S.

Twenty drops to be taken four times daily. The patient was instructed verbally by Dr. Meyer to increase the dose until he attained a maximum of sixty drops per day.

The doses which the man actually took, and the time of taking them, are conveniently thrown into a tabular form as follows:—

No.	1.	March 14,	7	p.m.,	5	drops	equal to	aconitine nitrate,	.4	mgrm.
,,	2.	,,	9	p.m.,	20	,,	,,	,,	1.6	,,
,,	3.	March 15,	8	a.m.,	20	,,	,,	,,	1.6	,,
,,	4.	,,	11	a.m.,	20	,,	,,	,,	1.6	,,
,,	5.	,,	4	p.m.,	20	,,	,,	,,	1.6	,,
,,	6.	,,	9	p.m.,	20	,,	,,	,,	1.6	,,
,,	7.	March 16,	10	p.m.,	10	,,	,,	,,	.8	,,

In the whole seven doses, which were distributed over forty-eight hours, he took 9.2 mgrms. (.14 grain) of aconitine nitrate.

On taking dose No. 1, he experienced a feeling of constriction (*Zusammenziehung*), and burning spreading from the mouth to the stomach, but this after a little while subsided. Two hours afterwards he took No. 2, four times the quantity of No. 1. This produced the same immediate symptoms, but soon he became cold, and felt very ill. He had an anxious oppressive feeling about the chest, with a burning feeling about the throat; the whole body was covered with a cold sweat, his sight failed, he became giddy, there was excessive muscular weakness, he felt as if he had lost power over his limbs, he had great difficulty in breathing. During the night he passed no water, nor felt a desire to do so. About half an hour after he had taken the medicine, he began to vomit violently, which relieved him much; he then fell asleep.

Dose No. 3, equal as before to 1.6 mgrm., he took in the morning. He experienced almost exactly the same symptoms as before, but convulsions were added, especially of the face; the eyes were also prominent; twenty minutes after he had taken the dose, vomiting came on, after which he again felt better.

He took dose No. 4, and had the same repetition of symptoms, but in the interval between the doses he felt weaker and weaker; he had no energy, and felt as if paralysed. No. 5 was taken, and produced, like the others, vomiting, after which he felt relieved. Neither he nor his wife seemed all this time to have had any suspicion that the medicine was really doing harm, but thought that the effects were due to its constant rejection by vomiting, so, in order to prevent vomiting with No. 6, he drank much cold water. After thus taking the medicine, the patient

479 *Intoxicationsfälle durch Aconitin Nitricum Gallicum, nebst Sections Bericht*, von Dr. Albert Busscher; *Berl. klinische Wochenschrift*, 1880, No. 24, pp. 338, 356.

seemed to fall into a kind of slumber, with great restlessness; about an hour and a half afterwards he cried, "I am chilled; my heart, my heart is terribly cold. I am dying; I am poisoned." His whole body was covered with perspiration; he was now convulsed, and lost sight and hearing; his eyes were shut, his lips cracked and dry, he could scarcely open his mouth, and he was extremely cold, and thought he was dying. The breathing was difficult and rattling; from time to time the muscular spasms came on. His wife now made a large quantity of hot strong black tea, which she got him to drink with great difficulty; although it was hot, he did not know whether it was hot or cold. About five minutes afterwards he vomited, and did so several times; this apparently relieved him, and he sank into a quiet sleep; during the night he did not urinate. In the morning the wife went to Dr. Carl Meyer, described the symptoms, and accused the medicine. So convinced was Dr. Meyer that the medicine did not cause the symptoms, that he poured out a quantity of the same, equal to 4 mgrms. of aconitine nitrate, and took it himself in some wine, to show that it was harmless, and ordered them to go on with it. The unhappy physician died of aconitine poisoning five hours after taking the medicine.[480] In the meantime, the woman went home, and her husband actually took a seventh, but smaller dose, which produced similar symptoms to the former, but of little severity; no more was taken.

The absence of diarrhœa, and of the pricking sensations so often described, is in this case noteworthy. Both diarrhœa and formication were also absent in a third case reported by Dr. Busscher in the same paper.

§ 436. The most important criminal case is undoubtedly that of Lamson:—At the Central Criminal Court, in March, 1882, George Henry Lamson, surgeon, was convicted of the murder of his brother-in-law, Percy Malcolm John. The victim was a weakly youth of eighteen years of age, paralysed in his lower limbs from old standing spinal disease. The motive for perpetrating the crime was that Lamson, through his wife (Malcolm John's sister), would receive, on the death of his brother-in-law, a sum of £1500, and, according to the evidence, it is probable that there had been one or more previous attempts by Lamson on the life of the youth with aconitine given in pills and in powders. However this may be, on November 24, 1880, Lamson purchased 2 grains of aconitine, came down on Dec. 3 to the school where the lad was placed, had an interview with his brother-in-law, and, in the presence of the head-master, gave Malcolm John a capsule, which he filled then and there with some white powder, presumed at the time to be sugar. Lamson only stayed altogether twenty minutes in the house, and directly after he saw his brother-in-law swallow the capsule, he left. Within fifteen minutes Malcolm John became unwell, saying that he felt as if he had an attack of heart-burn, and then that he felt the same as when his brother-in-law had on a former occasion given him a quinine pill. Violent vomiting soon set in, and he complained of pains in his stomach, a sense of constriction in his throat, and of being unable to swallow. He was very restless—so much so that he had to be restrained by force from injuring himself. There was delirium a few minutes before death, which took place about three hours and three-quarters after swallowing the fatal dose. The *post-mortem* appearances essentially consisted of redness of the greater curvature of the stomach, and the posterior portion of the same organ. In one part there was a little pit, as if a blister had broken; the rest of the viscera were congested, and the brain also slightly congested.[481]

§ 437. The symptoms of poisoning by the tincture, extract, or other preparation, do not differ from those detailed. As unusual effects, occasionally seen, may be noted profound unconsciousness lasting for two hours (Topham's case), violent twitching of the muscles of the face, opisthotonos, and violent convulsions. It is important to distinguish the symptoms which are not constant from those which are constant, or nearly so. The tingling and creeping sensations about the tongue, throat, lips, &c., are not constant; they certainly were not present in the remarkable German case cited earlier. Speaking generally, they seem more likely to occur after taking the root or the ordinary medicinal preparations. A dilated state of the pupil is by no means constant, and not to be relied upon. Diarrhœa is seen after taking the root or tincture by the stomach, but is often absent. In short, the only constant

---

[480] The symptoms suffered by Dr. Meyer are to be found in *Neder. Tijdschrift van Geneeskunde*, 1880, No. 16.

[481] To these cases of poisoning by the alkaloid aconitine may be added one recorded in Bouchardat's *Annuaire de Thérapeutie*, 1881, p. 276. The case in itself is of but little importance, save to illustrate the great danger in permitting the dispensing of such active remedies of varying strength. A gentleman suffering from "angina pectoris" was prescribed "Hottot's aconitine" in granules, and directed carefully to increase the dose up to four granules, according to the effect produced. The prescription was taken to a pharmacist, who, instead of supplying Hottot's aconitine, supplied some other of unknown origin. The medicine was taken daily, and the dose raised to four granules, which were taken with benefit until the whole was exhausted. He then went to Hottot's establishment, and had a fresh supply, presumably of the same substance, but a very little time after he had taken his usual dose of four granules, he suffered from symptoms of aconitine poisoning, headache, vertigo, feebleness of the voice, and muscular weakness, and was alarmingly ill. He recovered after some hours of medical treatment.

symptoms are difficulty of breathing, progressive muscular weakness, generally vomiting, and a weak intermittent pulse.

§ 438. **Physiological Action.**—Aconitine, according to Dr. S. Ringer, is a protoplasmic poison, destroying the functions of all nitrogenous tissue—first of the central nervous system, next of the nerves, and last of the muscles. Aconitine without doubt acts powerfully on the heart, ultimately paralysing it; there is first a slowing of the pulse, ascribed to a central excitation of the vagus; then a quickening, due to paralysis of the peripheral termination of the vagus in the heart; lastly, the heart's action becomes slow, irregular, and weak, and the blood-pressure sinks. The dyspnœa and convulsions are the usual result, seen among all warm-blooded animals, of the heart affection. Plugge found that the motor nerves, and more especially their intra-muscular terminations, were always paralysed; but if the dose was small the paralysis might be incomplete. Bœhm and Wartmann, on the other hand, considered that the motor paralysis had a central origin, a view not supported by recent research. The action of aconitine in this way resembles curare. The muscles themselves preserve their irritability, even after doses of aconitine which are five to ten times larger than those by which the nerve terminations are paralysed.

§ 439. **Post-mortem Appearances.**—Among animals (mammals) the appearances most constantly observed have been hyperæmia of the cerebral membranes and brain, a fulness of the large veins, the blood generally fluid—sometimes hyperæmia of the liver, sometimes not. When aconitine has been administered subcutaneously, there have been no inflammatory appearances in the stomach and bowels.

In the case of Dr. Carl Meyer, who died in five hours from swallowing 4 mgrms. of aconitine nitrate, the corpse was of a marble paleness, the pupils moderately dilated. The colour of the large intestine was pale; the duodenum was much congested, the congestion being most intense the nearer to the stomach; the mucous membrane of the stomach itself was strongly hyperæmic, being of an intense red colour; the spleen was enlarged, filled with much dark blood. The liver and kidneys were deeply congested, the lungs also congested; the right ventricle of the heart was distended with blood; in the pericardium there was a quantity of bloody serum. The brain was generally blood-red; in the cerebral hemispheres there were several large circumscribed subarachnoid extravasations. The substance of the brain on section showed many red bloody points.

In a case recorded by Taylor, in which a man died in three hours from eating a small quantity of aconitine root, the only morbid appearance found was a slight reddish-brown patch on the cardiac end of the stomach, of the size of half a crown; all the other organs being healthy.

§ 440. **Separation of Aconitine from the Contents of the Stomach or the Organs.**—It would appear certain that in all operations for the separation of aconite alkaloids (whether from the organic matters which make up the plant, or from those constituting animal tissues), mineral acids and a high heat should be avoided. A 1 per cent. sulphuric acid does not, however, hydrolyse, if acting in the cold, so that the process already given, may be followed.

The chemical examination in the Lamson case was entrusted to Dr. Stevenson, assisted by Dr. Dupré, and was conducted on the principles detailed. The contents of the stomach were treated with alcohol, and digested at the ordinary temperature of the atmosphere; the contents were already acid, so no acid in this first operation was added. The mixture stood for two days and was then filtered. The insoluble portion was now exhausted by alcohol, faintly acidulated by tartaric acid, and warmed to 60°; cooled and filtered, the insoluble part being washed again with alcohol. The two portions—that is, the spirituous extract acid from acids pre-existing in the contents of the stomach, and the alcohol acidified by tartaric acid—were evaporated down separately, exhausted by absolute alcohol, the solutions filtered, evaporated, and the residue dissolved in water. The two aqueous solutions were now mixed, and shaken up with ether, which, as the solution was acid, would not remove any alkaloid, but might remove various impurities; the residue, after being thus partially purified by ether, was alkalised by sodic carbonate, and the alkaloid extracted by a mixture of chloroform and ether. On evaporation of the chloroform and ether, the resulting extract was tested physiologically by tasting, and also by injections into mice. By means analogous to those detailed, the experts isolated aconitine from the vomit, the stomach, liver, spleen, and urine, and also a minute quantity of morphine, which had been administered to the patient to subdue the pain during his fatal attack. When tasted, the peculiar numbing, tingling sensation lasted many hours. These extracts were relied upon as evidence, for their physiological effect was identical with that produced by aconitine. For example, the extract obtained from the urine caused symptoms to commence in a mouse in two minutes, and death in thirty minutes, and the symptoms observed by injecting a mouse with known aconitine coincided in every particular with the symptoms produced by the extraction from the urine.

With regard to the manner of using "*life tests*," since in most cases extremely small quantities of the active principle will have to be identified, the choice is limited to small animals, and it is better to use mice or birds, rather than reptiles. In the Lamson case, subcutaneous injections were employed, but it is a question whether there is not less error in administering it by the mouth. If two healthy mice are taken, and the one fed with a little meal, to which a weighed quantity of the extract under experiment has been added, while to the other some meal mixed with a supposed equal dose of aconitine is given, then the symptoms may be compared; and several objections to any operative proceeding on such small animals are obviated. It is certain that any extract which causes distinct numbness of the lips will contain enough of the poison to kill a small bird or a mouse, if administered in the ordinary way.[482]

VI.—The Mydriatic Group of Alkaloids—Atropine—Hyoscyamine—Solanine—Cytisine.

1. ATROPINE.

§ 441. **Atropine (Daturine)**, $C_{17}H_{23}NO_3$.—This important alkaloid has been found in all parts of the *Atropa belladonna*, or deadly nightshade, and in all the species of *Datura*.

The *Atropa belladonna* is indigenous, and may be found in some parts of England, although it cannot be said to be very common. It belongs to the *Solanaceæ*, and is a herbaceous plant with broadly ovate entire leaves, and lurid-purple axillary flowers on short stalks; the berries are violet-black, and the whole of the plant is highly poisonous. The juice of the leaves stains paper a purple colour. The seeds are very small, kidney-shaped, weighing about 90 to the grain; they are covered closely with small, round projections, and are easily identified by an expert, who may be supposed to have at hand (as is most essential) samples of different poisonous seeds for comparison. The nightshade owes its poisonous properties to *atropine*.

The yield of the different parts of belladonna, according to Gunther,[483] is as follows:—

TABLE SHOWING THE ALKALOIDAL CONTENT OF VARIOUS PARTS OF THE BELLADONNA PLANT.

	Quantity of Alkaloids in the Fresh Substance, per cent.		Quantity of Alkaloids in the Dry Substance, per cent.	
	(*a*.) By Weighing.	(*b*.) By Titration.	(*a*.) By Weighing.	(*b*.) By Titration.
Leaves,	0 .2022	0 .20072	0 .838	0 .828
Stalk,	0 .0422	...	0 .146	...
Ripe fruit,	0 .2128	0 .20258	0 .821	0 .805
Seed,	0 .26676	...	0 .407	...
Unripe fruit,	0 .1870	0 .1930	0 .955	0 .955
Root,	0 .0792	...	0 .210	...

Atropine appears to exist in the plant in combination with malic acid. According to a research by Ladenburg, hyoscyamine is associated with atropine, both in the Belladonna and Datura plants.[484]

From a research by W. Schütte,[485] it appears that the younger roots of wild belladonna contain hyoscyamine only, whilst the older roots contain atropine as well as hyoscyamine, but only in small proportion; the same was observed to be the case in the older cultivated roots.

The ripe berries of cultivated *Atropa belladonna nigra* contain atropine and hyoscyamine; those of the wild plant contain atropine only; the ripe fruit of *Atropa belladonna lutea* contains only atropine and another base, perhaps identical with atropamine; the unripe fruit of wild *Atropa belladonna nigra* contains hyoscyamine, with only a small quantity of atropine.

---

482 Dr. A. Langaard has described a species of aconite root, named by the Japanese *Kŭsa-ūsū*. From his experiments on frogs and rabbits, its physiological action seems not to differ from that of aconitine generally.—*Ueber eine Art Japanische Akonit-knollen, Kŭsa-ūsū genannt, u. über das in denselben vorkommende Akonitin. Virchow's Archiv*, B. 79, 1880, p. 229.

483 *Pharm. Zeitschr. f. Russl.*, Feb., 1869; Dragendorff, *Die chemische Werthbestimmung einiger starkwirkenden Droguen*, St. Petersburg, 1874.

484 *Ber. der deutsch. Chem. Ges.*, Bd. 13.

485 *Arch. Pharm.*, ccxxix., 492-531; *Journ. Chem. Soc.* (abstract), February 1892, 231.

The leaves of the yellow and black-fruited wild *Atropa belladonna* contain hyoscyamine and atropine, the latter being in small quantity only.

Fresh and old seeds of *Datura Stramonium* contain chiefly hyoscyamine; small quantities of atropine and scopolamine are also present.

§ 442. **The Datura Stramonium or Thorn-apple** is also indigenous in the British Islands, but, like belladonna, it cannot be considered a common plant. Datura belongs to the Solanaceæ; it grows from 1 to 2 feet in height, and is found in waste places. The leaves are smooth, the flowers white; the fruit is densely spinous (hence the name thorn-apple), and is divided into four dissepiments below, two at the top, and containing many seeds.

The *Datura*, or the *Dhatura*-plants, of India have in that country a great toxicological significance, the white-flowered datura, or *Datura alba*, growing plentifully in waste places, especially about Madras. The purple-coloured variety, or *Datura fastuosa*, is also common in certain parts. There is a third variety, the *Datura atrox*, found about the coast of Malabar. The seeds of the white datura have been mistaken in India for those of capsicum. The following are some of the most marked differences:—

Seeds of the Common or White Datura.	Seeds of Capsicum.
(1.) Outline angular.	Outline rounded.
(2.) Attached to the placenta by a large, white, fleshy mass separating easily, leaving a deep furrow along half the length of the seed's concave border.	Attached to the placenta by a cord from a prominence on the concave border of the seed.
(3.) Surface scabrous, almost reticulate, except on the two compressed sides, where it has become almost glaucous from pressure of the neighbouring seeds.	Uniformly scabrous, the sides being equally rough with the borders.
(4.) Convex border thick and bulged with a longitudinal depression between the bulgings, caused by the compression of the two sides.	Convex border thickened, but uniformly rounded.
(5.) A suitable section shows the embryo curved and twisted in the fleshy albumen.	The embryo, exposed by a suitable section, is seen to resemble in outline very closely the figure 6.
(6.) The taste of the datura seeds is very feebly bitter. The watery decoction causes dilatation of the pupil.	The taste of capsicum is pungent; a decoction irritates the eye much, but does not cause dilatation of the pupil.

The identity of the active principle in both the datura and belladonna tribes is now completely established.[486]

§ 443. **Pharmaceutical Preparations.**—(*a.*) *Of the leaves. Extract of Belladonna.*—This contains, according to Squire,[487] from 0.73 to 1.7 per cent. of total alkaloids. *Belladonna Juice* (*succus belladonnæ*).—Strength in alkaloid about 0.05 per cent. *Tincture of Belladonna.*—Half the strength of the juice, and therefore yielding about 0.025 per cent. of alkaloid.

(*b.*) *Belladonna Root.*—*Belladonna plaster* contains 20 per cent. of alcoholic extract of belladonna. *Alcoholic Extract of Belladonna.*—This extract, according to Squire,[488] contains from 1.6 to 4.45 per cent. of alkaloid. *Belladonna liniment* is an alcoholic extract with the addition of camphor; its strength is about equal to 0.2 per cent. of alkaloid. *Belladonna ointment* contains about 10 per cent. of the alcoholic extract.

(*c.*) *The Alkaloid.*—*Atropine Discs* (*lamellæ atropinæ*).—These are discs of gelatin, each weighing about $^1/_{50}$

[486] See a research by Ernst Schmidt, "Ueber die Alkaloide der Belladonna-Wurzel u. des Stechapfel-Samens," *Lieb. Annl.*, Bd. 208, 1881.

[487] *Companion to the British Pharmacopœia*, 1894.

[488] *Companion to the British Pharmacopœia*, 1894.

grain, and containing for ophthalmic use $^{1}/_{5000}$ grain of atropine sulphate. Similar discs are made for hypodermic use, but stronger; each containing $^{1}/_{120}$ grain. *Solution of Atropine Sulphate.*—Strength about 1 per cent. *Atropine Ointment.*—Strength about 1 in 60, or 1.60 per cent. of atropine.

(*d.*) *Stramonium.*—An extract of the seeds is officinal in Britain; the alkaloidal content is from 1.6 to 1.8 per cent. There is also a tincture which contains about 0.06 per cent. of alkaloid.

§ 444. **Properties of Atropine,** $C_{17}H_{23}NO_3$.—Atropine, hyoscyamine, and hyoscine have all the same formula, but differ in their molecular constitution. Atropine by hydrolysis, either by heating it with hydrochloric acid or baryta water, is decomposed into tropine and tropic acid:—

$$\underset{\text{Atropine.}}{C_{17}H_{23}NO_3} + H_2O = \underset{\text{Tropine.}}{C_8H_{15}NO} + \underset{\text{Tropic acid.}}{C_9H_{10}O_3}.$$

On the other hand, by heating tropic acid and tropine together, atropine is regenerated. Hence it is proved by analysis and synthesis, that atropine is tropic acid-tropine, just as aconitine is benzoyl-aconine. Tropic acid has been produced synthetically by boiling β-chlorphenyl-propionic acid with potash, which at once shows its constitutional formula, viz.:—

$$C_6H_5CH\begin{cases} CH_2OH \\ COOH \end{cases}$$

Tropic acid has a melting-point of 117° to 118°. Tropine is a four-fold hydrated oxethyl-methyl-pyridine, and has the constitutional formula of $C_5H_3(H_4)(C_2H_4OH)N(CH_3)$; hence the constitutional formula of atropine is—

$$C_6H_5—CH\begin{cases} CH_2(OH) \\ CO—O(C_2H_4—C_5H_7=N—CH_3) \end{cases}$$

Tropine is a white, crystalline, strongly alkaline mass, melting at 60°, and volatilising at 230° undecomposed. It is soluble in water, alcohol, and ether, and gives precipitates with tannic acid, iodised hydriodic acid, Mayer's reagent, gold chloride, and mercuric chloride. Tropine gold chloride melts at 210° to 212°. Atropic acid ($C_9H_8O_2$), melting-point 198° to 200°, and isatropic acid ($C_9H_8O_2$), may also be obtained by the action of hydrochloric acid—the first, in radiating crystals, melting at 106°, and capable of distillation; the second, in thin rhombic plates, melting about 200°, and not volatile. Picric acid also gives a precipitate of beautiful plates. To obtain this the carbazotic acid must be in excess, and time must be given for the precipitate to form.

Atropine forms colourless crystals (mostly in groups or tufts of needles and prisms), which are heavier than water, and possess no smell, but an unpleasant, long-enduring, bitter taste. The experiments of E. Schmidt place the melting-point between 115° and 115.5°. It is said to sublime scantily in a crystalline form, but the writer has been unable to obtain any crystals by sublimation; faint mists collect on the upper disc, at about 123°, but they are perfectly amorphous.

Its reaction is alkaline; one part requires, of cold water, 300; of boiling, 58; of ether, 30; of benzene, 40; and of chloroform, 3 parts for solution. In alcohol and amyl alcohol it dissolves in almost every proportion. It turns the plane of polarisation weakly to the left.

§ 445. **Tests.**—Atropine mixed with nitric acid exhibits no change of colour. The same is the case with concentrated sulphuric acid in the cold; but on heating, there ensues the common browning, with development of a peculiar odour, likened by Gulielmo to orange flowers, by Dragendorff to the flowers of the *Prunus padus*, and by Otto to the *Spiræa ulmaria*—a sufficient evidence of the untrustworthiness of this as a distinctive test. The odour, indeed, with small quantities, is certainly not powerful, nor is it strongly suggestive of any of the plants mentioned. A far more intense odour is given off if a speck of atropine is evaporated to dryness with a few drops of strong solution of baryta, and heated strongly; the scent is decidedly analogous to that of hawthorn-blossom, and unmistakably agreeable.

By boiling a small quantity of atropine, say 1 mgrm., with 2 mgrms. of calomel and a very little water, the calomel blackens, and crystals may be obtained of a double salt; this reaction is, however, given also by hyoscyamine and homatropine. Mercuric potassium iodide solution, and mercuric bromide solution give amorphous precipitates, which, after a time, become crystalline, and have characteristic forms.

A solution of iodine in potassium iodide gives a precipitate with acidulated solutions of atropine in even a dilution of 1 : 10,000. Tannin precipitates, and the precipitate is soluble in excess of the reagent. If atropine be dissolved in dilute hydrochloric acid, and a 5 per cent. of gold chloride solution be added, a precipitate of a gold compound ($C_{17}H_{23}NO_3HClAuCl_3$) separates. The precipitate is in the form of rosettes or needles; melting-point 137°. On boiling it with water, however, it melts into oily drops, and this peculiar behaviour distinguishes it from the analogous salt of hyoscyamine, which does not melt in boiling water. The percentage of gold left on a combustion of atropine gold chloride is 31.35 per cent. 100 parts of the gold salt are equal to 46.2 of atropine. A platinum salt may also be obtained, $(C_{17}H_{23}NO_3HCl)_2,PtCl_4$, containing 29.5 per cent. of platinum.

Vitali's test is important; it consists in the production of a violet colour with alcoholic potash after oxidation.

The test may be applied as follows:—Equal parts, say 1 mgrm., of nitrate of sodium and of the substance to be tested, are rubbed together with a glass rod on a porcelain slab, and to this mixture 1 drop of sulphuric acid is added; the mixture is spread out in a thin film; upon this is strewn a little powdered potassium hydrate, and finally 1 drop of alcohol added; a violet colour is produced which passes into a fine red; according to the author of the test, 0.001 mgrm. of atropine sulphate can by this test be detected. Strychnine obscures this reaction.

Atropine, homatropine, and hyoscyamine show an alkaline reaction with phenolphthalein: atropine and homatropine give a precipitate with $HgCl_2$. Hyoscyamine, not cocaine, precipitates $HgCl_2$, and is alkaline to litmus, but not to phenolphthalein. Atropine behaves as follows:—(1) Sodium nitrate, sulphuric acid, and afterwards sodium hydroxide, gives a violet colour; (2) the test as before, but with nitrite instead of nitrate, gives orange colour, which, on dilution with sodium hydroxide solution, changes to red, violet, or lilac; (3) when heated with glacial acetic acid and sulphuric acid for a sufficient time, a greenish-yellow fluorescence is produced.—*Flückiger, Pharm. Journ. Trans.* (3), vol. xvi. p. 601-602.

The two alkaloids, strychnine and atropine, are not likely to be often together in the human body, but that it may sometimes occur is shown by a case recorded by L. Fabris.[489] A patient in the hospital at Padua had for some time been treated with daily injections of 3 mgrms. of strychnine nitrate; unfortunately, one day, instead of the 3 mgrms. of strychnine, the same quantity of atropine sulphate was injected, and the patient died after a few hours, with symptoms of atropine poisoning.

On chemical treatment of the viscera, a mixture of alkaloids was obtained which did not give either the reactions of strychnine or of atropine. To test the possibility of these alkaloids obscuring each other's reactions, mixtures of 3 per cent. solutions (the strength of the injections) of atropine sulphate and strychnine nitrate were mixed together, and strychnine tested for by the dichromate and sulphuric acid test.

A mixture of equal parts gave the strychnine reaction very clearly, but the atropine reaction not at all; 1 strychnine with 3 of atropine gave strychnine reaction, but not that of atropine; 1 strychnine with 4 atropine gave indistinct reaction for both alkaloids; 1 of strychnine with 5 of atropine gave a momentary atropine reaction, the violet was, however, almost immediately replaced by a red colour. Vitali's reaction was not clearly shown until the mixture was in the proportion of 9 of atropine to 1 of strychnine, but mixtures in the proportion of 3 strychnine and 1 atropine will give distinct mydriasis.

In such a case, of course, the strychnine should be separated from the atropine; this can be effected by precipitating the strychnine as chromate, filtering and recovering from the filter the atropine by alkalising and shaking it out with ether.

The atropine may be farther purified by converting it into oxalate, dissolving the oxalate in as small a quantity of alcohol as possible, and precipitating the oxalate out with ether; the precipitate is collected, dissolved in as small a quantity of water as possible, the water made alkaline, and the base shaken out with ether.

The most reliable test for atropine, or one of the mydriatic alkaloids, is its action on the iris; a solution of atropine, even so weak as 1 : 130,000, causing dilatation.[490] This action on the iris has been studied by Ruyter,[491] Donders, and von Graefe.

The action is local, taking effect when in dilute solution only on the eye to which it has been applied; and it has been produced on the eyes of frogs, not only in the living subject, but after the head has been severed from the body and deprived of brain. The thinner the cornea, the quicker the dilatation; therefore, the younger the person or animal, the more suitable for experiment. In frogs, with a solution of 1 : 250, dilatation commences in about five minutes; in pigeons, seven minutes; and in rabbits, ten minutes. In man, a solution of 1 : 120 commences to act in about six to seven minutes, reaches its highest point in from ten to fifteen minutes, and persists more or less for six to eight

[489] *Gazzetta*, xxii., i. 347-350.

[490] *De Actione Atropæ Belladonnæ in Iridem*, Traj. ad Rhen., 1852.

[491] *Arch. Ophthal.*, ix. 262, 1864.

days. A solution of 1 : 480 acts first in fifteen to twenty minutes, and reaches its greatest point in twenty minutes; a solution of 1 : 48,000 requires from three-quarters of an hour to an hour to show its effect. Dogs and cats are far more sensible to its influence than man, and therefore more suitable for experiment. If the expert chooses, he may essay the proof upon himself, controlling the dilatation by Calabar bean; but it is seldom necessary or advisable to make personal trials of this nature.[492]

§ 446. **Statistics of Atropine Poisoning.**—Since atropine is the active principle of belladonna and datura plants, and every portion of these—root, seeds, leaves, and fruit—has caused toxic symptoms, poisoning by any part of these plants, or by their pharmaceutical or other preparations, may be considered with strict propriety as atropine poisoning. Our English death statistics for the ten years ending 1892, record 79 deaths (50 males and 29 females) from atropine (for the most part registered under the head of belladonna); 29 (or 36.7 per cent.) were suicidal, the rest accidental.

The greatest number of the accidental cases arise from mistakes in pharmacy; thus, belladonna leaves have been supplied for ash leaves; the extract of belladonna has been given instead of extract of juniper; the alkaloid itself has been dispensed in mistake for theine;[493] a more curious and marvellously stupid mistake is one in which it was dispensed instead of assafœtida (Schauenstein, *op. cit.*, p. 652). Further, valerianate of atropine has been accidentally substituted for quinine valerianate, and Schauenstein relates a case in which atropine sulphate was administered subcutaneously instead of morphine sulphate; but the result was not lethal. Many other instances might be cited. The extended use of atropine as an external application to the eye naturally gives rise to a few direct and indirect accidents. Serious symptoms have arisen from the solution reaching the pharynx through the lachrymal duct and nose. A curious indirect poisoning, caused by the use of atropine as a collyrium, is related by Schauenstein.[494] A person suffered from all the symptoms of atropine poisoning; but the channel by which it had obtained access to the system was a great mystery, until it was traced to some coffee, and it was then found that the cook had strained this coffee through a certain piece of linen, which had been used months before, soaked in atropine solution, as a collyrium, and had been cast aside as of no value.

§ 447. **Accidental and Criminal Poisoning by Atropine.**—External applications of atropine are rapidly absorbed, *e.g.*, if the foot of a rat be steeped for a little while in a solution of the alkaloid, and the eyes watched, dilatation of the pupils will soon be observed. If the skin is broken, enough may be absorbed to cause death. A case is on record in which .21 grm. of atropine sulphate, applied as an ointment to the abraded skin, was fatal.[495] Atropine has also been absorbed from the bowel; in one case, a clyster containing the active principles of 5.2 grms. (80 grains) of belladonna root was administered to a woman twenty-seven years of age, and caused death. Allowing the root to have been carefully dried, and to contain .21 per cent. of alkaloid, it would seem that so little as 10.9 mgrms. (.16 grain) may even prove fatal, if left in contact with the intestinal mucous membrane. Belladonna berries and stramonium leaves and seeds are eaten occasionally by children. A remarkable series of poisonings by belladonna berries occurred in London during the autumn of 1846.

Criminal poisoning by atropine in any form is of excessive rarity in Europe and America, but in India it has been frightfully prevalent. In all the Asiatic cases the substance used has been one of the various species of datura, and mostly the bruised or ground seeds, or a decoction of the seeds. In 120 cases recorded in papers and works on Indian toxicology, I find no less than 63 per cent. of the cases criminal, 19 per cent. suicidal, and 18 per cent. accidental. In noting these figures, however, it must be borne in mind that known criminal cases are more certain to be recorded than any other cases. The drug has been known under the Sanscrit name of *dhatoora* by the Hindoos from most remote times. It was largely used by the Thugs, either for the purpose of stupefying their victim or for killing him; by loose wives to ensure for a time the fatuity of their husbands; and, lastly, it seems in Indian history to have played the peculiar *rôle* of a state agent, and to have been used to induce the idiocy or insanity of persons of high rank, whose mental integrity was considered dangerous by the despot in power. The Hindoos, by centuries of practice, have attained such dexterity in the use of the "datura" as to raise that kind of poisoning to an art, so that

---

[492] A. Ladenburg (*Compt. Rend.*, xc. 92), having succeeded in reproducing atropine by heating tropine and tropic acid with hydrochloric acid, by substituting various organic acids for the tropic acid, has obtained a whole series of compounds to which he has given the name of *tropeines*. One of these, hydroxytoluol (amygdalic) tropeine, he has named *homatropine*. It dilates the pupil, but is less poisonous than atropine.

[493] Hohl, *De Effectu Atropini. Diss. Halle*, 1863.

[494] Maschka's *Handbuch*.

[495] Ploss, *Zeitschr. f. Chir.*, 1863.

Dr. Chevers, in his *Medical Jurisprudence for India*,[496] declares that "there appears to be no drug known in the present day which represents in its effects so close an approach to the system of slow poisoning, believed by many to have been practised in the Middle Ages, as does the datura."

§ 448. **Fatal Dose.**—It is impossible to state with precision the exact quantity which may cause death, atropine being one of those substances whose effect, varying in different cases, seems to depend on special constitutional tendencies or idiosyncracies of the individual. Some persons take a comparatively large amount with impunity, while others scarcely bear a very moderate dose without exhibiting unpleasant symptoms. Eight mgrms. (⅛ grain) have been known to produce poisonous symptoms, and .129 grm. (2 grains) death. We may, therefore, infer that about .0648 grm. (1 grain) would, unchecked by remedies, probably act fatally; but very large doses have been recovered from, especially when treatment has been prompt.

Atropine is used in veterinary practice, from 32.4 to 64.8 mgrms. (½ to 1 grain) and more being administered subcutaneously to horses; but the extent to which this may be done with safety is not yet established.

§ 449. **Action on Animals.**—The action of atropine has been studied on certain beetles, on reptiles (such as the salamander, triton, frogs, and others), on guinea-pigs, hedgehogs, rats, rabbits, fowls, pigeons, dogs, and cats. Among the mammalia there is no essential difference in the symptoms, but great variation in the relative sensibility; man seems the most sensitive of all, next to man come the carnivora, while the herbivora, and especially the rodents, offer a considerable resistance. According to Falck the lethal dose for a rabbit is at least .79 mgrm. per kilo. It is the general opinion that rabbits may eat sufficient of the belladonna plant to render their flesh poisonous, and yet the animals themselves may show no disturbance in health; but this must not be considered adequately established. Speaking very generally, the higher the animal organisation the greater the sensibility to atropine. Frogs are affected in a peculiar manner. According to the researches of Fraser,[497] the animal is first paralysed, and some hours after the administration of the poison lies motionless, the only signs of life being the existence of a slight movement of the heart and muscular irritability. After a period of from forty-eight to seventy-two hours, the fore limbs are seized with tetanic spasms, which develop into a strychnine-like tetanus.

§ 450. **Action on Man.**—When atropine is injected subcutaneously, the symptoms, as is usually the case with drugs administered in this manner, may come on immediately, the pupil not unfrequently dilating almost before the injection is finished. This is in no way surprising; but there are instances in which decoctions of datura seeds have been administered by the stomach, and the commencement of symptoms has been as rapid as in poisoning by oxalic or even prussic acid. In a case tried in India in July 1852, the prosecutor declared that, while a person was handing him a *lota* of water, the prisoner snatched it away on pretence of freeing the water from dirt or straws, and then gave it to him. He then drank only two mouthfuls, and, complaining of the bitter taste, fell down insensible within forty yards of the spot where he had drunk, and did not recover his senses until the third day after. In another case, a man was struck down so suddenly that his feet were scalded by some hot water which he was carrying.—*Chevers.*

When the seeds, leaves, or fruit of atropine-holding plants are eaten, there is, however, a very appreciable period before the symptoms commence, and, as in the case of opium poisoning, no very definite rule can be laid down, but usually the effects are experienced within half an hour. The first sensation is dryness of the mouth and throat; this continues increasing, and may rise to such a degree that the swallowing of liquids is an impossibility. The difficulty in swallowing does not seem to be entirely dependent on the dry state of the throat, but is also due to a spasmodic contraction of the pharyngeal muscles. Tissore[498] found in one case such constriction that he could only introduce emetics by passing a catheter of small diameter. The mucous membrane is reddened, and the voice hoarse.[499] The inability to swallow, and the changed voice, bear some little resemblance to hydrophobia—a resemblance heightened to the popular mind by an inclination to bite, which seems to have been occasionally observed; the pupils are early dilated, and the dilatation may be marked and extreme; the vision is deranged, letters and figures often

[496] Dr. Chevers's work contains a very good history of datura criminal poisoning.

[497] *Transact. of Edin. Roy. Soc.*, vol. xxv. p. 449. *Journ. of Anat. and Physiol.*, May 1869, p. 357.

[498] *Gaz. hebd.*, 1856.

[499] A friend of the author's was given, by a mistake in dispensing, 16 minims of a solution of atropine sulphate, equivalent to ⅐ grain of atropine (or 9.3 mgrms). Ten minutes after taking the dose there was dilatation of the pupil, indistinctness of vision, with great dryness of the throat and difficulty in swallowing; he attempted to eat a biscuit, but, after chewing it, he was obliged to spit it out, as it was not possible to swallow; the throat was excessively sore, and there was a desire to pass urine, but only a few drops could be voided. In forty-five minutes he was unable to stand or walk. There was a bright rash on the chest. In two hours he became insensible, and was taken to the Middlesex Hospital, recovering under treatment in about eight hours.

appear duplicated; the eyeballs are occasionally remarkably prominent, and generally congested; the skin is dry, even very small quantities of atropine arresting the cutaneous secretion; in this respect atropine and pilocarpine are perfect examples of antagonism. With the dryness of skin, in a large percentage of cases, occurs a scarlet rash over most of the body. This is generally the case after large doses, but Stadler saw the rash produced on a child three months old by .3 mgrm. of atropine sulphate. It appeared three minutes after the dose, lasted five hours, and was reproduced by a renewed dose.[500] The temperature of the body with large doses is raised; with small, somewhat lowered. The pulse is increased in frequency, and is always above 100—mostly from 115 to 120, or even 150, in the minute. The breathing is at first a little slowed, and then very rapid. Vomiting is not common; the sphincters may be paralysed so that the evacuations are involuntary, and there may be also spasmodic contractions of the urinary bladder. The nervous system is profoundly affected; in one case there were clonic spasms,[501] in another,[502] such muscular rigidity, that the patient could with difficulty be placed on a chair. The lower extremities are often partly paralysed, there is a want of co-ordination, the person reels like a drunken man, or there may be general jactitation. The disturbance of the brain functions is very marked; in about 4 per cent. only of the recorded cases has there been no delirium, or very little—in the majority delirium is present. In adults this generally takes a garrulous, pleasing form, but every variety has been witnessed. Dr. H. Giraud describes the delirium from datura (which it may be necessary to again repeat is *atropine* delirium) as follows:—"He either vociferates loudly or is garrulous, and talks incoherently; sometimes he is mirthful, and laughs wildly, or is sad and moans, as if in great distress; generally he is observed to be very timid, and, when most troublesome and unruly, can always be cowed by an angry word, frequently putting up his hands in a supplicating posture. When approached he suddenly shrinks back as if apprehensive of being struck, and frequently he moves about as if to avoid spectra. But the most invariable accompaniment of the final stage of delirium, and frequently also that of *sopor*, is in the incessant picking at real or imaginary objects. At one time the patient seizes hold of parts of his clothes or bedding, pulls at his fingers and toes, takes up dirt and stones from the ground, or as often snatches at imaginary objects in the air, on his body, or anything near him. Very frequently he appears as if amusing himself by drawing out imaginary threads from the ends of his fingers, and occasionally his antics are so varied and ridiculous, that I have seen his near relatives, although apprehensive of danger, unable to restrain their laughter."[503] This active delirium passes into a somnolent state with muttering, catching at the bedclothes, or at floating spectra, and in fatal cases the patient dies in this stage. As a rule, the sleep is not like opium coma; there is complete insensibility in both, but in the one the sleep is deep, without muttering, in the other, from atropine, it is more like the stupor of a fever. The course in fatal cases is rapid, death generally taking place within six hours. If a person live over seven or eight hours, he usually recovers, however serious the symptoms may appear. On waking, the patient remembers nothing of his illness; mydriasis remains some time, and there may be abnormality of speech and weakness of the limbs, but within four days health is re-established. In cases where the seeds have been swallowed, the symptoms may be much prolonged, and they seem to continue until all the seeds have been voided—perhaps this is due to the imperfect but continuous extraction of atropine by the intestinal juices.

Chronic poisoning by atropine may, from what has been stated, be of great importance in India. It is probable that its continuous effect would tend to weaken the intellect, and there is no reason for any incredulity with regard to its power as a factor of insanity. Rossbach has ascertained that if dogs are, day after day, dosed with atropine, they become emaciated; but a certain tolerance is established, and the dose has to be raised considerably after a time to produce any marked physiological effect.

§ 451. **Physiological Action of Atropine.**—From the numerous experiments on animals which have been performed for the purpose of elucidating the action of atropine, it is clear that the terminations of the vagus in the heart muscle are first excited, and then paralysed. The excitor-motor ganglion is also paralysed, and finally the heart itself; death resulting from heart paralysis. The respiratory disturbance is also to be ascribed to the vagus; the terminations in the lung are paralysed, and, at the same time, the poison circulating through the respiratory nervous centre stimulates it first, and then it also becomes finally paralysed. The small vessels are generally widened after a previous transitory narrowing. Organs containing unstriped muscular fibre are generally paralysed, as well as the

[500] *Med. Times*, 1868.

[501] *Lancet*, vol. i., 1881, p. 414.

[502] *Ibid.*, vol. i., 1876, p. 346.

[503] In an English case of belladonna poisoning, the patient, a tailor, sat for four hours, moving his hands and arms as if sewing, and his lips as if talking, but without uttering a word.

ends of the nerves regulating secretion—hence the dryness of the skin. The action on the iris is not thoroughly elucidated.

§ 452. The *diagnosis* of atropine poisoning may be very difficult unless the attention of the medical man be excited by some suspicious circumstance. A child suffering from belladonna rash, with hot dry skin, quick pulse, and reddened fauces, looks not unlike one under an attack of scarlet fever. Further, as before mentioned, some cases are similar to rabies; and again, the garrulous delirium and the hallucinations of an adult are often very similar to those of *delirium tremens*, as well as tomania.

§ 453. **Post-mortem Appearances.**—The *post-mortem* appearances do not seem to be characteristic, save in the fact that the pupils remain dilated. The brain is usually hyperæmic, and in one case the absence of moisture seems to have been remarkable. The stomach and intestines may be somewhat irritated if the seeds, leaves, or other parts of the plant have been eaten; but the irritation is not constant if the poisoning has been by pure atropine, and still less is it likely to be present if atropine has been administered subcutaneously.

§ 454. **Treatment.**—The great majority of cases recover under treatment. In 112 cases collected by F. A. Falck, 13 only were fatal (11.6 per cent.). The greater portion of the deaths in India are those of children and old people—persons of feeble vitality. The Asiatic treatment, which has been handed down by tradition, is the application of cold water to the feet; but the method which has found most favour in England is treatment by pilocarpine, a fifth of a grain or more being injected from time to time. Pilocarpine shows as perfect antagonism as possible; atropine dries, pilocarpine moistens the skin; atropine accelerates, pilocarpine slows the respiration. Dr. Sydney Ringer and others have published a remarkable series of cases showing the efficacy of this treatment, which, of course, is to be combined where necessary with emetics, the use of the stomach-pump, &c.[504]

§ 455. **Separation of Atropine from Organic Tissues, &c.**—From the contents of the stomach, atropine may be separated by acidulating strongly with sulphuric acid (15 to 20 c.c. of dilute H_2SO_4 to 100 c.c.), digesting for some time at a temperature not exceeding 70°, and then reducing any solid matter to a pulp by friction, and filtering, which can generally be effected by the aid of a filter-pump. The liver, muscles,[505] and coagulated blood, &c., may also be treated in a precisely similar way. The acid liquid thus obtained, is first, to remove impurities, shaken up with amyl alcohol, and after the separation of the latter in the usual manner, it is agitated with chloroform, which will take up any of the remaining amyl alcohol,[506] and also serve to purify further. The chloroform is then removed by a pipette (or the separating flask before described), and the fluid made alkaline, and shaken up with ether, which, on removal, is allowed to evaporate spontaneously. The residue will contain atropine, and this may be farther purified by converting it into oxalate, as suggested earlier.

From the urine,[507] atropine may be extracted by acidifying with sulphuric acid, and agitation with the same series of solvents. Atropine has been separated from putrid matters long after death, nor does it appear to suffer any decomposition by the ordinary analytical operations of evaporating solutions to dryness at 100°. In other words, there seems to be no necessity for operations *in vacuo*, in attempts at separating atropine.

TABLE SHOWING THE ALKALOIDAL CONTENT OF VARIOUS PARTS OF THE HENBANE PLANT.

	Plant Destitute of Flowers.				Plant in Flower.				Plant in Fruit.			
	Hyosc.-Albus.		Hyosc.-Niger.		Hyosc.-Albus.		Hyosc.-Niger.		Hyosc.-Albus.		Hyosc.-Niger.	
	1868.	1869.	1868.	1869.	1868.	1869.	1868.	1869.	1868.	1869.	1868.	1869.
Seeds,	...	...	...	...	...	...	...	...	0.162	0.172	0.075	0.118
Leaves,	0.588	0.469	0.154	0.192	0.359	0.329	0.147	0.206	0.211	0.153	0.065	0.110
Stalk,	0.012	...	0.070	0.017	0.036	0.048	0.032	0.030	0.027	0.029	0.009	0.010
Root,	0.128	0.176	0.027	0.080	0.146	0.262	0.127	0.138	0.106	0.086	0.028	0.056

[504] See, for Dr. Ringer's cases, *Lancet*, vol. i., 1876, p. 346. Refer also to *Brit. Med. Journ.*, vol. i., 1881, p. 594; *ib.*, p. 659.

[505] Neither amyl alcohol nor chloroform removes atropine from an *acid* solution.

[506] Atropine goes into the blood, and appears to be present in the different organs in direct proportion to the quantity of blood they contain. Dragendorff has found in the muscles of rabbits fed upon belladonna sufficient atropine for quantitative estimation.

[507] Dragendorff has found atropine in the urine of rabbits fed with belladonna; the separation by the poison is so rapid that it often can only be recognised in the urine during the first hour after the poison has been taken.

2. HYOSCYAMINE.

§ 456. This powerful alkaloid is contained in small quantities in datura and belladonna, and also is found in the common lettuce (.001 per cent.),[508] and in *Scopola carmolica*, a solanaceous plant indigenous to Austria and Hungary;[509] but its chief source is the *Hyoscyamus niger* and *Hyoscyamus alba* (black and white henbane): it is also found in the *Duboisia myoporoides*. The latter plant was considered to contain a new alkaloid, "*Duboisine*," but duboisine is a mixture of hyoscyamine and hyoscine. Ladenburg's hyoscine accompanies hyoscyamine, and is an isomeride of both atropine and hyoscyamine; its chemical reactions are similar to those of hyoscyamine, as well as its physiological effects.[510]

Hyoscyamine ($C_{17}H_{23}NO_3$), as separated in the course of analysis, is a resinoid, sticky, amorphous mass, difficult to dry, and possessing a tobacco-like odour. It can, however, be obtained in well-marked odourless crystals, which melt at 108°-109°, a portion subliming unchanged. It liquefies under boiling water without crystallisation. According to Thorey,[511] hyoscyamine crystallises out of chloroform in rhombic tables, and out of benzene in fine needles; but out of ether or amyl alcohol it remains amorphous. When perfectly pure, it dissolves with difficulty in cold, but more readily in hot, water; if impure, it is hygroscopic, and its solubility is much increased. In any case, it dissolves easily in alcohol, ether, chloroform, amyl alcohol, benzene, and dilute acids. Hyoscyamine neutralises acids fully, and forms crystallisable salts, which assume for the most part the form of needles. It is isomeric with atropine, and is converted into atropine by heating to 110°, or warming with alcoholic potash. The gold salt melts at 159°, and does not melt in boiling water like the atropine gold salt.

§ 457. **Pharmaceutical and other Preparations of Henbane.**—The leaves are alone officinal in the European pharmacopœias; but the seeds and the root, or the flowers, may be met with occasionally, especially among herbalists. The table[512] will give an idea of the alkaloidal content of the different parts of the plant.

In order to ascertain the percentage of the alkaloid in any part of the plant, the process followed by Thorey has the merit of simplicity. The substance is first exhausted by petroleum ether, which frees it from fat; after drying, it is extracted with 85 per cent. alcohol at a temperature not exceeding 40°. The alcoholic extracts are then united, the alcohol distilled off, and the residue filtered. The filtrate is now first purified by agitation with petroleum ether, then saturated by ammonia, and shaken up with chloroform. The latter, on evaporation, leaves the alkaloid only slightly impure, and, after washing with distilled water, if dissolved in dilute sulphuric acid, a crystalline sulphate may be readily obtained.

A tincture and an extract of henbane leaves and flowering tops are officinal in most pharmacopœias; an extract of the seeds in that of France.

An oil of hyoscyamus is officinal in all the Continental pharmacopœias, but not in the British.

Henbane juice is recognised by the British pharmacopœia; it is about the same strength as the tincture.

An ointment, made of one part of the extract to nine of simple ointment, is officinal in the German pharmacopœia.

The tincture (after distilling off the spirit) and the extracts (on proper solution) may be conveniently titrated by Mayer's reagent which, for this purpose, should be diluted one-half; each c.c. then, according to Dragendorff, equalling 6.98 mgrms. of hyoscyamine. Kruse found 0.042 per cent. of hyoscyamine in a Russian tincture, and .28 per cent. in a Russian extract. Any preparation made with extract of henbane will be found to contain nitrate of potash, for Attfield has shown the extract to be rich in this substance. The ointment will require extraction of the fat by petroleum ether; this accomplished, the determination of its strength is easy.

The oil of hyoscyamus is poisonous, and contains the alkaloid. An exact quantitative research is difficult; but if 20 grms. of the oil are shaken up for some time with water acidified by sulphuric acid, the fluid separated from the oil, made alkaline, shaken up with chloroform, and the latter removed and evaporated, sufficient will be obtained to test successfully for the presence of the alkaloid, by its action on the pupil of the eye.

§ 458. **Dose and Effects.**—The dose of the uncrystalline hyoscyamine is 6 mgrms. ($^1/_{10}$ grain), carefully

508 T. S. Dymond, *Journ. Chem. Soc. Trans.*, 1892, 90.

509 W. R. Dunstan and A. E. Chaston. *Pharm. Journ. Trans.* (3), xx. 461-464.

510 See *Ber. der deutsch. Chem. Gesell.*, 13, 1549 to 1554. By boiling hyoscine hydrochloride with animal charcoal, and then precipitating with auric chloride, a good crystalline compound, melting at 198°, can be obtained.

511 *Pharm. Zeitschr. f. Russl.*, 1869.

512 This table, taken from Dragendorff's *Chemische Werthbestimmung einiger starkwirkenden Droguen*, embodies the researches of Thorey.

increased. I have seen it extensively used in asylums to calm violent or troublesome maniacs. Thirty-two mgrms. (½ grain) begin to act within a quarter of an hour; the face flushes, the pupils dilate, there is no excitement, all muscular motion is enfeebled, and the patient remains quiet for many hours, the effects from a single dose not uncommonly lasting two days. 64.8 mgrms. (1 grain) would be a very large, and possibly fatal, dose. The absence of delirium or excitement, with full doses of hyoscyamine, is a striking contrast to the action of atropine, in every other respect so closely allied; yet there are cases on record showing that the henbane root itself has an action similar to that of belladonna, unless indeed one root has been mistaken for another; *e.g.*, Sonnenschein relates the following ancient case of poisoning:—In a certain cloister the monks ate by error the root of henbane. In the night they were all taken with hallucinations, so that the pious convent was like a madhouse. One monk sounded at midnight the matins, some who thereupon came into chapel could not read, others read what was not in the book, others sang drinking songs—in short, there was the greatest disturbance.

§ 459. **Separation of Hyoscyamine from Organic Matters.**—The isolation of the alkaloid from organic tissues or fluids, in cases where a medicinal preparation of henbane, or of the leaves, root, &c., has been taken, is possible, and should be carried out on the principles already detailed. Hyoscyamine is mainly identified by its power of dilating the pupil of the eye. It is said that so small a quantity as .0083 mgrm. ($^1/_{4000}$ grain) will in fifteen minutes dilate the eye of a rabbit. It is true that atropine also dilates the pupil; but if sufficient of the substance should have been isolated to apply other tests, it can be distinguished from atropine by the fact that the latter gives no immediate precipitate with platinic chloride, whilst hyoscyamine is precipitated by a small quantity of platinic chloride, and dissolved by a larger amount, and also by the characters of the gold salt.

3. HYOSCINE.

§ 460. **Hyoscine**, $C_{17}H_{23}NO_3$.—According to E. Schmidt[513] the formula is $C_{17}H_{21}NO_4 + H_2O$, and the alkaloid is identical with scopolamine. Scopolamine has a m.p. of 59°, gives an aurochloride, crystallising in needles, the m.p. of which is 212° to 214°; when boiled with baryta water, it splits up into atropic acid and scopoline, a base ($C_8H_{13}NO$), m.p. 110°, boiling-point, 241° to 243°; scopoline forms an aurochloride, m.p. 223°-225°; and a platinochloride, m.p. 228°-230°; but Ladenburg,[514] in answer to Schmidt, asserts that hyoscine exists, and is not identical with scopolamine. A sample of commercial hyoscine hydrobromide Nagelvoort found to melt, water-free, at 198°; other commercial samples of hydrobromide melted at 179° and 186°; the latter sample giving an aurochloride which melted at 192°. Pure hyoscine gold chloride is stated to melt at 198°. Its reactions are much the same as those of atropine, but it does not blacken calomel. It is very poisonous.

According to experiments on animals, the heart is first slowed, then quickened; the first effect being due to a stimulation of the inhibitory nervous apparatus, the second to a paralysing action on the same. The temperature is not altered. The pupils are dilated, the saliva diminished. The irritability of the brain is lessened.[515]

4. SOLANINE.

§ 461. **Distribution of Solanine.**—Solanine is a poisonous nitrogenised glucoside found in all parts of the plants belonging to the nightshade order. The English common plants in which solanine occurs are the edible potato plant (*Solanum tuberosum*), the nightshade (*Solanum nigrum*), and the *Solanum dulcamara*, or bitter-sweet. The berries of the *Solanum nigrum* and those of *S. dulcamara* contain about 0.3 per cent. Mature healthy potatoes appear to contain no solanine, but from 150 grms. of diseased potatoes G. Kassner[516] separated 30 to 50 mgrms.

R. Firbas,[517] in a research on the active substances or young shoots of the *S. tuberosum* found two products—one crystalline, *Solanine*; the other amorphous, *Solaneine*. He gives the following formula to solanine—$C_{52}H_{93}NO_{18}4\frac{1}{2}H_2O$; when dried at 100° it becomes anhydrous. From a solution in 85 per cent. alcohol it crystallises in colourless needles, m.p. 244°; these are almost insoluble in ether and alcohol, but are readily dissolved in dilute hydrochloric acid. On hydrolysis solanine breaks up into solanidine and a sugar, according to the equation—

$$C_{52}H_{93}NO_{18} = C_{40}H_{61}NO_2 + 2C_6H_{12}O_6 + 4H_2O.$$

§ 462. **Properties of Solanine.**—The reaction of the crystals is weakly alkaline; the taste is somewhat bitter and pungent. Solanine is soluble in 8000 parts of boiling water, 4000 parts of ether, 500 parts of cold, and 125 of boiling alcohol. It dissolves well in hot amyl alcohol, but is scarcely soluble in benzene. An aqueous solution froths

[513] *Arch. Pharm.*, ccxxx. 207-231.

[514] *Ber.*, xxv. 2388-2394.

[515] Parloff, *St Petersburg Med. Chem. Acad.*, Dissert. No. 9, 1889-90.

[516] *Arch. Pharm.* (3), xxv. 402, 403.

[517] *Monatsh.*, x. 541-560; *Journ. Chem. Soc.* (Abst.), Jan. 1890.

on shaking, but not to the degree possessed by saponine solutions.

The amyl alcohol solution has the property of gelatinising when cold. It does this if even so little as 1 part of solanine is dissolved in 2000 of hot amyl alcohol. The jelly is so firm that the vessel may be inverted without any loss. This peculiar property is one of the most important tests for the presence of solanine. The hot ethylic alcohol solution will, on cooling, also gelatinise, but a stronger solution is required. From very dilute alcoholic solutions (and especially with slow cooling) solanine may be obtained in crystals. In dilute mineral acids solanine dissolves freely, and forms salts, which for the most part have an acid reaction and are soluble in alcohol and in water, but with difficulty in ether. The compounds with the acids are not very stable, and several of them are broken up on warming the solution, solanine separating out from the aqueous solutions of the solanine salts. The alkaloid may be precipitated by the fixed and volatile alkalies, and by the alkaline earths. Solanine will stand boiling with strongly alkaline solutions without decomposition; but dilute acids, on warming, hydrolyse. By heating solanine in alcoholic solution with ethyl iodide in closed tubes, and then treating the liquid with ammonia, ethyl solanine in well-formed crystals can be obtained. Solanine is precipitated by phosphomolybdic acid, but by very few other substances. It gives, for example, no precipitate with the following reagents:—Platinic chloride, gold chloride, mercuric chloride, potassic bichromate, and picric acid. Tannin precipitates it only after a time. Sodic phosphate gives a crystalline precipitate of solanine phosphate, if added to a solution of solanine sulphate. Both solanine and solanidine give with nitric acid at first a colourless solution, which, on gentle warming, passes into blue, then into light red, and lastly becomes weakly yellow. Solanine, dissolved in strong sulphuric acid, to which a little Fröhde's reagent is added, at first colours the fluid light brown; after standing some time the edges of the drop becomes reddish-yellow, and finally the whole a beautiful cherry-red, which gradually passes into dark violet when violet-coloured flocks separate.

§ 463. **Solanidine.**—Solanidine has stronger basic properties than solanine. Its formula is $C_{40}H_{61}NO_2$. It is obtained from an alcoholic solution in amorphous masses interspersed with needles; m.p. 191°. It dissolves readily in hot alcohol, with difficulty in ether. With hydrochloric acid it forms a hydrochloride—$3(C_{40}H_{61}NO_2HCl)HCl + H_2O$ or $1\frac{1}{2}H_2O$. This hydrochloride is a slightly yellow powder, only sparingly soluble in water, and carbonising without melting when heated to 287°. Solanidine also forms a sulphate, $3(C_{40}H_{61}NO_2H_2SO_4)H_2SO_4 + 8H_2O$; this salt is in the form of scaly plates, melting at 247°; it dissolves readily in water.

The sugar obtained from the hydrolysis of solanidine is a yellow amorphous mass dissolving readily in water and wood spirit, and has a specific rotatory power of $[\alpha]_D = + 28.623$. With Phenylhydrazine hydrochloride and sodium acetate in aqueous solution it forms a glucosazone, melting at 199°. It is probably a mixture of sugars.

Solaneine is the name that has been given to the amorphous substance accompanying solanine; on hydrolysis it yields solanidine and the same sugar as solanine. Its formula is $C_{52}H_{82}NO_{13}$ with $4H_2O$.

§ 464. **Poisoning from Solanine.**—Poisoning from solanine has been, in all recorded cases, induced, not by the pure alkaloid (which is scarcely met with out of the laboratory of the scientific chemist), but by the berries of the different species of *Solanum*, and has for the most part been confined to children. The symptoms in about twenty cases,[518] which may be found detailed in the medical literature of this century, have varied so greatly that the most opposite phenomena have been witnessed as effects of poisoning by the same substance. The most constant phenomena are a quick pulse, laboured respiration, great restlessness, and hyperæsthesia of the skin. Albumen in the urine is common. Nervous symptoms, such as convulsions, aphasia, delirium, and even catalepsy, have been witnessed. In some cases there have been the symptoms of an irritant poison—diarrhœa, vomiting, and pain in the bowels: in many cases dilatation of the pupil has been observed.

Rabbits are killed by doses of .1 grm. per kilo. The symptoms commence in about ten minutes after the administration, and consist of apathy and a low temperature; the breathing is much slowed. Convulsions set in suddenly before death, and the pupils become dilated. The *post-mortem* appearances in animals are intense redness and injection of the meninges of the cerebellum, of the medulla oblongata, and the spinal cord. Dark red blood is found in the heart, and the kidneys are hyperæmic. The intestinal mucous membrane is normal.

§ 465. **Separation of Solanine from the Tissues of the Body.**—Dragendorff has proved the possibility of separating solanine from animal tissues by extracting it from a poisoned pig. The best plan seems to be to extract

---

[518] See "Death of Three Children by *S. nigrum*"; Hirtz., *Gaz. Med. de Strasbourg*, 1842; Maury, *Gaz. des Hôp.*, 1864; J. B. Montane, *Chim. Med.*, 1862; Magne, *Gaz. des Hôp.*, 1869; Manners, *Edin. Med. Journ.*, 1867. Cases of poisoning by bitter-sweet berries are recorded in *Lancet*, 1856; C. Bourdin, *Gaz des Hôpitaux*, 1864; Bourneville, the berries of *S. tuberosum*, *Brit. Med. Journ.*, 1859.

with cold dilute sulphuric acid water, which is then made alkaline by ammonia, and shaken up with warm amyl alcohol. This readily dissolves any solanine. The peculiar property possessed by the alkaloid of gelatinising, and the play of colours with Fröhde's reagent, may then be essayed on the solanine thus separated.

5. CYTISINE.

§ 466. **The Cytisus Laburnum.**—The laburnum tree, *Cytisus laburnum*, so common in shrubberies, is intensely poisonous. The flowers, bark, wood, seeds, and the root have all caused serious symptoms. The active principle is an alkaloid, to which the name of Cytisine has been given. The best source is the seeds. The seeds are powdered and extracted with alcohol containing hydrochloric acid, the alcohol distilled off, the residue treated with water and filtered through a wet filter to remove any fatty oil, the filtrate treated with lead acetate; and, after separating the precipitated colouring matter, made alkaline with caustic potash, and shaken with amyl alcohol. The amyl alcohol is shaken with dilute hydrochloric acid, the solution evaporated, the crude crystals of hydrochloride thus obtained treated with alcohol to remove colouring matters, and recrystallised several times from water; it then forms well-developed, colourless, transparent prisms. From the hydrochloride the free base is readily obtained.

Cytisine, $C_{11}H_{14}N_2O$.—To cytisine used to be ascribed the formula $C_{20}H_{27}N_3O$, but a study of the salt and new determinations appear to prove that it is identical with ulexine.[519] Cytisine is in the form of white radiating crystals, consisting, when deposited from absolute alcohol, of anhydrous prisms, which melt at from 152° to 153°. Cytisine has a strong alkaline reaction; it is soluble in water, alcohol, and chloroform, less so in benzene and amyl alcohol, almost insoluble in cold light petroleum, and insoluble in pure ether. The specific rotatory power in solution is $[\alpha]_D 17° = -119.57$.

It is capable of sublimation in a current of hydrogen at 154.5°; the sublimate is in the form of very long needles and small leaflets; at higher temperatures it melts to a yellow oily fluid, again becoming crystalline on cooling. Cytisine is a strong base; it precipitates the earths and oxides of the heavy metals from solutions of the chlorides, and, even in the cold, expels ammonia from its combinations.

Cytisine forms numerous crystalline salts, among which may be mentioned two platinochlorides, $C_{11}H_{14}N_2OH_2PtCl_6 + 2\frac{1}{2}H_2O$ and $(C_{11}H_{14}N_2O)_2H_2PtCl_6$, crystallising in golden yellow needles, which are tolerably soluble in water; and the aurochloride, $C_{11}H_{14}N_2OHAuCl_4$, crystallising in short, red-brown, hook-shaped needles; m.p. 212° to 213°, without evolution of gas.

§ 467. **Reactions of Cytisine.**—Concentrated sulphuric acid dissolves cytisine without colour; if to the solution is added a drop of nitric acid, it becomes orange-yellow, and on addition of a crystal of potassic bichromate, first yellow, then dirty brown, and lastly green. Concentrated nitric acid dissolves the base in the cold without colour, but, on warming, it becomes orange-yellow. Picric, tannic, and phosphomolybdic acids, potassic, mercuric, and potass. cadmium iodides, and iodine with potassic iodide, all give precipitates. Neither potassic bichromate nor mercuric chloride precipitates cytisine, even though the solution be concentrated. The best single test appears to be the reaction discovered by Magelhaes; this consists in adding thymol to a solution of cytisine in concentrated sulphuric acid, when a yellow colour, finally passing into an intense red, is produced.

§ 468. **Effects on Animals.**—W. Marmé found subcutaneous doses of from 30 to 40 mgrms. fatal to cats; death was from paralysis of the respiration, and could be avoided by artificial respiration. Cattle are sometimes accidentally poisoned by laburnum. An instance of this is recorded in the *Veterinarian* (vol. lv. p. 92). In Lanark a storm had blown a large laburnum tree down to the ground; it fell into a field in which some young heifers were grazing, and they began to feed on the leaves and pods. Two or three died, and three more were ill for some time, but ultimately recovered.

The laburnum, however, does not always have this effect, for there is a case related in the *Gardeners' Chronicle*, in which five cows browsed for some time on the branches and pods of an old laburnum tree that had been thrown aside. Rabbits and hares are said to feed eagerly, and without injury, on the pods and branches.

§ 469. **Effects on Man.**—The sweet taste of many portions of the laburnum tree, as well as its attractive appearance, has been the cause of many accidents. F. A. Falck has been able to collect from medical literature no less than 155 cases—120 of which were those of the accidental poisoning of children: only 4 (or 2.6 per cent.), however, died, so that the poison is not of a very deadly character.

[519] A. W. Gerrard and W. H. Symons dispute this; they ascribe to ulexine the formula of $C_{11}H_{14}N_2O$, to cytisine $C_{20}H_{27}N_3O$. Ulexine is very hygroscopic, cannot be sublimed, even in a vacuum, without decomposition, and dissolves readily in chloroform; on the contrary, cytisine is not hygroscopic, sublimes completely, and is almost insoluble in chloroform, *Pharm. J.* (3), xx. 1017. A. Partheil, *Ber.*, xxiii. 3201-3203; *Arch. Pharm.*, ccxxx. 448-498.

One of the earliest recorded cases is by Christison.[520] A servant-girl of Inverness, in order to excite vomiting in her fellow-servant (the cook), boiled some laburnum bark in soup; very soon after partaking of this soup, the cook experienced violent vomiting, which lasted for thirty-six hours; she had intense pain in the stomach, much diarrhœa, and great muscular weakness; she appears to have suffered from gastro-intestinal catarrh for some time, but ultimately recovered.

Vallance[521] has described the symptoms observed in the poisoning of fifty-eight boys, who ate the root of an old laburnum tree, being allured by its sweet taste. All were taken ill with similar symptoms, differing only in severity; two who had eaten half an ounce (nearly 8 grms.) suffered with especial severity. The symptoms were first vomiting, then narcosis, with convulsive movements of the legs and strange movements of the arms: the pupils were dilated. This dilatation of the pupil Sedgwick also saw in the poisoning of two children who ate the root. On the other hand, when the flower, seeds, or other portions of the laburnum have been eaten, the symptoms are mainly referable to the gastro-intestinal tract, consisting of acute pain in the stomach, vomiting, and diarrhœa. On these grounds it is therefore more than probable that there is another active principle in the root, differing from that which is in those portions of the tree exposed to the influence of sunlight.[522]

The *post-mortem* appearances are, so far as known, in no way characteristic.

VII.—The Alkaloids of the Veratrums.

§ 470. The alkaloids of the veratrums have been investigated by Dr. Alder Wright, Dr. A. P. Luff, and several other chemists.[523]

The method which Wright and Luff adopted to extract and separate these alkaloids from the root of *V. album* and *V. viride*, essentially consisted in exhausting with alcohol, to which a little tartaric acid has been added, filtering, distilling off the alcohol, dissolving the residue in water, alkalising with caustic soda, and shaking up with ether. The ethereal solution was next separated, and then washed with water containing tartaric acid, so as to obtain a solution of the bases as tartrates: in this way the same ether could be used over and over again. Ultimately a rough separation was made by means of the different solubilities in ether, pseudo-jervine being scarcely soluble in this medium, whilst jervine, veratralbine, veratrine, and cevadine are very soluble in it.

The yield of Wright and Luff's alkaloids was as follows:—

TABLE SHOWING THE ALKALOIDS IN THE VERATRUMS.

	V. album. Per Kilo.	V. viride. Per Kilo.
Jervine,	1.3 grm.	.2 grm.
Pseudo-jervine,	.4 „	.15 „
Rubi-jervine,	.25 „	.02 „
Veratralbine,	2 .2 „	Traces.
Veratrine,	.05 „	Less than .004 grm.
Cevadine,	Absent.	„ .43 „

From whence it appears that *V. album* has only a very small quantity of veratrine, that it is almost absent in *V. viride*; on the other hand, *V. viride* contains a fair quantity of cevadine, an alkaloid absent in *V. album*.

Besides the six principles enumerated, G. Salzberger has recently separated two other crystalline substances, to which he has given the names of *protoveratrine* and *protoveratridine*, and Pehkschen has also separated a ninth substance, to which he has given the name of *veratroidine*.

The formulæ of the nine bodies which have been separated from hellebore root are as follows:—

---

[520] *Ed. Med. Journ.*, 1843.

[521] *Brit. Med. Journ.*, 1875.

[522] See also a case related by Dr. Popham, in which ten children ate laburnum seeds; the pupils were dilated. They all recovered. *B. and F. Med. Chir. Review*, Ap. 1863; also a case reported by H. Usher, *Med. Times and Gazette*, Sept. 15, 1862.

[523] "The Alkaloids of the Veratrums," by C. R. Alder Wright, D.Sc., and A. P. Luff, *Journ. Chem. Soc.*, July 1879; "The Alkaloids of *Veratrum viride*," by C. Alder Wright, D.Sc., *ib.*, 1879.

			Melting-point.
1.	Veratrine,	$C_{37}H_{53}NO_{11}$,	...
2.	Cevadine,	$C_{32}H_{49}NO_9$,	205°-206°
3.	Protoveratrine,	$C_{32}H_{51}NO_{11}$,	245°-250°
4.	Pseudo-jervine, -	$C_{29}H_{43}NO_7$ (*Wright*),	299°-300°
		$C_{29}H_{49}NO_{12}$ (*Pehkschen*),	...
5.	Veratralbine,	$C_{28}H_{43}NO_5$,	...
6.	Protoveratridine,	$C_{26}H_{45}NO_8$,	265°
7.	Rubi-jervine, -	$C_{26}H_{43}NO_2$ (*Wright* and *Luff*),	236°
		(*Salzberger*),	240°-245°
8.	Jervine,	$C_{26}H_{37}NO_3 2H_2O$,	237°-239°
9.	Veratroidine,	$C_{32}H_{53}NO_9$,	149°

Three of these alkaloids possess powerful sternutatory properties, the least quantity applied to the nostrils exciting sneezing; the three are veratrine, cevadine, and protoveratrine.

Protoveratrine, $C_{32}H_{51}NO_{11}$, has been obtained by G. Salzberger[524] from powdered hellebore root, by the following process:—

The powdered root is first freed from fatty and resinous matters by treatment with ether, and then the fat-free powder is exhausted with alcohol. The alcohol is evaporated off in a vacuum, the extract mixed with much acetic acid water, filtered from the insoluble residue, and treated with metaphosphoric acid; the voluminous precipitate contains much amorphous matter, with insoluble compounds of jervine and rubi-jervine. The precipitate is filtered off, and the filtrate treated with excess of ammonia and shaken up with ether. On separating the ether and distilling, protoveratrine crystallises out, and can be obtained pure by recrystallisation from strong alcohol.

Protoveratrine crystallises in four-sided plates, which melt with charring at 245° to 250°. The base is insoluble in water, benzene, and light petroleum; chloroform and boiling 96 per cent. alcohol dissolve it somewhat; cold ether scarcely touches it, boiling ether dissolves it a little.

Concentrated sulphuric acid dissolves the alkaloid slowly with the production of a greenish colour, which passes to cornflower blue, and, after some hours, becomes violet. Sulphuric acid and sugar gives a different colour to that produced by commercial veratrine. There is first a green colour which darkens into olive green, then becomes dirty green, and finally dark brown. When warmed with strong sulphuric, hydrochloric, or phosphoric acids, there is a strong odour of isobutyric acid developed. Dilute solutions of the salts are precipitated by ammonia, Nessler's reagent, gold chloride, potassium mercury iodide, cadmium iodide, phosphotungstic acid, and picric acid; no precipitate is produced by tannin, platinum chloride, or mercuric chloride.

§ 471. **Veratrine** ($C_{37}H_{53}NO_{11}$) is a crystallisable alkaloid, which is a powerful irritant of the sensory nerves of the mucous membrane, and excites violent sneezing. Treated with concentrated sulphuric acid, it dissolves with a yellow colour, deepening into orange, then into blood-red, and finally passing into carmine-red. If the freshly-prepared sulphuric acid solution is now treated with bromine water, a beautiful purple colour is produced. Concentrated hydrochloric acid dissolves veratrine without the production of colour, but, with careful warming, it becomes beautifully red. This reaction is very delicate, occurring with .17 mgrm. On saponification veratrine yields veratric acid.

Veratric acid is procatechu-dimethylether acid, and has the constitutional formula,

$$C_6H_3\left\langle\begin{matrix}COOH\\(OCH_3)_2\end{matrix}\right.$$

Veratric acid forms colourless needles and four-sided prisms which have a marked acid reaction; it melts on heating to a colourless fluid, and sublimes without decomposition; it is easily soluble in hot alcohol, but insoluble in ether. If dissolved in nitric acid, water separates nitro-veratric acid, $C_9H_9(NO_2)O_4$ which crystallises out of alcohol

[524] *Arch. Pharm.*, ccxxviii. 462-483.

in small yellow scales. Veratric acid unites with bases forming crystalline salts; the silver salt has the composition of $C_9H_9AgO_4$ = 37.37 per cent. silver, and may assist in identification. It is crystalline with a melting point of 205° to 206°.

Cevadine, $C_{32}H_{49}NO_9$ (Merck's veratrine).—It has powerful sternutatory properties, and, under the influence of alcoholic potash, yields tiglic[525] acid and cevine, $C_{27}H_{43}NO_8$.

According to Ahrens, angelic acid is first formed, and then converted into tiglic acid. When the alkaloid is boiled with hydrochloric acid, tiglic acid is formed, and a ruby red mass. Nitric acid oxidises cevadine completely; with potassic permanganate it yields acetic and oxalic acids; with chromic acid it forms acetaldehyde and carbon dioxide.[526]

The Continental authorities always give to cevadine the name of veratrine. Cevadine forms a crystalline aurochloride, a crystalline mercurochloride, $C_{32}H_{49}NO_9HHgCl_3$, and a crystalline picrate, $C_{32}H_{49}NO_9C_6H_3N_8O_7$. The mercury salt crystallises in small silvery plates, and melts with decomposition at 172°. The picrate forms stable crystals blackening at 225°; both of the latter salts are but little soluble in water, but are soluble in alcohol. Cevadine also unites with bromine, forming a tetrabromide, an amorphous yellow powder insoluble in water, but readily soluble in alcohol, ether, and chloroform.

§ 472. **Jervine**, ($C_{26}H_{37}NO_32H_2O$) (*Wright* and *Luff*), $C_{14}H_{22}NO_2$ (*Pehkschen*),[527] crystallises in white needles, and, when anhydrous, melts at 237.7°. It is slightly lævorotatory. At 25° one part of the base dissolves in 1658 benzene, 268 ether, 60 chloroform, and 16.8 absolute alcohol. It is insoluble in light petroleum, and but slightly soluble in ethyl acetate, water, or carbon bisulphide. It forms a very insoluble sulphate, and a sparingly soluble nitrate and hydrochloride. Jervine gives, with sulphuric acid and sugar, a violet colour, passing to blue. Treated with strong sulphuric acid it dissolves to a yellow fluid, which becomes successively dark yellow, brownish yellow, and then greenish. The green shade is immediately developed by diluting with water. Jervine does not produce sneezing.

§ 473. **Pseudo-jervine**, $C_{29}H_{43}NO_7$ (*Wright*), m.p. 299°; $C_{29}H_{49}NO_{12}$, m.p. 259° (*Pehkschen*), may be obtained in a crystalline state. One part is soluble in 10.9 parts of light petroleum, 372 parts of benzene, 1021 parts of ether, 4 of chloroform, and 185 of absolute alcohol. The pure base gives no colour with sulphuric, nitric, or hydrochloric acids. It does not produce sneezing.

§ 474. **Protoveratridine**, $C_{26}H_{45}NO_8$, is probably derived from protoveratrine. Salzberger[528] isolated it from powdered hellebore roots by treating the powder with barium hydroxide and water, and extracting with ether. The ether extract was separated and freed from ether in a current of hydrogen at a low temperature.

From the dark green syrup obtained jervine crystallised out, and from the mother liquor ultimately protoveratridine was separated.

Protoveratridine crystallises in colourless four-sided plates, which melt at 265°. It is almost insoluble in alcohol, chloroform, methyl alcohol, and acetone, and insoluble in benzene, light petroleum, and ether. Concentrated sulphuric acid gives a violet, then a cherry-red colour. Its solution in concentrated hydrochloric acid becomes light red on warming, and there is an odour of isobutyric acid. It is readily soluble in dilute mineral acids, and the solution, on the addition of ammonia, yields the alkaloid in a crystalline condition. The sulphuric acid solution gives precipitates with phosphotungstic, picric, and tannic acids, and with potassium mercury iodide; but gives no precipitate with platinum chloride, potassium-cadmium iodide, or with Millon's reagent.

It forms a platinum salt, $(C_{26}H_{45}NO_8)_2H_2PtCl_6 + 6H_2O$, which is precipitated in large six-sided plates on adding alcohol to a mixed solution of platinum chloride and a salt of the base.

Protoveratridine is not poisonous, and does not cause sneezing. Its solutions are very bitter.

§ 475. **Rubi-jervine**, $C_{26}H_{43}NO_2$, is a crystallisable base wholly different from jervine, yet probably closely allied to it. It forms a light yellow, indistinctly crystalline gold salt ($C_{26}H_{43}NO_2$,HCl,$AuCl_3$): it gives a different play of colours from jervine with sulphuric acid. The concentrated acid dissolves rubi-jervine to a clear yellow fluid, becoming successively dark yellow, brownish yellow, and brownish blood-red, changing after several hours to a brownish purple. On diluting slightly with water the brownish-red liquid, it becomes successively crimson, purple, dark lavender, dark violet, and ultimately light indigo. Its hydrochloride and sulphate are both more soluble than

[525] Tiglic acid, $C_5H_8O_2$, is a volatile acid, m.p. 64°, boiling point, 198.5°; it forms a soluble barium salt, and an insoluble silver salt.

[526] *Ber.*, xxiii. 2700-2707.

[527] *Jour. Pharm.* (5), xxii. 265-269.

[528] *Arch. Pharm.*, ccxxviii. 462-483.

either of the corresponding salts of jervine or pseudo-jervine.

§ 476. **Veratralbine,** $C_{28}H_{43}NO_5$, an amorphous non-sternutatory base, gives, when a speck of the substance is dissolved in sulphuric acid, a play of colours, becoming successively yellow, dark yellow, brownish orange, and brownish blood-red, with a strong green fluorescence. It yields no acid on saponification.

§ 477. **Veratroidine,** $C_{32}H_{53}NO_9$, is another base which has been separated by C. Pehkschen.[529] Its melting point is 149°. One part dissolves in 13 of benzene, 59 of chloroform, and 9 of ether. It yields amorphous salts with the mineral acids, and with oxalic and acetic acids. It is precipitated by most of the group reagents. With 11 per cent. solution of hydrochloric acid it gives a beautiful rose colour.

§ 478. **Commercial Veratrine.**—Commercial veratrine is a mixture of alkaloids, and has usually fairly constant properties, one of which is its intense irritant action on the nostrils. Placed on moist blue-red litmus paper it gives a blue spot. It is but little soluble in water, 1 : 1500; but readily dissolves in alcohol and chloroform; it is but little soluble in amyl alcohol, benzene, and carbon disulphide.

When a very small quantity is treated with a drop of sulphuric acid, the acid in the cold strikes a yellow colour; on warming, the colour becomes violet, slowly changing to orange and cherry red. Sensible to 100th of mgrm. If this test is performed in a test-tube, a green-yellow fluorescence is also seen on the sides of the test-tube.

Commercial veratrine strikes a pink-red colour with hydrochloric acid in the cold if a long time is allowed to elapse, but it at once appears if the acid is warmed, and is permanent. The solution becomes fluorescent if two drops of acetic acid are added.

If a small quantity of commercial veratrine is added to melted oxalic acid and the warming continued, a blood-red colour is obtained.

Veratrine, warmed with syrupy phosphoric acid, develops an odour of butyric acid.

A dark green colour, followed by reddish purple and blue colours, is obtained by adding a sprinkling of finely-powdered sugar to a solution of veratrine in sulphuric acid. This is best seen with a solution of 1 to 10,000; if in dilution of 1 to 100,000 a grass-green colour is produced, followed by purple and blue colours, quickly changing to brown or black.[530]

When two or three drops of sulphuric acid and furfur aldehyde (5 drops to 10 c.c. of acid) are added to minute particles of alkaloids, a more or less characteristic colour makes its appearance; this is particularly the case with veratrine. A few particles rubbed with a glass rod, and moistened with the reagent, gives first a yellowish-green, then an olive-green mixture, the edges afterwards becoming a beautiful blue. On warming, the mixture gradually acquires a purple-violet colour. The blue substance obtained in the cold is insoluble in alcohol, ether, or chloroform. The least amount of water decolorises the solution, and, on adding much water, a fairly permanent yellow solution is obtained.[531]

§ 479. **Pharmaceutical Preparations.**—The alkaloid is officinal in the English, American, and Continental pharmacopœias. There is also an *unguentum veratrinæ*—strength about 1.8 per cent. In the London pharmacopœia of 1851 there used to be a wine of white hellebore, the active principle of 20 parts of the root by weight being contained in 100 parts by measure of the wine. Such a wine would contain about 0.084 per cent. of total alkaloids. Of the green hellebore there is a tincture (*tinctura veratri viridis*), to make which four parts by weight of the root are exhausted by 20 parts by measure of spirits; the strength varies, but the average is 0.02 per cent. of total alkaloids.

§ 480. **Fatal Dose.**—The maximum dose of the commercial alkaloid is laid down as 10 mgrms. (.15 grain), which can be taken safely in a single dose, but nothing sufficiently definite is known as to what is a lethal dose. 1.3 grm. of the powdered rhizome has caused death, and, on the other hand, ten times that quantity has been taken with impunity, so that at present it is quite an open question.

§ 481. **Effects on Animals—Physiological Action.**—Experiments on animals have proved that the veratrums act on the sensory nerves of the skin, and those of the mucous membranes of the nose and intestinal canal; they are first excited, afterwards paralysed. When administered to frogs, sugar and lactic acid appear in the urinary excretion.[532] It exercises a peculiar influence on voluntary muscle; the contractility is changed, so that, when excited, there is a long-continuing contraction, and from a single stimulus more heat is disengaged than with healthy muscle; the motor nerves are also affected. The respiration, at first quickened, is then slowed, and finally paralysed. The

[529] *Op. cit.*

[530] *Flückiger's Reactions*, 1893.

[531] A. Wender, *Chem. Zeitung*, xvii. 950, 951.

[532] *Zeit. Phys. Chem.*, xvi. 453-459.

heart's action is also first quickened, the blood-pressure at the same time is raised, and the small arteries narrowed in calibre; later follow sinking of the pressure, slowing of the heart, and dilatation of the vessels, and the heart becomes finally paralysed.

§ 482. **Effects on Man.**—Poisoning by veratrum, sabadilla, or pharmaceutical preparations containing veratrine, is not common. Plenk witnessed a case in which the external application of sabadilla powder to the head caused delirium, and Lentin also relates a case in which an infant at the breast seems to have died from an external application made for the purpose of destroying lice. In both instances, however, there is a possibility that some of the medicament was swallowed.

Blas recorded, in 1861, the case of two children who drank a decoction of white hellebore, the liquid being intended as an external application to an animal. They showed serious symptoms, but ultimately recovered.

A scientific chemist took 3.8 grms. (58 grains) of the tincture of green hellebore for the purpose of experiment. There followed violent symptoms of gastric irritation, vomiting, and diarrhœa, but he also recovered.[533]

Casper relates the poisoning of a whole family by veratrum; from the stomach of the mother (who died) and the remains of the repast (a porridge of lentils) veratrine was separated.

Faber[534] recorded the poisoning of thirty cows by veratrum; eight died, and it is noteworthy that violent poisonous symptoms were produced in animals partaking of their flesh and milk.

§ 483. The symptoms appear soon after the ingestion, and consist of a feeling of burning in the mouth, spreading downwards to the stomach, increased secretion of saliva, and difficulty of swallowing; then follow violent vomiting and diarrhœa, with great pain in the bowels, often tenesmus; there is also headache, giddiness, a feeling of anxiety, and the pupils are dilated. The consciousness is ordinarily intact; the pulse is weak and slow, and the breathing embarrassed; the skin is benumbed. There may be also formicating feelings, and twitchings in the muscles with occasionally the tetanic cramps, which are constantly seen in frogs. In cases which end fatally, the disturbance of the breathing and circulation increases, and death takes place in collapse.

An important case of slow poisoning is on record,[535] in which two brothers, aged twenty-one and twenty-two years, died after nine and eleven weeks of illness, evidently from repeated small doses of the powder of *Veratrum album*. They became very weak and thin, suffered from diarrhœa and bloody stools, sleeplessness, disturbance of the intellect, and delirium.

§ 484. The *post-mortem* signs do not appear distinctive; even in the case just mentioned—in which one would expect to find, at all events, an extensive catarrh of the intestinal canal—the results seem to have been negative.

§ 485. **Separation from Organic Matters.**—The method of Stas (by which the organic matters, whether the contents of the stomach or the tissues, are treated with alcohol, weakly acidified by tartaric acid) is to be recommended. After filtering, the alcoholic extract may be freed from alcohol by careful distillation, and the extract taken up with water. By now acidifying gently the watery extract, and shaking it up with ether and chloroform, fatty matters, resinous substances, and other impurities, are removed, and it may then be alkalised by soda or potash, and the veratrine extracted by ether. The residue should be identified by the hydrochloric acid and by the sulphuric acid and bromine reactions; care should also be taken to ascertain whether it excites sneezing.

A ptomaine, discovered by Brouardel,[536] was described by him as both chemically and physiologically analogous to veratrine. A. M. Deleziniere[537] has since investigated this substance. Only when in contact with air does the analogy to veratrine obtain, and Deleziniere, to ascertain its reactions, studied it when in an atmosphere of nitrogen. It appears to be a secondary monamine, $C_{32}H_{31}N$, and is in the form of a colourless, oily liquid, with an odour like that of the hawthorn. It is insoluble in water, but alcohol, ether, toluene, and benzene dissolve it readily. It oxidises in the presence of air. The salts are deliquescent.

VIII.—Physostigmine.

§ 486. The ordeal bean of Calabar (*Physostigma faba*) is a large, all but tasteless, kidney-shaped bean, about an inch in length, and half an inch thick; its convex edge has a furrow with elevated ridges, and is pierced by a small

533 *Med. Times and Gazette*, Jan. 3, 1863.

534 *Zeitschr. f. Staatsarzneik.*, 1862.

535 Nivet and Géraud, *Gaz. Hebdom.*, 1861.

536 *Moniteur Scient.* (3), 10, 1140.

537 *Bull. Soc. Chim.* (3), 1, 178-180.

hole at one extremity. The integuments are coffee-brown in colour, thin, hard, and brittle; they enclose two white cotyledons, easily pulverisable, and weighing on an average 3.98 grms. (61 grains). The seed contains at least one alkaloid, termed *Physostigmine* (first separated in 1864 by Jobst and Hesse), and possibly a second, according to Harnack and Witkowsky, who have discovered in association with physostigmine a new alkaloid, which they call *Calabarine*, and which differs from physostigmine in being insoluble in ether and soluble in water. It is also soluble in alcohol; and further, the precipitate produced by potassium iodo-hydrargyrate in calabarine solutions is insoluble in alcohol.

§ 487. **Physostigmine**, or **eserine**, is not easily obtained in a crystalline state, being most frequently extracted as a colourless varnish, drying into brittle masses. It is, however, quite possible to obtain it in the form of partially-crystalline crusts, or even rhombic plates, by care being taken to perform the evaporation, and all the operations, at as low a temperature as possible, and preferably in a dimly-lit room; for, if the temperature rises to 40°, much of the alkaloid will be decomposed. Hesse recommends that the beans be extracted, alcohol by the alcoholic solution alkalised by sodic carbonate, and the liquid shaken up with ether, which will retain the alkaloid. The ether solution is now separated, and acidified slightly with very dilute sulphuric acid; the fluid, of course, separates into two layers, the lower of which contains the alkaloid as a sulphate, the upper is the ether, which is withdrawn, and the acid fluid passed through a moist filter. The whole process is then repeated as a purification.

Again, Vee, who has repeatedly obtained the alkaloid in a crystalline condition, directs the extraction of the beans by alcohol, the alcoholic solution to be treated as before with sodic carbonate, and then with ether; the ethereal solution to be evaporated to dryness, dissolved in dilute acid, precipitated by sugar of lead, and the filtrate from this precipitate alkalised by potassic bicarbonate, and then shaken up with ether. The ethereal solution is permitted to evaporate spontaneously, the crystalline crusts are dissolved in a little dilute acid, and the solution is lastly alkalised by potassic bicarbonate, when, after a few minutes, crystalline plates are formed.

The formula ascribed to physostigmine is $C_{15}H_{21}N_3O_2$. It is strongly alkaline, fully neutralising acids and forming tasteless salts. It is easily melted, and perhaps partly decomposed, at a temperature of 45°; at 100° it is certainly changed, becoming of a red colour, and forming with acids a red solution. It dissolves easily in alcohol, ether, chloroform, and bisulphide of carbon, but is not easily soluble in water.

The salts formed by the alkaloid with the acids are generally hygroscopic and uncrystallisable, but an exception is met with in the hydrobromide, which crystallises in stellate groups.[538] If CO_2 is passed into water containing the alkaloid in suspension, a clear solution is obtained; but the slightest warmth decomposes the soluble salt and reprecipitates the alkaloid. The hydrarg-hydroiodide ($C_{15}H_{21}N_3O_2$,HI,2HgI) is a white precipitate, insoluble in water, becoming yellow on drying, soluble in ether and alcohol, and from such solutions obtained in crystalline prismatic groups. A heat of 70° melts the crystals, and they solidify again in the amorphous condition.

It gives a precipitate with gold chloride, reducing the gold; also one with mercuric chloride easily soluble in hydrochloric acid. It gives no precipitate with platinum chloride.

§ 488. **Tests.**—Da Silva's[539] test for eserine is as follows:—A minute fragment of eserine or one of its salts is dissolved in a few drops of fuming nitric acid; this makes a yellow solution, but evaporated to complete dryness it is pure green. The green substance, called by others chloreserine, dissolves to a non-fluorescent green solution; in water and also in strong alcohol it shows a band in the red between λ670 and λ688, a broader but more nebulous band in the blue and violet between λ400 and λ418, and a very feeble band in the orange.

J. B. Nagelvoort[540] has recommended the following tests:—(*a*) An amorphous residue of a permanent blue colour is obtained if a trace of the alkaloid, or one of its salts, is evaporated in the presence of an excess of ammonia; this blue alkaloid dissolves in dilute acids with a red colour; sensitiveness 0.00001 gm. (1 : 100000). The solution has beautiful red fluorescence in reflected light; when evaporated, it leaves a residue that is green at first, changing to blue afterwards, the blue residue being soluble in water, alcohol, and chloroform, but not in ether. Chloroform extracts the blue colour from the watery ammoniacal solution only partially. The blue solutions are reddened at first by H_2S, and discoloured afterwards. The blue colour is restored by expelling the H_2S on the water-bath. (*b*) A red fluid is obtained when 0.010 gm. eserine or its salicylate, 0.050 gm. of slacked lime, and 1 c.c. of water are added together. Warmed in a water-bath, it turns green, and a piece of red litmus-paper suspended in the test-tube turns blue; a glass rod moistened with HCl gives off the well-known white clouds characteristic of an ammonia reaction.

---

[538] M. Duquesnel, *Pharm. J. Trans.* (3), v. 847.

[539] S. J. Ferreira da Silva, *Compt. Rend.*, cxvii. 330, 331.

[540] *Flückiger's Reactions*, 1893.

The green solution does not lose its colour by evaporation. Baryta water, added to an eserine solution, gives a white precipitate that turns red when strongly agitated, sensitive to 0.01 mgrm. (1 : 100000).

§ 489. **Pharmaceutical Preparations.**—The only preparations officinal in this country are a spirituous extract (*Extractum physostigmatis*), used principally for external application, the dose of which is not more than 18.1 mgrms. (.18 grain), and gelatine discs for the purpose of the ophthalmic surgeon, each disc weighing about $\frac{1}{50}$th grain, and containing $\frac{1}{1000}$ gr. of the alkaloid.

§ 490. **Effects on Animals.**—A large number of experiments have been made upon animals with physostigmine, most of them with the impure alkaloid, which is a mixture of calabarine and physostigmine. Now, the action of calabarine seems to be the opposite to that of physostigmine—that is, it causes tetanus. Hence, these experiments are not of much value, unless the different proportions of the alkaloids were known. Harnack and Witkowsky[541] made, however, some researches with pure physostigmine, of which the following are the main results:—The smallest fatal dose for rabbits is 3 mgrms. per kilo.; cats about the same; while dogs take from 4 to 5 mgrms. per kilo. Frogs, under the influence of the alkaloid, lie paralysed without the power of spontaneous movement, and the sensibility is diminished; later, the breathing ceases, and the reflex irritability becomes extinguished. The activity of the heart is through .5 mgrm. slowed, but at the same time strengthened.

The warm-blooded animals experimented upon show rapid paralysis of the respiratory centre, but the animal by artificial respiration can be saved. Fibrillar muscular twitching of all the muscles of the body are observed. Death follows in all cases from paralysis of the respiration. Experiments (first by Bexold, then by Fraser and Bartholow, and lastly by Schroff) have amply shown that atropine is, to a certain extent, an antidote for physostigmine poisoning. Fraser also maintains an antagonism between strychnine and physostigmine, and Bennet that chloral hydrate is antagonistic to physostigmine.

Effects on Man.—The bean has long been used by the superstitious tribes of the West Coast of Africa as an ordeal, and is so implicitly believed in that the innocent, when accused of theft, will swallow it, in the full conviction that their innocency will protect them, and that they will vomit up the bean and live. In this way, no doubt, life has often been sacrificed. Christison experimented upon himself with the bean, and nearly lost his life. He took 12 grains, and was then seized with giddiness and a general feeling of torpor. Being alarmed at the symptoms, he took an emetic, which acted. He was giddy, faint, and seemed to have lost all muscular power; the heart and pulse were extremely feeble, and beat irregularly. He afterwards fell into a sleep, and the next day he was quite well.

In August 1864 forty-six children were poisoned at Liverpool by eating some of the beans, which had been thrown on a rubbish heap, being part of the cargo of a ship from the West Coast of Africa. A boy, aged six, ate six beans, and died. In April of the same year, two children, aged six and three years, chewed and ate the broken fragments of one bean; the usual symptoms of gastric irritation and muscular weakness followed, but both recovered. Physostigmine contracts the iris to a point; the action is quite local, and is confined to the eye to which it is applied. When administered internally, according to some, it has no effect on the eyes, but according to others, it has a weak effect in contracting the pupil. In any case, the difference of opinion shows that the effect, when internally administered, is not one of a marked character.

§ 491. **Physiological Action.**—The physiological action of physostigmine is strikingly like that of nicotine, which it resembles in being a respiratory poison, first exciting, afterwards paralysing the vagus. Like nicotine, also, it produces a great loss of muscular power; it first excites, and then paralyses the intra-muscular terminations of the nerves; and, again, like nicotine, it induces a tetanus of the intestine. A difference between physostigmine and nicotine exists in the constant convulsive effects of the former, and in the greater influence on the heart of the latter.

§ 492. **Post-mortem Appearances.**—But little is known relative to the *post-mortem* appearances likely to be found in human poisoning; redness of the stomach and intestines is probably the chief sign.

§ 493. **Separation of Physostigmine.**—For the extraction of physostigmine from the fluids of the body, Dragendorff recommends benzene: the alcoholic filtered extract (first acidified) may be agitated with such solvents as petroleum and benzene, in order to remove colouring matter; then alkalised and shaken up with benzene, and the latter allowed to evaporate spontaneously—all the operations being, as before stated, carried on under 40°. If much coloured, it may be purified according to the principles before mentioned. In cases where enough of the extract (or other medicinal preparation) has been taken to destroy life, the analyst, with proper care, would probably not have much difficulty in separating a small quantity of the active principle. It is rapidly eliminated by the saliva and other secretions. In most cases it will be necessary to identify physostigmine by its physiological activity, as well as by

[541] *Arch. f. Pathol. u. Pharm.*, 1876, Bd. v.

its chemical characters. For this purpose a small quantity of the substance should be inserted in the eye of a rabbit; if it contains the alkaloid in question, in twenty minutes, at the very latest, there will be a strong contraction of the pupil, and a congested state of the conjunctival vessels. Further researches may be made with a small quantity on a bird or frog. The chief symptoms observed will be those of paralysis of the respiratory and voluntary muscles, followed by death. If a solution is applied to the web of a frog's foot, the blood-vessels become dilated. Physostigmine appears, according to Dragendorff and Pander, to act as an irritant, for they always observed gastro-enteritis as a result of the poison, even when injected subcutaneously. The enhanced secretion from all mucous surfaces, and the enlargement of the blood-vessels, are also very constant symptoms. But of all these characteristics, the contraction of the pupil is, for the purposes of identification, the principal. A substance extracted from the tissue or other organic matters, in the manner mentioned, strongly contracting the pupil and giving the bromine reaction, would, in the present state of our knowledge, be indicative of physostigmine, and of that alone.

§ 494. **Fatal Dose of Physostigmine.**—One mgrm. (.015 grain) as sulphate, given by Vee to a woman subcutaneously, caused vomiting, &c., after half an hour. A disciple of Gubler's took 2 mgrms. without apparent effect; but another mgrm., a little time after, caused great contraction of the pupil and very serious symptoms, which entirely passed off in four hours. It would thus seem that three times this (*i.e.*, 6 mgrms.) would be likely to be dangerous. If so, man is far more sensitive to physostigmine than dogs or cats; and 3 mgrms. per kilo.—that is, about 205 mgrms. (3 grains)—would be much beyond the least fatal dose.

IX.—Pilocarpine.

§ 495. From the leaves of the jaborandi, *Pilocarpus pennatafolius* (Nat. Ord. *Rutaceæ*), two alkaloids have been separated—*jaborandi* and *pilocarpine.*

Jaborandi ($C_{10}H_{12}N_2O_3$) is a strong base, differing from pilocarpine in its sparing solubility in water, and more ready solubility in ether; its salts are soluble in water and alcohol, but do not crystallise. P. Ghastaing,[542] by treating pilocarpine with a large quantity of nitric acid, obtained nitrate of jaborandi, and operating in the same way with hydrochloric acid, obtained the hydrochlorate of jaborandi; hence, it seems that jaborandi is derived from pilocarpine.

§ 496. **Pilocarpine** ($C_{11}H_{16}N_2O_2$) is a soft gelatinous mass, but it forms with the mineral acids crystallisable salts. The solutions are dextra-rotatory. On boiling with water, it decomposes into trimethylamine and m-pyridine lactic acid,

$$C_{11}H_{16} + H_2O = N(CH_3)_3 + C_5H_4NCHO\left\langle\begin{matrix} CH_3 \\ COOH \end{matrix}\right. ;$$

hence it is a pyridine derivative, and its graphic formula probably

$$\begin{array}{c} \quad\quad\quad\quad CO-O \\ \quad\quad\quad\quad | \\ C_5H_4N-C-N(CH_3)_3 \\ \quad\quad\quad\quad | \\ \quad\quad\quad\quad CH_3 \end{array}$$

The nitrate and hydrochloride are at present much used in pharmacy. Pilocarpine gives a precipitate with phosphomolybdic acid, potassio-mercuric iodide, and most general alkaloidal reagents, but none that are very distinctive. When a solution of gold chloride is added to one of pilocarpine, a salt falls, having the composition $C_{11}H_{16}N_2O_2,HCl + AuCl_3$. It is not very soluble in water (about 1 in 4600), and has been utilised for the estimation of pilocarpine. Pilocarpine fused with potash yields trimethylamine, carbon dioxide, butyric, and traces of acetic acid. Pilocarpine dissolves without the production of colour in sulphuric acid; but, with bichromate of potash and sulphuric acid, a green colour is produced. It may be extracted from an aqueous solution made alkaline by ammonia, by shaking up with chloroform or benzene.

§ 497. **Tests.**—When a little of the alkaloid is mixed with ten times its weight of calomel, and rubbed, and moistened by the breath, the calomel is blackened; cocaine also acts similarly; but the two could not be mistaken

[542] *Compt. Rend.*, vol. xciv. p. 223.

for each other. If a solution of mercur-potassium iodide is added to a solution of the hydrochloride, the amorphous precipitate becomes, in the course of a day or two, oily drops. "A solution of iodine in potassium iodide gives in pilocarpine solutions a brown precipitate that often crystallises to feathery brown crystals (microscopically), and of serrated form, something like the blade of a scroll-saw, when the crystallisation is incomplete."—*Flückiger's Reactions.*

§ 498. **Effects.**—Pilocarpine, given subcutaneously in doses of about 32 mgrms. (½ grain), causes within five minutes a profuse perspiration and salivation, the face becomes flushed, and the whole body sweats; at the same time, the buccal secretion is so much increased that in a few hours over a pint may be secreted. The tears, the bronchial secretion, and the intestinal secretions are also augmented; there are generally headache and a frequent desire to pass water; the pulse is much quickened, and the temperature falls from 1°.4 to 4°: the symptoms last from two to five hours. Langley has shown that the over-action of the submaxillary gland is not affected by section either of the *chorda tympani* or of the sympathetic supplying the gland. Although pilocarpine quickens the pulse of man, it slows, according to Langley,[543] the heart of the warm-blooded animals, and that of the frog. With regard to the frog, Dr. S. Ringer's researches are confirmatory. With large doses the heart stops in diastole. If to the heart thus slowed, or even when recently stopped, a minute quantity of atropine be applied, it begins to beat again. There is also a most complete antagonism between atropine and pilocarpine in other respects, atropine stopping the excessive perspiration, and relieving the headache and pain about the pubes, &c. Pilocarpine, given internally, does not alter the size of the pupil, but the sight may, with large doses, be affected. If a solution is applied direct to the eye, then the pupil contracts. No fatal case of its administration has occurred in man. The probable dangerous dose would be about 130 mgrms. (2 grains) administered subcutaneously. Pilocarpine must be classed among the heart poisons.

X.—Taxine.

§ 499. **Properties of Taxine.**—The leaves and berries, and probably other portions of the yew tree (*Taxus baccata*), are poisonous. The poison is alkaloidal, and was first separated by Marmé.

Taxine ($C_{37}H_{52}O_{10}N$).—Taxine cannot be obtained in crystals, but as a snow-white amorphous powder, scarcely soluble in water, but dissolving in alcohol, in ether, and in chloroform; insoluble in benzene. It melts at 82°, gives an intense purple-red, with sulphuric acid, and colours Fröhde's reagent reddish-violet.

A slightly acid aqueous solution of the alkaloid gives precipitates with all the group reagents and with picric acid.

The salts are soluble in water; the hydrochloride may be obtained by passing gaseous HCl into anhydrous ether. The platinichloride forms a yellow micro-crystalline powder $(C_{37}H_{52}O_{10}N)_2H_2PtCl_6$. The salts are generally difficult to crystallise.[544]

§ 500. **Poisoning by Yew.**—Falck has been able to collect no less than 32 cases of poisoning by different parts of the yew—9 were from the berries, and the rest from the leaves. They were all accidental; 20 persons died, or 62.5 per cent.

§ 501. **Effects on Animals—Physiological Action.**—From the researches of Marmé-Borchers, it appears that taxine acts upon the nervous centres—the nervous trunks themselves and the muscles remaining with their excitability unimpaired, even some time after death. Taxine kills through paralysis of the respiration, the heart beating after the breathing has stopped. The leaves contain much formic acid, and their irritant action on the intestine is referred to this cause.

§ 502. **Effects on Man.**—Several deaths from yew have resulted in lunatic asylums from the patients chewing the leaves. For example, a few years ago, at the Cheshire County Asylum, a female, aged 41, was suddenly taken ill, apparently fainting, her face pale, her eyes shut, and pulse almost imperceptible. Upon the administration of stimulants, she somewhat revived, but in a little while became quite unconscious. The pupils were contracted, and there were epileptiform convulsions, succeeded by stertorous breathing. These convulsions returned from time to time, the action of the heart became weaker, and there was a remarkable slowing of the respirations, with long intervals between the breathing. The woman died within an hour from the time when her illness was first observed, and within two hours of eating the leaves. Yew leaves were found in her stomach. In another case that occurred at

[543] "The Action of Jaborandi on the Heart," by J. N. Langley, B.A., *Journ. Anat. and Physiol.*, vol. x. p. 187.

[544] A. Hilger and F. Brande, *Ber.*, xxiii. 464-468.

the Parkside Asylum,[545] the patient died suddenly in a sort of epileptic fit. Yew leaves were again found in the stomach. In a case quoted by Taylor, in which a decoction of the leaves was drunk by a girl, aged 15, for the purpose of exciting menstruation, she took the decoction on four successive mornings. Severe vomiting followed, and she died eight hours after taking the last dose. In another case there were also no symptoms except vomiting, followed by rapid death. Mr. Hurt, of Mansfield, has recorded a case of poisoning by the berries. The child died in convulsions before it was seen by any medical man.

From these and other recorded cases, the symptoms seem generally to be a quick pulse, fainting or collapse, nausea, vomiting, convulsions, slow respiration, and death, as a rule sudden and unexpected. We may suppose that the sudden death is really due to a rapid paralysis of the respiration, and suffocation.

§ 503. **Post-Mortem Appearances.**—In the case of the girl who drank the decoction, nothing unusual was observed in the stomach or organs of the body; but when the leaves have been eaten, usually more or less congestion of the mucous membrane of the stomach, as well as of the bowels, is apparent. In the case of the child who ate the berries (Hurt's case), the stomach was filled with mucous and half-digested pulp of the berries and seeds. The mucous membrane was red in patches and softened, and the small intestines were also inflamed.

XI.—Curarine.

§ 504. Commercial curare is a black, shining, resinoid mass, about 83 per cent. of which is soluble in water, and 79 in weak spirit. It is a complicated mixture of vegetable extracts, from which, however, a definite principle possessing basic characters (*curarine*) has been separated.

The extract is an arrow poison[546] prepared by different tribes of Indians in South America, between the Amazon and the Orinoco; therefore, samples are found to vary much in their poisoning properties, although it is noticeable that qualitatively they are the same, and produce closely analogous symptoms. It is supposed that some of the curare is derived from different species of strychnos. This is the more probable, because, as before stated, the South American strychnines paralyse, and do not tetanise. It is not unlikely that the active principles of curare (or woorari) may be methyl compounds similar to those which have been artificially prepared, such as methyl strychnine and methyl brucine, both of which have a curare-like action.

Curarine was first separated by Preyer in a crystalline form in 1865. He extracted curare with boiling alcohol, to which a few drops of soda solution had been added, evaporated off the alcohol, took up the extract with water, and, after filtration, precipitated by phosphomolybdic acid, which had been acidified with nitric acid. The precipitate was dried up with baryta water, exhausted with boiling alcohol, and curarine precipitated from the alcoholic solution by anhydrous ether. It may also be obtained by precipitating with mercuric chloride solution, and throwing out the mercury afterwards by means of hydric sulphide, &c.

Curarine, when pure, forms colourless, four-sided, very hygroscopic prisms of bitter taste, and weakly alkaline reaction; soluble in water and alcohol in all proportions, but with difficulty soluble in amyl alcohol and chloroform, and not at all in anhydrous ether, bisulphide of carbon, or benzene. The base forms crystallisable salts with hydrochloric, nitric, and acetic acids. Curarine strikes a purple colour with strong nitric acid. Concentrated solutions of curarine mixed with dilute glycerin, give an amorphous precipitate with potassic bichromate, and the precipitate

---

545 *Pharm. Journ.* (3), No. 294.

546 A constituent of the Borneo arrow poison is "derrid," a toxic principle obtained from a leguminous plant, the *Derris elliptica*; it is a resinous substance, which has not yet been obtained in the pure state. It is said not to be a glucoside, nor to contain any nitrogen (Greshoff, *Ber.*, xxiii. 3537-3550).

The Comalis on the east coast of Africa prepare an arrow poison from the aqueous extract of the root of Oubaion, a tree closely related to *Carissa Schimperii.*

Oubain is prepared by treating the aqueous extract with lead acetate, getting rid of excess of lead by SH_2, and concentrating in a vacuum. The syrup is boiled with six times its volume of alcohol of 85°, and allowed to cool in shallow vessels; crystals are obtained which are recrystallised, first from alcohol, and afterwards from water.

Oubain, $C_{30}H_{46}O_{12}$, forms thin white nacreous lamellæ. It is tasteless, odourless, and neutral, almost insoluble in cold water, and soluble in boiling water; it dissolves readily in moderately concentrated alcohol, is almost insoluble in absolute alcohol, and insoluble in ether and chloroform. Its melting-point is 200°. The solution of oubain in water is lævorotatory $[\alpha]_D = -340$. It is a glucoside, yielding on boiling with dilute acids a sugar. It is very poisonous; 2 mgrms. will kill a dog of 12 kilos. weight in a few minutes, if subcutaneously injected; but, taken by the stomach, it produces no effect.—Arnaud, *Compt. Rend.*, cvi. 1011-1014.

treated with sulphuric acid strikes a beautiful blue colour. Curarine chromate is distinguished from strychnine chromate by its amorphous character, and by its comparatively easy solubility. If the chromates of strychnine and curarine be mixed, and the mixed chromates be treated with ammonia, strychnine will be precipitated, and curarine pass into solution, thus forming a ready method of separating them.

§ 505. **Physiological Effects.**—According to Voisin and Liouville's experiments, subcutaneous injections of curare on man cause, in small doses, strong irritation at the place of application, swelling, and pain. The temperature of the body is raised from 1° to 2°, and the number of respirations increased from 4 to 8 per minute. The pulse becomes somewhat stronger and more powerful. The urine is increased, and contains sugar. Large doses administered to warm-blooded animals cause, after a short time, complete paralysis of voluntary motion and of reflex excitability, and the animal dies in asphyxia, the heart continuing to beat.

This state is best produced for the purpose of experiment on frogs, and, indeed, is the best test for the poison. A very minute dose injected beneath the skin of a frog soon paralyses both the voluntary and respiratory muscles; the animal continues to breathe by the skin; the heart beats normally, or, perhaps, a little weakly, and the frog may remain in this motionless condition for days and yet recover. Only curare and its congeners have this effect. By tying the femoral artery of one of the frog's legs before administering the poison, an insight into the true action of the drug is obtained. It is then found that the reflex excitability and power of motion in the leg are retained, although all the rest of the body is paralysed. The only explanation of this is that curare does not act centrally, but paralyses the intramuscular ends of the motor nerves. Curare is eliminated partly through the liver and partly through the kidneys. Dragendorff found it in the fæces, while a striking proof that it is excreted by the kidneys is given by the experiment of Bidder,[547] in which the urine of a frog poisoned by curare was made to poison a second, and the urine of the second, a third. The easy excretion of curare through the kidneys furnishes an explanation of the relatively large dose of curare which can be taken by the stomach without injury. A dose which, given by subcutaneous injection, would produce violent symptoms, perhaps death, may yet be swallowed, and no ill effects follow. It is hence presumed that, in the first case, the poison is, comparatively speaking, slowly absorbed, and almost as fast separated, and put, as it were, outside the body by going into the urine; while, in the other case, the whole dose is thrown suddenly into the circulation.

§ 506. **Separation of Curarine.**—It is hardly probable that the toxicologist will have to look for curarine, unless it has entered the body by means of a wound or by subcutaneous injection; so that in all cases the absorbed poison alone must be sought for. The seat of entry, the liver, the kidneys, and the urine are the only parts likely to be of any use. Dragendorff recommends the extraction of the tissues with water feebly acidulated with a mineral acid, to precipitate albuminous matters, &c., by strong alcohol, and separate, by means of benzene, fatty matters. The liquid is then made alkaline, and shaken up with petroleum ether, which removes certain alkaloidal matters. It is now evaporated to dryness, mixed with finely-powdered glass, and extracted with absolute alcohol. The alcohol is evaporated to dryness, and any curarine extracted from this residue with water. By very careful drying up of this last extract, and taking it up in alcohol, the alkaloid is said to be obtained so pure as to respond to chemical tests. The identification may be by the colour reaction of sulphuric acid described *ante*, in all cases supplemented by its physiological action on frogs.[548]

[547] *Arch. f. Anat. u. Physiol.*, 1879, p. 598.

[548] It is known that curare may cause slight symptoms of excitation before the paralysis comes on. M. Couty has succeeded in isolating these symptoms by employing feeble extracts of *Strychnos triplinervia*, or small doses of certain native preparations. By these means, in dogs, a new phase of intoxication may be present for ten or even twenty minutes. In the first instance the animal is agitated, jumping, scratching, barking, as if in a state of general hyperæsthesia. Then it presents half choreic shocks or tremors; the pupils dilate, and are alternately dilated and contracted. The heart's action is increased or diminished in frequency; sometimes there is vomiting, micturition, or defecation; and there is always salivation. Finally, the central and peripheral temperature are raised, and the excitability of the muscles and nerves becomes highly increased. With the native preparation of curare, it is impossible to prolong this stage, and symptoms of paralysis soon become associated with those of excitement. The choreic shocks were found to be arrested by section of the sciatic nerve. Other experiments proved that the spasms originated from the spinal cord, and were influenced by its preceding functional condition. If the cord was tied in the mid-dorsal region, and the curare injected, the spasms were still produced in the hind legs; but if, after the operation, the excitability of the posterior segment became lowered, the spasm was no longer produced in the hind legs. This dependence on a perfect functional activity is a point of difference of these spasms from those produced by strychnine, and by asphyxia. The action of small doses of curare is not, however, limited to the spinal cord. The diminished frequency of the heart continues after section of the pneumogastrics,

XII.—Colchicine.

§ 507. The whole of the *Colchicum autumnale*, or common meadow-saffron, is poisonous, owing to the presence of an alkaloid (discovered by Pelletier and Caventou) called *Colchicine*.

According to Johannson's experiments, the dried colchicum seeds contain 1.15 per cent. of colchicine; the leaves, 1.459 per cent.; the bulbs, from 1.4 to 1.58 per cent.; and the roots, 0.634 per cent. The frequent poisoning of cattle in the autumn by colchicum, its use in quack pills for rheumatism, and its supposed occasional presence in beer, give it an analytical importance.

§ 508. **Colchicine** ($C_{22}H_{25}NO_6$) may be extracted from the seeds, &c., in the manner recommended by Hübler:—The seeds are treated, without crushing, by hot 90 per cent. alcohol, and the alcoholic solution evaporated to a syrup, which is diluted with twenty times its bulk of water and filtered; the liquid is next treated with acetate of lead, again filtered, and the lead thrown out by phosphate of soda. Colchicine is now precipitated as a tannate.[549] The precipitation is best fractional, the first and last portions being rejected as containing impurities. The tannate is decomposed in the usual way with litharge and extracted by alcohol.

A simpler method is, however, extraction by chloroform from an aqueous solution, feebly acidified, as recommended by Dragendorff. The parts of the plant are digested in very dilute acid water, and the resulting solution concentrated and shaken up with chloroform, which is best done in a separating tube.

Colchicine contains four methoxyl groups, and its constitutional formula is considered to be $C_{15}H_9[NH(CH_3CO)](COOCH_3)(OCH_3)_3$.

Its melting-point is 143°-147°. It is usually a white, gummy mass. It is easily soluble in cold water, in alcohol, and in chloroform. The solutions are lævorotatory. It is hardly soluble in ether. Boiling with dilute acids or alkalies in closed tubes yields colchiceine.

Colchiceine contains three methoxyl groups. It melts at 150°, dissolves but little in cold, copiously in boiling water. Colchiceine appears to be an acid, forming salts with the alkalies.

Zeisel[550] has formed acetotrimethylcolchicinamide ($NHAcC_{15}H_9(OMe)_3CONH_3$) by heating colchicine with alcoholic ammonia in closed tubes for four hours at 100°. The amide is crystallised from hot alcohol; it is readily soluble in dilute HCl, almost insoluble in water; when a strong hydrochloric acid solution of the amide is treated with a small amount of potassium nitrite a splendid violet colour is produced.

§ 509. **Tests.**—Ferric chloride, if added to an alcoholic solution of the alkaloid, strikes a garnet red; if to an aqueous solution a green or brownish-green; nitric acid added to the solid substance gives a violet colour. Erdmann's reagent (nitrosulphuric acid) gives in succession green, dark blue, and violet colours, ultimately turning yellow, changed, on addition of an alkali, to raspberry-red. Mandelin's reagent (1 grm. of ammonium vanadate in 200 grms. of sulphuric acid) gives a green colour.

§ 510. **Pharmaceutical Preparations.**—Colchicine itself is officinal in Austria—the wine in the British, French, and Dutch, and the seeds themselves in all the pharmacopœias. The wine of colchicum, officinal in nearly all the pharmacopœias, is made with very different proportions of seeds or bulbs.

The tincture of colchicum is officinal in our own and in all the Continental pharmacopœias; in the British, one part of seeds is exhausted by eight parts of proof spirit.

A tincture of colchicum seeds, examined by Johannson, contained .18 per cent. of colchicine, and a tincture prepared from the bulbs .14 per cent.

Colchicum vinegar is not officinal in Britain, but one containing 5.4 per cent. of acetic acid is so in the Netherlands, Germany, and France; the strength appears to be about .095 per cent. of colchicine.

An extract of colchicum is officinal in Britain and France; and an acetic extract in Britain. The latter is the most active of all the pharmaceutical preparations of colchicum.

Lastly, an oxymel of colchicum is in use in Germany, France, and the Netherlands.

---

and will even occur if the pneumogastrics have been previously divided. From these facts M. Couty considers that curare must not be regarded as entirely destitute of a "convulsant" action, nor of an action on the central nervous system.

[549] The purest tannic acid must be used. The commercial tannin may be purified by evaporating to dryness with litharge, exhausting the tannate of lead repeatedly with boiling alcohol and water, and, lastly, suspending in water, and separating the lead by SH_2.

[550] *Monatsh.*, ix. 1-30.

Quack and Patent Medicines.—In all specifics for gout the analyst will naturally search for colchicum. Most gout pills contain the extracts; and liquids, such as "Reynolds' gout specific," the wine or the tincture, variously flavoured and disguised.

The strength of the different pharmaceutical preparations may be ascertained by dissolving in chloroform, evaporating off the chloroform, dissolving in water (which is finally acidified by from 7 to 10 per cent. of sulphuric acid), and titrating with Mayer's reagent. If the solution is diluted so that there is about one part of colchicine in 600 of the solution, then each c.c. of Mayer's reagent equals 31.7 mgrms. colchicine.

§ 511. **Fatal Dose.**—In Taylor's *Principles of Medical Jurisprudence* is mentioned an instance in which 3½ drachms of colchicum wine, taken in divided doses, caused death on the fourth day. The quantity of the active principle in the colchicum wine, as found by Johannson (*Dragendorff*), being 0.18 per cent., it follows that 24.4 mgrms. (.378 grain) were fatal, though not given as one dose, so that this quantity may be considered as the least fatal one. Casper puts the lethal dose of colchicine at from 25 to 30 mgrms. (.385 to .463 grain). It is, however, incontestable that there are cases of recovery from as much as 70 mgrms. (1.08 grain). The lethal dose of the pharmaceutical preparations of colchicum may, on these grounds, be predicted from their alkaloidal contents, and, since the latter is not constant, in any medico-legal inquiry, it may be necessary, where facility is given, to ascertain the strength of the preparation administered.

§ 512. **Effects of Colchicine on Animals.**—The researches of Rossbach show that the carnivoræ are more sensitive to colchicine than any other order of mammals. Frogs show a transitory excitement of the nervous system, then there is loss of sensation, paralysis of motion, and of the respiratory apparatus; the heart beats after the respiration has ceased. Death follows from paralysis of the respiration. The mucous membrane of the intestine is much congested and swollen.

I have seen cattle die from the effects of eating the meadow-saffron; the animals rapidly lose condition, suffer great abdominal pain, and are generally purged. The farmers, in certain parts of the country, have had extensive losses from want of care and knowledge with regard to colchicum poisoning.

§ 513. **Effects of Colchicum on Man.**—Colchicum poisoning in man[551] is not very common: 2 deaths (accidental) are recorded in England and Wales during the ten years ending 1892. F. A. Falck was able to collect from medical literature, prior to 1880, 55 cases, and he gives the following analysis of the cases:—In 2, colchicum was taken for suicidal purposes; of the unintentional poisonings, 5 were from too large a medicinal dose of colchicum wine, syrup, or extract, given in cases of rheumatism; in 13 cases, colchicum was used as a purgative; 42 cases were owing to mistaking different preparations for drinks, or cordials—the tincture in 5, and the wine in 14, being taken instead of orange tincture, quinine wine, schnapps or Madeira; in 1 case the corms were added to mulled wine, in another, the leaves consumed with salad; in 16 cases (all children), the seeds of colchicum were eaten. Forty-six of the 55 died—that is, 83.7 per cent.

In the remarkable trial at the Central Criminal Court, in 1862, of Margaret Wilson (*Reg.* v. *Marg. Wilson*), who was convicted of the murder of a Mrs. Somers, the evidence given rendered it fairly probable that the prisoner had destroyed four people at different dates by colchicum. The symptoms in all four cases were—burning pain in the throat and stomach, intense thirst, violent vomiting and purging, coldness and clamminess of the skin, excessive depression, and great weakness. One victim died on the second day, another on the fifth, a third on the eighth, and the fourth on the fourteenth day. Schroff witnessed a case in which a man took 2 grms. (nearly 31 grains) of the corms; in one and a half hours he experienced general *malaise*; on the next day there were flying muscular pains, which at length were concentrated in the diaphragm, and the breathing became oppressed; there was also pain in the neighbourhood of the duodenum, the abdomen was inflated with gas; there was a sickly feeling and faintness. Then came on a sleepy condition, lasting several hours, followed by fever, with excessive pain in the head, noises in the ears, and delirium; there was complete recovery, but the abdomen continued painful until the fifth day.

In another instance, a gentleman, aged 50,[552] had taken twenty-eight of Blair's gout-pills in four and a half days for the relief of a rheumatic affection. He suffered from nausea, griping pains in the belly, considerable diarrhœa, vomiting, and hiccough; towards the end there was stupor, convulsive twitchings of the muscles, paralysis, and death. The fatal illness lasted fourteen days; he was seen by three medical men at different dates—the first seems to have considered the case one of diarrhœa, the second one of suppressed gout; but Dr. C. Budd was struck with

[551] For the curious epidemic of diarrhœa which broke out in the Rhone Gorge in 1785, and was referred to colchicine, see "Foods," p. 287.

[552] See *Lancet*, vol. i., 1881, p. 368.

the similarity of the symptoms to those from an acrid poison, and discovered the fact that the pills had been taken. These pills I examined; they were excessively hard, and practically consisted of nothing else than the finely-ground colchicum corms; six pills yielded 8 mgrms. of colchicine, so that the whole twenty-eight would contain 39 mgrms. (3⁄5 grain). Dr. Budd considered that the whole of the pills, which were of a stony hardness, remained in the bowels for some time undigested, so that the ultimate result was the same as if the whole had been taken in one dose.

§ 514. The general symptoms produced by colchicum are—more or less burning pain in the whole intestinal tract, vomiting, diarrhœa, with not unfrequently bloody stools; but sometimes diarrhœa is absent. In single cases tenesmus, dysuria, and, in one case, hæmaturia have been noted. The respiration is usually troubled, the heart's action slowed, the pulse small and weak, and the temperature sinks. In a few cases there have been pains in the limbs; cerebral disturbance is rare; but in two cases (one described *ante*) there was stupor. Muscular weakness has been observed generally. In a few cases there have been cramps in the calves and in the foot, with early collapse and death.

Post-mortem Appearances.—Schroff found in rabbits poisoned with from .1 to 1.0 grm. of colchicine, tolerably constantly enteritis and gastritis, and always a thick, pitch-like blood in the heart and veins. Casper has carefully recorded the *post-mortem* appearances in four labourers, ages ranging from fifteen to forty years, who, finding a bottle of colchicum-wine, and supposing it to be some kind of brandy, each drank a wine-glassful. They all died from its effects. In all four there was great hyperæmia of the brain membranes and of the kidneys. The large veins were filled with thick, dark, cherry-red blood, very similar to that seen in sulphuric acid poisoning. There was an acid reaction of the contents of the stomach. The lungs were moderately congested. The mucous membrane of the stomach of the one who died first was swollen and scarlet with congestion; with the second there was some filling of the vessels at the small curvature; while the stomachs of the third and fourth were quite normal. In 5 cases described by Roux there was also hyperæmia of the brain and kidneys, but no gastritis or enteritis. It is, therefore, evident that there are in man no constant pathological changes from colchicine poisoning.

§ 515. **Separation of Colchicine from Organic Matters.**—W. Obolonski[553] has recommended the following process:—The finely divided viscera are triturated with powdered glass and digested for twelve hours with alcohol. The liquid is squeezed out and the dry residue washed with alcohol. The extract is concentrated at a temperature not exceeding 80°, and the cooled residue made up to the original volume with alcohol. The filtered liquid is evaporated as before, and this operation repeated until no more clots separate on addition of water. The residue is then dissolved in water, the solution purified by shaking with light petroleum, and the colchicine finally extracted with chloroform.

In cases of poisoning by colchicum at Berlin, Wittstock used the following process:—The contents of the stomach were mixed with a large amount of alcohol, a few drops of HCl added, and the whole well shaken; the fluid was then filtered, and the filtrate evaporated to a syrupy consistence at 37°. The resulting residue was dissolved in distilled water, the fat, &c., filtered off, and the liquid carefully evaporated. From the extract foreign matter was again separated by treatment with alcohol and filtration, and the last filtrate was evaporated to a syrupy consistence. The syrupy fluid was taken up by distilled water, filtered, evaporated to 30 grms., and 2 grms. of calcined magnesia with 90 grms. of ether were added. After a time, the ether was removed, and allowed to evaporate spontaneously. The residue was once more taken up with water, filtered from fat, &c., and evaporated. This final residue gave all the reactions of colchicine. In medico-legal researches, it must be remembered that colchicine is absorbed but slowly, a not insignificant portion remaining in the bowels, with the fæces.

XIII.—Muscarine and the Active Principles of Certain Fungi.

§ 516. **The Amanita Muscaria**, or fly-blown agaric, is a very conspicuous fungus, common in fir-plantations, about the size and shape of the common mushroom; but the external surface of the pileus is of a bright red, or sometimes of a yellowish cast, and studded over with warts. The common name of the fungus denotes that it was used in former times as a popular insecticide; the fungus was bruised, steeped in milk, and the milk exposed, in the same way as we now expose arsenical fly-papers.

Some peculiar properties of the agaric have long been known to the natives of Kamschatka, and of the north-eastern part of Asia generally. They collect the fungi in the hottest months, and hang them up to dry. The fungus is then rolled up in a kind of bolus, and swallowed without chewing. One large, or two small, fungi will produce a

[553] *Zeit. anal. Chem.*, xxix. 493.

kind of intoxication, which lasts a whole day. It comes on in about two hours' time, and is very similar to that of alcohol. There is a giddy feeling, the spirits are exalted, the countenance becomes flushed, involuntary actions and words follow, and sometimes loss of consciousness. It renders some persons remarkably active, and proves highly stimulant to muscular exertion; by too large a dose violent spasmodic effects are produced. "So very exciting to the nervous system in many individuals is this fungus, that the effects are often very ludicrous. If a person under its influence wishes to step over a straw or small stick, he takes a stride or a jump sufficient to clear the trunk of a tree. A talkative person cannot keep silence or secrets, and one fond of music is perpetually singing. The most singular effect of the amanita is the influence which it has over the urine. It is said that from time immemorial the inhabitants have known that the fungus imparts an intoxicating quality to that secretion, which continues for a considerable time after taking it. For instance, a man moderately intoxicated to-day will, by the next morning, have slept himself sober, but (as is the custom) by taking a teacup of his urine he will be more powerfully intoxicated than he was the preceding day. It is, therefore, not uncommon for confirmed drunkards to preserve their urine as a precious liquor against a scarcity of the fungus. The intoxicating property of the urine is capable of being propagated; for every one who partakes of it has his urine similarly affected. Thus, with a very few amanitas, a party of drunkards may keep up their debauch for a week. Dr. Langsdorf mentions that by means of the second person taking the urine of the first, the third of the second, and so on, the intoxication may be propagated through five individuals."[554]

§ 517. A few cases of poisoning by the fly-blown agaric from time to time have occurred in Europe, where it has been eaten in mistake for the edible fungi, or taken by children allured by the bright attractive colours. In these cases the poisonous symptoms noticed have been those of gastro-intestinal irritation, as shown by vomiting and diarrhœa, *dilated*[555] pupils, delirium, tetanic convulsions, slow pulse, stertorous breathing, collapse, and death. In a few cases epileptic attacks and trismus have been observed. The course is usually a rapid one, the death occurring within twelve hours. In cases of recovery, convalescence has been prolonged.

The post-mortem characteristics are not distinctive, a fluid condition of the blood, hyperæmia of the brain, liver, and kidneys has been noticed.

§ 518. **Muscarine.**—These effects are partly due to an undiscovered, toxic substance—which seems to be destroyed at the temperature of boiling water, and is probably of rather easy destructibility—and of a very definite poisonous alkaloid (*muscarine*) first separated by a complex process by Schmiedeberg and Koppe in 1869.[556] It is a trimethylammonium base, and has lately been formed synthetically by Schmiedeberg and Harnack,[557] by treating cholin with nitric acid. Muscarine is isomeric with betain and oxycholin, from which it is separated by its fluorescence and poisonous properties.

The structural formula of muscarine, and its connection with choline, is as follows:—

$$\begin{array}{l} CH_2OH \\ | \\ CH_2 \\ | \\ N(CH_3)_3OH \end{array}$$

Choline.

$$\begin{array}{l} CH_2OH \\ | \\ CHOH \\ | \\ N(CH_3)_3OH \end{array}$$

Muscarine.

[554] Lindley's *Vegetable Kingdom.*

[555] This is the more curious, for muscarine strongly contracts the pupil. It, however, tends to prove what is stated in the text—viz., that there is more than one poisonous substance in *Amanita.*

[556] *Das Muscarin, das giftige Alkaloid des Fliegenpilzes.* Leipzig, 1869.

[557] *Arch. f. exper. Path.*, Bd. 4 u. 5.

An atom of hydrogen from the choline, CH_2, group, being replaced by hydroxyl.

Muscarine is a colourless, strongly alkaline, syrupy fluid, which, if allowed to stand over sulphuric acid, becomes gradually crystalline, but liquefies again on exposure to the atmosphere. It dissolves in water in every proportion, and also in alcohol, but is very little soluble in chloroform, and insoluble in ether. It is not precipitated by tannin: it forms salts with acids, and gives precipitates with auric chloride, phosphotungstic, and phosphomolybdic acids, and also with potassio-mercuric iodide. The last precipitate is at first amorphous, but it gradually becomes crystalline. This was the compound used by the discoverers to separate the base. With many other general alkaloidal reagents muscarine forms no compound that is insoluble, and therefore gives no precipitate, such, *e.g.*, as iodine with potassic iodide, picric acid, and platinic chloride. Muscarine is a stronger base than ammonia, and precipitates copper and iron oxides from solutions of their salts. Muscarine is very poisonous; 2 to 4 mgrms. are sufficient in subcutaneous injection to kill cats in from two to twelve hours—larger doses in a few minutes; but with rabbits the action is less intense. Cats become salivated, their pupils contract, they vomit, and are purged, the breathing becomes frequent, and there is marked dyspnœa. At a later stage the respirations are slower, and there are convulsions, and death.

The alkaloid has also been tried on man. Doses of from 3 to 5 mgrms., injected subcutaneously, cause, after a few minutes' profuse salivation, increased frequency of the pulse, nausea, giddiness, confusion of thought and myosis, but no vomiting, and no diarrhœa. Small quantities applied to the eye cause, after a few minutes, a derangement of the accommodation, but no change in the size, of the pupil; larger quantities cause also myosis, which depends upon an excitement of the sphincter iridis, or of the oculomotorius.

§ 519. The actions of muscarine and atropine are to a great extent antagonistic. This is especially and beautifully demonstrated by the effects of the two substances on the frog's heart. The action of muscarine upon the heart is to excite the inhibitory nerve apparatus, while the action of atropine is to paralyse the same system. One mgrm. of muscarine, injected subcutaneously into a frog, arrests the heart *in diastole*, but if a suitable dose of atropine is applied to the heart thus arrested, it begins to beat again; or, if atropine is first given, and then muscarine, the heart does not stop. The muscarine heart, when it has ceased to beat, may be successfully stimulated by galvanism. Muscarine at first excites the respiratory centre, and then paralyses it.

§ 520. **Detection of Muscarine in the Body.**—Muscarine itself is not likely to be taken as a poison or administered; but if it is sought for in the fly-blown agaric, or in the tissues or organs of persons who have been poisoned by the fungus, the process of Brieger appears the best. The process depends upon the fact that muscarine gives a soluble mercuric chloride compound, and is not precipitated by chloride of platinum, whilst most other substances accompanying it give more or less insoluble precipitates. The substances are treated with water acidulated with hydrochloric acid, and the acidulated extract concentrated (best in a vacuum) to a syrup. The syrupy residue is now treated with water, and the solution precipitated by means of mercuric chloride solution and any precipitate filtered off; the filtrate is freed from mercury by SH_2, and evaporated to a syrup; the syrup is repeatedly extracted with alcohol, and the alcoholic solution precipitated with platinum chloride and any precipitate filtered off. The filtrate is freed from alcohol, and all the platinum thrown out of solution by SH_2; the aqueous filtrate is now concentrated to a small volume, and again platinum chloride added, any precipitate which forms is filtered off, and the final filtrate allowed to crystallise. If muscarine be present, a crystalline compound of muscarine platinum chloride will form.

The crystals are usually octahedral in form, and have the composition $(C_5H_{14}NO_2Cl)_2PtCl_4$; the percentage of platinum is 30.41.

It would probably be necessary to identify farther, by the action of the poison on a frog.

§ 521. **The Agaricus phalloides**, a common autumn fungus, has been several times mistaken for mushrooms, and has proved fatal; of some 53 cases collected by Falck, no less than 40, or 75 per cent., were fatal; the real mortality is much lower than this, for it is only such cases that are pronounced and severe which are likely to be recorded. The fungus contains a toxalbumin which has been named "phallin." The action of this toxalbumin is to dissolve the blood corpuscles; according to Kobert, even one 250,000th dilution produces "polycholie," with all its consequences, such as the escape of hæmoglobin and its decomposition products in the blood and urine, multiple blood coagulation through the fibrin ferment becoming free, and serious cerebral disturbance. If into a dog, cat, or rabbit, only 0.5 mgrm. of phallin be injected intravenously, within from twenty to thirty minutes blood from a vein shows that the serum has a red colour.

The symptoms in man first appear in from three to forty-eight hours; there is mostly diarrhœa, violent vomiting, with cramp in the legs, cyanosis, and collapse. There are also nervous phenomena, convulsions, trismus, and, in a few cases, tetanic spasms. The pulse, in seven cases described by Maschka, was very small, thready, and quick, but in others, again, small and slow. The pupils have in some cases been dilated, in others unchanged. Death is generally rapid. In two of Maschka's cases from sixty to sixty-eight hours after the investigation, but in the rest from twelve to eighteen hours. Life may, however, be prolonged for several days. In a case recorded by Plowright,[558] in which a boy had eaten a piece of the pileus, death occurred on the fourth day.

§ 522. **The post-mortem appearances** observed in Maschka's seven cases were—absence of cadaveric rigidity, dilatation of the pupil, a dark red fluid condition of the blood, numerous ecchymoses in the pleura, in the substance of the lungs, the pericardium, the substance of the heart, the liver, kidneys, and spleen. The mucous membrane of the digestive canal presented nothing characteristic. In two cases there were a few ecchymoses, and in one the mucous membrane of the stomach was softened, red, and easily detached. In one case only were any remnants of the fungus found, by which the nature of the substance eaten could be determined. The bladder in each case was full. In three cases a fatty degeneration of the liver had commenced. The same appearance was met with in some of the older cases related by Orfila.

§ 523. **The Agaricus pantherinus** is said to be poisonous, although Hertwig found it to have no action when given to dogs.

The Agaricus ruber, a bright-hued fungus, growing profusely on the Hampshire coast, of a purple-red colour—the colouring-matter not only covering the pileus, but also extending down the stipe—is poisonous, and has recently been chemically investigated by Phipson,[559] who has identified a colouring-matter *ruberine*, and an alkaloid *agarythrine*. Agarythrine is separated by macerating the fungus (from which the skin containing the colouring-matter has been removed) as completely as possible in water acidulated with 8 per cent. of hydrochloric acid. The filtered solution is neutralised by sodic carbonate, and the alkaloid shaken up with ether. On evaporation the ether leaves a white, somewhat greasy-looking substance, having a bitter burning taste, and easily fusible into yellow globules, giving forth an odour like quinoleine; it is soluble in alcohol and ether. From Phipson's observations it would appear probable that the red colouring-matter is derived from a decomposition of this alkaloidal substance. A rose-red colour is produced by the action of nitric acid, and chlorinated lime first reddens and then bleaches it. Buchwald[560] has recorded three cases of poisoning by this fungus; the patients were labourers, who, after eating the fungus, suffered from vomiting, thirst, a "drunken" condition, cramp, albuminuria, and disturbance of the sensory functions. The fungus causes in cats myosis, but is said not to affect rabbits.

§ 524. **The Soletus satanas, or luridus (Lenz)**, is poisonous; very small quantities of the uncooked fungus caused in Lenz, who experimented upon its properties, violent vomiting. In cases in which this fungus has been eaten accidentally, the symptoms have been very similar to cholera.

§ 525. **The Common Morelle** seems under certain conditions to be poisonous. From six to ten hours after ingestion there have appeared depression, nausea, jaundice, dilated pupils, and in the worst cases at the end of the first day, delirium, somnolence, and muscular cramps, followed by collapse and death. In a case observed by Kromholz, the *post-mortem* appearances were jaundice, a dark fluid state of the blood, and hyperæmia of the brain and liver. Boström fed a dog with 100 grms. of the fresh young morelle; the animal died on the third day, and the canaliculi of the kidney were found filled with hæmoglobin, partly amorphous, and partly crystalline.[561]

DIVISION II.—GLUCOSIDES.

I.—Digitalis Group.

§ 526. **The Digitalis purpurea**, or foxglove, is a plant extremely common in most parts of England, and poisoning may occur from the accidental use of the root, leaves, or seeds. The seeds are very small and pitted; they weigh 1126 to a grain (*Guy*), are of a light brown colour, and in form somewhat egg-shaped. The leaves are large,

[558] *Lancet*, 1879.
[559] *Chem. News*, p. 199, 1882.
[560] *Industr. Bl.*, 1876.
[561] See Casper's *Viertelj.*, 1844; Keber, *Preuss. Vereinszeitg.* 1846; Boström, *Ber. d. Phys. Med. Soc.*, Erlangen, 1880; Schauenstein, "Giftige Schwämme" in Maschka's *Handbuch*, &c.

ovate, crenate, narrowed at the base, rugous, veined, and downy, especially on the under surface. Their colour is a dull green, and they have a faint odour and a bitter, nauseous taste. The leaf is best examined in section. Its epidermis, when fresh, is seen to consist of transparent, hexagonal, colourless cells, beneath which, either singly or in groups, there are round cells of a magenta tint, and beneath these again a layer of columnar cells, and near the lower surface a loose parenchyma. The hairs are simple, appearing scantily on the upper, but profusely on the lower, surface; each is composed of from four to five joints or cells, and has at its base a magenta-coloured cell. The small leaves just below the seed-case, and the latter itself, are studded with glandular hairs. The root consists of numerous long slender fibres.

§ 527. **Chemical Composition.**—It is now generally accepted that there exist in the foxglove, at least, four distinct principles—*digitalin, digitonin, digitoxin*, and *digitalein*. Besides these there are several others of more or less definite composition, which are all closely related, and may be derived from a complex glucoside by successive removals of hydrogen in the form of water.

The following is the theoretical percentage composition of the digitalins, the identity of which has been fairly established. They are arranged according to their percentage in carbon:—

TABLE SHOWING THE COMPOSITION OF THE DIGITALINS.

Name.	Formula.	Percentage Composition.	
Digitalein,	$C_{21}H_{46}O_{11}$	C. 53.16 per cent.	H. 8.08 per cent.
Digitonin,[562]	$C_{31}H_{52}O_{17}$	C. 53.44 ,,	H. 7.46 ,,
Digitalin,	$C_{54}H_{84}O_{27}$	C. 58.16 ,,	H. 3.65 ,,
Digitaletin,	$C_{44}H_{30}O_{18}$	C. 62.41 ,,	H. 3.54 ,,
Digitoxin,	$C_{21}H_{32}O_{7}$	C. 63.63 ,,	H. 8.08 ,,
Digitaleretin,	$C_{44}H_{38}O_{18}$	C. 66.05 ,,	H. 4.58 ,,
Paradigitaletin,	$C_{44}H_{34}O_{14}$	C. 67.17 ,,	H. 4.3 ,,

§ 528. **Digitalein** is a colourless, amorphous body, easily soluble in water and in cold absolute alcohol. It may be precipitated from an alcoholic solution by the addition of much ether. It is with difficulty soluble in chloroform, and insoluble in ether. It is precipitated from a watery solution by tannin, or by basic lead acetate; saponification by dilute acids splits it up into glucose and digitaleretin. It has a sharp, acrid taste, and the watery solution froths on shaking.

§ 529, **Digitonin**, a white amorphous body, has many of the characters of saponin. Like saponin, it is easily soluble in water, and the solution froths, and, like saponin again, it is precipitated by absolute alcohol, by baryta water, and by basic lead acetate. It may be readily distinguished from saponin by treating a watery solution with sulphuric or hydrochloric acid. On saponifying, it is split up into digitogenin, galactose, and dextrose. On heating, a beautiful red colour develops. It does not give the bromine reaction.

Digitogenin is insoluble in water and aqueous alkalies; it is somewhat soluble in alcohol, chloroform, and glacial acetic acid; it forms a crystalline compound with alcoholic potash, which is strongly alkaline, and not very soluble in alcohol.

§ 530. **Digitalin**, when perfectly pure, forms fine, white, glittering, hygroscopic needles, or groups of crystalline tufts; it is without smell, but possesses a bitter taste, which is at once of slow development and of long endurance. On warming, it becomes soft under 100°, and, above that temperature, is readily decomposed with evolution of white vapours. It is insoluble in water, in dilute soda solution, in ether, and in benzene. It is soluble in chloroform, especially in chloroform and alcohol, and dissolves easily in warm acetic acid; twelve parts of cold and six of boiling alcohol of 90 per cent. dissolve one of digitalin. Dilute hydrochloric or sulphuric acid decompose it into glucose and digitaletin ($C_{44}H_{30}O_{18}$); if the action is prolonged, digitaleretin ($C_{44}H_{38}O_{18}$), and finally dehydrated digitaleretin, are formed. Concentrated sulphuric acid dissolves it with the production of a green colour, which by bromine passes

[562] According to Kiliani, digitonin has the composition of $C_{27}H_{44}O_{13}$, and it breaks up, when heated with hydrochloric acid, as follows:—

$$\underset{\text{Digitonin.}}{C_{27}H_{44}O_{13}} + 2H_2O = \underset{\text{Digitogenin.}}{C_{16}H_{24}O_3} + \underset{\text{Dextrose.}}{2C_6H_{12}O_6}.$$

—*Ber.*, xxiii. 1555-1568.

into violet-red, but on the addition of water becomes green again. Hydrochloric acid dissolves it with the production of a greyish-yellow colour, passing gradually into emerald green; water precipitates from this solution a resinous mass.

§ 531. **Digitaletin.**—A substance obtained by Walz on treating his digitalin by dilute acids. It is crystalline, and its watery solution tastes bitter. It melts at 175°, and decomposes, evolving an acid vapour at about 206°. It dissolves in 848 parts of cold, and 222 of boiling, water; in 3.5 parts of cold, and in from 2 to 4 of boiling, alcohol. It is with difficulty soluble in ether. It dissolves in concentrated sulphuric acid, developing a red-brown colour, which, on the addition of water, changes to olive-green. On boiling with dilute acids, it splits up into sugar and digitaleretin.

§ 532. **Digitoxin** always accompanies digitalin in the plant, and may by suitable treatment be obtained in glittering needles and tabular crystals. It is insoluble in water and in benzene. It dissolves with some difficulty in ether, and is readily dissolved by alcohol or by chloroform. On boiling with dilute acids, it is decomposed into an amorphous, readily soluble body,—*Toxiresin*. Digitoxin, according to Schmiedeberg, only exists in the leaves of the digitalis plant, and that in the proportion of 1 part in 10,000. Digitalin and digitoxin are *par excellence* the poisonous principles of the plant. Toxiresin is also intensely poisonous. It may be obtained in crystals by extracting the dry exhausted leaves with alcohol of 50 per cent., precipitating with lead acetate, and washing the precipitate first with a dilute solution of sodium carbonate (to remove colouring-matter), and then with ether, benzene, and carbon disulphide, in all of which it is insoluble; on decomposing the lead compound, digitoxin may be obtained in colourless scales or needle-shaped crystals.

§ 533. **Digitaleretin**, the origin of which has been already alluded to, is a yellowish-white, amorphous powder, possessing no bitter taste, melting at 60°, soluble in ether or in alcohol, but insoluble in water.

Paradigitaletin is very similar to the above, but it melts at 100°, and is insoluble in ether.

§ 534. Several other derivatives have been obtained and described, such as the inert *digitin*, *digitalacrin*, *digitalein*, and others, but their properties are, as yet, insufficiently studied. Digitalin, as well as digitoxin, may now be obtained pure from certain firms, but the ordinary digitalin of commerce is, for the most part, of two kinds, which may be distinguished as French and German digitalin. The French digitalin, or the digitalin of Homolle, is prepared by treating an aqueous extract of the digitalis plant with lead acetate, and freeing the filtrate from lead, lime, and magnesia, by successive additions of alkaline carbonate, oxalate, and phosphate, and then precipitating with tannin. The tannin precipitate is treated with litharge, and the digitalins boiled and extracted from the mass by means of alcohol, and lastly, purifying with animal charcoal. Crystals are in this way obtained, and by removing all substances soluble in ether by that solvent, digitalin may be separated. The German digitalin is prepared according to the process of Walz, and is extracted from the plant by treatment with alcohol of .852. The alcohol is removed by evaporation, and the alcoholic extract taken up with water; the watery extract is treated with lead acetate and litharge, filtered, the filtrate freed from lead by hydric sulphate, and the excess of acid neutralised by ammonia, and then tannin added to complete precipitation. The precipitate is collected and rubbed with hydrated oxide of lead, and the raw digitalin extracted by hot alcohol. The alcohol, on evaporation, leaves a mixture of digitalin mixed with other principles and fatty matter. If sold in this state, it may contain from 2 to 3 per cent. of digitalein and digitonin. On treating the mixture with ether, digitalin with some digitaletin is left behind, being almost insoluble in ether. Since, however, digitaletin is very insoluble in cold water, by treating the mixture with eight parts of its weight of cold water, digitalin is dissolved out in nearly a pure state. It may be further purified by treating the solution with animal charcoal, recrystallisation from spirit, &c.

§ 535. **Reactions of the Digitalins.**—Digitonin is dissolved by dilute sulphuric acid (1 : 3) without colour, and the same remark applies to hydrochloric acid; on warming with either of these acids, a violet-red colour appears; this reaction thus serves to distinguish digitonin from the three other constituents, as well as from saponin.

Sulphuric and gallic acids colour the glucosides of digitalin, digitalein, and digitonin, red, but not digitoxin, which can be identified in this way.

Sulphuric acid and bromine give with digitalin a red, and with digitalein a violet coloration, which, on the addition of water, change respectively into emerald and light green. This, the most important chemical test we possess, is sometimes called *Grandeau's test*; it is not of great delicacy, the limit being about .1 mgrm.

§ 536. **Pharmaceutical Preparations of Digitalin.**—Digitalin itself is officinal in the French, Belgium, Portuguese, Russian, Spanish, and Austrian pharmacopœias. It is prepared in our own by making a strong tincture of the leaves at 120° F.; the spirit is then evaporated off, and the extract heated with acetic acid, decolorised by animal charcoal, and filtered. After neutralisation with ammonia, the digitalin is precipitated with tannin, and the tannate of digitalin resolved into tannate of lead and free digitalin, by rubbing it with oxide of lead and spirit.

Digitalis leaf is officinal in most of the pharmacopœias.

Tincture of digitalis is officinal in our own and all the Continental pharmacopœias, and an ethereal tincture is used in France and Germany.

An *Acetum digitalis* is officinal in the Netherlands and Germany; an extract and infusion are also used to some extent.

With regard to the nature of the active principle in these different preparations, according to Dragendorff, digitonin and digitalein are most plentiful in the acetic and aqueous preparations; whilst in the alcoholic, digitalin, digitoxin, and digitalein are present.

According to Schmiedeberg, commercial digitalin contains, in addition to digitoxin, digitonin, digitalin, and digitalein; of these, digitonin is greatest in amount.[563]

§ 537. **Fatal Dose.**—The circumstance of commercial digitalin consisting of varying mixtures of digitoxin, digitalin, and digitalein, renders it difficult to be dogmatic about the dose likely to destroy life. Besides, with all heart-poisons, surprises take place; and very minute quantities have a fatal result when administered to persons with disease of the heart, or to such as, owing to some constitutional peculiarity, have a heart easily affected by toxic agents. Digitoxin, according to Kopp's[564] experiments, is from six to ten times stronger than digitalin or digitalein. Two mgrms. caused intense poisonous symptoms. Digitoxin is contained in larger proportions in Nativelle's digitalin than in Homolle's, or in the German digitalin. The digitalin of Homolle is prescribed in 1 mgrm. (.015 grain) doses, and it is thought dangerous to exceed 6 mgrms.

Lemaistre has, indeed, seen dangerous symptoms arise from 2 mgrms. (.03 grain), when administered to a boy fifteen years old. It may be predicated from recorded cases and from experiment, that digitoxin would probably be fatal to an adult man in doses of 4 mgrms. (1/16 grain), and digitalin, or digitalein, in doses of 20 mgrms. (.3 grain). With regard to commercial digitalin, as much as from 10 to 12 mgrms. (.15 to .18 grain) have been taken without a fatal result; on the other hand, 2 mgrms. gave rise to poisonous symptoms in a woman (Battaille). Such discrepancies are to be explained on the grounds already mentioned. It is, however, probable that 4 mgrms. (or 1/16 grain) of ordinary commercial digitalin would be very dangerous to an adult.

It must also, in considering the dose of digitalin, be ever remembered that it is a cumulative poison, and that the same dose—harmless if taken once—yet, frequently repeated, becomes deadly: this peculiarity is shared by all poisons affecting the heart. When it is desired to settle the maximum safe dose for the various tinctures, extracts, and infusions of digitalis used in pharmacy, there is still greater difficulty, a difficulty not arising merely from the varying strength of the preparations, but also from the fact of the vomiting almost invariably excited by large doses. Individuals swallow quantities without death resulting, simply because the poison is rapidly expelled; whereas, if the œsophagus was ligatured (as in the experiments on the lower animals formerly favoured by the French school of toxicologists), death must rapidly ensue. The following table is a guide to the maximum single dose, and also the amount safe to administer in the twenty-four hours in divided doses. As a general rule, it may be laid down that double the maximum dose is likely to be dangerous:—

TABLE SHOWING THE MAXIMUM SINGLE DOSE, AND MAXIMUM QUANTITY OF THE DIFFERENT PREPARATIONS OF DIGITALIS, WHICH CAN BE ADMINISTERED IN A DAY.

	Single Dose.		Per Day.	
	Grains or Minims.	Grammes or c.c's.	Grains or Minims.	Grammes or c.c's.
Powdered Leaves,	4 ½ grns.	.3 grm.	15 .4 grns.	1 .0 grm.
Infusion,	480 m.	28.3 c.c.	1440 m.	84.9 c.c.
Tincture,	45 m.	3 c.c.	135 m.	9 c.c.
Digitalin,	.03 grn.	.002 grm.	.09 grn.	.006 grm.
Extract,	3 .0 ,,	.2 ,,	12 .0 ,,	.8 ,,

§ 538. **Statistics.**—The main knowledge which we possess of the action of digitalis is derived from experiments on animals, and from occasional accidents in the taking of medicines; but in comparison with certain toxic agents

[563] H. Kiliani, *Ber.*, xxiii.

[564] *Archiv f. exp. Pathol. u. Pharm.*, vol. iii. p. 284, 1875.

more commonly known, the number of cases of death from digitalis is very insignificant. Of 42 cases of digitalis-poisoning collected by Husemann, 1 was criminal (murder); 1 the result of mistaking the leaves for those of borage; 42 were caused in medicinal use—in 33 of these last too large a dose had been given, in 3 the drug was used as a domestic remedy, in 2 of the cases the prescription was wrongly read, and in 1 digitalis was used as a secret remedy. Twenty-two per cent. of the 45 were fatal.

§ 539. **Effects on Man.**—It was first distinctly pointed out by Tardieu that toxic doses of digitalis, or its active principles, produced not only symptoms referable to an action on the heart, but also, in no small degree, gastric and intestinal irritation, similar to that produced by arsenic. Tardieu also attempted to distinguish the symptoms produced by the pharmaceutical preparations of digitalis (the tincture, extract, &c.), and the glucoside digitalin; but there does not appear a sufficient basis for this distinction. The symptoms vary in a considerable degree in different persons, and are more or less tardy or rapid in their development, according to the dose. Moderate doses continued for some time (as, for example, in the persistent use of a digitalis medicine) may produce their first toxic effects even at the end of many days; but when a single large dose is taken, the symptoms are rarely delayed more than three hours. They may commence, indeed, in half an hour, but have been known to be retarded for more than twenty-four hours, and the longer periods may be expected if digitalis is given in hard, not easily soluble pills. There is commonly a feeling of general *malaise*, and then violent retching and vomiting. The pulse at first may be accelerated, but it soon is remarkably slowed—it sinks commonly down to 50, to 40, and has even been known as low as 25. To these symptoms, referable to the heart and to the digestive tract, are added nervous troubles; there are noises in the ears, and disturbances of vision. In a case related by Taylor, a red-coal fire seemed to the patient to be of a blue colour; in another, related by Lersch,[565] there was blindness for eighteen hours, and for some time a confusion in the discrimination in colours; quiet delirium has also been noticed. As the case proceeds, the gastric symptoms also increase in severity; the tongue Christison, in one case, noticed to be enormously swollen, and the breath fœtid. Diarrhœa is commonly present, although also sometimes absent. The action of the kidneys is suppressed. Hiccough and convulsions close the scene.

In the cumulative form, the symptoms may suddenly burst out, and the person pass into death in a fainting-fit without any warning. As a rare effect, hemiplegia may be mentioned.

This brief *résumé* of the symptoms may be further illustrated by the following typical cases:—A recruit, aged 22, desiring to escape from military service, went to a so-called "*Freimacher*" who gave him 100 pills, of which he was to take eight in two doses daily. Eleven days after the use of the pills, he became ill, and was received into hospital, where he suddenly died after three weeks' treatment. His malady was at first ascribed to gastric catarrh; for he suffered from loss of appetite, nausea, and constipation. He complained of pain in the head, and giddiness. His breath smelled badly, and the region of the stomach was painful on pressure. The pulse was slow (56), the temperature of the body normal. Towards the end, the pulse sank to 52; he suffered from vomiting, noise in the ears, troubles of vision, great weakness, and later, hiccough and swelling in the neck. The mere act of standing up in order to show his throat caused him to faint; on the same day on which this occurrence took place, he suddenly died on the way to the nightstool. Thirteen of the pills were found in the patient's clothes, and from a chemical and microscopical examination it was found that they contained digitalis leaf in fine powder. The quantity which the unfortunate man took in the four weeks was estimated at 13.7 grms. (= about 211 grains).

Two of his comrades had also been to the "*Freimacher*," and had suffered from the same symptoms, but they had left off the use of the medicine before any very serious effect[566] was produced.[567]

An instructive case of poisoning by digitoxin occurred in the person of Dr. Koppe, in the course of some experiments on the drug. He had taken 1.5 mgrm. in alcohol without result; on the following day (May 14) he took 1 mgrm. at 9 A.M., but again without appreciable symptoms. Four days later he took 2 mgrms. in alcoholic solution,

[565] *Rhen. West. Corr. Bl.*, 15, 1848; Husemann in Maschka's *Handbuch*.

[566] Köhnhorn, *Vierteljahrsschr. f. ger. Med.*, 1876, n. F. xxiv. p. 402.

[567] There is an interesting case on record, in which a woman died from the expressed juice of digitalis. She was twenty-seven years of age, and took a large unknown quantity of the freshly expressed juice for the purpose of relieving a swelling of the limbs. The symptoms came on almost immediately, she was very sick, and was attacked by a menorrhagia. These symptoms continued for several days with increasing severity, but it was not until the fifth day that she obtained medical assistance. She was then found semi-comatose, the face pale, pulse slow, epigastrium painful on pressure, diarrhœa, and hiccough were frequent. She died on the twelfth day. The *post-mortem* appearances showed nothing referable to digitalis save a few spots of inflammation on the stomach.—Caussé, *Bull. de Thérapeutique*, vol. lvi. p. 100; *Brit. and For. Med. Chir. Review*, vol. xxvi., 1860, p. 523.

and an hour afterwards felt faint and ill, with a feeling of giddiness; the pulse was irregular, of normal frequency, 80 to 84. About three hours after taking the digitoxin, Dr. Koppe attempted to take a walk, but the nausea, accompanied with a feeling of weakness, became so intense that he was obliged to return to the house. Five hours after the dose, his pulse was 58, intermittent after about every 30 to 50 beats. Vomiting set in, the matters he threw up were of a dark green colour; after vomiting he felt better for a quarter of an hour, then he again vomited much bilious matter; the pulse sank to 40, and was very intermittent, stopping after every 2 or 3 beats. Every time there was an intermission, he felt a feeling of constriction and uneasiness in the chest. Six and a quarter hours after the dose there was again violent vomiting and retching, with paleness of the face. The muscular weakness was so great that he could not go to bed without assistance. He had a disorder of vision, so that the traits of persons well-known to him were changed, and objects had a yellow tint. He had a sleepless night, the nausea and vomiting continuing. During the following day the symptoms were very similar, and the pulse intermittent, 54 per minute. He passed another restless night, his short sleep being disturbed by terrible dreams. On the third day he was somewhat better, the pulse was 60, but irregular and still intermittent; the nausea was also a little abated. The night was similar in its disturbed sleep to the preceding. He did not regain his full health for several days.[568]

A third case may be quoted, which differs very markedly from the preceding, and shows what a protean aspect digitalin poisoning may assume. A woman, twenty-three years old, took on June 26th, at 7 A.M., for the purpose of suicide, 16 granules of digitalin. Two hours later there was shivering and giddiness, so that she was obliged to go to bed. In the course of the day she had hallucinations. In the evening at 8 P.M., after eating a little food, she had a shivering fit so violent that her teeth chattered; there was cold sweat, and difficulty in breathing; she became gradually again warm, but could not sleep. At 1 A.M. the difficulty of breathing was so great that she dragged herself to the window, and there remained until 3 A.M., when she again went back to bed, slept until 7 A.M., and woke tolerably well. Since this attempt of self-destruction had failed, she took 40 granules. After one hour she became giddy, had hallucinations, chilliness, cold sweats, copious vomiting, and colicky pains; there was great muscular weakness, but no diarrhœa. Towards evening the vomiting became worse. There was no action of the bowels, nor was any urine passed; she felt as if her eyes were prominent and large. The sufferings described lasted during the whole night until five o'clock the following day, when the vomiting ceased, whilst the hallucinations, chilliness, and cold sweat continued; and the thirst, sick feeling, and weakness increased. The next morning, a physician found her motionless in bed, with pale face, notable double exophthalmus, dilated pupils, and cold skin, covered with sweat; the pulse was small and intermittent, sometimes scarcely to be felt (46 to 48 per minute); the epigastrium was painful on pressure. She passed this second night without sleep, and in the morning the pulse had risen from 56 to 58 beats, but was not quite so intermittent. There was some action of the bowels, but no urine was passed, nor had any been voided from the commencement; the bladder was not distended. The following (third) day some red-coloured, offensive urine was passed; the skin was warmer, and the pulse from 60 to 64, still somewhat intermittent—from this time she began to improve, and made a good recovery.[569]

§ 540. **Physiological Action of the Digitalins.**—Whatever other physiological action this group may have, its effect on the heart's action is so prominent and decided, that the digitalins stand as a type of *heart poisons*. The group of heart poisons has been much extended of late years, and has been found to include the following:—Antiarin, an arrow poison; helleborin, a glucoside contained in the hellebore family; a glucoside found in the *Apocynaceæ*, *Thevatii neriifolia*, and *Thevatia iccotli*; the poisonous principle of the *Nerium oleander* and *N. odorum*; the glucoside of *Tanghinia venenifera*; convallamarin, derived from the species of *Convallaria*; scillotoxin, from the squill; superbin, from the Indian lily; and the alkaloid erythrophlœin from the *Erythrophlœum judiciale*. This list is yearly increasing.

§ 541. **Local Action.**—The digitalins have an exciting or stimulating action if applied to mucous membranes—*e.g.*, if laid upon the nasal mucous surface, sneezing is excited; if applied to the eye, there is redness of the conjunctivæ with smarting; if to the tongue, there is much irritation and a bitter taste. The leaves, the extract, and the tincture all have this directly irritating action, for they all redden and inflame mucous membranes.

§ 542. **Action on the Heart.**—The earlier experimenters on the influence of digitalis on the heart were Stannius and Traube. Stannius[570] experimented on cats, and found strong irregularity, and, lastly, cessation in diastole, in which state it responded no longer to stimuli. Rabbits and birds—especially those birds which lived on plants—

[568] *Arch. f. exp. Path. u. Pharm.*, vol. iii. p. 289, 1875.

[569] Related by Ducroix: *De l'Empoisonnement par la Digitale et la Digitaline.* Paris, 1864.

[570] *Arch. f. Physiol.*

were not so susceptible, nor were frogs.

Traube[571] made his researches on dogs, using an extract, and administering doses which corresponded to from .5 to 4.0 grms. He divided the symptoms witnessed into four stages:—

1st Stage.—The pulse frequently diminishes, while the pressure of the blood rises.

2nd Stage.—Not seen when large doses are employed; pulse frequency, as well as blood pressure, abnormally low.

3rd Stage.—Pressure low, pulse beats above the normal frequency.

The slowing of the heart[572] is attributed to the stimulus of the inhibitory nerves, but the later condition of frequency to their paralysis. After the section of the vagi the slow pulse frequently remains, and this is explained by the inhibitory action of the cardiac centre. The vagus, in point of time, is paralysed earlier than the muscular substance of the heart.

The increased blood pressure Traube attributed to increased energy of the heart's contraction, through the motor centre being stimulated later; the commencing paralysis explains the abnormally low pressure.

There is, however, also an influence on vaso-motor nerves. What Dr. Johnson has described as the "stop-cock" action of the small arteries comes into play, the small arteries contract and attempt, as it were, to limit the supply of poisoned blood. Ackermann,[573] indeed, witnessed this phenomenon in a rabbit's mesentery, distinctly seeing the arteries contract, and the blood pressure rise after section of the spinal cord. This observation, therefore, of Ackermann's (together with experiments of Böhm[574] and L. Brunton[575]) somewhat modifies Traube's explanation, and the views generally accepted respecting the cause of the increased blood pressure may be stated thus:—The pressure is due to prolongation of the systolic stroke of the cardiac pump, and to the "stop-cock" action of the arteries; in other words, there is an increase of force from behind (*vis a tergo*), and an increased resistance in front (*vis a fronte*).

§ 543. **Action of the Digitalins on the Muco-Intestinal Tract and other Organs.**—In addition to that on the heart, there are other actions of the digitalins; for example, by whatever channel the poison is introduced, vomiting has been observed. Even in frogs this, in a rudimentary manner, occurs. The diuretic action which has been noticed in man is wanting in animals, nor has a lessened diminution of urea been confirmed.

Ackermann found the temperature during the period of increased blood pressure raised superficially, but lowered internally. According to Boeck[576] there is no increase in the decomposition of the albuminoids.

§ 544. **The Action of Digitalin on the Common Blow-fly.**—The author has studied the effects of digitalin, made up into a thin paste with water, and applied to the head of the common blow-fly. There are at once great signs of irritation, the sucker is extruded to its full length, and the fly works its fore feet, attempting to brush or remove the irritating agent. The next symptom is a difficulty in walking up a perpendicular glass surface. This difficulty increases, but it is distinctly observed that weakness and paralysis occur in the legs before they are seen in the wings. Within an hour the wings become paralysed also, and the fly, if jerked from its support, falls like a stone. The insect becomes dull and motionless, and ultimately dies in from ten to twenty-four hours. A dose, in itself insufficient to destroy life, does so on repetition at intervals of a couple of hours. The observation is not without interest, inasmuch as it shows that the digitalins are toxic substances to the muscular substance of even those life-forms which do not possess a heart.

§ 545. **Action of the Digitalins on the Frog's Heart.**—The general action of the digitalins is best studied on the heart of the frog. Drs. Fagge and Stevenson have shown[577] that, under the influence of digitalin, there is a peculiar form of irregularity in the beats of the heart of the frog; the ventricle ultimately stops in the white contracted state, the voluntary power being retained for fifteen to twenty minutes afterwards; in very large doses there is,

---

571 *Ann. d. Charité-Krankenhauses*, vol. ii. p. 785.

572 Slowing of the pulse was mentioned first by Withering (*An Account of the Foxglove*, Lond., 1785). Beddoes afterwards observed that digitalis increased the force of the circulation, the slowing of the pulse not being always observed; according to Ackermann, if the inhibitory apparatus is affected by atropine, or if the patient is under deep narcosis, the slowing is absent.

573 *Deutsch. Arch. f. klin. Med.*, vol. xix. p. 125.

574 *Archiv f. d. Ges. Phys.*, vol. v. p. 153.

575 *On Digitalis, with Some Observations on the Urine*, Lond., 1868.

576 *Intoxication*, p. 404.

577 *Guy's Hospl. Reports*, 3rd ver., vol. xii. p. 37.

however, at once paralysis. Lauder Brunton[578] considers the action on the heart to essentially consist in the prolongation of the systole.

Atropine or curare have no influence on the heart thus poisoned. If the animal under the influence of digitalin be treated with muscarine, it stops in diastole instead of systole. On the other hand, the heart poisoned by muscarine is relieved by digitalin, and a similar influence appears to be exercised by atropine. The systolic stillness of the heart is also removed by substances which paralyse the heart, as delphinin, saponin, and apomorphin.

Large doses of digitalin, thrown suddenly on the circulation by intravenous injection, cause convulsions and sudden death, from quick palsy of the heart. With frogs under these circumstances there are no convulsions, but a reflex depression, which, according to Weil[579] and Meihuizen,[580] disappears on decapitation. The central cerebral symptoms are without doubt partly due to the disturbance of the circulation, and there is good ground for attributing them also to a toxic action on the nervous substance. The arteries are affected as well as the heart, and are reduced in calibre; the blood pressure is also increased.[581] This is essentially due to the firm, strong contraction of the heart, and also to the "stop-cock" action of the small arteries.[582]

§ 546. **Post-mortem Appearances.**—In the case of the recruit poisoned by digitalis leaf, the blood was found dark and fluid; the right ventricle and auricle of the heart were filled with blood, the left empty; the brain and its membranes were anæmic; the stomach and mucous membrane of the intestines were in parts ecchymosed, and there were patches of injection. In the case of the widow De Pauw, poisoned with digitalin by the homœopath (Conty de la Pommerais), the only abnormality discovered was a few hyperæmic points in the mucous membrane of the stomach and small intestines. It is then certain that although more or less redness of the lining membrane of the intestine track may be present, yet, on the other hand, the active principle of the digitalis may destroy life, and leave no appreciable sign.

§ 547. **Separation of the Digitalins from Animal Tissues, &c.**—It is best to make an alcoholic extract after the method of Stas, the alcohol being feebly acidulated by acetic acid, and all operations being carried on at a temperature below 60°. The alcoholic extract is dissolved in water feebly acidulated by acetic acid, and shaken up, first with petroleum ether to remove impurities (the ether will not dissolve any of the digitalins), then with benzene, and, lastly, with chloroform. The benzene dissolves digitalein, and the chloroform, digitalin and digitoxin. On allowing these solvents to evaporate spontaneously, residues are obtained which will give the reactions already detailed. Neither the bromine nor any other chemical test is sufficient to identify the digitalins; it is absolutely necessary to have resource to physiological experiment. The method used by Tardieu in the classical Pommerais case may serve as a model, more especially the experiments on frogs. Three frogs were properly secured, the hearts exposed, and the beats counted. The number of beats was found to be fairly equal. Frog No. 1 was placed under such conditions that the heart was constantly moist. Frog No. 2 was poisoned by injecting into the pleura 6 drops of a solution in which 10 mgrms. of digitalin were dissolved in 5 c.c. of water. The third frog was poisoned by a solution of the suspected extract. The number of beats per minute were now counted at definite intervals of time as follows:—

TABLE SHOWING THE ACTION OF DIGITALIN ON THE FROG'S HEART.

Frog No. 1. Unpoisoned.	Frog No. 2. Poisoned by a known quantity of digitalin.	Frog No. 3. Poisoned by the suspected extract.
No. of beats per minute.	No. of beats per minute.	No. of beats per minute.
After 6 minutes, 42	20	26

[578] *On Digitalis, with Some Observations on the Urine*, Lond., 1868.

[579] *Archiv f. Anat. u. Physiol.*, 1871, p. 282.

[580] *Archiv f. d. Ges. Physiol.*, vol. vii. p. 201.

[581] The following is a brief summary of observations on the blood pressure; four stages may be noticed—(1) Rise of normal blood pressure, not necessarily accompanied with a diminution of pulse frequency; (2) continuation of heightened blood pressure, the pulse being raised beyond the normal rate; (3) continued high pressure, with great irregularity of the heart and intermittent pulse; (4) quick depression of pressure, sudden stopping of the heart, and death.

[582] According to Boehm (*Arch. f. d. Ges. Physiol.*, Bd. v. S. 189) and to Williams (*Arch. f. exper. Pathol.*, Bd. xiii. S. 2), the rise of pressure is due entirely to the heart, and not to the contractions of the small arteries; but I fail to see how the small arteries can contract, and yet not heighten the pressure.

,,	10,,	40	16	irregular.	24	irregular.
,,	20,,	40	15		20	,,
,,	28,,	38	0		12	very irregular.
,,	31,,	36	0		0	

In operating in this way—which is strictly comparative, and, with care, has few sources of error—if the heart of the frog poisoned with the unknown extract behaves in the number and irregularity of its contractions similarly to that of the digitalin-poisoned heart, it is a fair inference that, at all events, a "heart-poison" has been separated; but it is, of course, open to question whether this is a digitalin or one of the numerous groups of glucosides acting in the same way. If sufficient quantity has been separated, chemical reactions, especially the bromine test (Grandeau's test), may decide, but with the larger number (yearly increasing) of substances acting similarly on the heart, great caution in giving an opinion will be necessary.

II.—Other Poisonous Glucosides Acting on the Heart.

§ 548. Several members of these glucosides have been studied by Schmiedeberg,[583] and his convenient divisions will be followed here:—

1. CRYSTALLISABLE GLUCOSIDES.

Antiarin ($C_{14}H_{20}O_5$).—Antiarin is an arrow poison obtained from the milky juice of the *Antiaris toxicaria* growing in Java. Antiarin is obtained in crystals, by first treating the inspissated milky juice with petroleum ether to remove fatty and other matters, and then dissolving the active principle out with absolute alcohol. The alcoholic extract is taken up with water, precipitated with lead acetate, filtered, and from the filtrate antiarin obtained by freeing the solution from lead, and then evaporating. De Vry and Ludwig obtained about 4 per cent. from the juice. Antiarin is crystalline, the crystals containing 2 atoms of water. Its melting-point is given as 220.6°; the crystals are soluble in water (254 parts cold, 27.4 parts boiling), they are not soluble in benzene, and with difficulty in ether; 1 part of antiarin requiring 2792 parts of ether.

The watery solution is not precipitated by metallic salts. On warming with dilute mineral acids, antiarin splits up into a resin and sugar. Concentrated sulphuric acid gives with antiarin a yellow-brown solution, hydrochloric and nitric acids strike no distinctive colours.

§ 549. **Effects.**—Antiarin is essentially a muscular and a heart poison. When given in a sufficient dose, it kills a frog in from half an hour to an hour. Its most marked effect is on the cardiac muscle, the heart beats more and more slowly, and at last stops, the ventricle being firmly contracted. As with digitalin, there is a very marked prolongation of the systole, and as with digitalin, after the beats have ceased, a forcible dilatation of the ventricle will restore them (Schmiedeberg). It is doubtful whether by physiological experiment antiarin could be differentiated from digitalin.

§ 550. **Separation of Antiarin.**—In any case of poisoning by antiarin, it would be best to extract with alcohol, evaporate, dissolve the alcoholic extract in water, precipitate with lead acetate, filter, free the filtrate from lead, and then, after alkalising with ammonia, shake the filtrate successively with petroleum ether, benzene, and a small quantity of ether in the manner recommended earlier. The liquid, now freed from all fatty, resinous, and alkaloidal bodies, is neutralised and evaporated to dryness in a vacuum, and the dry residue taken up with absolute alcohol, filtered, the alcohol evaporated at a very low temperature, and finally the extract dissolved in a small quantity of water, and submitted to physiological tests.

§ 551. **The Active Principles of the Hellebores.**—The Christmas rose (*Helleborus niger*), as well as *H. viridis*, *H. fœtidus*, and, in short, all the species of hellebore, are poisonous, and if the root is treated with alcohol, from the alcoholic extract may be separated two glucosides, *helleborin* and *helleborein*.

Helleborin is in the form of white, glittering needles, which, if placed on the tongue, are almost tasteless, but if dissolved in alcohol, and then tasted, give a burning, numbing sensation. By boiling with zinc chloride, helleborin splits up into sugar and a resin—*helleboresin*. Concentrated sulphuric acid dissolves the crystals with the production of a beautiful red colour; on standing, the solution after a while becomes colourless, and a white powder separates.

Helleborein forms colourless crystals, mostly consisting of fine needles; they have a bitter taste, excite

[583] *Beiträge zur Kentniss der pharmakol. Gruppe des Digitalins.*

sneezing, and are very hygroscopic. The crystals easily dissolve in water and dilute alcohol, but are with difficulty soluble in absolute alcohol, and not soluble in ether. They dissolve in fatty oils. Helleborein splits by the action of mineral acids into sugar and amorphous *helleboretin.*

Helleboretin is in the moist condition of a beautiful violet-blue colour, becoming, when dried at 100°, dirty green. Concentrated sulphuric acid dissolves it with the production of a brown-yellow colour, which on standing passes into violet and then into brown.

Marmé separated from *H. fœtidus*, in addition, a white, intensely odorous substance, but too small in quantity to thoroughly investigate its properties.

§ 552. There is little doubt that hellebore owes its properties to the glucosides just described. There are several instances of poisoning by hellebore root,[584] and by the pharmaceutical preparations, but none of poisoning by the pure active principles. Morgagni mentions a case in which 2 grms. (nearly 31 grains) of the watery extract of *H. Niger* caused death within eight hours; and Ferrari saw, after the use of the wine in which the root had been boiled, two persons poisoned with a like result. A more recent case was recorded by Felletar, in 1875, in which a person died from an infusion of hellebore; there was, however, old standing heart-disease, so that there may be a doubt as to the real cause of death in this instance. Schauenstein mentions a case in which the roots of hellebore were accidentally used in soup, but the bitter taste prevented any quantity being eaten. The physiological action, especially of helleborein, is that of an intense heart poison, and the symptoms produced by the hellebores are so strikingly like those of the digitalins that it might be difficult to distinguish clinically between them. In any case of poisoning, the active principle must be separated in the form of an alcoholic extract, and identified as a heart poison by physiological experiment.

§ 553. **Euonymin** is found in a resin obtained from the *Euonymus atropurpureus*; it is crystalline, crystallising in colourless, cauliflower-like masses consisting of groups of stellate needles, which are soluble in water, but with difficulty in alcohol. It is a glucoside, and a powerful heart poison, 1 mgrm. causing the heart of a frog to cease in diastole.[585]

§ 554. **Thevetin** ($C_{54}H_{48}O_2$).—A glucoside which has been separated from the Thevetia nereifolia, and perhaps also from the *Cerbera Odallam*. It is soluble in 124 parts of water at 14°, and is easily soluble in spirit, but not in ether. It is coloured by sulphuric acid red-brown, passing into cherry-red, and then, in a few hours, into violet. On boiling with diluted acids, it splits up into sugar and theveresin. Both thevetin and theveresin are powerful heart poisons.[586]

2. SUBSTANCES PARTLY CRYSTALLISABLE BUT WHICH ARE NOT GLUCOSIDES.

§ 555. **Strophantin** is a very poisonous substance which belongs physiologically to this group, but does not seem to be a glucoside. It is soluble in water and in alcohol, less so in ether and chloroform. It is found in the *kombé*, *manganja*, *inée*, or *onaje*, a West African poison derived from the *Strophanthus hispidus* of the family of *Apocynaceæ*. The poison has been investigated by several observers.[587]

Dr. Fraser considers, from his experiments, (1) That strophantin acts primarily on the heart, producing, as an end result, heart paralysis, with permanence of the ventricular systole. (2) He found the pulmonary respiration to continue in cold-blooded animals many minutes after the heart was paralysed. (3) The striped muscles of the body are affected, and twitches occur in them; their tonicity is exaggerated, and finally their functional activity is destroyed. This change is referred to an action on the muscular structure itself, independent of that upon the heart, and also independent of the cerebro-spinal nervous system. (4) The reflex action of the spinal cord is suspended after the heart is paralysed, but the motor conductivity of the spinal cord and of the nerve trunks continue after the striped muscles of the body are paralysed. (5) The lymph-hearts of the frog continue to contract for many minutes after the blood-heart has been paralysed.

§ 556. **Apocynin.**—In the root of *Apocynum cannabinum* a non-crystallisable substance, soluble in alcohol and ether, but not soluble easily in water, has been separated and found to have a physiological activity similar to that

[584] There used to be a tincture officinal in our pharmacopœia; the root of *H. viridis* is officinal in the German pharmacopœia, maximum single dose, .3 grm.; maximum total quantity in twenty-four hours, 1.2 grm. The tincture is also officinal on the Continent.

[585] Schmiedeberg, *op. cit.*, from unpublished researches of Professor H. Meyer, Dorpat.

[586] Husemann, *Archiv f. exper. Path. u. Pharmakol.*, Bd. v., S. 228, 1876.

[587] *Digitoxin* (see *ante*) belongs to this group.

of the digitalins.[588]

3. NON-CRYSTALLISABLE GLUCOSIDES ALMOST INSOLUBLE IN WATER.

§ 557. **Scillain, or Scillitin**, a glucoside which has been separated from the bulbs of the common squill. It is insoluble or nearly so in water, but easily dissolves in alcohol. It is little soluble in ether. It acts upon the heart, and is poisonous.

Adonidin, a very similar substance, has been separated from the root of the *Adonis vernalis* (Nat. Ord. *Ranunculaceæ*), to which the name of adonidin has been given.[589] It is an amorphous, colourless substance, without odour; soluble in alcohol, but with difficulty soluble in ether and water. It is precipitated by tannin, and on saponification by mineral acids, splits up into sugar and a substance soluble in ether. The effects on animals are identical with those of digitalin. The root has been used recently in medicine, and found to slow the heart and increase the urinary secretion; in this also it is like digitalis.

§ 558. **Oleandrin.**—Oleander leaves contain two chemically-different, nitrogen-free substances. The one is probably identical with digitalein; but as this is not certain, Schmiedeberg proposes to call it provisionally *neriin*. The other active substance is essentially the same as the oleandrin of Lukomske[590] and Betelli.[591] Oleandrin has basic properties, and is separated in the form of an amorphous mass, soluble in alcohol, ether, and chloroform, and slightly soluble in water. Schmiedeberg obtained a third product from African leaves, which he calls *nerianthin*. This, on treatment with sulphuric acid and bromine, gives a beautiful colour peculiar to oleander leaves. It is very similar in physiological and chemical properties to digitalin, and is probably derived by decomposition from one of the principles already described. There is also a product similar to digitaliresin.

The active principles of the oleander are separated by digestion of the leaves with alcohol of 50 per cent., and precipitating the alcoholic extract with lead acetate and ammonia. The first precipitate is yellow, and is probably composed of a tannin-like substance; the next precipitate is white, consisting of the lead compound of neriin. The precipitates are filtered off, and the filtrate concentrated; nerianthin, after a while, separates in light flocks, and the filtrate from this contains some of the other products.

§ 559. **Neriin or Oleander Digitalin.**—Neriin is, in the presence of much free mineral acid, precipitated by potass-bismuth iodide, a reaction first pointed out by Marmé,[592] as useful in the isolation of the helleborins; or it may be precipitated by tannin, and then the precipitate decomposed by dissolving in alcohol, and evaporating it to dryness with zinc oxide on the water-bath. It is next extracted by absolute alcohol, and precipitated by the addition of much ether. The further purification consists of resolution in alcohol, and fractional precipitation by ether. If, however, the potass-bismuth iodide process is used, the liquid must be acidified strongly with sulphuric acid, and the precipitate washed with diluted sulphuric acid. The precipitate may be decomposed by baryta, filtered, and the filtrate freed from baryta by carbon dioxide; the filtrate from this contains neriin with baric iodide; it is therefore treated with silver sulphate, then again with baryta, next with carbon dioxide, and also with SH_2 to get rid of the last trace of silver.

The filtrate will also contain some oleandrin which, by evaporating slowly in a vacuum, separates gradually in the form of a clear, resinous mass. It can be filtered off, and the neriin then may be precipitated pure by fractional precipitation. Its physiological action is the same as that of digitalein.

§ 560. The nerium oleander has several times caused grave symptoms of poisoning, and they have usually fairly agreed with those produced by foxglove. For example, Maschka[593] relates the case of a boy, two years old, who ate two handfuls of the nerium oleander. The effects commenced in ten minutes, the child was uneasy, and vomited. In six hours a sleepy condition came on; the face was pale, the skin cold, the pupils contracted, and the pulse slow and irregular. After the sickness the boy woke up, but again fell asleep, and this occurred frequently; coffee was given, which appeared to do good. The pulse was intermittent. On the following day the child was still ill, with an

---

[588] Hardy et Callois, "*Sur la matière active du Strophanthus Hispidus ou Inée*," *Gaz. Med. de Paris*; Pelikan, *Compt. Rend.*, t. 60, p. 1209, 1815; Sharpey, *Proc. Roy. Soc.*, May, 1865; Fagge and Stevenson, *Pharm. Journ.*, p. 11, 1865-66; Fraser, *Journ. of Anatom. and Phys.*, also *Proc. of Roy. Soc. of Edin.*; Poillo and Carville, *Arch. de Physiol. Norm. et Pathol.*, 1872; G. Valentin, *Zeitschr. et. Biologie.*, x. 133, 1874.

[589] Cervello, *Archiv für exp. Path. Pharm.*, 1882, p. 338.

[590] *Repert. de Chimie de Wurtz et Bareswill*, t. iii. p. 77, 1861.

[591] *Bull. Med. di Bologna*, t. xix. p. 321, 1865.

[592] *Zeitschr. f. rat. Med.* (3 R.), Bd. xxvi., S. 1, 1866.

[593] *Vierteljahrsschrift f. gericht. Med.*, Bd. ii., No. 17, 1860. *Brit. and For. Med. Chir. Review*, vol. xxvi. p. 523, 1860.

intermittent pulse, frequent vomiting, feebleness, sleeplessness, and dilatation of the pupil; there was no diarrhœa, on the contrary, the bowels were confined. On the third day recovery followed.

In an Indian case,[594] the symptoms were altogether peculiar, and belonged rather to the convulsive order. A wood-cutter, aged thirty-five, near Kholapore, took, for the purpose of suicide, a little over an ounce of the expressed juice of the oleander. The symptoms began so rapidly that he had not time to walk five yards before he fell insensible; he was brought to the hospital in this state; the face on his arrival was noticed to be flushed, the breathing stertorous, there were violent spasmodic contractions of the whole body, more marked on the left than on the right side. The effect of this was remarkable. During the intervals of the spasm, the patient lay evenly on his back, and when the convulsions commenced the superior contraction of the left side threw him on to the right, in which position he remained during the paroxysm, after the subsidence of which he fell back into his old position. The evacuations were involuntary and watery; the man was insensible, with frequent convulsions of the kind described, for two days, but on the third day became conscious, and made a good recovery.

In any case of poisoning, the methods by which neriin and oleandrin are separated from the plant can be applied to separate them from the tissues with more or less success. Here, as in all the other digitalin-like glucosides, physiological tests are alone of value in the final identification.

§ 561. **The Madagascar Ordeal Poison.**—To this group may also belong the poison of the *Tanghinia venenifera*, a tree in the Island of Madagascar, the fruit of which is used as an ordeal poison. It may be obtained in crystals; it is insoluble in water, and very poisonous. The upas of Singapore is also said to contain with strychnine a glucoside similar to antiarin.

4. SUBSTANCES WHICH, WITH OTHER TOXIC EFFECTS, BEHAVE LIKE THE DIGITALIS.

§ 562. **Erythrophlein** is an alkaloid, not a glucoside, and is obtained from the bark of the *Erythrophlœum guineense* (West Africa). It acts on the heart like digitalis, and has also effects similar to picrotoxin.

III.—Saponin—Saponin Substances.

§ 563. The term "saponin" of late years has been applied to a class of glucosides which possess the common property of being poisonous, and, when dissolved in water, forming solutions which froth on shaking like soap-suds.

The substances which have these properties are not all of the same series chemically, but those of the general formula, $C_nH_{2n-8}O_{10}$, are most numerous, and the following is a list:—

Name.	Formula.
Saponin, senegin,	
Quillaja-sapotoxin,	
Sapindus-sapotoxin,	$C_{17}H_{26}O_{10}$.
Grypsophila-sapotoxin,	
Agrostemma-sapotoxin,	
Saponin II., digitonin, saporubrin, assamin,	$C_{18}H_{28}O_{10}$.
Saponin III., quillajic acid, polygalic acid,	$C_{19}H_{30}O_{10}$.
Herniari-saponin,	
Cyclamin, sarsaparilla-saponin,	$C_{20}H_{32}O_{10}$.
Sarsa-saponin,	$C_{22}H_{36}O_{10}$.
Parillin,	$C_{26}H_{44}O_{10}$.
Melanthin,	$C_{29}H_{50}O_{10}$.

Possibly also dulcamarin $C_{22}H_{34}O_{10}$ and syringen $C_{17}H_{26}O_{10}$ may belong to this series.

There are some 150 distinct plants which thus yield saponins; a few of these plants are as follows:—*Saponaria officinalis*, *Gypsophila struthium*, *Agrostemma githago* (corn cockle), *Polygala senega*, *Monimia polystachia*, the

[594] *Transac. of Med. and Phys. Soc. of Bombay*, 1859.

bark of *Quillaja saponaria*, and *Chrysophyllum glycyphleum*.

The saponin separated from *Saponaria*, and from the corn cockle will be here described.

§ 564. **Properties.**—Saponin is a white amorphous powder, very soluble in water, to which it gives the curious property of frothing just like soap solution. To obtain this effect there must be at least 1 mgrm. in 1 c.c. of liquid. Saponin is neutral in reaction, it has no odour, but causes sneezing if applied to the mucous membrane of the nose; the taste is at first sweet, and then sharp and acrid. It is almost entirely insoluble in absolute alcohol, but dissolves in hot alcohol of 83° to separate again nearly completely on cooling. It is precipitated by basic lead acetate, and also by baryta water, but in each case it is advisable to operate on concentrated solutions. Picric acid, mercuric chloride, and alkaloidal "group reagents" give no precipitate. When a little of the solid substance is treated with "Nessler" reagent, there is a greenish or yellow colour produced. A drop of strong sulphuric acid, mixed with a minute quantity of saponin, strikes slowly a bright red colour, which, on heating, deepens to maroon-brown. Nordhausen sulphuric acid shows this better and more rapidly. If saponin is boiled with dilute acid it breaks up into sapogenin and sugar, and therefore the liquid after neutralisation reduces "Fehling." This reaction is probably after the following equation:—

$$2C_{17}H_{26}O_{10} + 2H_2O = 2C_8H_{11}O_2 + 3C_6H_{12}O_6.$$

Sapogenin may be separated by evaporating the neutralised liquid to dryness, treating the dry residue with ether, which dissolves out the sapogenin, and finally recovering the substance from the ethereal solution, and crystallising it from hot alcohol. Crystals are readily obtained if the alcoholic solution is allowed to evaporate spontaneously. A solution of saponin exposed to the air gets turbid, and develops carbon dioxide; not unfrequently the solution becomes mouldy.

§ 565. **Effects.**—Pelikan[595] has studied the effects of various saponins on frogs. One to two drops of a saturated watery solution of saponin applied subcutaneously to the leg, caused, in from five to six minutes, great weakness, accompanied by a loss of sensibility; but strong mechanical, chemical, or electrical stimuli applied to the foot excited reflex action, for the ischiatic nerve still retained its functions. Nevertheless, from the commencement, the excitability of the poisoned muscles was much weakened, and just before death quite disappeared. Section of the ischiatic nerve delayed the phenomena. Curarine did not seem to have any effect on the poisonous action. A concentrated solution applied to the heart of a frog soon arrests its beats, but weaker doses first excite, and then retard.[596]

The author has studied the general action of saponin on kittens, insects, and infusoria. Small doses, such as from 13 to 32 mgrms. ($^1/_5$ to $^1/_2$ grain), were injected beneath the loose skin of the back of the neck of a kitten, when there were immediate symptoms of local pain. In from five to ten minutes the respiration notably quickened, and the animal fell into a lethargic state, with signs of general muscular weakness; just before death the breathing became very rapid, and there were all the signs of asphyxia. The pathological appearances after death were fulness in the right side of the heart, and intense congestion of the intestinal canal, the stomach generally being perfectly normal in appearance, and the kidneys and other organs healthy. The least fatal dose for a kitten seems to be 13 mgrms., or .04 grm. to a kilogram.[597]

§ 566. **Action on Man.**—The effects of saponin on man have been but little studied; it has been administered by the mouth in doses of from .1 to .2 grm., and in those doses seems to have distinct physiological effects. There is increased mucous secretion, and a feeling of nausea; but neither diaphoresis nor diuresis has been observed. From the foregoing study it may be predicated that 2.6 grms. (40 grains), if administered subcutaneously to an adult, would endanger life. The symptoms would be great muscular prostration, weakness of the heart's action, and probably diarrhœa. In fatal cases, some signs of an irritant or inflammatory action on the mucous membranes of the stomach and intestines would be probable.

§ 567. **Separation of Saponin.**—Saponin is separated from bread, flour, and similar substances by the process given at p. 153, "Foods." The process essentially consists in extracting with hot spirit, allowing the saponin to separate as the spirit cools, collecting the precipitate on a filter, drying, dissolving in cold water, and precipitating with absolute alcohol. In operating on animal tissues, a more elaborate process is necessary. The author has

[595] *Berl. klin. Wochschr.*, 36, 186.

[596] J. Hoppe, *Nervenwirkung der Heilmittel*, H. 4, 37.

[597] The action of saponin when applied in concentrated solution to flies is that of an intense irritant. There is protrusion of the sucker, and progressive paralysis. The common infusoria live for some time in dilute solutions of saponin—this is also true of some of the higher forms; for example, a *Cyclops quadricornis* seemed in no way affected by a 2 per cent. solution.

successfully proceeded as follows:—The finely divided organ is digested in alcohol of 80 to 90 per cent. strength, and boiled for a quarter of an hour; the alcohol is filtered hot and allowed to cool, when a deposit forms, consisting of fatty matters, and containing any saponin present. The deposit is filtered off, dried, and treated with ether to remove fat. The insoluble saponin remaining is dissolved in the least possible quantity of water, and precipitated with absolute alcohol. It is also open to the analyst to purify it by precipitating with baryta water, the baryta compound being subsequently decomposed by carbon dioxide. Basic lead acetate may also be used as a precipitant, the lead compound being, as usual, decomposed by hydric sulphide; lastly, a watery solution may be shaken up with chloroform, which will extract saponin. By some one of these methods, selected according to the exigencies of the case, there will be no difficulty in separating the glucoside in a fairly pure state. The organ best to examine for saponin is the kidney. In one of my own experiments, in a cat poisoned with a subcutaneous dose of saponin (.2 grm.), evidence of the glucoside was obtained from the kidney alone. The time after death at which it is probable that saponin could be detected is unknown; it is a substance easily decomposed, and, therefore, success in separating it from highly putrid matters is not probable.

§ 568. **Identification of Saponin.**—An amorphous white powder, very soluble in water, insoluble in cold alcohol or ether, having glucosidal reactions, striking a red colour with sulphuric acid, imparting a soap-like condition to water, and poisonous to animals, is most probably a saponin.

DIVISION III.—CERTAIN POISONOUS ANHYDRIDES OF ORGANIC ACIDS.

I.—Santonin.

§ 569. Santonin ($C_{15}H_{18}O_3$) is a neutral principle extracted from the unexpanded heads of various species of *Artemisia* (Nat. Ord. *Compositæ*). The seeds contain, according to Dragendorff, 2.03 to 2.13 per cent. of santonin, and about 2.25 per cent. of volatile oil, with 3 per cent. of fat and resin. Santonin forms brilliant, white, four-sided, flat prisms, in taste feebly bitter. The crystals become yellow through age and exposure to light; they melt at 169°, and are capable of being sublimed; they are scarcely soluble in cold water, but dissolve in 250 parts of boiling water, freely in alkaline water, in 3 parts of boiling alcohol, and in 42 parts of boiling ether. Santonin is the anhydride of santonic acid ($C_{15}H_{20}O_4$). Santonin unites with alkalies to form santonates. Sodic santonate ($C_{15}H_{19}NaO_4 + 3\frac{1}{2}H_2O$) is officinal on the Continent; it forms colourless rhombic crystals, soluble in 3 parts of cold water.

§ 570. **Poisoning by Santonin.**—Eighteen cases of poisoning, either by santonin or santonin-holding substances, which F. A. Falck has been able to collect, were nearly all occasioned by its use as a remedy for worms. A few were poisonings of children who had swallowed it by accident. With one exception those poisoned were children of from two to twelve years of age; in five the flower heads, and in thirteen santonin itself was taken. Of the eighteen cases, two only died (about 11 per cent.).

§ 571. **Fatal Dose.**—So small a number of children have died from santonin, that data are not present for fixing the minimum fatal dose. .12 grm. of santonin killed a boy of five and a half years of age in fifteen hours; a girl, ten years old, died from a quantity of flower heads, equal to .2 grm. of santonin. The maximum dose for children is from 65 to 194 mgrms. (1 to 3 grains), and twice the quantity for adults.

§ 572. **Effects on Animals.**—Experiments on animals with santonin have been numerous. It has first an exciting action on the centres of nerves from the second to the seventh pairs, and then follows decrease of excitability. The medulla is later affected. There are tetanic convulsions, and death follows through asphyxia. Artificial respiration lessens the number and activity of the convulsions, and chloroform, chloral hydrate, or ether, also either prevent or shorten the attacks.

§ 573. **Effects on Man.**—One of the most constant effects of santonin is a peculiar aberration of the colour-sense, first observed by Hufeland in 1806. All things seem yellow, and this may last for twenty-four hours, seldom longer. According to Rose, this apparent yellowness is often preceded by a violet hue over all objects. If the lids are closed while the "yellow sight" is present, the whole field is momentarily violet. De Martiny,[598] in a few cases, found the "yellow sight" intermit and pass into other colours, *e.g.*, after .3 grm. there was first the yellow perception, then giving the same individual .6 grm., all objects seemed coloured red, after half an hour orange, and then again yellow. In another patient the effect of the drug was to give "green vision," and in a third blue.

[598] *Gaz. des Hôpit.*, 1860.

Hufner and Helmholtz explain this curious effect as a direct action on the nervous elements of the retina, causing them to give the perception of violet; they are first excited, then exhausted, and the eye is "violet blind." On the other hand, it has been suggested that santonin either colours the media of the eye yellow, or that there is an increase in the pigment of the *macula lutea*. I, however, cannot comprehend how the two last theories will account for the intermittency and the play of colours observed in a few cases. To the affections of vision are also often added hallucinations of taste and smell; there is headache and giddiness, and in fourteen out of thirty of Rose's observations vomiting occurred. The urinary secretion is increased. In large and fatal doses there are shivering of the body, clonic, and often tetanic convulsions; the consciousness is lost, the skin is cool, but covered with sweat, the pupils dilated, the breathing becomes stertorous, the heart's action weak and slow, and death occurs in collapse—in the case observed by Grimm in fifteen hours, in one observed by Linstow in forty-eight hours. In those patients who have recovered, there have also been noticed convulsions and loss of consciousness. Sieveking[599] has recorded the case of a child who took .12 grm. (1.7 grain) santonin; an eruption of nettle rash showed itself, but disappeared within an hour.

§ 574. **Post-mortem Appearances.**—The *post-mortem* appearances are not characteristic.

§ 575. **Separation of Santonin from the Contents of the Stomach, &c.**—It is specially important to analyse the fæces, for it has been observed that some portion goes unchanged into the intestinal canal. The urine, also, of persons who have taken santonin, possesses some important peculiarities. It becomes of a peculiar yellow-green, the colour appearing soon after the ingestion of the drug, and lasting even sixty hours. The colour may be imitated, and therefore confused with that which is produced by the bile acids; a similar colour is also seen after persons have been taking rhubarb. Alkalies added to urine coloured by santonin or rhubarb strike a red colour. If the urine thus reddened is digested on zinc dust, santonin urine fades, rhubarb urine remains red. Further, if the reddened urine is precipitated by excess of milk of lime or baryta water and filtered, the filtrate from the urine reddened by rhubarb is colourless, in that reddened by santonin the colour remains. Santonin may be isolated by treating substances containing it with warm alkaline water. The water may now be acidified and shaken up with chloroform, which will dissolve out any santonin. On driving off the chloroform, the residue should be again alkalised, dissolved in water, and acidified with hydrochloric acid, and shaken up with chloroform. In this way, by operating several times, it may be obtained very pure. Santonin may be identified by its dissolving in alcoholic potash to a transitory carmine-red, but the best reaction is to dissolve it in concentrated sulphuric acid, to which a very little water has been added, to warm on the water-bath, and then to add a few drops of ferric chloride solution to the warm acid; a ring of a beautiful red colour passing into purple surrounds each drop, and after a little time, on continuing the heat, the purple passes into brown. A distinctive reaction is also the production of "iso-santonin"; this substance is produced by warming santonin on the water-bath with sulphuric acid for a few hours, and then diluting with water; iso-santonin is precipitated, and may be crystallised from boiling alcohol. Iso-santonin melts at 138°; it has the same composition as santonin. It is distinguished from santonin by giving no red colour when treated with sulphuric or phosphoric acids.

II.—Mezereon.

§ 576. **The Daphne Mezereum** (L.).—Mezereon, an indigenous shrub belonging to the *Thymeleaceæ*, is rather rare in the wild state, but very frequent in gardens. The flowers are purple and the berries red. Buckheim isolated by means of ether an acrid resin, which was converted by saponifying agents into *mezereic acid*; the acrid resin is the anhydride of the acid. The resin is presumed to be the active poisonous constituent of the plant, but the subject awaits further investigation. There are a few cases of poisoning on record, and they have been mostly from the berries. Thus, Linné has recorded an instance in which a little girl died after eating twelve berries. The symptoms observed in the recorded cases have been burning in the mouth, gastroenteritis, vomiting, giddiness, narcosis, and convulsions, ending in death. The lethal dose for a horse is about 30 grms. of powdered bark; for a dog, the œsophagus being tied, 12 grms.; but smaller doses of the fresh leaves may be deadly.

[599] *Brit. Med. Journ.*, 1871.

DIVISION IV.—VARIOUS VEGETABLE POISONOUS PRINCIPLES—NOT ADMITTING OF CLASSIFICATION UNDER THE PREVIOUS THREE DIVISIONS.

I.—Ergot of Rye.

§ 577. Ergot is a peculiar fungus attacking the rye and other graminaceous plants;[600] it has received various names, *Claviceps purpurea* (Tulasne), *Spermœdia clavus* (Fries), *Sclerotium clavus* (D.C.), &c. The peculiar train of symptoms arising from the eating of ergotised grain (culminating occasionally in gangrene of the lower limbs), its powerful action on the pregnant uterus, and its styptic effects, are well known.

The very general use of the drug by accoucheurs has, so to speak, popularised a knowledge of its action among all classes of society, and its criminal employment as an abortive appears to be on the increase.[601]

The healthy grain of rye, if examined microscopically in thin sections, is seen to be composed of the seed-coating, made up of two layers, beneath which are the gluten-cells, whilst the great bulk of the seed is composed of cells containing starch. In the ergotised grain, dark (almost black) cells replace the seed-coat and the gluten-cells, whilst the large starch-containing cells are filled with the small cells of the fungus and numerous drops of oil.

§ 578. **The chemical constituents of ergot** are a fixed oil, trimethylamine, certain active principles, and colouring-matters.

The **fixed oil** is of a brownish-yellow colour, of aromatic flavour and acrid taste; its specific gravity is 0.924, and it consists chiefly of palmitin and olein; it has no physiological action.

Trimethylamine is always present ready formed in ergot; it can also be produced by the action of potash on ergot.

With regard to the **active principles of ergot** considerable confusion still exists, and no one has hitherto isolated any single substance in such a state of purity as to inspire confidence as to its formula or other chemical characters. They may, however, be briefly described.

C. Tamet[602] has separated an alkaloid, which appears identical with Wenzel's *ergotinine*. To obtain this the ergot is extracted by alcohol of 86°, the spirit removed by distillation, and the residue cooled; a resin (which is deposited) and a fatty layer (which floats on the surface) are separated from the extractive liquor and washed with ether; the ethereal solution is filtered and shaken with dilute sulphuric acid, which takes up the alkaloid; the aqueous solution of the substance is then filtered, rendered alkaline by KHO, and agitated with chloroform. The ergotinine is now obtained by evaporating the chloroform solution, care being taken to protect it from contact with the air. It gives precipitates with chloride of gold, potassium iodohydrargyrate, phosphomolybdic acid, tannin, bromine water, and the chlorides of gold and platinum. With moderately concentrated SO_4H_2, it gives a yellowish-red coloration, changing to an intense violet, a reaction which does not occur if the alkaloid has been exposed to the air. The composition of the base is represented by the formula $C_{70}H_{40}N_4O_{12}$, and a crystalline sulphate and lactate have been obtained.[603]

Wenzel's **Ecboline** is prepared by precipitating the cold watery extract of ergot with sugar of lead, throwing out the lead in the usual way by hydric sulphide, concentrating the liquid, and adding mercuric chloride, which only precipitates the ecboline. The mercury salt is now decomposed with hydric sulphide, and after the mercury precipitate has been filtered off, the filtrate is treated with freshly precipitated phosphate of silver, and refiltered; lastly, the liquid is shaken up with milk of lime, again filtered, and the lime thrown out by CO_2. The last filtrate contains ecboline only, and is obtained by evaporation at a gentle heat. It is an amorphous, feebly bitter substance, with an alkaline reaction, forming only amorphous salts.

The most recent research by Dragendorff on ergot tends to show that Wenzel's alkaloids, ergotinine and ecboline, are inactive. Dragendorff describes also (*a.*) *Scleromucin*, a slimy substance which goes into solution upon extraction of the ergot with water, and which is again precipitated by 40 to 45 per cent. alcohol. It is colloidal and soluble with difficulty in water. It contains nitrogen, but gives no albuminoid reaction, nor any reaction of an alkaloidal or glucosidal body; it yields to analysis—

---

600 Some of the *Cyperaceæ* are also attacked.

601 The Russian peasantry use the drug for the same purpose. *Vide* Mackenzie Wallace's "Russia," i. p. 117.

602 *Compt. Rendus*, vol. xxxi. p. 896.

603 *Compt. Rendus*, April 1878.

8 .26 per cent.	Water.
26.8 „	Ash.
39.0 „	Carbon.
6 .44„	Hydrogen.
6 .41„	Nitrogen.

(*b.*) **Sclerotic Acid.**—A feebly-acid substance, easily soluble in water and dilute and moderately concentrated alcohol. It passes, in association with other constituents of the ergot extract, into the diffusate, when the extract is submitted to dialysis; but after its separation in a pure state it is, like scleromucin, colloidal. It is precipitated by 85 to 90 per cent. alcohol, together with lime, potash, soda, silica, and manganese; but after maceration with hydrochloric acid, the greater part of the ash constituents can be separated by a fresh precipitation with absolute alcohol. The sample gave 40.0 per cent. of carbon, 5.2 per cent. hydrogen, 4.2 per cent. nitrogen, 50.6 per cent. oxygen, with 3.4 per cent. of ash. Sclerotic acid forms with lime a compound that is not decomposed by carbonic acid, and which upon combustion leaves from 19 to 20 per cent. of calcium carbonate. Both these substances are active, although evidently impure. Sclerotic acid is sold in commerce, and has been employed subcutaneously in midwifery practice in Russia and Germany for some time.

The inert principles of ergot are—(1.) A red colouring matter, *Sclererythrin*, insoluble in water, but soluble in dilute and strong alcohol, ether, chloroform, dilute solutions of potash, ammonia, &c. It can be obtained by dissolving in an alkali, neutralising with an acid, and shaking up with ether. Alcoholic solution of sclererythrin gives with aluminium sulphate, and with zinc chloride, a splendid red mixture; with salts of calcium, barium, and many of the heavy metals, it gives a blue precipitate; the yield is only .1 to .05 in a thousand parts.

(2.) Another colouring-matter, dissolving in concentrated sulphuric acid with the production of a fine blue violet colour, the discoverer has named *Scleroidin*. This is not soluble in alcohol, ether, chloroform, or water, but dissolves in alkaline solutions, potash producing a splendid violet colour; yield about 1 per 1000.

(3, 4.) Two crystalline substances, which may be obtained from ergot powder, first treated with an aqueous solution of tartaric acid, and the colouring-matters extracted by ether. One Dragendorff names *Sclerocrystallin* ($C_{10}H_{10}O_4$); it is in colourless needles, insoluble in alcohol and water, with difficulty soluble in ether, but dissolving in ammonia and potash solutions. The other crystalline substance is thought to be merely a hydrated compound of sclerocrystallin. Both are without physiological action.

Kobert recognises two active substances in ergot, and two alone; the one he calls *sphacelic acid*, the other *cornutin*.

§ 579. **Detection of Ergot in Flour** (see "Foods").—The best process is to exhaust the flour with boiling alcohol. The alcoholic solution is acidified with dilute sulphuric acid, and the coloured liquid examined by the spectroscope in thicker or thinner layers, according to the depth of colour. A similar alcoholic solution of ergot should be made, and the spectrum compared. If the flour is ergotised, the solution will be more or less red, and show two absorption bands, one in the green, and a broader and stronger one in the blue. On mixing the original solution with twice its volume of water, and shaking successive portions of this liquid with ether, amyl alcohol, benzene, and chloroform, the red colour, if derived from ergot, will impart its colour to each and all of these solvents.

§ 580. **Pharmaceutical Preparations.**—Ergot itself is officinal in all the pharmacopœias, and occurs in grains from ⅓ to 1 inch in length, and about the same breadth, triangular, curved, obtuse at the ends, of a purple colour, covered with a bloom, and brittle, exhibiting a pinkish interior, and the microscopical appearances already detailed. Ergot may also occur as a brown powder, possessing the unmistakable odour of the drug. A liquid extract of the B.P. is prepared by digesting 16 parts of ergot in 80 parts of water for twelve hours, the infusion is decanted or filtered off, and the digestion repeated with 40 parts of water; this is also filtered off, and the residue pressed, and the whole filtrate united and evaporated down to 11 parts; when cold, 6 parts of rectified spirit are added, and, after standing, the liquid is filtered and made up to measure 16. A tincture and an infusion are also officinal; the latter is very frequently used, but seldom sold, for it is preferable to prepare it on the spot. The tincture experience has shown to be far inferior in power to the extract, and it is not much used. Ergotin is a purified extract of uncertain strength; it is used for hypodermic injection; it should be about five times more active than the liquid extract.

§ 581. **Dose.**—The main difficulties in the statement of the medicinal dose, and of the minimum quantity which will destroy life, are the extreme variability of different samples of ergot, and its readiness to decompose. A full medicinal dose of ergot itself, as given to a woman in labour, is 4 grms. (61.7 grains), repeated every half hour. In this way enormous doses may be given in some cases without much effect. On the other hand, single doses of from 1 to 4 grms. have caused serious poisonous symptoms. The extract and the tincture are seldom given in larger doses than that of a drachm as a first dose, to excite uterine contraction. In fact, the medical practitioner has in many cases to experiment on his patient with the drug, in order to discover, not only the individual susceptibility, but the activity of the particular preparation used. From the experiments of Nikitin, it is probable that the least fatal dose of sclerotic acid for an adult man is 20 mgrms. per kilogrm.

§ 582. **Ergotism.**—Ergotised cereals have played a great part in various epidemics, probably from very early times, but the only accurate records respecting them date from the sixteenth century. According to Dr. Tissot,[604] the first recorded epidemic was in 1596, when a strange, spasmodic, convulsive disease broke out in Hessia and the neighbouring regions. It was probably due to spurred rye. In Voigtländer, the same disease appeared in 1648, 1649, and 1675; in 1702 the whole of Freiberg was attacked. In Germany and in France successive epidemics are described throughout the eighteenth century. In France, in 1710, Ch. Noel, physician at the *Hôtel Dieu*, had no less than fifty cases under treatment at the same time.

It is generally said that in 1630, Thuillier, in describing an ergot epidemic which broke out in Cologne, first referred the cause of the disease to spurred rye.

It is interesting to inquire into the mortality from this disease. In 1770, in an epidemic described by Taube, in which 600 were affected, 16 per cent. died. In a nineteenth-century epidemic (1855), in which, according to Husemann, 30 were ill, 23.3 per cent. died. In other epidemics, according to Heusinger, out of 102, 12 per cent. died; according to Griepenkerl, out of 155, 25 or 16 per cent. died; and, according to Meyer, of 283 cases, 6 per cent. died.

There are two forms of chronic poisoning by ergot—one a spasmodic form, the other the gangrenous form.

§ 583. **The convulsive form of ergotism** mostly begins with some cerebral disturbance. There are sparks before the eyes, giddiness, noises in the ears, and a creeping feeling about the body. There is also very commonly anæsthesia of the fingers and toes, and later of the extremities, of the back, and even of the tongue. Diarrhœa, vomiting, colic, and other signs of intestinal irritation seldom fail to be present; there are also tetanic spasms of the muscles, rising in some cases to well-marked tetanus; epilepsy, faintings, aberrations of vision, amaurosis, and amblyopia are frequent; the skin becomes of a yellow or earthy colour, and is covered with a cold sweat; boils and other eruptions may break out; blebs, like those caused by burns or scalds, have in a few cases been noticed. Death may occur in from four to twelve weeks after the eating of the spurred grain from exhaustion. In those individuals who recover, there remain for some time weakness, contractions of groups of muscles, anæmia, or affections of vision.

§ 584. **The Gangrenous Form of Ergotism.**—In this form there is generally acute pain in the limb or limbs which are to mortify; and there may be prodromata, similar to those already described. The limb swells, is covered with an erysipelatous blush, but at the same time feels icy cold; the gangrene is generally dry, occasionally moist; the mummified parts separate from the healthy by a moist, ulcerative process; and in this way the toes, fingers, legs, and even the nose, may be lost. During the process of separation there is some fever, and pyæmia may occur with a fatal result.

Fontenelle described a case in which a rustic lost all the toes of one foot, then those of the other; after that, the remnant of the first foot, and lastly the leg. But probably the most extraordinary case of gangrene caused by the use of ergot is that which occurred at Wattisham, Suffolk, in the family of a labouring man named John Downing. He had a wife and six children of various ages, from fifteen years to four months. On Monday, January 10, 1762, the eldest girl complained of a pain in the calf of her left leg; in the evening, her sister, aged 10, also experienced the same symptoms. On the following Monday, the mother and another child, and on Tuesday, all the rest of the family except the father became affected. The pain was very violent. The baby at the breast lived a few weeks, and died of mortification of the extremities. The limbs of the family now began to slough off, and the following are the notes on their condition made by an observer, Dr. C. Wollaston, F.R.S., on April 13:—

"The mother, aged 40. Right foot off at the ankle, the left leg mortified; a mere bone left, but not off.

"Elizabeth, aged 13. Both legs off below the knees.

"Sarah, aged 10. One foot off at the ankle.

[604] Dr. Tissot in *Phil. Trans.*, vol. lv. p. 106, 1765. This is a Latin letter by Dr. Baker, and gives a good history of the various epidemics of ergotism.

"Robert, aged 8. Both legs off below the knees.
"Richard, aged 4. Both feet off at the ankle.
"Infant, four months old, dead."

The father was also attacked a fortnight after the rest of the family, and in a slighter degree—the pain being confined to the fingers of his right hand, which turned a blackish colour, and were withered for some time, but ultimately got better.

As a remarkable fact, it is specially noted that the family were in other respects well. They ate heartily, and slept soundly when the pain began to abate. The mother looked emaciated. "The poor boy in particular looked as healthy and florid as possible, and was sitting on the bed, quite jolly, drumming with his stumps." They lived as the country people at the time usually lived, on dried peas, pickled pork, bread and cheese, milk, and small beer. Dr. Wollaston strictly examined the corn with which they made the bread, and he found it "very bad; it was wheat that had been cut in a rainy season, and had lain in the ground till many of the grains were black and totally decayed."[605]

§ 585. **Symptoms of Acute Poisoning by Ergot.**—In a fatal case of poisoning by ergot of rye, recorded by Dr. Davidson,[606] in which a hospital nurse, aged 28, took ergot, the symptoms were mainly vomiting of blood, the passing of bloody urine, intense jaundice, and stupor. But in other cases, jaundice and vomiting of blood have not been recorded, and the general course of acute poisoning shows, on the one hand, symptoms of intense gastro-intestinal irritation, as vomiting, colicky pains, and diarrhœa; and, on the other, of a secondary affection of the nervous system, weakness of the limbs, aberrations of vision, delirium, retention of urine, coma, and death.

§ 586. **Physiological Action as shown by Experiments on Animals.**—In spite of numerous experiments on animals and man, the action of the ergot principles remains obscure. It has been found in medicine to exert a specific action on the uterus,[607] causing powerful contractions of that organ, especially in labour. It is also a hæmostatic, and is used to check bleeding from the lungs and other internal organs of the body. This hæmostatic action, as well as the extraordinary property possessed by ergot, of producing an arrest or disturbance of the circulation inducing gangrene has naturally led to the belief that ergot causes a narrowing in the calibre of the small arteries, but this has not received the necessary experimental sanction. Holmes,[608] Eberty, Köhler,[609] and Wernick,[610] all observed a contraction in the part to which the ergot was applied, both in frogs and in warm-blooded animals; but L. Hermann,[611] although he made many experiments, and used the most different preparations, never succeeded in observing a contraction. It would also seem reasonable to expect that with a narrowing of the vessels, which means a peripheral obstruction, the blood-pressure would rise, but on the contrary the pressure sinks, a fact on which there is no division of opinion.

Nikitin has made some researches with pure sclerotic acid, which certainly possesses the most prominent therapeutic effects of ergot; but since it is not the only *toxic* substance, it may not represent the collective action of the drug, just in the same way that morphine is not equivalent in action to opium. Cold-blooded animals are very sensitive to sclerotic acid; of the warm-blooded the carnivoræ are more sensitive than the herbivoræ. The toxic action is specially directed to the central nervous system—with frogs, the reflex excitability is diminished to full paralysis; with warm-blooded animals reflex excitability is only diminished, and continues to exist even to death.

The temperature falls, the breathing is slowed, and the respiration stops before the heart ceases to beat; the peristaltic action of the intestines is quickened, and the uterus (even of non-pregnant animals) is thrown into

---

605 In the *Phil. Trans.* for 1762 there are two strictly concordant accounts of this case; and in the parish church of Wattisham, there is said to be a memorial tablet, which runs as follows:—"This inscription serves to authenticate the truth of a singular calamity which suddenly happened to a poor family in this parish, of which six persons lost their feet by a mortification not to be accounted for. A full narrative of their case is recorded in the Parish Register and *Philosophical Transactions* for 1762."

606 *Lancet*, Sept. 30, 1882.

607 In a case in which the author was engaged, a dabbler in drugs, having seduced a young woman, administered to her a dose of ergot which produced a miscarriage, and for this offence he was convicted. The defence raised was that ergot is a common medicine used by physicians in the treatment of amenorrhœa, and other uterine affections. Although in itself this statement was perfectly true, as a defence it was invalidated by the large dose given, the fact of the seduction, and the other circumstances of the case.

608 *Archiv d. Physiol. Norm. u. Pathol.*, iii. p. 384.

609 *Ueber die Wirkungen des Secale Cornutum*, Dissert. Halle, 1873.

610 *Arch. f. pathol. Anat.*, lvi. p 505.

611 *Lehrbuch der exper. Toxicologie*, Berlin, 1874, p. 386.

contraction. The terminations of the sensory nerves are paralysed by the direct action of sclerotic acid, but they remain intact with general poisoning. The heart of frogs is slowed by sclerotic acid. Eberty observed that this slowing of the heart (he used ergotin) was produced even after destruction of the spinal cord; he therefore considered it as acting on the inhibitory nerve apparatus of the heart itself. Rossbach, using Wenzel's ecbolin, has also studied its action on the heart of the frog, and observed that the slowing affected the ventricles rather than the auricles, so that for one ventricle-systole there were two contractions of the auricles; besides which, the contractions themselves were peculiar and abnormal in character. The cause of death from sclerotic acid seems to be paralysis of the respiration. It is said not to affect animal fœtal life. With regard to the effects produced by feeding animals with ergotised grain, experiments made during the last century have proved that it produces a gangrenous disease, *e.g.*, C. Salerné mixed one part of spurred rye with two of good barley, and fed pigs with the mixture; a few days afterwards the pigs perished with dilated, hard, and black bellies, and offensively ulcerated legs; another pig fed entirely on the rye, lost its four feet and both ears.

Kobert[612] has investigated the effects produced on animals by "sphacelic acid," and by "cornutin." Sphacelic acid appears to cause gangrene, like ergot, and Kobert believes that in "sphacelic acid" is to be found the gangrene-producing substance. In cases of death putrefaction is rapid, the mucous membrane of the intestine is swollen, and the spleen enlarged. If the mucous membrane of the intestine is examined microscopically, a large quantity of micro-organisms are found in the vessels, in the villi, between the muscular bundles and in the deeper layers of the intestinal walls; this is evidence that the protective epithelial cells have been destroyed. The mesentery of cats, pigs, and fowls, contains numerous small extravasations of blood. The organs generally, and especially the subcutaneous cellular tissue, are tinged with the colouring matters of the bile; this Kobert considers as evidence of weakened vitality of the red blood corpuscles. The walls of the blood-vessels show hyaline degeneration, and give with iodine a quasi-amyloid reaction. The vessels are often partly filled with a hyaline mass, in which, at a later date, a fine black pigment appears. These pigmented hyaline masses probably occlude the vessels, and hence cause gangrene.

Cornutin, according to Kobert, first excites the vagus; consequently there is slow pulse and heightened blood pressure; then it paralyses the vaso-motor centre, and the pulse is accelerated. Severe convulsions, preceded by formication, follow. Paralysis of the extensor muscles, with permanent deformity, may result. Cornutin stimulates the uterus to contraction, but it does not act so well in this respect alone as when given with sphacelic acid. In animals poisoned with cornutin, no special pathological changes of a distinctive nature have been described.

§ 587. **Separation of the Active Principles of Ergot from Animal Tissues.**—There has been no experience in the separation of the constituents of ergot from the organs of the body; an attempt might be made on the principles detailed earlier, but success is doubtful.

II.—Picrotoxin, the Active Principle of the Cocculus indicus (Indian Berry, Levant Nut).

§ 588. The berries of the *Menispermum cocculus* comprise at least three definite crystalline principles: *menispermine*,[613] *paramenispermine* (nitrogen containing bases), and *picrotoxin*, which possesses some of the characters of an acid.

§ 589. **Picrotoxin** ($C_{30}H_{34}O_{13}$) was discovered in 1820 by Boullay. It is usually prepared by extracting the berries with boiling alcohol, distilling the alcohol off, boiling the alcoholic residue with a large quantity of water, purifying the watery extract with sugar of lead, concentrating the colourless filtrate by evaporation, and crystallising

[612] *Lehrbuch der Intoxicationen*, by Dr. Rudolph Kobert, Stuttgart, 1893.

[613] *Menispermine* ($C_{18}H_{24}N_2O_2$?), discovered in 1834 by Pelletier and Courbe, is associated with a second named *paramenispermine*. The powdered berries are extracted by alcohol of 36°; the picrotoxin removed by hot water from the alcoholic extract; the menispermine and paramenispermine dissolved out together by acidulated water, and from this solution precipitated by ammonia. The brown precipitate is dissolved by acetic acid, filtered, and again precipitated by ammonia. This precipitate is dried, treated with cold alcohol, to separate a yellow resinous substance, and lastly with ether, which dissolves out the menispermine, but leaves the paramenispermine.

Menispermine forms white semi-transparent, four-sided, truncated prisms, melting at 120°, decomposed at a higher temperature, insoluble in water, but dissolving in warm alcohol and ether. Combined with 8 atoms of water it crystallises in needles and prisms. The crystals are without any taste; in combination with acids, salts may be formed.

Paramenispermine forms four-sided prisms, or radiating crystalline masses, melting at 250°, and subliming undecomposed. The crystals are soluble in absolute ether, insoluble in water, and scarcely soluble in ether.

Paramenispermine dissolves in acids, but apparently without forming definite salts.

the picrotoxin out of water.

Picrotoxin crystallises out of water, and also out of alcohol, in colourless, flexible, four-sided prisms, often arborescent, and possessing a silky lustre. They are unalterable in the air, soluble in 150 parts of cold, and 25 parts of boiling water, dissolving easily in acidified water, in spirit, in ether, in amyl alcohol, and chloroform. They are without smell, but have an extremely bitter taste. Caustic ammonia is also a solvent.

The crystals are neutral in reaction. They melt at 192°-200° C. to a yellow mass; at higher temperatures giving off an acid vapour, with a caramel-like odour, and lastly carbonising. Picrotoxin in cold concentrated sulphuric acid dissolves with the production of a beautiful gold-yellow to saffron-yellow colour, which becomes on the addition of a trace of potassic bichromate, violet passing into brown. An alcoholic solution turns a ray of polarised light to the left $[\alpha]_D = -28.1°$.

Picrotoxin behaves towards strong bases like a weak acid. Its compounds with the alkalies and alkaline earths are gummy and not easily obtained pure. Compounds with quinine, cinchonine, morphine, strychnine, and brucine can be obtained in the crystalline condition. Dilute sulphuric acid transforms it, with assimilation of water, into a weak gummy-like acid, which corresponds to the formula $C_{12}H_{16}O_6$. Nitric acid oxidises it to oxalic acid. Nitropicrotoxin and bromopicrotoxin, $C_{30}H_{33}(NO_2)O_{13}$, and $C_{30}H_{32}Br_2O_{13}$, can by appropriate treatment be obtained.

Concentrated aqueous solutions of alkalies and ammonia decompose picrotoxin fully on warming. It reduces alkaline copper solution, and colours bichromate of potash a beautiful green. The best test for its presence is, however, as follows:—The supposed picrotoxin is carefully dried, and mixed with thrice its bulk of saltpetre, the mixture moistened with sulphuric acid, and then decomposed with soda-lye in excess, when there is produced a transitory brick-red colour. For the reaction to succeed, the picrotoxin should be tolerably pure.

Solutions of picrotoxin are not precipitated by the chlorides of platinum, mercury, and gold, iodide of potassium, ferro- and ferri-cyanides of potassium, nor by picric nor tannic acids.

§ 590. **Fatal Dose.**—Vossler killed a cat in two hours with a dose of .12 grm. (1.8 grain); and another cat, with the same dose, died in 45 minutes. Falck destroyed a young hound with .06 grm. (.92 grain) in 24 to 26 minutes. Given by subcutaneous or intravenous injection, it is, as might be expected, still more lethal and rapid in its effects. In an experiment of Falck's, .03 grm. (.46 grain), injected into a vein, destroyed a strong hound within 20 minutes; .016 grm. (.24 grain) injected under the skin, killed a guinea-pig in 22 minutes; and .012 grm. (.18 grain) a hare in 40 minutes. Hence it may be inferred that from 2 to 3 grains (12.9 to 19.4 centigrms.) would in all probability, be a dangerous dose for an adult person.

§ 591. **Effects on Animals.**—The toxic action of picrotoxin on fish and frogs has been proposed as a test. The symptoms observed in fish are mainly as follows:—The fish, according to the dose, show uncertain motions of the body, lose their balance, and finally float to the surface, lying on one side, with frequent opening of the mouth and gill-covers. These symptoms are, however, in no way distinguishable from those induced by any poisonous substance in the water, or by many diseases to which fish are liable. Nevertheless, it may be conceded that in certain cases the test may be valuable—if, *e.g.*, beer be the matter of research, none of the methods used for the extraction of picrotoxin will be likely to extract any other substance having the poisonous action described on fish, so that, as a confirmatory test, this may be of use.

Frogs, under the influence of picrotoxin, become first uneasy and restless, and then somewhat somnolent; but after a short time tetanic convulsions set in, which might lead the inexperienced to imagine that the animal was poisoned by strychnine. There is, however, one marked distinction between the two—viz., that in picrotoxin poisoning an extraordinary swelling of the abdomen has been observed, a symptom which, so far as known, is due to picrotoxin alone. The frog is, therefore, in this instance, the most suitable object for physiological tests.

Beer extract containing picrotoxin is fatal to flies; but no definite conclusion can be drawn from this, since many bitter principles (notably quassia) are in a similar manner fatal to insect life.

§ 592. **Effects on Man.**—Only two fatal cases of poisoning by picrotoxin are on record. In 1829 several men suffered from drinking rum which had been impregnated with *Cocculus indicus*; one died, the rest recovered. In the second case, a boy, aged 12, swallowed some of a composition which was used for poisoning fish, the active principle of which was *Cocculus indicus*; in a few minutes the boy experienced a burning taste, he had pains in the gullet and stomach, with frequent vomiting, and diarrhœa. A violent attack of gastro-enteritis supervened, with fever and delirium; he died on the nineteenth day. The *post-mortem* signs were those usual in peritonitis: the stomach was discoloured, and its coats thinner and softer than was natural; there were also other changes, but it is obvious that, as the death took place so long after the event, any pathological signs found are scarcely a guide for future cases.

§ 593. **Physiological Action.**—The convulsions are considered to arise from an excitation of the medulla oblongata; the vagus centre is stimulated, and causes spasm of the glottis and slowing of the heart's action during the attack. Röhrig also saw strong contraction of the uterus produced by *picrotoxin*. According to the researches of Crichton Browne, *chloral hydrate* acts in antagonism to picrotoxin, and prevents the convulsions in animals if the dose of picrotoxin is not too large.

§ 594. **Separation from Organic Matters.**—Picrotoxin is extracted from aqueous acid solutions by either chloroform, amyl alcohol, or ether; the first is the most convenient. Benzene does not extract it, if employed in the same manner. On evaporation of the solvent the crude picrotoxin can be crystallised out of water, and its properties examined.

R. Palm[614] has taken advantage of the fact that picrotoxin forms a stable compound with freshly precipitated lead hydroxide, by applying this property as follows:—the solution supposed to contain picrotoxin is evaporated to dryness, and the extract then taken up in a very little water, acidified and shaken out with ether. The ether is evaporated, the ethereal extract dissolved in a little water, the aqueous solution filtered through animal charcoal, and precipitated by means of lead acetate, avoiding excess. The solution is filtered and shaken with freshly prepared lead hydroxide. The lead hydroxide is dried and tested direct for picrotoxin; if it does contain picrotoxin then on adding to it concentrated H_2SO_4 a beautiful saffron yellow is produced as bright as if the substance was pure picrotoxin.

III.—The Poison of Illicium Religiosum—A Japanese Plant.

§ 595. A new poison belonging to the picrotoxin class has been described by Dr. A. Langaard. In 1880, 5 children in Japan were poisoned by the seeds of the *Illicium religiosum*; 3 of the children died. Dr. Langaard then made various experiments on animals with an active extract prepared by exhaustion with spirit, and ultimate solution of the extract in water. Eykmann has also imperfectly examined the chemistry of the plant, and has succeeded in isolating a crystalline body which is not a glucoside; it is soluble in hot water, in chloroform, ether, alcohol, and acetic acid, but it is insoluble in petroleum ether; it melts at 175°, and above that temperature gives an oily sublimate. Langaard's conclusions are that all parts of the plant are poisonous. The poison produces excitation of the central apparatus of the medulla oblongata and clonic convulsions analogous to those produced by picrotoxin, toxiresin, and cicutoxin. Before the occurrence of convulsions, the reflex excitability of frogs is diminished, the respiratory centre is stimulated, hence frequency of the respiration. Small doses cause slowing of the pulse through stimulation of the vagus and of the peripheral terminations of the vagus; in the heart the functional activity is later diminished. Small doses kill by paralysing the respiratory centre, large by heart paralysis. The proper treatment seems to be by chloral hydrate, for when animals are poisoned by small lethal doses it appears to save life, although when the dose is large it has no effect.—*Ueber die Giftwirkung von Japanischem Sternanis* (*Illicium religiosum*, Sieb.), *Virch. Archiv*, Bd. lxxxvi., 1881, S. 222.

IV.—Picric Acid and Picrates.

§ 596. **Picric Acid**, $C_6H_3N_3O_7$, or $C_6H_2\left\langle^{OH}_{(NO_2)_3}\right.$ is trinitrophenol; it forms a number of salts, all of which are more or less poisonous. Picric acid is much used in the arts, especially as a dye. The pure substance is in the form of pale yellow crystals, not very soluble in cold water, but readily soluble in hot water, and readily soluble in benzene, ether, and petroleum ether. The solution is yellow, tastes bitter, and dyes animal fibres, such as wool; but it can be washed out of plant fibres such as cotton.

§ 597. **Effects of Picric Acid.**—Picric acid and its salts have a tendency to decompose the elements of the blood, and to produce methæmoglobin; picric acid is also an excitor of the nervous system, producing convulsions. To these two effects must be added a third; in acid solution it has a strong affinity for albumin, so that if it meets with an acid tissue it combines with the tissue, and in this way local necroses are set up. The action on albumin is somewhat weakened by the reduction in the body of part of the picric acid to picraminic acid $C_6H_2(NO_2)_2NH_2OH$, a substance that does not so readily form compounds with albuminous matters. Doses of 0.5 to 0.9 grm. (about 8 to

[614] *J. Pharm.*, (5), xvii. 19-20.

14 grains) may be taken several days in succession without marked symptoms. Ultimately, however, what is known as "picric jaundice" appears, the conjunctiva and the whole skin being stained more or less yellow. The urine, at first of a dark yellow, is later of a red brown colour. Dyspepsia, with flatulence and an inclination to diarrhœa have been noticed. A single dose of a gramme (15.4 grains) caused in a case described by Adler[615] pain in the stomach, headache, weakness, diarrhœa, vomiting of yellow matters, quickening and afterwards slowing of the pulse; the skin was of a brown yellow colour, and there were nervous symptoms. The urine was ruby red. In both fæces and urine picric acid could be recognised. The excretion of picric acid continued for six days. A microscopical examination of the blood showed a diminution of the red blood corpuscles, an increase in the white. Chéron[616] has described a case in which the application of 0.45 grm. (6.9 grains) to the vagina produced yellowness of the skin in an hour, and the urine was also coloured red. Erythema, somnolence, burning and smarting in the stomach and in the kidneys were also noticed.

§ 598. **Tests.**—Picric acid is easily separated from either tissues or other organic matters. These are acidified with sulphuric acid and then treated with 95 per cent. alcohol; the alcohol is filtered off, distilled, and the residue treated with ether; this last ethereal extract will contain any picric acid that may be present.

If the ether extract contains much impurity, it may be necessary to drive off the ether, and to take up the residue with a little warm water, then to cool, filter through a moistened filter paper, and test the aqueous solution. Picric acid, warmed with KCN and KHO gives a blood-red colour, from the production of iso-purpurate of potash. Ammoniacal copper sulphate forms with picric acid yellow-green crystals which strongly refract the light. If a solution of picric acid be reduced by the addition of a hydrochloric acid solution of stannous chloride, the subsequent addition of ferric chloride produces a blue colour, due to the formation of amidoimidophenol hydrochloride $C_6H_2OH(NH_2)(NH)_2HCl$.

V.—Cicutoxin.

§ 599. The *Cicuta virosa*, a not very common umbelliferous plant growing in moist places, is extremely poisonous. It is from 3 to 4 feet in height, with white flowers; the umbels are large, the leaves are tripartite, the leaflets linear lanceolate acute, serrate decurrent; the calyx has five leaf-like teeth, the petals are obcordate with an inflex point; the carpels have five equal broad flattened ridges with solitary stripes. Böhm[617] succeeded, in 1876, in separating an active principle from this plant. The root was dried, powdered, and exhausted with ether; on evaporation of the ether the extract was taken up with alcohol, and after several days standing the filtrate was treated with petroleum ether; after removing the petroleum, the solution was evaporated to dryness in a vacuum; it was found to be a resinous mass, to which was given the name *cicutoxin*. It was fully soluble in alcohol, ether, or chloroform, and was very poisonous, but what its exact chemical nature may be is still unknown.

§ 600. **Effects on Animals.**—Subcutaneously injected into frogs, cicutoxin acts something like picrotoxin, and something like the barium compounds. Ten to fifteen minutes after the injection the animal assumes a peculiar posture, holding the legs so that the thigh is stretched out far from the trunk, and the leg at right angles with the thigh; voluntary motion is only induced by the strongest stimuli, and when the frog springs, he falls down plump with stiffly stretched-out limbs. The frequency of breathing is increased, the muscles of the abdomen are thrown into contraction, and the lungs being full of air, on mechanical irritation there is a peculiar loud cry, depending upon the air being forced under the conditions detailed through the narrow glottis. Tetanic convulsions follow, gradually paresis of the extremities appears, and, lastly, full paralysis and death; these symptoms are seen after doses of from 1 to 2 mgrms. The lethal dose for cats is about 1 centigrm. per kilo. Diarrhœa, salivation, and frequent breathing are first seen, and are followed by tonic and clonic convulsions, then there is an interval, during which there is heightened excitability of reflex action, so that noises will excite convulsions. Small doses by exciting the vagus slow the pulse; larger doses quicken the pulse, and raise the arterial pressure. Cicutoxin is supposed to act specially on the medulla oblongata, while the spinal cord and the brain are only secondarily affected.

§ 601. **Effects on Man.**—F. A. Falck was able to collect thirty-one cases of poisoning by cicuta; of these 14 or 45.2 per cent. died. The symptoms are not dissimilar to those described in animals. There are pain and burning in the stomach, nausea, vomiting, headache, and then tetanic convulsions. These, in some cases, are very severe, and

[615] *Wiener. med. Woch.*, 1880, 819.

[616] J. Chéron, *Journ. de Thêr.*, 1880, 121.

[617] *Arch. f. exp. Path.*, Bd. v., 1876.

resemble those induced by strychnine; but in a few cases there is early coma without convulsions. There is also difficulty or absolute impossibility of swallowing. In fatal cases the respiration becomes stertorous, the pulse small, the pupils dilated, and the face cyanotic, and death occurs within some four hours, and in a few cases later. The *fatal dose* is unknown.

§ 602. **Separation of Cicutoxin from the Body.**—An attempt might be made to extract cicutoxin from the tissues on the same principles as those by which it has been separated from the plant, and identified by physiological experiments. In all recorded cases, identification has been neither by chemical nor physiological aids, but by the recognition of portions of the plant.

VI.—Æthusa Cynapium (Fool's Parsley).

§ 603. This plant has long been considered poisonous, and a number of cases are on record in which it is alleged that death or illness resulted from its use. Dr. John Harley,[618] however, in an elaborate paper, has satisfactorily proved the innocence of this plant, and has analysed the cases on record. He has experimented on himself, on animals, and on men, with the expressed juice and with the tincture. The results were entirely negative: some of the published cases he refers to conium, and others to aconite.

VII.—Œnanthe Crocata.

§ 604. **The Water Hemlock.**[619]—This, a poisonous umbelliferous plant, indigenous to England, and growing in moist places such as ditches, &c., is in flower in the month of August. It resembles somewhat celery, and the root is something like the parsnip, for which it has been eaten. All parts of the plant are said to be poisonous, but the leaves and stalks only slightly so, while the root is very deadly. We unfortunately know nothing whatever about the active principles of the plant, its chemistry has yet to be worked out. M. Toulmouche (*Gaz. Méd.*, 1846) has recorded, as the expert employed in the case, an attempt to murder by using the *œnanthe* as a poison; a woman scraped the root into her husband's soup with evil intent, but the taste was unpleasant, and led to the detection of the crime. The root has been mistaken several times for parsnip and other edible roots, and has thus led to poisonings. The case of 36 soldiers poisoned in this way, in 1758, has been recorded by Orfila; there was one death. In 1803 three soldiers were poisoned at Brest—1 died. In Woolwich Bossey witnessed the poisoning of 21 convicts who ate the roots and leaves of the plant—6 died. In 1858 there were several sailors poisoned in a similar way—2 died; while there have been numerous cases in which the plant has been partaken of by children.

§ 605. The effects of the poison may be gathered from a case of poisoning[620] which occurred in 1882 at Plymouth; a Greek sailor, aged thirty, found on the coast what he considered "wild celery," and ate part of the root and some of the stem. Two hours after this he ate a good meal and felt perfectly well, but fifteen minutes later he suddenly and violently vomited; the whole contents of the stomach were completely evacuated. In five minutes he was completely unconscious, and had muscular twitchings about the limbs and face. There was a copious flow of a thick tenacious mucus from the mouth which hung about the lips and clothing in viscid strings. Twenty-four hours after the poisoning he was admitted into the South Devon Hospital apparently semi-comatose; his legs dragged, and he had only feeble control of them; the extremities were cold, but there was general free sweating. He could be roused only with difficulty. There were no spasms, the pupils were dilated and sluggish, the respiration only 14 per minute. Twelve hours after admission he became warmer, and perspired freely; he slept continuously, but could easily be roused. On the following day he was quite conscious, and made a good recovery. Two companions who had also eaten a smaller quantity of the hemlock dropwort, escaped with some numbing sensations, and imperfect control over the extremities. In the Woolwich cases the symptoms seem to have been something similar; in about twenty minutes, one man, without any apparent warning, fell down in strong convulsions, which soon ceased, although he looked wild; a little while afterwards his face became bloated and livid, his breathing stertorous and

[618] *St. Thomas' Hospital Reports*, N.S., 1875.

[619] The earliest treatise on poisoning by the water-hemlock is by Wepfer. *Cicutæ Aquat. Historia et Noxæ*, 1679; for cases see Trojanowsky, *Dorp. med. Ztg.*, 1875; Meyer, *Med. Zeitg. f. Preussen*, 1842; Schlesier in Casper's *Wochenschrift*, 1843; Maly, *Œster. med Wochenschr.*, 1844; Badgeley, *Montreal med. Gaz.*, 1844; Lender, *Viertelj. f. ger. Med.*, 1865; Gampf, *Cöln. Pharm. Zeitg.*, 1875; and the treatises of Taylor and others.

[620] *Lancet*, Dec. 18, 1882.

convulsive, and he died in five minutes after the first symptoms had set in. A second died with similar symptoms in a quarter of an hour; a third died in about an hour, a fourth in a little more than an hour; two other cases also proved fatal, one in nine days, the other in eleven. In the two last cases there were signs of intestinal irritation. The majority of the others fell down in a state of insensibility with convulsions, the after-symptoms being more or less irritation of the intestinal canal.

§ 606. **Post-mortem Appearances.**—It was noticed in the Woolwich cases that those who died quickly had congestion of the cerebral vessels, and, in one instance, there was even extravasation of blood, but the man who died first of all had no congestion of the cerebral vessels. The lining membrane of the wind-pipe and air tubes was intensely injected with blood, and the lungs were gorged with fluid blood; the blood in the heart was black and fluid. The stomach and intestines were externally of a pink colour. The mucous membrane of the stomach was much corrugated, and the follicles particularly enlarged. In the two protracted cases the stomach was not reddened internally, but the vessels of the brain were congested.

VIII.—Oil of Savin.

§ 607. The leaves of the *Sabina communis* (*Juniperus Sabina*), or common savin, an evergreen shrub to be found in many gardens, contains a volatile oil, which has highly irritant properties. Savin leaves are occasionally used in medicine, maximum dose 1 grm. (15.4 grains). There is also a tincture—maximum dose 3 c.c. (about 45 mins.)—and an ointment made by mixing eight parts of savin tops with three of yellow wax and sixteen parts of lard, melting and digesting for twenty minutes, and then straining through calico. The oil, a tincture, and an ointment, are officinal pharmaceutical preparations.

The oil of savin is contained to the extent of about 2 per cent. in the leaves and 10 per cent. in the fruit. It has a peculiar odour, its specific gravity is .89 to .94, and it boils at 155° to 160°. An infusion of savin leaves (the leaves being drunk with the liquid) is a popular and very dangerous abortive.

It is stated by Taylor that oil of savin has no abortive effect, save that which is to be attributed to its general effect upon the system, but this is erroneous. Röhrig found that, when administered to rabbits, it had a very evident effect upon the pregnant uterus, throwing it into a tetanic contraction. The action was evident after destruction of the spinal cord. The plant causes great irritation and inflammation, whether applied to the skin or taken internally. The symptoms are excruciating pain, vomiting, and diarrhœa, and the person dies in a kind of collapse.

In a case in which the author was engaged some years ago, a woman, pregnant by a married man, took an unknown quantity of infusion of savin tops. She was violently sick, suffered great pain, with diarrhœa, and died in about 26 hours. The pharynx was much reddened, and the gullet even congested; the stomach was inflamed, and contained some greenish matter, in which the author was able to detect savin tops, as well as to separate by distillation a few drops of a strong savin-like smelling oil. The time which would elapse between the swallowing of the poison and the commencement of the pain was an important factor in this case, for the man was accused of having supplied her with the infusion. From the redness of the pharynx, and, generally, the rapid irritation caused by ethereal oils, the author was of opinion that but a few minutes must have passed between the taking of the liquid and the sensation of considerable burning pain, although it is laid down in some works, as for example Falck's *Toxicologie*, that commonly the symptoms do not commence for several hours. Symptoms which have been noticed in many cases are—some considerable irritation of the urinary organs, such as strangury, bloody urine, &c.; in a few cases vomiting of blood, in others anæsthesia, convulsions, and coma. Death may occur within 12 hours, or may be postponed for two or three days.

§ 608. **Post-mortem Appearances.**—More or less inflammation of the bowels, stomach, and intestinal tract, with considerable congestion of the kidneys, are the signs usually found.

§ 609. **Separation of the Poison and Identification.**—Hitherto reliance has been placed entirely on the finding of the savin tops, or on the odour of the oil. There is no reliable chemical test.

IX.—Croton Oil.

§ 610. Croton oil is an oil expressed from the seeds of *Croton tiglium*, a plant belonging to the natural order *Euphorbiaceæ*, growing in the West Indies. The seeds are oval in shape, not unlike castor-oil seeds, and about three-eighths of an inch in length. Both the seeds and the oil are very poisonous. The chemical composition of croton oil can scarcely be considered adequately settled. The most recent view, however, seems to be that it contains a fixed oil ($C_9H_{14}O_2$) with certain glycerides.[621] On saponifying and decomposing the soap a series of volatile fatty acids can be distilled over, the principal of which are methyl crotonic acid, with small quantities of formic, acetic, iso-butyric, valeric, and perhaps propionic, and other acids.[622] The peculiar properties of croton are due rather to the fixed oil than to the volatile principles. The only officinal preparation in the British pharmacopœia is a "*croton oil liniment*," containing one part of croton oil to seven of equal parts of oil of cajuput and rectified spirit.

§ 611. **Dose.**—The oil is given medicinally as a powerful purgative in doses up to 65 mgrms. (about a grain). It is used externally as an irritant or vesicant to the skin. A very dangerous dose would be from fifteen to twenty times the medicinal dose.

Effects.—Numerous cases of poisoning from large doses of croton oil are recorded in medical literature, but the sufferers have mostly recovered. The symptoms are pain, and excessive purging and vomiting.

In the case of a chemist,[623] who took half an ounce of impure croton oil instead of cod-liver oil, the purging was very violent, and he had more than a hundred stools in a few hours; there was a burning pain in the gullet and stomach, the skin was cyanosed, the pupils dilated, and great faintness and weakness were felt, yet the man recovered. A child, aged four, recovered from a teaspoonful of the oil given by mistake directly after a full meal of bread and milk. In five minutes there were vomiting and violent purging, but the child was well in two days. A death occurred in Paris, in 1839, in four hours after taking two and a half drachms of the oil. The symptoms of the sufferer, a man, were those just detailed, namely, burning pain in the stomach, vomiting, and purging. Singularly enough, no marked change was noticed in the mucous membrane of the stomach when examined after death. An aged woman died in 3 days from a teaspoonful of croton-oil embrocation; in this case there were convulsions.

In the case of *Reg.* v. *Massey and Ferraud*,[624] the prisoners were charged with causing the death of a man, by poisoning his food with jalap and six drops of croton oil. The victim, with others who had partaken of the food, suffered from vomiting and purging; he became better, but was subsequently affected with inflammation and ulceration of the bowels, of which he died. In this case it was not clear whether the inflammation had anything to do with the jalap and croton oil or not, and the prisoners were acquitted. In a criminal case in the United States, a man, addicted to drink, was given, when intoxicated, 2 drachms of croton oil in a glass of whisky. He vomited, but was not purged, and in about twelve hours was found dead. The mucous membrane of the stomach and small intestines proved to be much inflamed, and in some parts eroded, and croton oil was separated from the stomach.

§ 612. **Post-mortem Appearances.**—Inflammation of the stomach and intestines are the signs usually found in man and animals.

§ 613. **Chemical Analysis.**—The oil may be separated from the contents of the stomach by ether. After evaporation of the ether, the blistering or irritant properties of the oil should be essayed by placing a droplet on the inside of the arm.

X.—The Toxalbumins of Castor-Oil Seeds and of Abrus.

§ 614. **The Toxalbumin of Castor-Oil Seeds.**—In castor-oil seeds, besides the well-known purgative oil, there exists an albuminous body intensely poisonous, which has been carefully investigated by Stillmark,[625] under the direction of Kobert.[626] Injected into the circulation it is more poisonous than strychnine, prussic acid, or arsenic; and since the pressed seeds are without taste or smell, this poison has peculiar dangers of its own.

It is essentially a blood poison, coagulating the blood.

The blood, if carefully freed from all fibrin, is yet again brought to coagulation by a small amount of this body.

If castor-oil seeds are eaten, a portion of the poison is destroyed by the digestive processes; a part is not thus destroyed, but is absorbed, and produces in the blood-vessels its coagulating property. Where this takes place, ulcers

[621] G. Schmidt, *Arch. Pharm.* [3] 13, 213-229. Schlippe, Liebig's *Annalen*, 105, 1. Geuther and Fröhlich, *Zeitschrift f. Chem.*, 1870, 26 and 549; *Journ. Chem. Society*, March 1879, p. 221.

[622] Benedikt has found 0.55 per cent. of unsaponifiable matter in croton oil. Lewkowitsch gives the iodine value 101.7 to 104.7, and solidifying point as 18.6°-19.0°. (*Cheml. Analysis of the Oils, Fats, and Waxes*, by R. Benedikt, translated and enlarged by J. Lewkowitsch, London, 1895.)

[623] *Revue de Thérapeut.*, May 1881.

[624] *Orfila*, t. i. p. 108.

[625] H. Stillmark, *Dorp. Arb.*, Bd. iii., 1889.

[626] Kobert's *Lehrbuch*, 453-456.

naturally form, because isolated small areas are deprived of their blood supply. These areas thus becoming dead, may be digested by the gastric or intestinal fluids, and thus, weeks after, death may be produced. The symptoms noted are nausea, vomiting, colic, diarrhœa, tenesmus, thirst, hot skin, frequent pulse, sweats, headache, jaundice, and death in convulsions or from exhaustion. Animals may be made immune by feeding them carefully with small doses, gradually increased.

The *post-mortem* appearances are ulceration in the stomach and intestines. In animals the appearances of hæmorrhagic gastro-enteritis, with diffuse nephritis, hæmorrhages in the mesentery and so forth have been found.

§ 615. **Toxalbumin of Abrus.**—A toxalbumin is found in the *Abrus precatorius* (Jequirity) which causes quite similar effects and symptoms. That it is not identical is proved by the fact that, though animals may become immune by repeated doses of Jequirity against "Abrin," the similar substance from castor-oil seeds only confers immunity against the toxalbumin of those seeds, and not against abrin; and similarly abrin confers no immunity against the castor albumin. Either of these substances applied to the conjunctiva produces coagulation in the vessels and a secondary inflammation, to which in the case of jequirity has been given the name of "jequirity-ophthalmia."[627]

The general effect of these substances, and, above all, the curious fact that a person may acquire by use a certain immunity from otherwise fatal doses is so similar to poisonous products evolved in the system of persons suffering from infectious fevers, that they have excited of late years much interest, and a study of their methods of action will throw light upon many diseased processes.

At present there are no chemical means of detecting the presence of the toxalbumins mentioned. Should they be ever used for criminal purposes, other evidence will have to be obtained.

XI.—Ictrogen.

§ 616. **Ictrogen.**—Various lupins, *e.g.*, *Lupinus luteus*, *L. angustifolius*, *L. thermis*, *L. linifolius*, *L. hirsutus*, contain a substance of which nothing chemically is known, save that it may be extracted by weakly alkaline water, and which has been named "ictrogen"; this must not be confused with the alkaloid of lupins named "lupinine," a bitter tasting substance. In large doses a nerve poison. Ictrogen has the unusual property of acting much like phosphorus. It causes yellow atrophy of the liver, and produces the following symptoms:—Intense jaundice; at first enlargement of the liver, afterwards contraction; somnolence, fever, paralysis. The urine contains albumen and the constituents of the bile. After death there is found to be parenchymatous degeneration of the heart, kidneys, muscles, and liver. If the animal has suffered for some time the liver may be cirrhotic.

Hitherto the cases of poisoning have been confined to animals. Many thousands of sheep and a few horses and deer have, according to Kobert, died in Germany from eating lupin seeds. Further information upon the active principles of lupins may be obtained by referring to the following treatises:—G. Schneidemuhl, *Die lupinen Krankheit der Schafe*; *Vorträge f. Thierärzte*. Ser. 6, Heft. 4, Leipzig, 1883. C. Arnold and G. Schneidemuhl, *Vierter Beitrag zur Klarstellung der Ursache u. des Wesens der Lupinose*, Luneburg, 1883; Julius Löwenthal, *Ueber die physiol. u. toxicol. Wirkungen der Lupinenalkaloide, Inaug.-Diss.*, Königsberg, 1888.

XII.—Cotton Seeds.

§ 617. Cotton seeds, used as an adulterant to linseed cake, &c., have caused the death of sheep and calves. Cotton seeds contain a poison of which nothing is chemically known, save that it is poisonous. It produces anæmia and cachexia in animals when given in small repeated doses.

After death the changes are, under these circumstances, confined to the kidney; these organs showing all the signs of nephritis. If, however, the animal has eaten a large quantity of cotton seeds, then there is gastro-enteritis, as well as inflammation of the kidneys.

XIII.—Lathyrus Sativus.

§ 618. Various species of vetchlings, such as *L. sativus*, *L. cicera*, *L. clymenum*, are poisonous, and have caused an epidemic malady in parts of Spain, Africa, France, and Italy, among people who have eaten the seeds. The

[627] Heinr. Hellin, *Der giftige Eiweisskorper-Abrin u. seine Wirkung auf das Blut. Inaug.-Diss.*, Dorpat., 1891.

symptoms are mainly referable to the nervous system, causing a transverse myelitis and paraplegia. In this country it is chiefly known as a poisonous food for horses; the last instance of horse-poisoning by lathyrus was that of horses belonging to the Bristol Tramways and Carriage Company.[628] The company bought some Indian peas; these peas were found afterwards to consist mainly of the seeds of *Lathyrus sativus*, for out of 335 peas no fewer than 325 were the seeds of *Lathyrus*. The new peas were substituted for the beans the horses had been having previously on the 2nd November, and the horses ate them up to the 2nd December. Soon after the new food had been given, the horses began to stumble and fall about, not only when at work, but also in their stalls; to these symptoms succeeded a paralysis of the larynx; this paralysis was in some cases accompanied by a curious weird screaming, which once having been heard could never be forgotten; there was also gasping for breath and symptoms of impending suffocation. A few of the horses were saved by tracheotomy. Some died of suffocation; one horse beat its brains out in its struggles for breath; 127 horses were affected; 12 died.

The above train of symptoms has also been recorded in similar cases; added to which paralysis of the lower extremities is frequent. After death atrophy of the laryngeal muscles, wasting of the nervus recurrens, and atrophy of the ganglion cells of the vagus nucleus as also of the multipolar ganglion cells in the anterior horns of the spinal cord have been found.

The active principle of the seeds has not been satisfactorily isolated. The symptoms suggest the action of a toxalbumin. Teilleux found a resin acid; Louis Astier a volatile alkaloid, and he explains the fact that the seeds, after being heated, are no longer poisonous by the dissipation of this alkaloid.

XIV.—Arum—Bryony—Locust Tree—Male Fern.

§ 619. **Arum maculatum**, the common cuckoo-pint, flowering in April and May, and frequent in the hedges of this country, is extremely poisonous. Bright red succulent attractive berries are seen on a single stalk, the rest of the plant having rotted away, and these berries are frequently gathered by children and eaten. The poison belongs to the class of acrid irritants, but its real nature remains for investigation.

Some of the species of the same natural order growing in the tropics are far more intensely poisonous.

§ 620. **The Black Bryony.**—*Tamus communis*, the black bryony, a common plant by the wayside, flowering in May and June, possesses poisonous berries, which have been known to produce death, with symptoms of gastro-enteritis. In smaller doses the berries are stated to produce paralysis of the lower extremities.[629]

§ 621. **The Locust Tree.**—The *Robinia pseudo-acacia*, a papilionaceous tree, contains a poison in the leaves and in the bark. R. Coltmann[630] has recorded a case in China of a woman, twenty-four years of age, who, at a time of famine, driven by hunger, ate the leaves of this tree. She became ill within forty-eight hours, with high fever; the tongue swelled and there was much erysipelatous-like infiltration of the tissues of the mouth; later the whole body became swollen. There was constipation and so much œdema of the eyelids that the eyeballs were no longer visible. Recovery took place without special treatment. Power and Cambier[631] have separated from the bark an albumose, which is intensely poisonous, and is probably the cause of the symptoms detailed.

§ 622. **Male Fern.**—An ethereal extract of *Aspidium Filix mas* is used as a remedy against tape worm.

Poullson[632] has collected up to the year 1891 sixteen cases of poisoning by male fern; from which it would appear that 7 to 10 grms. (103 to 154 grains) of the extract may be fatal to a child, and 45 grms. (rather more than 1½ oz.) to an adult. The active principle seems to be filicic acid and the ethereal oil. Filicic acid, under the influence of saponifying agencies, breaks up into butyric acid and phloroglucin.

The symptoms produced are pain, heaviness of the limbs, faintness, somnolence, dilatation of the pupil, albuminuria, convulsions, lock-jaw, and collapse. In animals there have also been noticed salivation, amaurosis, unsteady gait, dragging of the hind legs, dyspnœa, and paralysis of the breathing centres. The *post-mortem* appearances which have been found are as follows:—Redness and swelling with hæmorrhagic spots of the mucous membranes of the stomach and intestines; acute œdema of the brain and spinal cord with petechia in the meninges; the kidneys inflamed, the liver and spleen congested, and the lungs œdematous.

---

[628] Bristol Tramways and Carriage Company *v.* Weston & Co., *Times*, July 17, 1894.

[629] Contagne, *Lyon med.*, xlvi., 1884, 239.

[630] *Medical and Surgical Reporter*, lxi., 1889.

[631] *Pharm. Journ.*, 1890, 711.

[632] *Arch. exp. P.*, Bd. 29.

There is no characteristic reaction for male fern; the research most likely to be successful is to attempt to separate from an ethereal extract filicic acid, and to decompose it into butyric acid and phloroglucin; the latter tinges red a pine splinter moistened with hydrochloric acid.

PART VII.—POISONS DERIVED FROM LIVING OR DEAD ANIMAL SUBSTANCES.

DIVISION I.—POISONS SECRETED BY LIVING ANIMALS.

I.—Poisonous Amphibia.

§ 623. The glands of the skin of certain amphibia possess a secretion that is poisonous; the animal is unable to empty the poison glands by any voluntary act, but the secretion can readily be obtained by pressure. Zalesky found the juice in the skin glands of the *Salamandra maculosa*, milky, alkaline in reaction, and bitter in taste. He isolated from it an organic base, which he named *Salamandrine* ($C_{34}H_{60}N_2O_5$), it is soluble in water and in alcohol, and forms salts. Salamandrine is a strong poison; injected subcutaneously into rabbits it causes shivering, epileptiform convulsions, and salivation; then tetanus, followed by oppressed respiration, dilated pupils, and anæsthesia. Death occurs after a kind of paralytic state. When given to dogs, it causes vomiting. In frogs, tetanus occurs first and then paralysis—the result of all the experiments being that salamandrine acts on the brain and spinal cord, leaving the heart and muscular substance unaffected. A similar secretion obtained from the water salamander (*Triton cristatus*), causes, according to Vulpian, the death of dogs in from three to eighteen hours; the symptoms being progressive weakness, slowing of the respiration, and depression of the heart's action.

§ 624. The secretion of the skin of the common toad contains methylcarbylaminic acid, carbylamine, and, according to Fornara, an alkaloid which is soluble in alcohol, and to which the name of *phrynine* has been applied; its action is toxic on all animals experimented upon, save toads. Administered subcutaneously to frogs, it has a digitalis-like action, causing rapid paralysis of the heart, and the breathing soon after ceases; the muscles become early rigid.

II.—The Poison of the Scorpion.

§ 625. There are several species of scorpions. The small European variety (*Scorpio europæus*) is found in Italy, the south of France, and the Tyrol; the African scorpion (*Bothus afer*, L.), which attains the length of 16 cm., is found in Africa and the East Indies; *Androctonus bicolor* in Egypt; and the *Androctonus occitanus* in Spain, Italy, Greece, and North Africa.

In the last joint of the tail the scorpion is provided with a poisonous apparatus, consisting of two oval glands, the canal of which leads into a round bladder, and this last is connected with a sting. When the sting is inserted, the bladder contracts, and expels the poison through the hollow sting into the wound. The smaller kinds of scorpion sting with as little general effect as a hornet, but the large scorpion of Africa is capable of producing death. There is first irritation about the wound, and an erysipelatous inflammation, which may lead to gangrene. Vomiting and diarrhœa then set in, with general weakness and a fever, which may last from one to one and a half days; in the more serious cases there are fainting, delirium, coma, convulsions, and death. According to G. Sanarelli[633] the blood corpuscles of birds, fishes, frogs, and salamanders are dissolved by the poison; only the nucleus remaining intact; the blood corpuscles of warm-blooded animals are not affected.

Valentin made some experiments on frogs with the *Androctonus occitanus*. He found that soon after the sting the animal remains quiet, but on irritation it moves, and is thrown into a transitory convulsion; to this follow twitchings of single muscular bundles. The frog is progressively paralysed, and the reflex irritability is gradually extinguished from behind forwards; at first the muscles may be excited by electrical stimuli to the nerves, but later they are only capable of contraction by direct stimuli.

---

[633] G. Sanarelli, *Bollet. della Soc. della sez. dei cult. delle Scienze med.*, v., 1888, 202.

III.—Poisonous Fish.

§ 626. A large number of fish possess poisonous properties; in some cases the poison is local; in others the poison is in all parts of the body.

Many fish are provided with poison glands in connection with the fins or special weapons, and such are used for purposes of defence; for example, *Synanceia brachio* is provided with a back fin consisting of 13 spines, each of which has two poison reservoirs; the reservoirs are connected with 10 to 12 tubular glands which secrete the poison, a clear feebly acid bluish fluid, exciting in a concentrated condition, local gangrene; in a diluted one, paralysis of the nervous centres.

Another kind of localisation is the localisation in certain of the internal organs. Remy states, that there are twelve varieties of *Tetrodon* in Japanese waters, all of which are poisonous. M. Minra and K. Takesaki[634] find that the poison of the *Tetrodon* is confined to the sexual organs of the female, and at the time of activity of these glands, the poisonous properties are most intense; but, even in winter, when the glands are atrophied, Remy found the glands were so poisonous that he could prepare from them a fluid, which, administered subcutaneously, killed dogs within two hours. The symptoms in the dog are restlessness, salivation, vomiting of slimy masses, dilatation of the pupil, paralysis and great dyspnœa. Death occurs by the lung. After death the appearances are similar to those from asphyxia; in addition to which there are small ecchymoses in the stomach and intestines; the salivary glands and pancreas are also injected. The symptoms observed in man are similar, there is headache, dilated pupils, vomiting, sometimes hæmatamesis, convulsions, paralysis, dyspnœa and death.

Some fishes are poisonous on account of the food they live upon; the *Meletta venenosa* is only poisonous when it feeds upon a certain green monad; *Clupea thrissa*, *C. venenosa* and certain species of *Scarus*, neither possess poison glands nor poisonous ovaries; but also derive their poisonous properties from their food. In the West Indies it is well-known that fish caught off certain coral banks are unwholesome, while the same species caught elsewhere may be eaten with safety.

A good many shell-fish, especially mussels, occasionally cause intense poisonous symptoms; those usually noticed are high fever, nettle rash, dilated pupils, and diarrhœa. It may be that in these cases a ptomaine, the product of bacterial action, has been ingested. To the agency of bacteria has been ascribed illness produced in Russia by a good many fish of the sturgeon species. The symptoms are those of cerebro-spinal paralysis. The "Icthyismus gastricus" of Germany may belong to the same type. Prochorow[635] has described illness from ingestion of *Petromyzon fluviatilis* in Russia. Whether the fish was eaten raw or cooked, the effect was the same, producing a violent diarrhœa, dysenteric in character. Even the broth in which the fish had been boiled produced symptoms. Fresh blood of the eel is stated to be intensely poisonous; this property is apparently due to a toxalbumin; Pennavaria[636] relates the case of a man who took, in 200 c.c. of wine, 0.64 kilo. of fresh eel blood and suffered from diarrhœa with symptoms of collapse.

In the *Linnean Transactions* for November, 1860, is recorded a fatal accident, which took place on board the Dutch ship "Postillion" at Simon's Bay, Cape of Good Hope. The boatswain and purser's steward partook of the liver of the *toad* or *ball-bladder* (*Diodon*); within twenty minutes the steward died; in ten minutes the boatswain was violently ill; the face flushed, the eyes glistening, and the pupils contracted; there was cyanosis of the face, the pulse was weak and intermittent, and swallowing was difficult, the breathing became embarrassed, and the body generally paralysed. Death took place in seventeen minutes. The liver of one fish only is said to have been eaten. This might weigh 4 drachms. If the account given is literally correct, the intensity of the poison equals that of any known substance.

The poisonous nature of the goby has also led to several accidents, and we possess a few experiments made by Dr. Collas,[637] who fed chickens with different parts of the fish, and proved that all parts were alike poisonous. The effects were slow in developing; they commenced in about an hour or an hour and a half, and were well developed in five hours, mainly consisting of progressive muscular weakness and prostration. Death occurred without convulsions.

[634] Virchow's *Archiv*, 1890, Bd. 122.

[635] *Pharmac. Ztg.*, 1885.

[636] *Il Farmacista Italiano*, xii., 1888.

[637] *Soc. Sci. Rev.*, July 19, 1862; *Brit. and For. Med. Chir. Rev.*, Oct. 1862, p. 536.

IV.—Poisonous Spiders and Other Insects.

§ 627. It is probable that all spiders are poisonous; the only species, however, of which we have any definite information relative to their poisonous properties, are *Lycosa tarantula* and the *Latrodectus malmignatus*, to which may be added the New Zealand *katipo*. These spiders possess a poisonous gland connected with their masticatory apparatus, which secretes a clear, oily, bitter acid-reacting fluid; the acidity seems due to formic acid.

Zangrilli has observed several cases of tarantula bite; soon after the occurrence the part bitten is anæsthetic, after a few hours there are convulsive shiverings of the legs, cramps of the muscles, inability to stand, spasm of the pharyngeal muscles, quickening of the pulse, and a three days' fever, with vomiting of yellow, bilious matter; recovery follows after copious perspiration. In one case there was tetanus, and death on the fourth day. The extraordinary effects attributed to the bite of the tarantula, called *tarantism* in the Middle Ages, are well detailed by Hecker;[638] this excitement was partly hysterical and partly delirious, and has not been observed in modern times.

Dax has described the effects of the bite of the *L. malmignatus*; it occasioned headache, muscular weakness, pain in the back, cramps, and dyspnœa; the symptoms disappeared after several days.

§ 628. The *katipo* is a small poisonous spider confined to New Zealand. Mr. W. H. Wright has recorded the case of a person who, in 1865, was bitten by this spider on the shoulder. The part rapidly became swollen, and looked like a large nettle-rash wheal; in an hour the patient could hardly walk, the respiration and circulation were both affected, and there was great muscular prostration; but he recovered in a few hours. In other cases, if the accounts given are to be relied upon, the bite of the spider has produced a chronic illness, accompanied by wasting of the body, followed by death after periods varying from six weeks to three months.[639]

§ 629. **Ants.**—The various species of ants possess at the tail special glands which secrete *formic acid*. Certain exotic species of ants are provided with a sting, but the common ant of this country has no special piercing apparatus. The insect bites, and then squirts the irritating secretion into the wound, causing local symptoms of swelling and inflammation.

§ 630. **Wasps, &c.**—Wasps, bees, and hornets all possess a poison-bag and sting. The fluid secreted is as clear as water, and of an acid reaction; it certainly contains formic acid, with some other poisonous constituent. An erysipelatous inflammation generally arises round the sting, and in those cases in which persons have been attacked by a swarm of bees, signs of general poisoning, such as vomiting, fainting, delirium, and stupor, have been noticed. Death has occasionally resulted.

§ 631. **Cantharides.**—Commercial cantharides is either the dried entire, or the dried and powdered blister-beetle, or Spanish fly (*Cantharis vesicatoria*). The most common appearance is that of a greyish-brown powder, containing shining green particles, from which cantharidin is readily extracted by exhausting with chloroform, driving off the chloroform by distillation or evaporation, and subsequently treating the extract with bisulphide of carbon, which dissolves the fatty matters only. Finally, the cantharidin may be recrystallised from chloroform, the yield being .380 to .570 per cent. Ferrer found in the wings and their cases, .082 per cent.; in the head and antennæ, .088; in the legs, .091; in the thorax and abdomen, .240; in the whole insect, .278 per cent. Wolff found in the *Lytta aspera*, .815 per cent.; Ferrer in *Mylabris cichorei*, .1 per cent.; in *M. punctum*, .193; and in *M. pustulata*, .33 per cent. of *cantharidin.*

§ 632. **Cantharidin** ($C_{10}H_{12}O_4$) has two crystalline forms—(1) Right-angled four-sided columns with four surfaces, each surface being beset with needles; and (2) flat tables. It is the anhydride of a ketone acid (cantharidic acid), $C_8H_{13}O_2$-CO-COOH. It is soluble in alkaline liquids, and can be recovered from them by acidifying and shaking up with *ether*, *chloroform*, or *benzene*; it is almost completely insoluble in water. 100 parts of alcohol (99 per cent.) dissolve at 18° 0.125 part; 100 of bisulphide of carbon, at the same temperature, 0.06 part; ether, .11 part; chloroform, 1.2 part; and benzene, .2 part. Cantharidin can be completely sublimed, if placed in the subliming cell, floating on mercury; a scanty sublimate of crystals may be obtained at so low a temperature as 82.5°; at 85°, and above, the sublimation is rapid. If the cantharidin is suddenly heated, it melts; but this is not the case if the temperature is raised gradually. The tube melting-point is as high as 218°. Potassic chromate with sulphuric acid decomposes cantharidin with the production of the green oxide of chromium. An alkaline solution of permanganate, iodic acid, and sodium amalgam, are all without influence on an alcoholic solution of cantharidin. With bases,

[638] "The Epidemics of the Middle Ages," by J. F. C. Hecker, translated by B. G. Babington, M.D., F.R.S. (*The Dancing Mania*, chap, ii., &c.)

[639] *Transac. of the New Zealand Inst.*, vol. ii., 1869; *Brit. and For. Med. Chir. Review*, July 1871, p. 230.

cantharidin forms crystallisable salts, and, speaking generally, if the base is soluble in water, the "*cantharidate*" is also soluble; the lime and magnesic salts dissolve readily. From the soda or potash salt, mineral acid will precipitate crystals of cantharidin; on heating with pentasulphide of phosphorus, o-xylol is produced.

§ 633. **Pharmaceutical Preparations of Cantharides.**—The P.B. preparations of cantharides are—*Acetum cantharides*, or vinegar of cantharides, containing about .04 per cent. of cantharidin.

Tincture of cantharides, containing about .005 per cent. of cantharidin.

A solution of cantharides for blistering purposes, *Liquor epispasticus*, a strong solution of the active principle in ether and acetic acid, containing about .16 per cent. of cantharidin.

There are also—An *ointment*; a blistering paper, *Charta epispastica*; a blistering plaster, *Emplastrum cantharides*; and a warm plaster, *Emplastrum calefaciens*.

§ 634. **Fatal Dose.**—It is difficult to state the fatal dose of cantharidin, the unassayed powder or tincture having mostly been taken. A young woman died from 1.62 grm. (25 grains) of the powder, which is perhaps equivalent to 6.4 mgrms. (1 grain) of cantharidin, whilst the smallest dose of the tincture known to have been fatal is (according to Taylor) an ounce. This would be generally equivalent to 15 mgrms. (.24 grain). Hence the fatal dose of cantharidin may be approximately stated as from 6 mgrms. upwards. But, on the other hand, recovery has taken place from very large doses.

§ 635. **Effects on Animals.**—Certain animals do not appear susceptible to the action of cantharidin. For example, hedgehogs and swallows are said to be able to take it with impunity. Radecki[640] found that cantharidin might even be injected into the blood of fowls without any injury, and frogs also seem to enjoy the same impunity; while dogs, cats, and other animals are sensitive to the poison. Galippe ascertained that after the injection of 5 mgrms. into the veins of a dog, there was exaltation of the sexual desire; the pupils quickly dilated, the dog sought a dark place, and became sleepy. Animals when poisoned die in asphyxia from paralysis of the respiratory centre. Schachowa[641] made some observations on the effect of cantharides on the renal excretion of a dog fed daily with 1 grm. in powder. On the third day, pus corpuscles were noticed; on the fifth, bacteria; on the thirteenth, the urine contained a large quantity of fatty matters, and several casts; and on the seventeenth, red shrivelled blood corpuscles were observed.

Effects on Man.—Heinrich[642] made the following experiments upon himself:—Thirty living blister-beetles were killed, and digested, without drying, in 35 grms. of alcohol for fourteen days, of this tincture ten drops were taken. There ensued immediately a feeling of warmth in the mouth and stomach, salivation, the pulse was more frequent than in health, there was a pleasant feeling of warmth about the body, and some sexual excitement lasting three hours. In half an hour there was abdominal pain, diarrhœa, and tenesmus, and frequent painful micturition. These symptoms subsided in a few hours, but there was a want of appetite, and pain about the kidneys lasting until the following day. In the second experiment, on taking 1 cgrm. of cantharidin, there were very serious symptoms of poisoning. Blisters formed on the tongue, and there was salivation, with great difficulty in swallowing, and a general feeling of illness. Seven hours after taking the poison, there were frequent micturitions of bloody urine, diarrhœa, and vomiting. Twenty hours after the ingestion the face was red, the skin hot, the pulse twenty beats beyond the normal pulsation, the tongue was denuded to two-thirds of its extent of its epithelium, and the lips and mucous membrane were red and swollen; there was great pain in the stomach, intestines, and in the neighbourhood of the kidneys, continuous desire to micturate, burning of the urethra, and swelling of the glands. There was no sexual excitement whatever; the urine was ammoniacal, and contained blood and pus; the symptoms gradually subsided, but recovery was not complete for fourteen days.

§ 636. The foregoing is a fair picture of what may be expected in cantharides poisoning. It is remarkable that the popular idea as to the influence of cantharidin in exciting the sexual passion, holds good only as to the entire cantharides, and not with cantharidin. It is very possible that cantharidin is not the only poisonous principle in the insect. The symptoms in other cases, fatal or not, have been as follows:—Immediate burning in the mouth and throat, extending to the stomach and alimentary canal, and increasing in intensity until there is considerable pain. Then follow salivation, difficulty in swallowing, and vomiting, and generally diarrhœa, pain in the kidneys, irritation of the bladder, priapism, and strangury, are all present. The pulse is accelerated, the breathing disturbed, there are pains in the head, and often mydriasis, giddiness, insensibility, delirium, and convulsions; trismus has been noticed.

[640] *Die Cantharidin Vergift.*, Diss., Dorpat, 1806.

[641] *Unters. über die Nieren*, Diss., Bern, 1877; Cornil, *Gaz. Méd.*, 1880.

[642] Schroff, *Zeitschrift d. Ges. d. Aerzte in Wien*, 13, 56.

The desire to micturate frequently is urgent, the urine is generally bloody, and contains pus. Pregnant women have been known to abort. In a few of the cases in which a different course has been run, the nervous symptoms have predominated over those of gastro-intestinal irritation, and the patient has sunk in a kind of collapse. In a case of chronic poisoning by cantharides, extending over three months, and recorded by Tarchioni Bonfanti,[643] after the first dose appeared tetanic convulsions, which subsided in twenty-four hours, there was later cystitis, and from time to time the tetanic convulsions returned; gastro-enteritis followed with frequent vomiting, when, cantharides being found in the matters ejected, the otherwise obscure nature of the illness was shown.

In a case recorded by Sedgwick,[644] following the gastro-enteric symptoms, there were epileptic convulsions; in this instance also was noticed an unpleasant smell, recalling the notion formerly held that cantharides imparted a peculiar odour to the breath and urine. In a case of chronic poisoning related by Tardieu, six students, during several months, used what they thought was pepper with their food, but the substance proved to be really powdered cantharides. The quantity taken each day was probably small, but they suffered from pain about the loins, and also irritation of the bladder. There was no sexual excitement.

§ 637. **Post-mortem Appearances.**—In a French criminal case, in which a man poisoned his step-brother by giving cantharides in soup, the pathological signs of inflammation of the gastro-intestinal tract were specially evident, the mouth was swollen, the tonsils ulcerated, the gullet, stomach, and intestines were inflamed, and the mucous membrane of the intestines covered with purulent matter. In another case there was an actual perforation 3 inches from the pylorus. The inflammatory appearances, however, are not always so severe, being confined to swelling and inflammation without ulceration. In all cases there has been noted inflammation of the kidneys and urinary passages, and this is seen even when cantharidin is administered to animals by subcutaneous injection. In the urine will be found blood and fatty epithelial casts, as well as pus. The contents of the stomach or the intestines will probably contain some remnants of powdered cantharides, if the powder itself has been taken.

§ 638. **Tests for Cantharidin, and its Detection in the Tissues, &c.**—The tests for cantharidin are—(1.) Its form, (2.) its action in the subliming cell, and (3.) its power of raising a blister.

The most convenient method of testing its vesicating properties, is to allow a chloroformic solution of the substance supposed to be cantharidin to evaporate to dryness, to add to this a drop of olive oil (or almond oil), and to take a drop up on the smallest possible quantity of cotton wool, and apply the wool to the inside of the arm, covering it with good oilskin, and strapping the whole on by the aid of sticking-plaster. In about an hour or more the effect is examined. The thin skin of the lips is far more easily blistered than that of the arm, but the application there is inconvenient.

Dragendorff has ascertained that cantharidin is not present in the contents of a blister raised by a cantharides plaster, although it has been found in the urine of a person treated by one; and Pettenkofer has also discovered cantharidin in the blood of a boy to whose spine a blister had been applied.

The great insolubility of cantharidin in water has led to various hypotheses as to its absorption into the system. It is tolerably easily dissolved by potash, soda, and ammonia solutions, and is also taken up in small proportion by sulphuric, phosphoric, and lactic acids. The resulting compounds quickly diffuse themselves through animal membranes. Even the salts with lime, magnesia, alumina, and the heavy metals, are not quite insoluble. A solution of salt with cantharidin, put in a dialysing apparatus, separates in twenty-four hours enough cantharidin to raise a blister.

Cantharidin has actually been discovered in the heart, brain, muscles, contents of the stomach, intestines, and fæces (as well as in the blood and urine) of animals poisoned by the substance. A urine containing cantharidin is alkaline and albuminous. Cantharidin, although readily decomposed by chemical agents, is so permanent in the body that it has been detected in the corpse of a cat eighty-four days after death.

In any forensic case, the defence will not improbably be set up that some animal (*e.g.*, a fowl poisoned by cantharides) has been eaten and caused the toxic symptoms, for cantharides is an interesting example of a substance which, as before stated, for certain animals (such as rabbits, dogs, cats, and ducks), is a strong poison, whilst in others (*e.g.*, hedgehogs, fowls, turkeys, and frogs), although absorbed and excreted, it appears inert. Experiment has shown that a cat may be readily poisoned by a fowl saturated with cantharides; and in Algeria the military surgeons meet with cystitis among the soldiers, caused by eating frogs in the months of May and June, the frogs living in these months almost exclusively on a species of cantharides.

---

[643] *Gaz. Med. Ital. Lomb.*, 1863.
[644] *Med. Times*, 1864.

Dragendorff recommends the following process:—The finely-pulped substance is boiled in a porcelain dish with potash-lye (1 part of potash and 12 to 18 of water) until the fluid is of a uniform consistence. The fluid, after cooling, is (if necessary) diluted with an equal bulk of water, for it must not be too thick; then shaken with chloroform in order to remove impurities; and after separation of the chloroform, strongly acidified with sulphuric acid, and mixed with about four times its volume of alcohol of 90 to 95 per cent. The mixture is kept for some time at a boiling temperature, filtered hot, and the alcohol distilled from the filtrate. The watery fluid is now again treated with chloroform, as above described. The chloroform extract is washed with water, the residue taken up on some hot almond oil, and its blistering properties investigated. The mass, heated with potash in the above way, can also be submitted to dialysis, the diffusate supersaturated with sulphuric acid, and shaken up with chloroform.

In order to test further for cantharidin, it can be dissolved in the least possible potash or soda-lye. The solution, on evaporation in the water-bath, leaves crystals of a salt not easily soluble in alcohol, and the watery solution of which gives with chloride of calcium and baryta a white precipitate; with sulphate of copper and sulphate of protoxide of nickel, a green; with cobaltous sulphate, a red; with sugar of lead, mercury chloride and argentic nitrate, a white crystalline precipitate. With palladium chloride there occurs a yellow, hair-like, crystalline precipitate; later crystals, which are isomorphous with the nickel and copper salts.

If the tincture of cantharides has been used in considerable quantity, the urine may be examined; in such a case there will collect on the surface drops of a green oil, which may be extracted by petroleum ether; this oil is not blister-raising. Cantharides in powder may, of course, be detected by its appearance.

To the question whether the method proposed would extract any other blister-producing substance, the answer is negative, since ethereal oil of mustard would be decomposed, and the active constituents of the *Euphorbias* do not withstand the treatment with KHO. Oils of anemone and anemonin are dissolved by KHO, and again separated out of their solutions, but their blistering property is destroyed. They are volatile, and found in anemone and some of the *Ranunculaceæ*. In the *Aqua pulsatilla* there is an oil of anemone, which may be obtained by shaking with ether; but this oil is not permanent, and if the *Aqua pulsatilla* stand for a little time, it splits up into anemonic acid and anemonin, and then cannot be reobtained. A blistering substance, obtained from the *Anacardia orientalia* and the fruit of the *Anacardium occidentale* and *Semecarpus anacardium*, is not quite destroyed by a short action with potash, but is by one of long duration; this substance, however, cannot be confused with cantharidin, for it is oily, yellow, easily soluble in alcohol and ether, and differs in other respects.

V.—Snake Poison.

§ 639. The poisonous snakes belong chiefly to two classes, the *Proteroglypha* and the *Solenoglypha*.

Weir Mitchell and Ed. T. Reichert[645] have made some important experiments on snake poison, using the venom of some 200 snakes. Most of the snakes were rattlesnakes, a few were cobras and other species. They came to the conclusion that the active constituents are contained in the fluid part alone, the solid particles suspended in the fluid having no action. The poison they considered to consist of two toxalbumins, one a globulin, acting more particularly on the blood, the other, a peptone (albumose?), acting more particularly on the tissues. Differences in snake venom depend on the relative proportions of these two substances. The peptone, which acts more especially locally on the tissues, determines an inflammatory action, with much swelling and multiple extravasation of blood, which may proceed to a moist gangrene. The globulin has a paralysing influence on the heart, the vasomotor centres, the peripheral ends of the splanchnic nerves, as well as on the respiratory centres of both warm and cold-blooded animals. Feoktisow's[646] researches show that although the heart continues to beat after the respiration has ceased for a few minutes, it has no force. The blood pressure sinks immediately after the injection. Whether the globulin is injected subcutaneously or direct into the veins, there is commonly considerable extravasation of blood in the chest and abdomen; the intestine is often filled with blood as well as the pericardium; and the urine is bloody. The poison of *Vipera ammodytes* in watery solution may be boiled for six minutes, and yet is as active as before. According to Lewin, snake poison generally can be heated to 125° and yet preserve its poisonous properties. These last observations are not in accordance with the belief of some that the active principle of snake venom is a ferment, or, indeed, in harmony with the idea that it is a globulin or toxalbumin; for such bodies have not, so far as we know, the stability to withstand so high a degree of heat.

[645] *Smithsonian Contributions to Knowledge*, Washington, 1886.

[646] *Exp. Unters. über Schlangengift. Inaug. Diss.*, Dorpat, 1888.

§ 640. **The Poison of the Cobra.**—The poison excreted from the salivary glands of the cobra di capello is the most deadly animal fluid known. When first ejected, it is an amber-coloured, rather syrupy, frothy liquid, of specific gravity 1.046, and of feeble acid reaction; it dries rapidly on exposure to air to a yellow film, which readily breaks up into brilliant yellow granules, closely imitating crystals. The yellow powder is very acrid and pungent to the nostrils, and excites a painful (though transitory) inflammation, if applied to the mucous membrane of the eye; the taste is bitter, and it raises little blisters on the tongue. It is perfectly stable, and preserves its activity for an indefinite time. The dried poison as described is perfectly soluble in water, and if the water is added in proper proportions, the original fluid is without doubt reproduced, the solution usually depositing a sediment of epithelial *débris*, and often containing little white threads.

The poison has been examined by several chemists, but until of late years with a negative result. The writer was the first to isolate, in 1876, a crystalline principle, which appears to be the sole acting ingredient; the yellow granules were dissolved in water, the albumen which the venom so copiously contains coagulated by alcohol, and separated by filtration; the alcohol was then driven off at a gentle heat, the liquid concentrated to a small bulk, and precipitated with basic acetate of lead. The precipitate was separated, washed, and decomposed in the usual way by SH_2, and on removing the lead sulphide, crystals having toxic properties were obtained.

Pedler,[647] precipitating the albumen by alcohol, and then to the alcoholic solution adding platinic chloride, obtained a semi-crystalline precipitate, which from an imperfect combustion he thinks may have something like the composition $PtCl_4(C_{17}H_{25}N_4O_7HCl)_2$. I have examined the platinum compound, and made several combustions of different fractions, but was unable to obtain the compound in a sufficient state of purity to deduce a formula. My analysis agreed with those of Pedler for nitrogen—viz., 9.93 per cent. (Pedler, 9.69); hydrogen 4.17 (Pedler, 4.28); but were higher for carbon, 41.8 per cent. (Pedler, 33.42 per cent.); one fraction gave 7.3 per cent. of platinum, another double that amount. Material was insufficient to thoroughly investigate the compound, but it was evident that several double salts were formed. The blood of the cobra is also poisonous. A. Calmette[648] has found that 2 c.c. of fresh cobra blood, injected into the peritoneum of a rabbit weighing 1.5 kilo., causes death in six hours; the same dose of the defibrinated blood injected into the veins is fatal in three minutes.

§ 641. **Fatal Dose.**—From my experiments on cats, rabbits, and birds, it seems probable that the least fatal dose for cats and rabbits, lies between .7 and .9 mgrm. per kilo., and for birds somewhere about .7 mgrm. per kilo. of the dried poison; the venom contains about 60 per cent. of albuminous matter, and about 10 per cent. of poisonous substance; therefore, the lethal power is represented by something like .07 to .09 mgrm. per kilo., if the pure toxic principle free from albumen and diluting impurities be considered.

§ 642. **Effects on Animals.**—Almost immediately local pain or signs of uneasiness at the seat of injection are observed. There is then a variable interval, seldom exceeding 20 minutes (and generally much less), but in one of my experiments half an hour elapsed after the injection of a fatal dose before any effect was evident. The symptoms once produced, the course is rapid, and consists, first, of acceleration of the respirations, and then a progressive slowing, soon followed by convulsions. The convulsions are probably produced by the interference with the respiration and the deficient oxidation of the blood, and are therefore, the so-called "carbonic acid convulsions." There is paresis or paralysis of the limbs. Death seems to occur from asphyxia, and the heart beats for one or more minutes after the respirations have ceased. If the dose is so small as not to produce death, no after-effects have been observed; recovery is complete.

Sir J. Fayrer, and Dr. Lauder Brunton consider that the terminations of the motor nerves suffer; on the other hand, Dr. Wall would explain the phenomena by referring the action entirely to the central nervous system, and concludes that the effects of the cobra poison consist in the extinction of function extending from below upwards of the various nerve centres constituting the cerebro-spinal system. In addition to this, there is a special and rapid action on the respiratory and allied nuclei, and this it is that causes death.

§ 643. **Effects on Man.**—By far the best account hitherto published of the effects of the cobra poison is a paper by Dr. Wall,[649] in which he points out the very close similarity between the symptoms produced and those of glosso-pharyngeal paralysis. This is well shown in the following typical case:—A coolie was bitten on the shoulder about twelve at midnight by a cobra; he immediately felt burning pain at the spot bitten, which increased. In fifteen minutes

[647] *Proc. Roy. Soc.*, vol. xxvii. p. 17.

[648] *Compt. Rend., Soc. de Biol.*, 1894.

[649] "On the Difference of the Physiological Effects Produced by the Poison of Indian Venomous Snakes," by A. T. Wall, M.D., *Proc. Roy. Soc.*, 1881, vol. xxxii. p. 333.

afterwards he began, he said, to feel intoxicated, but he seemed rational, and answered questions intelligently. The pupils were natural, and the pulse normal; the respirations were also not accelerated. He next began to lose power over his legs, and staggered. In thirty minutes after the bite his lower jaw began to fall, and frothy viscid mucous saliva ran from his mouth; he spoke indistinctly, like a man under the influence of liquor, and the paralysis of the legs increased. Forty minutes after the bite, he began to moan and shake his head from side to side, and the pulse and respirations were somewhat accelerated; but he was still able to answer questions, and seemed conscious. There was no paralysis of the arms. The breathing became slower and slower, and at length ceased one hour and ten minutes after the bite, the heart beating for about one minute after the respiration had stopped.

There is often very little sign of external injury, merely a scratch or puncture being apparent, but the areolar tissue lying beneath is of a purple colour, and infiltrated with a large quantity of coagulable, purple, blood-like fluid. In addition, the whole of the neighbouring vessels are intensely injected, the injection gradually diminishing as the site of the poisoned part is receded from, so that a bright scarlet ring surrounds a purple area, and this in its turn fades into the normal colour of the neighbouring tissues. At the margin is also a purple blood-like fluid, replaced by a pinkish serum, which may often be traced up in the tissues surrounding the vessels that convey the poison to the system, and may extend a considerable distance. These appearances are to be accounted for in great part by the irritant properties of the cobra venom. The local hyperæmia and the local pain are the first symptoms. In man there follows an interval (which may be so short as a few minutes, or so long as four hours) before any fresh symptoms appear; the average duration of the interval is, according to Dr. Wall, about an hour. When once the symptoms are developed, then the course is rapid, and, as in the case quoted, a feeling like that of intoxication is first produced, and then loss of power over the legs. This is followed by a loss of power over the speech, over swallowing, and the movement of the lips; the tongue becomes motionless, and hangs out of the mouth; the saliva is secreted in large quantities, and runs down the face, the patient being equally unable to swallow it or to eject it, and the glosso-pharyngeal paralysis is complete.

§ 644. **Antidotes and Treatment.**—Professor Halford some years ago proposed ammonia, and M. Lacerda in recent times has declared potassic permanganate an antidote to the cobra poison. The ammonia theory has been long disproved, and before Lacerda had made his experiments I had published the chemical aspect of some researches,[650] which showed that mixing the cobra venom with an alkaline solution of potassic permanganate destroyed its poisonous properties. Other experiments were also made in every conceivable way with potassic permanganate, injecting it separately, yet simultaneously, into different parts of the same animal's body, but so long as it does not come into actual contact with the poison it has no antidotal power whatever over the living subject. Other observers, previous to the researches mentioned and since, all agree that permanganate is no true antidote.[651] It only acts when it comes directly into contact with the venom, but when the venom is once absorbed into the circulation potassic permanganate, whether acid, alkaline, or neutral, is powerless. That it is of great use when applied to a bite is unquestionable, for it neutralises or changes any of the venom hanging about the wound, and which, if allowed to remain, might yet be absorbed; but here it is obvious that the venom is, so to speak, outside the body. A. Galmette (*Annales de l'Institut Pasteur*, 25th March 1892) has found that gold chloride forms an insoluble compound with the cobra poison, which is not poisonous, and that animal living tissues impregnated with gold chloride will not absorb the poison. He even advances some evidence tending to show that gold chloride may overtake, as it were, the venom in the circulation, and thus act as a true antidote. This is improbable, and, until confirmed, the general treatment most likely to be successful is the immediate sucking of the wound, followed by the application of an alkaline solution of permanganate; and lastly, if the symptoms should nevertheless develop, an attempt should be made to maintain the breathing by galvanism and artificial respiration.[652]

---

[650] *Analyst*, Feb. 28, 1877.

[651] See Note on the effect of various substances in destroying the activity of the cobra poison. By T. Lauder Brunton and Sir J. Fayrer, *Proc. Roy. Soc.*, vol. xxvii. p. 17.

[652] Some of my experiments on the cobra poison may be briefly detailed, illustrating the general statement in the text:—

1. A quantity equal to 1 mgrm. of the dried venom was injected subcutaneously into a chicken. The symptoms began in two minutes with loss of power over both legs. In eight minutes the legs were perfectly paralysed. There were convulsive movements of the head and wings, slowing of the respiration, and death in ten minutes. The same quantity of poison was treated with a little tannin, and the clear liquid which separated from the precipitate injected into another chicken. The respiration became affected in ten minutes; in eighteen minutes the bird had become very quiet, and lay insensible; in twenty minutes it was dead, the respiration ceasing before the heart.

2. In seven experiments with cobra poison, first rendered feebly alkaline with an alkaline solution of potassic permanganate,

§ 645. **Detection of the Cobra Venom.**—In an experiment on a rabbit, the animal was killed by the subcutaneous injection of 8 mgrms. per kilo. of the cobra poison. Immediately after death, 2 c.c. of the blood were injected into a small rabbit; in fifteen minutes there was slow respiration with pains in the limbs; in thirty minutes this had, in a great measure, passed off, and in a little time the animal was well. In any case in which it is necessary to attempt to separate the cobra venom, the most likely method of succeeding would be to make a cold alcoholic extract, evaporate in a vacuum, take up the residue in a little water, and test its effect on small animals.

§ 646. **Duboia Russellii.**—The *Duboia russellii* or *Russell's viper* is one of the best known and most deadly of the Indian vipers. The effects of the poison of this viper are altogether different from those of the cobra. The action commences by violent general convulsions, which are often at once fatal, or may be followed by rapid paralysis and death; or these symptoms, again, may be recovered from, and death follow at a later period. The convulsions do not depend on asphyxia, and with a small dose may be absent. The paralysis is general, and may precede for some time the extinction of the respiration, the pupils are widely dilated, there are bloody discharges, and the urine is albuminous. Should the victim survive the first effects, then blood-poisoning may follow, and a dangerous illness result, often attended with copious hæmorrhages. A striking example of this course is recorded in the *Indian Med. Gaz.*, June 1, 1872.

A Mahommedan, aged 40, was bitten on the finger by Russell's viper; the bitten part was soon after excised, and stimulants given. The hand and arm became much swollen, and on the same day he passed blood by the rectum, and also bloody urine. The next day he was sick, and still passing blood from all the channels; in this state he remained eight days, losing blood constantly, and died on the ninth day. Nothing definite is known of the chemical composition of the poison; it is probably qualitatively identical with "viperin."

---

no effect followed. Three of the experiments were on chickens, four on rabbits.

3. A chicken was injected with 1 mgrm. of cobra poison in one leg, and in the other simultaneously with a solution of potassic permanganate. Death followed in sixteen minutes. Another chicken was treated in the same way, but with injections of potassic permanganate solution every few minutes. Death resulted in thirty-seven minutes. Four other similar experiments were made—two with feebly alkaline permanganate, two with permanganate made feebly acid with sulphuric acid—but death occurred with the usual symptoms.

4. Cobra poison was mixed with a weak solution of iodine, and a quantity equal to half a mgrm. was injected into a chicken. The symptoms began directly, were fully developed in ten minutes, and death took place in twenty-one minutes.

5. Equal volumes of cobra venom and aldehyde were mixed, and a quantity equivalent to 1 mgrm. of the cobra poison injected. The symptoms were immediate paralysis and insensibility, and the respiration rapidly fell. Death occurred in four minutes without convulsions.

6. The cobra venom was mixed with a feebly alkaline solution of pyrogallic acid, and injected subcutaneously into a chicken. In six minutes the usual symptoms commenced, followed in thirteen minutes by death.

7. One mgrm. was injected into a chicken. The respirations at the commencement were 120; in twenty-two minutes they sank to 96, in twenty-five minutes to 84, in twenty-seven minutes to 18, and then to occasional gasps, with slight movement of the wings and toes. There was death in thirty-two minutes after the injection.

8. A young rabbit was injected with .5 mg. (equal to 1 mgrm. per kilo.) of cobra poison. In two hours it was apparently moribund, with occasional short gasps. Artificial respiration was now attempted. There was considerable improvement, but it was intermitted during the night, and the animal was found dead in the morning, having certainly lived six hours.

9. A strong healthy kitten was injected with 1 mgrm. of cobra venom (equal to 5 mgrms. per kilo.). In twenty minutes the symptoms were well developed, and in an hour the animal was gasping—about twelve short respirations per minute. Artificial respiration was kept up for two hours, and the animal recovered, but there was great muscular weakness lasting for more than twenty-four hours.

10. A brown rabbit, weighing about 2 kilos., was injected with 12 mgrms. (6 per kilo.) of the cobra poison. The symptoms developed within ten minutes; ammonia was injected, and also given by the nostril. The heart's action, which, previous to the administration of the ammonia, had been beating feebly, became accelerated, but death followed within the hour, the heart beating two minutes after the respiration had ceased.

11. A brown rabbit, about 2 kilos. in weight, was injected with 1.5 mgrms. of cobra poison (.75 per kilo.). There were no symptoms for nearly an hour, then sudden convulsions, and death.

12. Another rabbit of the same size was treated similarly, but immediately after the injection made to breathe nitrous oxide; death took place in thirty minutes. A rabbit, a little over 2 kilos. in weight, was injected with 7 mgrms. of cobra venom per kilo., and then 10 mgrms. of monobromated camphor were administered. In fifteen minutes there was general paralysis of the limbs, from which in a few minutes the animal seemed to recover; thirty minutes after the injection there were no very evident symptoms, but within forty minutes there was a sudden accession of convulsions, and death. Experiments were also made with chloroform, morphine, and many other substances, but none seemed to exercise any true antidotal effect.

§ 647. **The Poison of the Common Viper.**—The common viper still abounds in certain parts of Great Britain, as, for example, on Dartmoor. The venom was analysed in a partial manner by Valentin. In 1843 Prince Lucien Bonaparte separated a gummy varnish, inodorous, glittering, and transparent, which he called *echidnin* or *viperin*; it was a neutral nitrogenous body without taste, it arrested the coagulation of the blood, and, injected into animals, produced all the effects of the bite of the viper. Phisalix and G. Bertrand have studied the symptoms produced in small animals after injection. A guinea-pig, weighing 500 grms., was killed by 0.3 grm. of the dried venom dissolved in 5000 parts of saline water; the symptoms were nausea, quickly passing into stupor. The temperature of the body fell. The autopsy showed the left auricle full of blood, the intestine, lungs, liver, and kidneys injected. The blood of the viper is also poisonous, and produces the same symptoms as the venom.[653] The same observers have shown (*Compt. rend.*, cxviii., Jan. 1894) that the blood of the water-snake (*Tropidonotus natrix*) and of the Thuringian adder (*Tropidonotus viperinus*) is poisonous, producing the same symptoms as that of the viper.

The Venom of Naja Haje (Cleopatra's Asp).—It has been stated that 20,000 persons annually die in Ceylon from the bite of Cleopatra's asp. Graziani (*Rif. Med.*, October 7, 1893) has undertaken a physiological study of the venom, which has already received attention at the hands of Calmette, Wall and Armstrong, Weir Mitchell, Reichardt, and others. The venom, when dried, appears as transparent scales, easily soluble in water, very slightly so in alcohol, ether, or chloroform; its aqueous solution has an unpleasant odour, and is neutral to test paper. Chemically it gives all the tests described by Weir Mitchell and others as characteristic of the venom of *Naja tripudians*. The physiological effects of this dried venom were tried on guinea-pigs, rabbits, and frogs, to all of which it proved fatal in extremely minute doses. The guinea-pig, a few seconds after injection, becomes paralysed in its hind limbs, it foams at the mouth, and makes violent attempts at vomiting. The eyes are half closed, but occasionally for short periods there is a partial disappearance of the paralysis, and the animal makes feeble attempts to support itself. Respiratory embarrassment is soon added to the foregoing symptoms, and the animal lies perfectly prone, devoting all its attention to breathing, which is rendered still more difficult by the vomiting and frothy saliva which is secreted in abundance. Finally death ensues from asphyxia. The *post-mortem* examination reveals the heart still feebly beating, the lungs pallid, and the blood in the organs very dark. The liver and kidneys are hyperæmic, but the brain and cord, with their coverings, are anæmic. In the rabbit the course of the poisoning is practically identical with that described above. Histologically, the following facts are made out in addition to the foregoing. The red blood-corpuscles are in great measure broken down, and there are also effusions into the muscular tissues. The kidneys are very hyperæmic, and there is marked degeneration of the epithelium lining the glomeruli and convoluted tubules. The glomerular capsules are much distended, and numerous leucocytes are discernible throughout the organ. The liver, also, is hyperæmic, and shows numerous broken-down blood-corpuscles, and partial necrosis of many of the liver cells. Examination of the central nervous system reveals no particular changes.

DIVISION II.—PTOMAINES—TOXINES.

§ 648. **Definition of a Ptomaine.**—A ptomaine may be considered as a basic chemical substance derived from the action of bacteria on nitrogenous substances. If this definition is accepted, a ptomaine is not necessarily formed in the dead animal tissue; it may be produced by the living, and, in all cases, it is the product of bacterial life. A ptomaine is not necessarily poisonous; many are known which are, in moderate doses, quite innocuous.

When Selmi's researches were first published there was some anxiety lest the existence of ptomaines would seriously interfere with the detection of poison generally, because some were said to be like strychnine, others like colchicine, and so forth. Farther research has conclusively shown that at present no ptomaine is known which so closely resembles a vegetable poison as to be likely in skilled hands to cause confusion.

Isolation of Ptomaines.

§ 649. **Gautier's[654] Process.**—The liquid is acidified with oxalic acid, warmed, filtered, and distilled in a vacuum.

In this way pyrrol, skatol, phenol, indol, and volatile fatty acids are separated and will be found in the distillate. The residue in the retort is treated with lime, filtered from the precipitate that forms, and distilled in a vacuum, the distillate being received in weak sulphuric acid. The bases accompanied with ammonia distil over. The distillate is

[653] *Compt. rend. Soc. de Biol.*, t. v. 997.

[654] *Ptomaines et Leucomaines*, E. J. A. Gautier, Paris, 1886.

now neutralised by sulphuric acid[655] and evaporated nearly to dryness, separating the mother liquid from sulphate of ammonia, which crystallises out. The mother liquids are treated with absolute alcohol, which dissolves the sulphates of the ptomaines. The alcohol is got rid of by evaporation, the residue treated with caustic soda, and the bases shaken out by successive treatment with ether, petroleum ether, and chloroform. The residue remaining in the retort with the excess of lime is dried, powdered, and exhausted with ether; the ethereal extract is separated, evaporated to dryness, the dry residue taken up in a little water, slightly acidulated, and the bases precipitated by an alkali.

§ 650. **Brieger's Process.**—Brieger[656] thus describes his process:—

"The matters are finely divided and boiled with water feebly acidulated with hydrochloric acid.

"Care must be taken that on boiling, the weak acid reaction must be retained, and that this manipulation only lasts a few minutes.

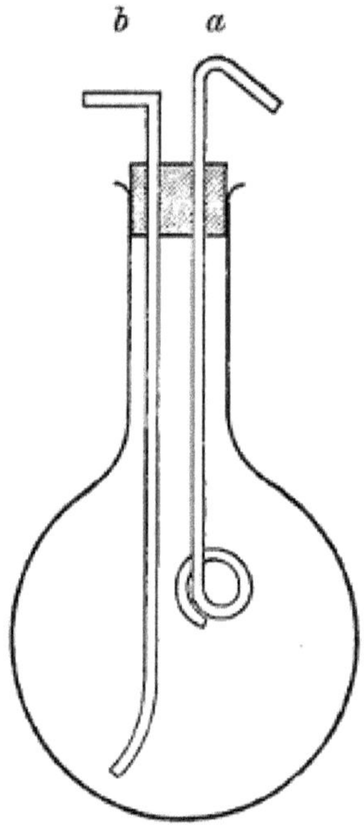

"The insoluble portion is filtered off, and the filtrate evaporated, either in the gas-oven or on the water-bath, to syrupy consistency. If the substances are offensive, as alcoholic and watery extracts of flesh usually are, the use of Bocklisch's simple apparatus (see diagram) is to be recommended. The filtrate to be evaporated is placed in a flask provided with a doubly perforated caoutchouc cork carrying two bent tubes; the tube *b* terminates near the bottom of the flask, while the tube *a* terminates a little above the level of the fluid to be evaporated. The tube *a* is connected with a water pump which sucks away the escaping steam. In order to avoid the running back of the condensed water forming in the cooler part of the tube, the end of the tube *a* is twisted into a circular form. Through the tube *b*, which has a fine capillary bore, a stream of air is allowed to enter, which keeps the fluid in constant agitation, continually destroying the scum on the surface, and avoiding sediments collecting at the bottom, which may cause fracture of the flask. According to the regulation of the air current, a greater or smaller vacuum can be produced. The fluid, evaporated to the consistency of a syrup, is treated with 96 per cent. alcohol, filtered, and the filtrate precipitated with lead acetate.

"The lead precipitate is filtered off, the filtrate evaporated to a syrup, and the syrup again treated with 96 per cent. alcohol. This is again filtered, the alcohol got rid of by evaporation, water added, the lead thrown down by SH_2, and the fluid, after the addition of a little hydrochloric acid, evaporated to the consistence of a syrup; this syrup

[655] The first acid apparently is so dilute that the distillate more than neutralises it, hence more sulphuric acid is added to complete neutralisation.

[656] *Untersuchungen über Ptomaine*, Theil iii., Berlin, 1886.

is exhausted with 96 per cent. alcohol, and precipitated with an alcoholic solution of mercury chloride. The mercury precipitate is boiled with water, and by the different solubility of the mercury salts of certain ptomaines some separation takes place. If it is suspected that some of the ptomaines may have been separated with the lead precipitate, this lead precipitate can be decomposed by SH_2 and investigated. I have only (says Brieger) in the case of mussels been able to extract from the lead precipitate small quantities of ptomaines.

"The mercury filtrate is freed from mercury and evaporated, the excess of hydrochloric acid being carefully neutralised by means of soda (for it must only be slightly acid); then it is again treated with alcohol, so as to separate as much as possible the inorganic constituents. The alcoholic extract is evaporated, dissolved in a little water, neutralised with soda, acidulated with nitric acid, and precipitated with phospho-molybdic acid. The phospho-molybdic acid precipitate is decomposed with neutral lead acetate, which process may be facilitated by heating on the water-bath. After getting rid of the lead by treatment with SH_2, the fluid is evaporated to a syrup and alcohol added, by which process many ptomaines may be eliminated as hydrochlorates; or they can be converted into double salts (of platinum or gold) for the purpose of separation. In the filtrate from phospho-molybdate, ptomaines may also be found by treating with lead acetate to get rid of the phospho-molybdic acid, and then adding certain reactives. Since it is but seldom that the hydrochlorates are obtained in a state of purity, it is preferable to convert the substance separated into a gold or platinum salt or a picrate, since the greater or less solubility of these compounds facilitates the purification of individual members; but which reagent is best to add, must be learned from experience. The melting-point of these salts must always be taken, so that an idea of their purity may be obtained. It is also to be noted that many gold salts decompose on warming the aqueous solution; this may be avoided by the addition of hydrochloric acid. The hydrochlorates of the ptomaines are obtained by decomposing the mercury, gold, or platinum combinations by the aid of SH_2, while the picrates can be treated with hydrochloric acid and shaken up with ether, which latter solvent dissolves the picric acid.

"Considerable difficulty in the purification of the ptomaines is caused by a nitrogenous, amorphous, non-poisonous, albumin-like substance, which passes into all solutions, and can only be got rid of by careful precipitation with an alcoholic solution of lead acetate, in which it is soluble in excess. This albuminoid forms an amorphous compound with platinum, and acts as a strongly reducing agent (the platinum compound contains 29 per cent. platinum). When this albuminoid is eliminated, then the hydrochlorates or the double salts of the ptomaines crystallise."

§ 651. **The Benzoyl Chloride Method.**—The fatty diamines in dilute aqueous solutions, shaken with benzoyl chloride and soda, are converted into insoluble dibenzoyl derivatives; these may be separated from benzamide and other nitrogenous products by dissolving the precipitate in alcohol, and pouring the solution into a large quantity of water.[657] Compounds which contain two amido groups combined with one and the same carbon atom, do not yield benzoyl derivatives when shaken with benzoyl chloride and soda. Hence this reaction can be utilised for certain of the ptomaines only. The solution must be dilute, because concentrated solutions of creatine, creatinine, and similar bodies also give precipitates with benzoyl chloride; no separation, however, occurs unless these bodies are in the proportion of five per thousand.

The process is specially applicable for the separation of ethylenediamine, pentamethylenediamine (cadaverine), and tetramethylenediamine (putrescine) from urine. In a case of cystinuria Udrànsky and E. Baumann[658] have found 0.24 grm. of benzoyltetramethylenediamine, 0.42 grm. of benzoylpentamethylenediamine in a day. Diamines are absent in normal fæces and urine. Stadthagen and Brieger[659] have also found, in a case of cystinuria diamines, chiefly pentamethylenediamine.

The operation is performed by making the liquid alkaline with soda, so that the alkalinity is equal to about 10 per cent., adding benzoyl chloride, shaking until the odour of benzoyl chloride disappears, and then filtering; to the filtrate more benzoyl chloride is added, the liquid shaken, and, if a precipitate appears, this is also filtered off, and the process repeated until all diamines are separated.

The precipitate thus obtained is dissolved in alcohol, and the alcoholic solution poured into a considerable volume of water and allowed to stand over night; the dibenzoyl compound is then usually found to be in a crystalline condition. The compound is crystallised once or twice from alcohol or ether, and its melting-point and properties studied. Mixtures of diamines may be separated by their different solubilities in ether and alcohol.

[657] L. V. Udrànsky and Baumann, *Ber.*, xxi. 2744.

[658] L. V. Udrànsky and Baumann, *Zeit. f. physiol. Chem.*, xiii. 562.

[659] *Arch. pathol. Anatom.*, cxv. p. 3.

A solution of 0.00788 grm. of pentamethylenediamine in 100 c.c. of water gave 0.0218 grm. of the dibenzoyl-derivative when shaken with benzoyl chloride (5 c.c.) and 40 c.c. of soda (10 per cent.) and kept for twenty-four hours. In a second experiment with a similar solution only 0.0142 grm. of dibenzoyl-derivative was obtained;[660] hence the process is not a good quantitative process, and, although convenient for isolation, gives, so far as the total amount recovered is concerned, varying results.

§ 652. **The Amines.**—The amines are bases originating from ammonia and built on the same type. Those that are interesting as poisons are monamines, diamines, and the quaternary ammonium bases.

Considered as compound ammonias, the amines are divided into primary or amide bases, secondary or imid bases, and tertiary or nitrile bases, according as to whether one, two, or three atoms of hydrogen have been displaced from the ammonia molecule by an alkyl; for instance, methylamine NH_2CH_3 is a primary or amide base, because only one of the three atoms of H in NH_3 has been replaced by methyl; similarly, dimethylamine is a secondary or imid base, and trimethylamine is a tertiary or nitrile base.

The quaternary bases are derived from the hypothetical ammonium hydroxide NH_4OH, as, for example, tetraethyl ammonium hydroxide $(C_2H_5)_4N,OH$.

The diamines are derived from two molecules of NH, and therefore contain, instead of one molecule of nitrogen, two molecules of nitrogen; in two molecules of ammonia there are six atoms of hydrogen, two, four, or six of which may be replaced by alkyls; as, for example,

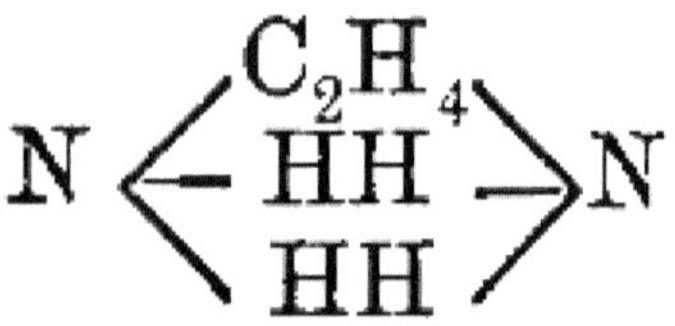

Ethylenediamine.

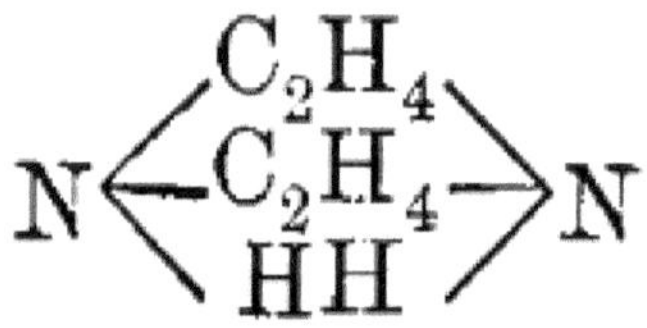

Diethylenediamine.

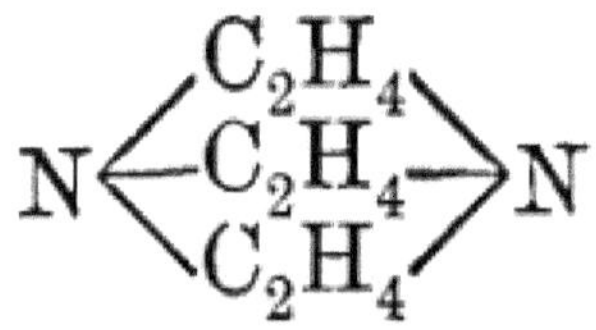

Triethylenediamine.

The monamines are similar to ammonia in their reactions; some of them are stronger bases; for instance, ethylamine expels ammonia from its salts. The first members of the series are combustible gases of pungent odour, and easily soluble in water; the higher homologues are fluids; and the still higher members solids.

The hydrochlorides are soluble in absolute alcohol, while chloride of ammonium is insoluble; this property is taken advantage of for separating amines from ammonia. The amines form double salts with platinic chloride; this is also utilised for recognition, for the purpose of separation, and for purification; for instance, ammonium-platinum-chloride on ignition yields 43.99 per cent. of platinum, and methylamine-platinum-chloride yields 47.4 of platinum. It is comparatively easy to ascertain whether an amine is primary, secondary, or tertiary.

The primary and secondary amines react with nitrous acid, but not the tertiary; the primary amines, for instance, are converted into alcohols, and there is an evolution of nitrogen gas; thus methylamine is decomposed into methyl alcohol, nitrogen, and water.

$CH_3NH_2 + (OH)NO = CH_3(OH) + N_2 + H_2O$.

The secondary amines, treated in the same way, evolve no nitrogen, but are converted into nitrosamines; thus dimethylamine, when treated with nitrous acid, yields nitrosodimethylamine,

$(CH_3)_2NH + (OH)NO = (CH_3)_2(NO)N + H_2O$;

and the nitrosamines respond to the test known as Lieberman's nitroso-reaction, which is thus performed:—The substance is dissolved in phenol and a few drops of concentrated sulphuric acid added. The yellow colour at first produced changes into blue by adding to the acid liquid a solution of potash.

The primary amines, and the primary amines alone, treated with chloroform and alcoholic potash, yield the peculiarly offensive smelling carbylamine or isonitrile (Hofmann's test),

V

$$NH_2(CH_3) + CHCl_3 + 3KOH = C{\equiv}N\text{-}CH_3 + 3KCl + 3H_2O.$$

Again the primary bases, when treated with corrosive sublimate and carbon disulphide, evolve sulphuretted

[660] *Ber.*, xxi. 2744.

hydrogen, and mustard oil is produced, *e.g.*,

$$NH_2(C_2H_5) + CS_2 = CS{=}N\text{-}C_2H_5 + H_2S.$$

Ethylamine. Ethylmustard oil.

Where a sufficient quantity of an amine is obtained, the primary, secondary, or tertiary character of the amine may be deduced with certainty by treating it with methyl or ethyl iodide.

A molecule of the base is digested with a molecule of methyl iodide and distilled with potash; the distillate is in the same manner again treated with methyl iodide and again distilled; and the process is repeated until an ammonium base is obtained, which will take up no more iodide. If three methyl groups were in this way introduced, the original substance was primary, if two, secondary, if one, tertiary.

The quaternary bases, such as tetraethyl ammoniumoxhydrate, decompose, on heating, into triethylamine and ethylene; the corresponding methyl compound in like manner yields trimethylamine and methyl-alcohol.

On the other hand, the primary, secondary, and tertiary bases do not decompose on heating, but volatilise without decomposition.

The chief distinctions between these various amines are conveniently put into a tabular form as follows:—

	Primary, NH_2R.	Secondary, NHR_2.	Tertiary, NR_3.	Quaternary, $NR_4(OH)$.
On treating with methyl iodide it takes up the following number of methyl groups,	3	2	1	...
Reaction with nitrous acid,	Decomposes with evolution of nitrogen gas.	Formation of nitrosamine.	...	...
Mustard oil, &c., on treatment with CS_2 and sublimate,	Mustard oil formed.	...	...	...
Chloroform and alcoholic potash,	Formation of carbylamine.	...	...	...
Effect of strong heat,	Sublimes.	Sublimes.	Sublimes.	Decomposes.
On addition of acids,	Combines to form salts.	Combines to form salts.	Combines to form salts.	...

§ 653. **Methylamine,** CH_3NH_2.—This is a gas at ordinary temperatures; it is inflammable, and possesses a strong ammoniacal odour. It has been found in herring brine, and is present in cultures of the comma bacillus; it has also been found in poisonous sausages, but it is not in itself toxic.

It forms crystalline salts, such as, for example, the hydrochloride, the platinochloride (Pt = 41.4 per cent.), and the aurochloride (Au = 53.3 per cent. when anhydrous). The best salt for estimation is the platinochloride, insoluble in absolute alcohol and ether.

§ 654. **Dimethylamine**, $(CH_3)_2NH$.—Dimethylamine is also a gas; it has been found in various putrefying substances. It forms crystalline salts, such as the hydrochloride, the platinochloride (Pt = 39.1 per cent.), and an aurochloride (Au = 51.35 per cent.). It is not poisonous.

In Brieger's process it may occur in both the mercuric chloride precipitate and filtrate. From cadaverine it may be separated by platinum chloride; cadaverine platinochloride is with difficulty soluble in cold water and crystallises from hot water, while dimethylamine remains in the mother liquor. From choline it may be separated by recrystallising the mercuric precipitate from hot water. From methylamine it may be separated by converting into chloride and extracting with chloroform; dimethylamine chloride is soluble, methylamine chloride insoluble in chloroform.

§ 655. **Trimethylamine**, $(CH_3)_3N$.—Trimethylamine in the free state is an alkaline liquid with a fishy odour, boiling at 9.3°; it is not toxic save in large doses.

It occurs in a great variety of plants, and is also found in putrefying substances. It is a product of the decomposition of choline, betaine, and neuridine, when these substances are distilled with potash.

In Brieger's process, if an aqueous solution of mercuric chloride is used as the precipitant, trimethylamine (if present) will be almost entirely in the filtrate, from which it can be obtained by getting rid of the mercury by SH_2, filtering, evaporating to dryness, extracting with alcohol, and precipitating the alcoholic solution with platinic chloride. It forms crystalline salts with hydrochloric acid, platinum chloride, and gold chloride; the platinum double salt yields 37 per cent. of platinum, the gold salt 49.4 per cent. gold. The gold salt is easily soluble, and this property permits its separation from choline, which forms a compound with gold chloride soluble with difficulty.

§ 656. **Ethylamine**, $C_2H_5NH_2$.—Ethylamine is in the free state an ammoniacal liquid boiling at 18.7°. It is a strong base, miscible with water in every proportion. It has been found in putrefying yeast, in wheat flour, and in the distillation of beet sugar residues. It is not poisonous; the hydrochloride forms deliquescent plates melting at 76°-80°; the platinochloride contains 39.1 per cent. of platinum, and the gold salt 51.35 per cent. of gold. In other words, the same percentages as the corresponding salts of dimethylamine, with which, however, it cannot be confused.

§ 657. **Diethylamine**, $(C_2H_5)_2NH$, is an inflammable liquid boiling at 57.5°; it forms salts with hydrochloric acid, platinum and gold, &c.; the gold salt contains 47.71 per cent. of gold, and its melting-point is about 165°.

§ 658. **Triethylamine**, $(C_2H_5)_3N$, is an oily base but slightly soluble in water, and boiling at 89°-89.5°. It gives no precipitate with mercuric chloride in aqueous solution; it forms a platinochloride containing 31.8 per cent. of platinum. It has been found in putrid fish.

§ 659. **Propylamine.**—There are two propylamines; one, normal propylamine, $CH_3CH_2.CH_2.NH_2$, boiling at 47°-48°, and iso-propylamine, $(CH_3)_2CH.NH_2$, boiling at 31.5°; both are ammoniacal fish-like smelling liquids. The hydrochloride of normal propylamine melts at 155°-158°, and iso-propylamine chloride melts at 139.5°.

It has been found in cultures of human fæces on gelatin. None of the above amines are sufficiently active in properties to be poisonous in the small quantities they are likely to be produced in decomposing foods.

§ 660. **Iso-amylamine**, $(CH_3)_2CH.CH_2.CH_2.NH_2$, is a colourless alkaline liquid, possessing a peculiar odour. It boils at 97°-98°. It forms a deliquescent hydrochloride. The platinochloride crystallises in golden yellow plates.

Iso-amylamine occurs in the putrefaction of yeast, and is a normal constituent of cod-liver oil. It is intensely poisonous, producing convulsions.

Diamines.

§ 661. **Rate of Formation of Diamines.**—Diamines are formed in putrefactive processes, generally where there is abundance of nitrogen. Garcia[661] has attempted to trace the rates at which they are formed by allowing meat extracts to decompose, precipitating by benzoyl chloride the dibenzoyl compound, and weighing; the following were the results obtained:—

Time.	Weight of benzoyl compound.

[661] *Zeit. f. physiol. Chemie*, xvii. 6. 571.

24 hours,	0.56	grm.
2 days,	0.75	„
3 days,	0.82	„
4 days,	0.73	„
5 days,	0.57	„
6 days,	0.58	„

§ 662. **Ethylidenediamine.**—Brieger found in putrid haddock, in the filtrate from the mercury chloride precipitate:—gadinine, neuridine, a base isomeric with ethylenediamine $C_2H_8N_2$ (but which Brieger subsequently more or less satisfactorily identified with ethylidenediamine), muscarine, and triethylamine; these bases were separated as follows:—

The filtrate from the mercury chloride solution was freed from mercury by SH_2, evaporated to a syrup, and then extracted with alcohol. From the alcoholic solution platinum chloride precipitated neuridine, this was filtered off, the filtrate freed from alcohol and platinum, and the aqueous solution concentrated to a small volume and precipitated with an aqueous solution of platinum chloride; this precipitated ethylidene platinum chloride. The mother liquor from this precipitate was concentrated on the water-bath, and, on cooling, the platinochloride of muscarine crystallised out. From the mother liquor (freed from the crystals), on standing in a desiccator, the gadinine double salt crystallised out, and from the mother liquor (freed from gadinine after removal of the platinum by SH_2) distillation with KHO recovered trimethylamine.

From the platinochloride of ethylenediamine, the chloride can be obtained by treating with SH_2, filtering, and evaporating; by distilling the chloride with a caustic alkali, the free base can be obtained by distillation.

Ethylidenediamine is isomeric with ethylenediamine, but differs from it in the following properties:—ethylidenediamine is poisonous, ethylenediamine is non-poisonous.

Ethylenediamine forms a platinochloride almost insoluble in hot water, while the ethylidene salt is more easily soluble. The properties of the gold salts are similar, ethylenediamine forming a difficultly soluble gold salt, ethylidene a rather soluble gold salt.

Ethylidenediamine forms a hydrochloride, $C_2H_8N_22HCl$, crystallising in long glistening needles, insoluble in absolute alcohol, rather soluble in water. The hydrochloride gives precipitates in aqueous solution with phospho-molybdic acid, phospho-antimonic acid, and potassium bismuth iodide; the latter is in the form of red plates.

The platinochloride, $C_2H_8N_22HCl.PtCl$ (Pt = 41.5 per cent.), is in the form of yellow plates, not very soluble in cold water.

Ethylidenediamine, when subcutaneously injected into guinea-pigs, produces an abundant secretion from the mucous membranes of the nose, mouth, and eyes. The pupils dilate, and the eyeballs project. There is acute dyspnœa; death takes place after some twenty-four hours, and the heart is stopped in diastole.

Trimethylenediamine is believed to have been isolated by Brieger from cultivations in beef broth of the comma bacillus.

It occurs in small quantity in the mercuric chloride precipitate, and is isolated by decomposing the precipitate with SH_2, evaporating the filtrate from the mercury sulphide to dryness, taking up the residue with absolute alcohol, and precipitating by an alcoholic solution of sodium picrate. The precipitate contains the picrate of trimethylenediamine, mixed with the picrates of cadaverine and creatinine. Cadaverine picrate is insoluble in boiling absolute alcohol, the other picrates soluble; so the mixed picrates are boiled with absolute alcohol, and the insoluble cadaverine filtered off. Next, the picrates of creatinine and trimethylenediamine are freed from alcohol, the solution in water acidified with hydrochloric acid, the picric acid shaken out by treatment with ether, and then the solution precipitated with platinum chloride; the platinochloride of trimethylenediamine is not very soluble, while creatinine easily dissolves; so that separation is by this means fairly easy.

It also gives a difficultly soluble salt with gold chloride.

The picrate consists of felted needles, melting-point 198°. Phospho-molybdic acid gives a precipitate crystallising in plates; potassium bismuth iodide gives dark coloured needles.

It produces in animals violent convulsions and muscular tremors; but the substance has hitherto been obtained in too small a quantity to be certain as to its identification and properties.

§ 663. **Neuridine**, $C_5H_{14}N_2$.—Neuridine is a diamine, and is apparently the most common basic product of putrefaction; it has been obtained from the putrefaction of gelatin, of horseflesh, of fish, and from the yelk of eggs.

It is usually accompanied by choline, from which it can be separated by converting the bases into hydrochlorides, choline hydrochloride being soluble in absolute alcohol, neuridine scarcely so. Brieger isolated neuridine from putrid flesh by precipitating the watery extract with mercuric chloride. He decomposed the mercury precipitate with SH_2, and, after having got rid of the sulphide of mercury by filtration, he concentrated the liquid to a small bulk, when a substance separated in crystals similar in form to urea; this was purified by recrystallisation from absolute alcohol, and converted into the platinum salt.

Another method which may be used for the separation and purification of neuridine is to dissolve it in alcohol and precipitate with an alcoholic solution of picric acid; the picrate may be decomposed by treatment with dilute mineral acid, and the picric acid removed by shaking with ether.

The free base has a strong seminal odour. It is gelatinous, and has not been crystallised. It is insoluble in ether and in absolute alcohol, and not readily soluble in amyl alcohol. It gives white precipitates with mercuric chloride, neutral and basic lead acetates. It does not give Hofmann's isonitrile reaction. When distilled with a fixed alkali, it yields di- and trimethylamine.

The hydrochloride, $C_5H_{14}N_22HCl$, crystallises in long needles, which are insoluble in absolute alcohol, ether, benzol, chloroform, petroleum ether, and amyl alcohol; but the hydrochloride is very soluble in water and in dilute alcohol.

The hydrochloride gives no precipitate with mercuric chloride, potass-mercuric iodide, potass-cadmium iodide, iodine and iodide of potassium, tannic acid, ferricyanide of potassium, ferric chloride, and it does not give any colour with Fröhde's reagent.

On the other hand, phosphotungstic acid, phospho-molybdic acid, picric acid, potass-bismuth iodide, platinum chloride, and gold chloride all give precipitates.

Neuridine hydrochloride is capable of sublimation, and at the same time it is decomposed, for the sublimed needles show red or blue colours.

Neuridine platinochloride, $C_5H_{14}N_22HCl.PtCl_4$, yields 38.14 per cent. of platinum; it crystallises in flat needles, soluble in water, from which it is precipitated on the addition of alcohol.

The aurochloride has the formula $C_5H_{14}N_22HCl2AuCl_3$; it is rather insoluble in cold water, and crystallises in bunches of yellow needles. On ignition, it should yield 41.19 per cent. of gold.

The picrate, $C_5H_{14}N_2,2C_6H_2(NO_2)_3OH$, is almost insoluble in cold water, and crystallises in needles. It is not fusible, but decomposes at about 230°.

Neuridine is not poisonous.

§ 664. **Cadaverine** (Pentamethylenediamine, $C_5H_{14}N_2$=NH_2CH_2-CH_2-CH_2-$CH_2CH_2NH_2$) is formed in putrid animal matters, and in cultures of the genus *Vibrio*. It has been found in the urine and fæces in cases of cystinuria, and Roos[662] has separated it by the benzoyl-chloride method from the fæces of a patient suffering from tertian ague. It may be formed synthetically by dissolving trimethylcyanide in absolute alcohol, and then reducing by sodium (Mendius' reaction).

Cadaverine is a thick, clear, syrupy liquid, with a peculiar coniine- as well as a semen-like odour. It absorbs eagerly CO_2 from the air, and ultimately is converted into a solid crystalline mass. It volatilises with the steam when boiled with water, and may be distilled in the presence even of the caustic alkalies and the alkaline earths without decomposition. It does not give oil of mustard when treated with CS_2 and mercuric chloride, nor does it give with chloroform and alcoholic potash, carbylamine (isonitrile). If dehydrated by KHO, it boils at from 115°-120° (*Brieger*).[663]

When cadaverine is treated with methyl iodide, two atoms of hydrogen may be replaced with methyl, forming the base $C_5H_{12}(CH_3)_2N_2$; the platinochloride of this last base crystallises in long red needles.

Cadaverine forms well-defined crystalline salts as well as compounds with metals.

Cadaverine hydrochloride, $C_5H_{14}N_22HCl$, crystallises in needles which are deliquescent, or it may be obtained from an alcoholic solution in plates. The crystals are insoluble in absolute alcohol, but readily soluble in 96 per cent. alcohol. Putrescine hydrochloride, on the other hand, is with difficulty soluble in alcohol of that strength; hence the two hydrochlorides can be separated by taking advantage of their difference in solubility in 96 per cent. alcohol; but the better method for separation is the benzoyl-chloride process. On dry distillation, cadaverine hydrochloride decomposes into NH_3,HCl and piperidine $C_5H_{11}N$. The compound with mercury chloride—$C_5H_{14}N_22HCl,4HgCl_2$

[662] *Zeit. f. physiol. Chemie*, xvi., 1892.

[663] Brieger has also given to the pure base a boiling-point of 175°.

($Hg = 63.54$ per cent.); melting-point, 214°-216°—is insoluble in alcohol and in cold water; this property is also useful to separate it from putrescine, the mercury compound of which is soluble in cold water. The platinochloride, $C_5H_{14}N_22HCl,PtCl_4$ ($Pt = 38.08$ per cent.), crystallises in dirty red needles; but, by repeated crystallisation, it may be obtained in clear chrome yellow, short, octahedral prisms; it is soluble with difficulty in hot water, insoluble in cold water. The salt decomposes at 235°-236°.

The aurochloride—$C_5H_{14}N_22HCl2AuCl$ ($Au = 50.41$ per cent.), melting-point 188°—crystallises partly in cubes and partly in needles, and is easily soluble in water.

Other salts are the picrate, $C_5H_{14}N_22C_6H_2(NO_2)_3OH$, melting-point 221° with decomposition; with difficulty soluble in cold, but dissolving in hot water, and insoluble in absolute alcohol. There are also a neutral oxalate, $C_5H_{14}N_2,H_2C_2O_4 + 2H_2O$, melting-point 160°; and an acid oxalate, $C_5H_{14}N_22H_2C_2O_4 + H_2O$, melting-point 143° with decomposition; both these oxalates are insoluble in absolute alcohol.

Cadaverine dibenzoyl—$C_5H_{10}(NHCOC_6H_5)_2$, melting-point 129°-130°—crystallises in needles and plates, soluble in alcohol and slightly soluble in ether, insoluble in water.

It is not acted on by hot dilute acids or alkalis, and when dissolved in concentrated hydrochloric acid and alcohol it is, only after prolonged boiling, decomposed into benzoic acid and the free base. The benzoic acid after getting rid of the alcohol by evaporation, can be removed by shaking up with ether; then the hydrochloride can be decomposed by an alkali and the free base obtained, or the platinum salt of cadaverine may be formed by precipitation with platinum chloride. Should cadaverine and putrescine be in the same liquid, the dibenzoyl compounds may be separated as follows:—the crystalline precipitate is collected on a filter, washed with water until the filtrate runs clear, and then dissolved in warm alcohol; this solution is poured into twenty times its volume of ether and allowed to stand; after a short time crystals form of the putrescine compound, which are far less soluble in alcohol than those of cadaverine dibenzoyl; these crystals are filtered off and repeatedly crystallised from alcohol until the melting-point is about 175°-176°. The filtrate contains the cadaverine compound; this latter is recovered by evaporating off the ether-alcohol.

§ 665. **Putrescine—Tetramethylenediamine**, $C_4H_{12}N_2{=}NH_2CH_2CH_2CH_2CH_2NH_2$.

The free base is a clear liquid, with a semen-like odour, boiling-point 135°. It is a common base in putrefying animal substances, and also occurs in the urine in cases of cystinuria. It can be obtained synthetically by reducing ethylene cyanide by the action of sodium in absolute alcohol.

The best method of separating putrescine is the benzoyl chloride method already given.

Putrescine forms crystalline salts, of which the following are the most important:—

Putrescine hydrochloride, $C_4H_{12}N_22HCl$, forms long colourless needles, insoluble in absolute alcohol, easily soluble in water.

The platinochloride, $C_4H_{12}N_22HCl.PtCl_4$ ($Pt = 39.2$ per cent.), is with difficulty soluble in cold water. When pure, the salt is in the form of six-sided plates.

The aurochloride, $C_4H_{12}N_22HCl.2AuCl_3 + 2H_2O$ ($Au = 51.3$ per cent.), is insoluble in cold water, in contradistinction to cadaverine aurochloride, which easily dissolves.

The picrate, $C_4H_{12}N_22C_6H_2(NO_2)_3OH$, is a salt of difficult solubility. It crystallises in yellow plates. It browns at 230°, and melts with evolution of gas at 250°.

Dibenzoylputrescine, $C_4H_8(NHCOC_6H_5)_2$, forms silky plates or long needles, melting-point 175°-176°. By boiling it for twelve hours with alcohol and strong hydrochloric acid the compound may be broken up into hydrochloride of putrescine and free benzoic acid. As stated before, it is less soluble in alcohol than the corresponding compound of cadaverine.

Putrescine is not poisonous. On the other hand, by repeated treatment with methyl iodide, it takes up four methyl radicals, and the tetramethyl compound, $C_4H_8(CH_3)_4N_2$, produces symptoms similar to those of muscarine poisoning.

§ 666. **Metaphenylenediamine**, $C_6H_4\left\langle\begin{matrix}NH_2{}^1\\NH_2{}^3\end{matrix}\right.$, is a crystalline substance, melting-point 63°, boiling-point 276°-277°. The crystals are easily soluble in alcohol or ether, with difficulty in water. The least trace of nitrous acid strikes a yellow colour from the formation of triamidobenzol.

§ 667. **Paraphenylenediamine,** $C_6H_4\begin{cases} NH_2^{1} \\ NH_2^{4} \end{cases}$, is in the form of tabular crystals, melting-point 140°, boiling-point 267°. If this substance is oxidised with ferric chloride or manganese binoxide and sulphuric acid, chinone is produced; if treated with SH_2 and ferric chloride, a violet sulphur-holding colouring matter, allied to methylene blue, is formed; these reactions are tests for the presence of the para-compound.

Both these diamines are poisonous. Metaphenylenediamine produces, in the dog, the symptoms of an aggravated influenza with continual sneezing and hoarse cough, which, if the dose is large enough, ends in coma and death. Paraphenylenediamine produces exophthalmia, the tissues of the eye undergoing complete alteration.[664]

Both compounds, in doses of 100 mgrms. per kilo., cause more or less salivation, with diarrhœa. The para-compound is more poisonous than the meta-compound. So far as the author is aware, neither of these diamines have been separated with certainty from the urine of sick persons, nor from products of decomposition.

§ 668. **Hexamethylenediamine,** $C_6H_{16}N_2$.—Hexamethylenediamine has been found by A. Garcia[665] in a putrefying mixture of horse-flesh and pancreas.

§ 669. **Diethylenediamine,** $C_4H_{10}N_2$, is a crystalline substance, melting-point 104°, boiling-point 145°-146°. After melting, it solidifies on cooling, forming a hard crystalline mass. It is extremely soluble in water, and is deposited from alcohol in large transparent crystals. A technical product called "spermin piperazidin" or "piperazine" has been found by A. W. v. Hoffmann[666] to be identical with diethylenediamine. The hydrochloride crystallises in colourless needles, insoluble in alcohol, readily soluble in water. The platinochloride, $C_4H_{10}N_2H_2PtCl_6$, is in small yellow needles, and is fairly easily soluble in hot water, but dissolves but slightly in hot alcohol. The mercuro-chloride, $C_4H_{10}N_2H_2HgCl_4$, crystallises in concentrically grouped needles, and is readily soluble in hot water, but is reprecipitated on adding alcohol. The picrate, $C_4H_{10}N_2,C_6H_2(NO_2)_3OH$, crystallises from water in yellow needles, almost insoluble in alcohol.[667]

§ 670. **Mydaleine** is a poisonous base discovered by Brieger in putrid animal matters. It is probably a diamine, but has not been obtained in sufficient quantity for accurate chemical study. The platinochloride is extremely soluble in water, and only comes down from an absolute alcohol solution. It has been obtained in a crystalline form, giving on analysis 38.74 per cent. of platinum, C. 10.83 per cent., H. 3.23 per cent.

Mydaleine is very poisonous. Small quantities injected into guinea-pigs cause dilatation of the pupil, an abundant secretion from the nose and eyes, and a rise of temperature. Fifty mgrms. cause death. The *post-mortem* appearances are not distinctive; the heart is arrested in diastole; the intestines and bladder are contracted. In cats it causes profuse diarrhœa and vomiting.

§ 671. **Guanidine.**—Guanidine may be considered to have a relation to urea; for, if the oxygen of urea is replaced by the imide group NH, guanidine originates thus:—

$$\text{Urea} = O{=}C\begin{cases} NH_2 \\ NH_2 \end{cases} \qquad \text{Guanidine} = NHC\begin{cases} NH_2 \\ NH_2 \end{cases}$$

Hence guanidine from its structural formula is a carbodiamidimide. Guanidine may be formed by the action of oxidising agents, such as potassic chlorate and hydrochloric acid, on guanine; or by heating amide cyanide with ammonium chloride, and so forming guanidine chloride. It is also produced from the oxidation of albumin. When boiled with baryta-water it decomposes into urea and ammonia. It combines with acids to form salts; the gold salt, $CH_5N_3HCl,AuCl_3$, is in the form of long yellow needles, with difficulty soluble in water. Guanidine nitrate, $CH_5N_3HNO_3$, is also almost insoluble in cold water and similar to urea nitrate. By dissolving equivalent parts of phenol and guanidine in hot alcohol, triphenylguanidine is formed; on adding picric acid to a solution of triphenylguanidine, phenylguanidine picrate, $CH_2Ph_3N_3C_6H_2(NO_2)_3OH$, is formed, and falls as a precipitate of slender needles, melting-point 208°; this picrate is very slightly soluble, 1 part dissolving in 12,220 parts of water

---

664 *Comptes Rend.*, cvii. 533-535.

665 *Zeit. f. physiol. Chemie*, xvii. 543-555.

666 *Ber.*, xxiii. 3297-3303.

667 Sieber, J., *Ber.*, xxiii. 326-327.

at 15°. Guanidine is poisonous.[668]

A method of separating guanidine from urine has been worked out by Gergers and Baumann.[669] The principle of the method is based upon the fact that guanidine is precipitated by mercurous oxide. The urine is precipitated by hydrate of baryta, the precipitate filtered off, the alkaline filtrate neutralised by hydrochloric acid, and the neutral filtrate evaporated to a syrup on the water-bath; the syrup is exhausted by absolute alcohol, and the alcoholic solution filtered; this filtrate is freed from alcohol by distillation, the alcohol-free residue dissolved in a little water, shaken up with freshly precipitated mercury oxide, and allowed to stand for two days in a warm place; the precipitate formed is collected, acidulated with HCl and treated with SH_2; the mercury sulphide thus obtained is separated by filtration, the filtrate evaporated, and the residue dissolved in absolute alcohol. This solution is precipitated by platinum chloride, filtered, separated from any platinum ammonium salt, and evaporated to a small volume. After long standing the guanidine salt crystallises out. The best method to identify it appears to be, to ascertain the absence of ammonia and of urea, and then to gently warm the supposed guanidine with an alkali, which breaks guanidine up into ammonia and urea, according to the following equation:—

$$NH{=}C(NH_2)_2 + H_2O = NH_3 + CO(NH_2)_2.$$

The physiological effects of guanidine are as follows:—

A centigrm. of guanidine salt injected into the lymph sac in the back of frogs produces, after a few minutes, muscular convulsions: first, there are fibrillar twitchings of the muscles of the back; next, these spread generally so that the whole surface of the frog seems to be in a wave-like motion. Irritation of the limbs produces tetanus. There is, at the same time, increased secretion from the skin. The breathing is irregular. In large doses there is paralysis and death. The heart is found arrested in diastole. The fatal dose for a frog is 50 mgrms.; but 1 mgrm. will produce symptoms of illness. In dogs there is paralysis, convulsions, vomiting, and difficult breathing.

§ 672. **Methylguanidine**, $NH{=}C\begin{cases}NH.CH_3\\NH_2\end{cases}$.—Methylguanidine has been isolated by Brieger from putrefying horse-flesh; it has also been found in impure cultures in beef broth of Finkler and Prior's *Vibrio proteus*. Bocklisch isolated it, working with Brieger's process, from the mercuric chloride precipitate, after removal of the mercury and concentration of the filtrate, by adding a solution of sodium picrate. The precipitate contained the picrates of cadaverine, creatinine, and methylguanidine; cadaverine picrate, insoluble in boiling absolute alcohol, was separated by filtering from a solution of the picrates of the bases in boiling absolute alcohol; the alcohol was evaporated from the filtrate and the residue taken up with water. From this aqueous solution the picric acid was removed and then the solution precipitated with gold chloride; methylguanidine was precipitated, while creatinine remained in solution.

Methylguanidine aurochloride, $C_2H_7N_3HCl.AuCl_3$ (Au = 47.7 per cent.), forms rhombic crystals easily soluble in alcohol and ether; melting-point 198°. The hydrochloride, $C_2H_7N_3HCl$, crystallises in needles insoluble in alcohol. The picrate, $C_2H_7N_3C_6H_2(NO_2)_3OH$, comes down at first as a resinous mass, but, after boiling in water, is found to be in the form of needles soluble in hot absolute alcohol; melting-point 192°. The symptoms produced by methylguanidine are rapid respiration, dilatation of the pupils, paralysis, and death, preceded by convulsions. The heart is found arrested in diastole.

§ 673. **Saprine**, $C_5H_{14}N_2$.—Saprine is isomeric with cadaverine and neuridine; it was found by Brieger in human livers and spleens after three weeks' putrefaction. Saprine occurs, in Brieger's process, in the mercury precipitate. Its reactions are very similar to those of cadaverine; the main difference being that cadaverine hydrochloride gives a crystalline aurochloride, saprine does not; the platinum salt is also more soluble in water than the cadaverine salt. It is not poisonous.

§ 674. **The Choline Group.**—The choline group consists of choline, neurine, betaine, and muscarine.

All these bodies can be prepared from choline; their relationship to choline can be readily gathered from the following structural formulæ:—

---

[668] O. Prelinger, *Monatsb.*, xiii. 97-100.

[669] Pflüger's *Archiv*, xii. 205.

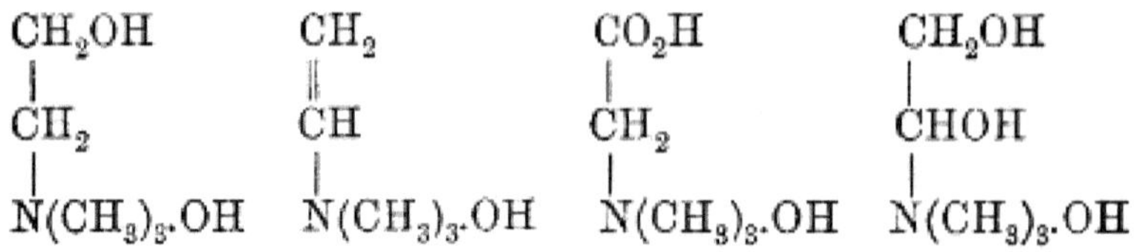

Choline. Neurine. Betaine. Muscarine.

Choline is a syrup with an alkaline reaction. On boiling with water, it decomposes into glycol and trimethylamine. It gives, when oxidised, muscarine. It forms salts. The hydrochloride is soluble in water and absolute alcohol; neurine hydrochloride and betaine hydrochloride are but little soluble in absolute alcohol, therefore this property can be utilised for their separation from choline. The platinochloride is insoluble in absolute alcohol; it melts at 225° with effervescence, and contains 31.6 per cent. of platinum. The mercurochloride is soluble with difficulty even in hot water. The aurochloride (Au = 44.5 per cent.) is crystalline, and with difficulty soluble in cold water; but is soluble in hot water and in alcohol; melting-point 264° with decomposition.

Choline is only poisonous in large doses.

§ 675. **Neurine** (Trimethyl-vinyl-ammonium hydrate), $C_2H_3N(CH_3)_3OH$.—Neurine is one of the products of decomposition of choline. It is poisonous, and has been separated by Brieger and others from decomposing animal matters. In Brieger's process, neurine, if present, will be for the most part in the mercuric chloride precipitate, and some portion will also be in the filtrate. The mercury precipitate is decomposed by SH_2, the mercury sulphide filtered off, and the filtrate, concentrated, treated with absolute alcohol and then precipitated by platinum chloride. It is usually accompanied by choline; the platinochloride of choline is readily soluble in water, neurine platinochloride is soluble with difficulty; this property is taken advantage of, and the platinochloride crystallised from water until pure. Neurine has a strong alkaline reaction.

Neurine chloride, $C_5H_{12}N.Cl$, crystallises in fine needles. The platinochloride, $(C_5H_{12}NCl)_2PtCl_4$ (Pt = 33.6 per cent.), crystallises in octahedra. The salt is soluble with difficulty in hot water.

The aurochloride, $C_5H_{12}NClAuCl_3$ (Au = 46.37 per cent.), forms flat prisms, which, according to Brieger, are soluble with difficulty in hot water.

Neurine is intensely poisonous, the symptoms being similar to those produced by muscarine.

Atropine is an antidote to neurine, relieving in suitable doses the effects, and even rendering animals temporarily immune against the toxic action of neurine.

When a fatal dose of neurine is injected into a frog there is in a short time paralysis of the extremities. The respiration stops first, and afterwards the heart, the latter in diastole.

The symptoms in rabbits are profuse nasal secretion and salivation with paralysis, as in frogs. Applied to the eye, neurine causes contraction of the pupil; to a less degree the same effect is produced by the ingestion of neurine.

Trimethyloxyammonium hydrochloride causes similar symptoms to neurine, but the action is less powerful.—V. Cervello, *Arch. Ital. Biol.*, vii. 232-233.

§ 676. **Betaine.**—Betaine may be separated from a solution in alcohol as large deliquescent crystals; the reaction of the crystals is neutral. Distilled with potash, trimethylamine and other bases are formed.

Betaine chloride, $C_5H_{12}NO_2Cl$, forms plates permanent in the air and insoluble in absolute alcohol. A solution of the chloride in water gives, with potassium mercuric iodide, a light yellow or whitish yellow precipitate, soluble in excess; but, on rubbing the sides of the tube with a glass rod, the oily precipitate crystallises as yellow needles; probably this is characteristic.

The aurochloride (Au = 43.1 percent.) forms fine cholesterine plates, soluble in water; melting-point 209°. Betaine is not poisonous.

§ 677. **Peptotoxine.**—Brieger submitted to the action of fresh gastric juice moist fibrin for twenty-four hours at blood heat. The liquid was evaporated to a syrup and boiled with ethylic alcohol, the ethylic alcohol was evaporated, the residue digested with amylic alcohol, and the amyl alcohol in its turn evaporated to dryness; the residue was a brown amorphous mass that was poisonous. It was farther purified by treating the extract with neutral lead acetate and then filtered; the filtrate was freed from lead by SH_2 and treated with ether, the ethereal extract being then separated and evaporated to dryness; this last residue was taken up with amyl alcohol, the alcohol evaporated to dryness, and the residue finally taken up with water and filtered. The filtrate is poisonous. The poisonous substance, to which Brieger gave the provisional name of peptotoxine, is a very stable substance, resisting the action of a boiling temperature, and even the action of strong alkalies. It gives precipitates with alkaloidal group reagents, and strikes a blue colour with ferric chloride and ferricyanide of potassium. The most characteristic test seems to be its action with Millon's reagent (a solution of mercury nitrate in nitric acid containing nitrous acid); this gives a white precipitate which, on boiling, becomes intensely red.

It is poisonous, killing rabbits in doses of 0.5 grm. per kilogrm., with symptoms of paralysis and coma. The nature of this substance requires further elucidation.

§ 678. **Pyridine Alkaloid from the Cuttle Fish.**—O. de Coninck[670] has obtained, by Gautier's process, an alkaloid from the cuttle fish, of the formula $C_8H_{11}N$, in the form of a yellow, mobile, strongly odorous liquid, very soluble in alcohol, ether, and acetone, boiling-point 202°. It quickly absorbs moisture from the air. It forms two mercuric chlorides, one of which has the formula $(C_8H_{11}N,HCl)_2HgCl_2$; this compound crystallises in small white needles, slightly soluble in water and dilute alcohol, but insoluble in absolute alcohol, and decomposing when exposed to moist air. The other salt is a sesqui-salt, forming long yellowish needles, insoluble in ordinary solvents, and decomposing when exposed to moist air. The alkaloid also forms deliquescent very soluble salts with hydrochloric and hydrobromic acids. A platinum salt is also formed, $(C_8H_{11}N)_2H_2PtCl_6$; it is of a deep yellow colour, almost insoluble in cold, but soluble in hot water; it is decomposed by boiling water, with the formation of a very insoluble compound in the shape of a brown powder, $(C_8H_{11}N)_2PtCl_4$. Coninck's alkaloid, on oxidation with potassic permanganate, yields a gummy acid; this acid, on purifying it by conversion into a potassium salt and then into a cupric salt, was found to be nicotinic acid; so that the alkaloid is undoubtedly a pyridine compound; indeed, the acid, distilled with lime, yields pyridine.

§ 679. **Poisons connected with Tetanus.**—Brieger, in 1887, isolated a base of unknown composition, to which he gave the name of "spasmotoxine." It was produced in cultures of the tetanus bacillus in beef broth.

Two more definite substances have also been discovered, viz., tetanine and tetanotoxine.

Tetanine, $C_{13}H_{30}N_2O_4$, is best isolated by the method of Kitasato and Weyl.[671] Their method of treating broth cultures of the tetanus bacillus is as follows:—

The broth is digested with 0.25 per cent. HCl for some hours at 460°, then rendered feebly alkaline, and distilled in a vacuum. The residue in the retort is then worked up for tetanine by Brieger's method; the distillate contains tetanotoxine, ammonia, indol, hydrogen sulphide, phenol, and butyric acid. On treating the contents of the retort by Brieger's mercury chloride method, the filtrate contains most of the poison. The mercury is removed by SH_2, the filtered solution evaporated and exhausted by absolute alcohol, in which the tetanine dissolves. Any ammonium chloride is thus separated, ammonium chloride being insoluble in absolute alcohol. The alcoholic solution, filtered from any insoluble substance, is next treated with an alcoholic solution of platinum chloride, which precipitates creatinine (and any ammonium salts), but does not precipitate tetanine. The platinum salt of tetanine may, however, be precipitated by the addition of ether to the alcoholic solution. The platinum salt, as obtained by precipitation from ether, is very deliquescent; it has, therefore, to be rapidly filtered off and dried in a vacuum. It can then be recrystallised from hot 96 per cent. alcohol, forming clear yellow plates; these plates, if dried in a vacuum, become with difficulty soluble in water.

Tetanine may be obtained as a free base by treating the hydrochloride with freshly precipitated moist silver oxide. It forms a strongly alkaline yellow syrup, and is easily decomposed in acid solution, but is permanent in alkaline solutions.

The platinochloride, as before observed, is precipitable by ether from alcoholic solution; it contains 28.3 per cent. of platinum, and decomposes at 197°.

The base produces tetanus.

§ 680. **Tetanotoxine** may be distilled, and be found in the distillate with other matters. It forms an easily soluble gold salt, melting-point 130°. The platinochloride is soluble with difficulty, and decomposes at 240°. The hydrochloride is soluble in alcohol and in water, melting-point about 205°.

Tetanotoxine produces tremor, then paralysis, and lastly, violent convulsions.

§ 681. **Mydatoxine**, $C_6H_{13}NO_2$.—A base obtained by Brieger from horse-flesh in a putrefactive condition and other substances. It is found in the mercury chloride precipitate. The free base is an alkaline syrup, isomeric with the base separated by Brieger from tetanus cultures. The hydrochloride is a deliquescent syrup, not forming any compound with gold chloride, but uniting with phospho-molybdic acid in forming a compound crystallising in

[670] *Comptes Rend.*, cvi. 858, 861; cviii. 58-59, 809-810; cvi. 1604-1605.

[671] *Zeit. f. Hygiene*, viii. 404.

cubes. It forms a double salt with gold chloride, sparingly soluble in water. The platinochloride (Pt = 29 per cent.) is very soluble in water, but not soluble in alcohol; melting-point 193° with decomposition.

The base in large doses is poisonous, causing lachrymation, diarrhœa, and convulsions.

§ 682. **Mytilotoxine,** $C_6H_{15}NO_2$.—This is believed to be the poison of mussels. Brieger isolated it as follows:—

The mussels were boiled with water acidified by hydrochloric acid; the liquid was filtered, and the filtrate evaporated to a syrup, and the syrup was repeatedly extracted with alcohol. It was found advisable to exhaust thoroughly with alcohol, otherwise much poison remained behind. The alcoholic solution was treated with an alcoholic solution of lead acetate. The filtrate was evaporated and the residue extracted with alcohol. The lead was removed by SH_2, the alcohol distilled off, water added to the remaining syrup, and the solution decolorised by boiling with animal charcoal. The solution was neutralised by sodium carbonate, acidulated with nitric acid, and precipitated with phosphomolybdic acid. The precipitate was then decomposed by warming with a neutral solution of lead acetate, and the filtrate (after the removal of the lead by the action of SH_2) was acidulated with HCl and evaporated to dryness. The residue was then extracted with absolute alcohol, filtered from any insoluble chloride, *e.g.*, betaine chloride, and precipitated by mercury chloride in alcohol.

The free base has a most peculiar odour, which disappears on exposure to air; at the same time, the poisonous properties also diminish. The base is destroyed by boiling with sodium carbonate; on the other hand, the hydrochloride may be evaporated to dryness or be boiled without decomposing.

The hydrochloride crystallises in tetrahedra; the aurochloride crystallises in cubes (Au=41.66 per cent.). Its melting-point is 182°.

§ 683. **Tyrotoxicon** (Diazobenzol, $C_6H_5N_2(OH)$).—It appears, from the researches of Vaughan and others, that diazobenzol is liable to be formed in milk and milk products, especially in summer time. It is confidently asserted by many that the summer diarrhœa of infants is due to this toxine; however that may be, it is well established that diazobenzol is a violent poison, causing sickness, diarrhœa, and, in large doses, an acute malady scarcely distinguishable from cholera, and which may end fatally. There will always be difficulty in detecting it, because of its instability. The following is the best process of extraction from milk. The milk will probably be acid from decomposition; if so, the whey must be separated by dilution and filtration; without dilution it may be found impracticable to get a clear filtrate. In order to keep the bulk down, 25 c.c. of the milk may be diluted up to 100 c.c., and, having obtained a clear filtrate from this 25 c.c. thus diluted, the filtrate is used to dilute another 25 c.c. of milk and so on. The acid filtrate is neutralised by sodium carbonate, agitated with an equal volume of ether, allowed to stand in a stoppered vessel for twenty-four hours, and the ether then separated and allowed to evaporate spontaneously. The residue is acidified with nitric acid and then treated with a saturated solution of potash, which forms a stable compound with diazobenzol, and the whole concentrated on the water-bath. On cooling, the tyrotoxicon compound forms six-sided plates. Before the whole of this process is undertaken, it is well to make a preliminary test of the milk as follows:—A little of the ether is allowed to evaporate spontaneously. Place on a porcelain slab two or three drops of a mixture of equal parts of sulphuric and carbolic acids, and add a few drops of the aqueous solution; if tyrotoxicon be present, a yellow to orange-red colour is produced. A similar colour is also produced by nitrates or nitrites, which are not likely to be present under the circumstances, milk having mere traces only of nitrates or nitrites; it may also be due to butyric acid, which, in a decomposed milk, may frequently be in solution. Therefore, if a colour occurs, this is not absolutely conclusive; if, however, no colour is produced, then it is certain that no diazobenzol has been separated. That is all that can be said, for the process itself is faulty, and only separates a fractional part of the whole.

§ 684. **Toxines of Hog Cholera.**—Toxines have been isolated by F. G. Novy[672] from a cultivation of Salmon's bacillus in pork broth. The fluid possessed a strong alkaline reaction. For the isolation, Brieger's method was used. The mercury chloride precipitate was amorphous and was converted into a chlorine-free platinum compound, to which was assigned the composition of $C_8H_{14}N_4PtO_8$. After separation of this compound, the mother liquor still contained a platinum salt crystallising in needles, and from this was obtained the chlorhydrate of a new base, to which was given the name of *susotoxine*; it had the composition of $C_{10}H_{26}N_22HCl,PtCl_4$. Susotoxine gives general alkaloidal reactions, and is very poisonous.

§ 685. **Other Ptomaines.**—Besides the ptomaines which have been already described, there are a number of others; the following may be mentioned: isoamylamine,[673] $(CH_3)_2CH.CH_2.CH_2NH_2$; butylamine,

[672] *Med. News*, September 1890.

[673] Hesse, *Chem. Jahresb.*, 1857, 403.

$CH_3CH_2CH_2CH_2NH_2$; dihydrolutidine,[674] $C_7H_{11}N$; hydrocollidine,[675] $C_8H_{13}N$; $C_{10}H_{15}N$ (a base isolated by Guareschi and Mosso[676] from ox-fibrin in a state of putrefaction by Gautier's method; it forms a crystalline hydrochloride and an insoluble platinochloride; its action is like that of curare but weaker); aselline,[677] $C_{25}H_{32}N_4$, isolated from cod-liver oil; typhotoxine,[678] $C_7H_{17}NO_2$, isolated from cultures of Eberth's bacillus. So far as the published researches go, it would appear that other crystalline substances have been isolated from the urine, from the tissues, and from the secretions of patients suffering from various diseases; the quantity obtained in each case has, however, been, under the most favourable circumstances, less than a gramme; often only a few milligrms. To specifically declare that a few milligrms. of a substance is a new body, requires immense experience and great skill; and, even where those qualifications are present, this is too often impossible. This being so, the long list of named ptomaines, such as erysipeline, varioline, and others, must have their existence more fully confirmed by more than one observer before they can be accepted as separate entities.

DIVISION III.—FOOD POISONING.

§ 686. A large number of cases of poisoning by food occur yearly; some are detailed in the daily press; the great majority are neither recorded in any journal, scientific or otherwise; nor, on account of their slight and passing character, is medical aid sought. The greatest portion of these cases are probably due to ptomaines existing in the food before being consumed; others may be due to the action of unhealthy fermentation in the intestinal canal itself; in a third class of cases, it is probable that a true zymotic infection is conveyed and develops in the sufferer; the latter class of cases, as, for instance, the Middlesborough epidemic of pleuro-pneumonia, is outside the scope of this treatise.

Confining the attention to cases of food poisoning in which the symptoms have been closely analysed and described, the reader is referred to thirteen cases of food poisoning, investigated by the medical officers of the Local Government Board between the years 1878 and 1891, as follows:—

1878. **A Case of Poisoning at Whitchurch from eating Roast Pork.**—Only the leg of pork was poisonous, other parts eaten without injury. Two persons died after about thirty hours' illness. The pork itself, on a particular Sunday, was innocuous; it became poisonous between the Sunday and the Monday; the toxicity appeared to gradually increase, for those who ate it for dinner on the Monday were not taken ill for periods of from seven to nineteen hours, while two persons who ate of it in the evening were attacked four hours after eating.

1880. **The Welbeck Epidemic**, due to eating cold boiled ham. Over fifty persons affected. Symptoms commenced in from twelve to forty-eight hours.

1881. **A Series of Poisoning from eating Baked Pork, Nottingham.**—Probably the gravy was the cause and not the pork itself. Many persons seriously ill. One died.

1881. **Tinned American Sausage.**—A man in Chester died from eating tinned American sausage. Poison found to be unequally distributed in the sausage.

1882. **Poisoning at Oldham by Tinned Pigs' Tongues.**—Two families affected. Symptoms commenced in about four hours. All recovered. After a few days' keeping it would appear that the poison had been decomposed.

1882. **A Family Poisoned by Roast Beef at Bishop Stortford.**—Only a particular piece of the ribs seemed to be poisonous, the rest of the carcase being innocuous. Symptoms did not commence until several hours after ingestion.

1882. **Ten different Families at Whitchurch Poisoned by eating Brawn.**—First symptoms after about four hours.

1884. **Tinned Salmon at Wolverhampton.**—Five persons, two being children, ate of tinned salmon at Wolverhampton. All suffered more or less. The mother's symptoms began after twelve hours, and she died in five days; the son died in three days, the symptoms commencing in ten hours. The *post-mortem* signs were similar to those from phosphorus poisoning, viz., fatty degeneration. Mice fed on the material also suffered, and their organs showed a similar degeneration.

[674] Gautier, A., and Morgues, *Compt. Rend.*, 1888.
[675] Gautier et Etard, *Bull. Soc. Chim.*, xxxvii., 1882.
[676] Guareschi et Mosso, *Les ptomaines*, 1883.
[677] Gautier, A., et Morgues, *Compt. Rend.*, 1888.
[678] Brieger, 1885, *Ptomaines*, iii.

1886. **The Carlisle A Case.**—At a wedding breakfast in Carlisle twenty-four persons were poisoned by food which had been kept in an ill-ventilated cellar. The articles suspected were an American ham, an open game pie, and certain jellies. The bride died. Symptoms commenced in from six to forty-three hours.

1886. **Poisoning by Veal Pie at Iron Bridge.**—Twelve out of fifteen ate of the pie; all were taken ill in from six to twelve hours.

1887. **Poisoning at Retford of Eighty Persons from eating Pork Pie or Brawn.**—Symptoms commenced at various intervals, from eight to thirty-six hours.

1889. **The Carlisle B Case.**—Poisoning by pork pies or boiled salt pork. Number of persons attacked, about twenty-five.

1891. **Poisoning by a Meat Pie at Portsmouth.**—Thirteen persons suffered from serious illness. Portions of the pies were poisonous to mice.

The symptoms in all these cases were not precisely alike; but they were so far identical as to show as great a similarity as in cases when a number of persons are poisoned by the same chemical substance. Arsenic, for instance, produces several types of poisoning; so does phosphorus.

Severe gastro-enteric disturbance, with more or less affection of the nervous system, were the main characteristics. These symptoms commenced, as before stated, at various intervals after ingestion of the food; but they came on with extreme suddenness. Rigors, prostration, giddiness, offensive diarrhœa, followed by muscular twitchings, dilatation of the pupil, drowsiness, deepening in bad cases to coma, were commonly observed. The *post-mortem* appearances were those of enteritis, with inflammatory changes in the kidney and liver. Convalescence was slow; sometimes there was desquamation of the skin.

In many of these cases Dr. Klein found bacteria which, under certain conditions, were capable of becoming pathogenic; but in no case does there seem to have been at the same time an exhaustive chemical inquiry; so that, although there was evidence of a poison passing through the kidney, the nature of the poison still remains obscure.

The deaths in England and Wales from unwholesome food during ten years were as follows:—

DEATHS IN ENGLAND AND WALES FROM UNWHOLESOME FOOD DURING THE TEN YEARS 1883-1892.

	1883.	1884.	1885.	1886.	1887.	1888.	1889.	1890.	1891.	1892.	Total.
Diseased meat,	1	...	...	...	...	...	...	...	...	...	1
Poisonous fish,	2	3	2	1	1	4	3	2	9	6	33
Unwholesome brawn,	...	1	...	...	...	...	...	...	...	...	1
Tinned salmon,	...	2	...	...	...	...	...	...	...	...	2
Putrid meat,	...	1	1	1	...	...	1	...	...	...	4
Diseased food,	...	1	...	...	...	...	...	...	...	...	1
Mussels,	...	1	...	...	...	...	1	...	...	...	2
Tinned foods,	...	...	...	...	2	...	...	...	...	...	2
Whelks,	...	...	...	...	1	...	...	...	...	...	1
Winkles,	...	...	...	...	...	...	...	1	...	...	1
Ptomaines,	...	...	...	...	...	...	...	...	1	...	1
	3	9	3	2	4	4	5	3	10	6	49

§ 687. **German Sausage Poisoning.**—A series of cases may be picked out from the accounts of sausage poisoning in Germany, all of which evidently depend upon a poison producing the same symptoms, and the essentially distinctive mark of which is extreme dryness of the skin and mucous membranes, dilatation of the pupil, and paralysis of the upper eyelids (ptosis). In an uncertain time after eating sausages or some form of meat, from one to twenty-four hours, there is a general feeling of uneasiness, a sense of weight about the stomach, nausea, and soon afterwards vomiting, and very often diarrhœa. The diarrhœa is not severe, never assumes a choleraic form, and is unaccompanied by cramps in the muscles. After a considerable interval there is marked dryness of the mucous membrane (a symptom which never fails), the tongue, pharynx, and the mouth generally seem actually destitute of secretion; there is also an absence of perspiration, the nasal mucous membrane participates in this unnatural want of secretion, the very tears are dried up. In a case related by Kraatzer,[679] the patient, losing a son, was much troubled, but wept no tear. This dryness leads to changes in the mucous membrane, it shrivels, and partly desquamates, aphthous swellings may occur, and a diffuse redness and diphtheritic-like patches have been noticed. There is obstinate constipation, probably from a dryness of the mucous lining of the intestines. The breath has an unpleasant odour, there is often a croupy cough, the urinary secretion alone is not decreased but rather augmented. Swallowing may be so difficult as to rise to the grade of aphagia, and the tongue cannot be manipulated properly, so that the speech may be almost unintelligible. At the same time, marked symptoms of the motor nerves of the face are present, the patient's sight is disturbed, he sees colours or sparks before his eyes; in a few cases there has been transitory blindness, in others diplopia. The pupil in nearly all the cases has been dilated, also in exceptional instances it has been contracted. The *levator palpebrae superioris* is paralysed, and the resulting ptosis completes the picture. Consciousness remains intact almost to death, there is excessive weakness of the muscles, perhaps from a general paresis. If the patient lives long enough, he gets wretchedly thin, and dies from marasmus. In more rapidly fatal cases, death follows from respiratory paralysis, with or without convulsions.

The post-mortem appearances which have been observed are—the mucous membranes of the mouth, gullet, and throat are white, hard, and parchment-like; that of the stomach is more or less injected with numerous hæmorrhages: the kidneys are somewhat congested, with some effusion of blood in the tubuli; the spleen is large and very full of blood, and the lungs are often œdematous, pneumonic, or bronchitic.

[679] Quoted by Husemann, *Vergiftung durch Wurstgift* (Maschka's *Handbook*).

Part VIII.—The Oxalic Acid Group Of Poisons.

§ 688. Oxalic acid is widely distributed both in the free state and in combination with bases throughout the vegetable kingdom, and it also occurs in the animal kingdom. In combination with potash it is found in the *Geranium acetosum* (L.), *Spinacia oleracea* (L.), *Phytolacca decandra* (L.), *Rheum palmatum* (L.), *Rumex acetosa*, *Atropa belladonna*, and several others; in combination with soda in different species of *Salsola* and *Salicornia*; and in combination with lime in most plants, especially in the roots and bark. Many lichens contain half their weight of calcic oxalate, and oxalic acid, either free or combined, is (according to the observations of Hamlet and Plowright[680]) present in all mature non-microscopic fungi. Crystals of oxalate of lime may be frequently seen by the aid of the microscope in the cells of plants. According to Schmidt,[681] this crystallisation only takes place in the fully mature cell, for in actively growing cells the oxalate of lime is entirely dissolved by the albumen of the plant.

In the animal kingdom oxalic acid is always present in the intestinal contents of the caterpillar. In combination with lime, it is constantly found in the allantois liquor of the cow, the urine of man, swine, horses, and cats. With regard to human urine, the presence or absence of oxalate of lime greatly depends upon the diet, and also upon the individual, some persons almost invariably secreting oxalates, whatever their food may be.

§ 689. **Oxalic Acid**, $H_2C_2O_42H_2O$ (90 + 36), specific gravity 1.64, occurs in commerce in prismatic crystals, very similar to, and liable to be mistaken for, either magnesic or zincic sulphates. The crystals are intensely acid, easily soluble in water (1 part requiring at 14.5° 10.46 parts of water); they are also soluble in parts of cold, and readily in boiling, alcohol. Oxalic acid is slightly soluble in cold absolute ether; but ether, although extracting most organic acids from an aqueous solution, will not extract oxalic acid.

Oxalic acid sublimes slowly at 100°, but rapidly and completely at 150°; the best means of obtaining the pure anhydride is to put a sufficient quantity of the acid into a strong flask, clamp it by suitable connections to a mercury pump, and sublime in a vacuum; in this way a sufficient quantity may be sublimed a little above 100°. It is well to remember, not only its low subliming temperature, but also that an aqueous solution, if kept at 100°, loses acid; hence all evaporating or heating operations must not exceed 98°, or there will be some loss. The effect of heat is first to drive off water, then, if continued up to about 190°, there is decomposition into carbon monoxide, carbon dioxide, water, and formic acid; the two reactions occurring simultaneously—

$C_2H_2O_4 = CO_2 + CO + H_2O.$

$C_2H_2O_4 = CO_2 + CH_2O_2.$

Heated with sulphuric acid to 110°, the following decomposition takes place:—

$H_2C_2O_4 = H_2O + CO_2 + CO.$

Oxalic acid decomposes fluor spar, the phosphates of iron, silver, zinc, copper, and the arseniates of iron, silver, and copper. It may be used to separate the sulphides of iron and manganese from the sulphides of zinc, cadmium, uranium, cobalt, mercury, and copper—dissolving the former, not the latter. Many minerals and other substances are also attacked by this acid.

If a solution of oxalic acid in water is boiled with ammonio or sodio terchloride of gold (avoiding direct exposure to light) the gold is precipitated—

$2AuCl_3 + 3H_2C_2O_4 = 6CO_2 + 6HCl + Au_2.$

When black oxide of manganese (free from carbonate) is mixed with an oxalate, and treated with dilute sulphuric acid, the oxalic acid is decomposed, and carbon dioxide evolved—

$MnO_2 + H_2C_2O_4 + H_2SO_4 = MnSO_4 + 2H_2O + 2CO_2.$

A similar reaction occurs with permanganate of potash.

If to a solution of oxalic acid, which may be neutralised with an alkali, or may contain free acetic acid, a solution

---

[680] *Chem. News*, vol. xxxvi. p. 93.

[681] *Ann. Chem. Pharm.*, vol. lxi. p. 297.

of acetate of lime be added, oxalate of lime is thrown down. This salt, important in an analytical point of view, it will be well to describe.

§ 690. **Oxalate of Lime** ($CaC_2O_4H_2O$), 1 part .863 crystallised oxalic acid. This is the salt which the analyst obtains for the quantitative estimation of lime or oxalic acid; it is not identical with that occurring in the vegetable kingdom, the latter containing $3H_2O$. Oxalate of lime cannot be precipitated for quantitative purposes from solutions containing chromium, aluminium, or ferric iron, since somewhat soluble salts are formed. It dissolves in solutions of magnesium and manganese,[682] and citrate of soda, and is also decomposed by boiling with solutions of copper, silver, lead, cadmium, zinc, nickel, cobalt, strontium, or barium. It is insoluble in solutions of chlorides of the alkalies and alkaline earths, and in water, in alkaline solutions, or in acetic acid; and is soluble in mineral acid only when the acid is strong and in considerable excess. It is unalterable in the air, and at 100°. When carefully and slowly ignited it may be wholly converted into carbonate of lime; if the heat is not properly managed (that is, if excessive), caustic lime may be formed in greater or smaller quantity.

§ 691. **Use in the Arts.**—Oxalic acid is chiefly used by dyers and calico-printers, but also by curriers and harness-makers for cleaning leather, by marble masons for removing iron stains, by workers in straw for bleaching, and it is applied to various household purposes,[683] such as the whitening of boards, the removing of iron-mould from linen, &c. The hydropotassic oxalate (binoxalate of potash), under the popular names of "*essential salt of lemons*" and salts of sorrel, is used for scouring metals and for removing ink-stains from linen.

§ 692. **Hydropotassic Oxalate, Binoxalate of Potash**, $KHC_2O_4(H_2O)$, is a white salt, acid in reaction, soluble in water, and insoluble in alcohol. Heated on platinum foil it leaves potassic carbonate, which may be recognised by the usual tests. Its aqueous solution gives, with a solution of acetate or sulphate of lime, a precipitate of calcic oxalate insoluble in acetic acid.

§ 693. **Statistics.**—Poisoning by oxalic acid is more frequent in England than in any other European country. In the ten years 1883-92, there were registered in England and Wales 222 deaths from oxalic acid—of these 199, or 89.6 per cent., were suicidal, the remainder accidental. The age and sex distribution of these cases is set out in the following table:—

POISONING BY OXALIC ACID IN ENGLAND AND WALES DURING THE TEN YEARS 1883-1892.

Accident or Negligence.

Ages,	0-1	1-5	5-15	15-25	25-65	65 and above	Total
Males,	1	...	...	2	...	14	17
Females,	...	...	...	1	5	...	6
Total,	1	...	...	3	5	14	23

Suicide.

Ages,	15-25	25-65	65 and above	Total
Males,	9	102	3	114
Females,	21	62	2	85
Total,	30	164	5	199

§ 694. **Fatal Dose.**—The smallest dose of oxalic acid known to have destroyed life is, according to Dr. Taylor, 3.88 grms. (60 grains); but recovery has taken place, on prompt administration of remedies, after eight times this quantity has been swallowed.

With regard to oxalate of soda, or binoxalate of potash, 14.2 grms. (half an ounce) have been taken without

[682] But it is reprecipitated unaltered by excess of alkaline oxalate.

[683] A "Liquid Blue," used for laundry purposes, contains much free oxalic acid.

fatal result, although the symptoms were very serious; and it may be held that about that quantity would usually cause death. Oxalic acid is not used in medicine, save as a salt, *e.g.*, oxalate of cerium.

§ 695. **Effects of Oxalic Acid and Oxalates on Animals.**—The first cases of poisoning by oxalic acid occurred early in the nineteenth century, a little more than fifty years after its discovery. Thompson[684] was the first who attempted, by experiment on animal life, to elucidate the action of the poison; he noted the caustic action on the stomach, and the effects on the heart and nervous system, which he attributed simply to the local injury through the sympathetic nerves. Orfila[685] was the next who took the matter up, and he made several experiments; but it was Robert Christison[686] who distinctly recognised the important fact that oxalic acid was toxic, quite apart from any local effects, and that the soluble oxalates, such as sodic and potassic oxalates, were violent poisons.

§ 696. Kobert and Küssner[687] have made some extended researches on the effects of sodic oxalate on rabbits, cats, dogs, guinea-pigs, hedgehogs, frogs, &c.—the chief results of which are as follows:—On injection of sodic oxalate solution in moderate doses into the circulation, the heart's action, and, therefore, the pulse, become arhythmic; and a dicrotic or tricrotic condition of the pulse may last even half a day, while at the same time the frequency may be uninfluenced. The blood-pressure also with moderate doses is normal, and with small atoxic doses there is no slowing of the respiration. On the other hand, toxic doses paralyse the respiratory apparatus, and the animal dies asphyxiated. With chronic and subacute poisoning the respiration becomes slower and slower, and then ceases from paralysis of the respiratory muscles. The first sign of poisoning, whether acute or chronic, is a sleepy condition; dogs lie quiet, making now and then a noise as if dreaming, mechanical irritations are responded to with dulness. The hind extremities become weak, and then the fore. This paresis of the hind extremities, deepening into complete paralysis, was very constant and striking. Take, for example, from the paper (*op. cit.*) the experiment in which a large cat received in six days five subcutaneous injections of 5 c.c. of a solution of sodic oxalate (strength 1 : 30), equalling .16 grm.; the cat died, as it were, gradually from behind forwards, so that on the sixth day the hinder extremities were fully motionless and without feeling. The heart beat strongly. The temperature of the poisoned animal always sinks below the normal condition. Convulsions in acute poisoning are common, in chronic quite absent; when present in acute poisoning, they are tetanic or strychnic-like. In all the experiments of Kobert and Küssner, lethal doses of soluble oxalates caused the appearance of sugar in the urine.

J. Uppmann[688] made forty-nine experiments on dogs, in which he administered relatively large doses by the stomach; no poisonous effect followed. Emil Pfeiffer[689] gave a dog in three successive days .2, .5, and lastly 1 grm. oxalic acid with meat, but no symptoms resulted. Yet that oxalic acid, as sodic oxalate, is poisonous to dogs, if it once gets into the circulation, cannot be disputed. The accepted explanation is that the large amount of lime phosphates in the digestive canal of dogs is decomposed by oxalic acid, and the harmless lime oxalate formed.

Oxalic acid is absorbed into the blood, and leeches have been known to die after their application to a person who had taken a large dose. Thus Christison[690] quotes a case related by Dr. Arrowsmith, in which this occurred:—"They were healthy, and fastened immediately; on looking at them a few minutes after, I remarked that they did not seem to fill, and on touching one it felt hard, and instantly fell off motionless and dead; the others were in the same state. They had all bitten, and the marks were conspicuous, but they had drawn scarcely any blood. They were applied about six hours after the acid had been taken."

§ 697. **Effects of Vaporised Oxalic Acid.**—Eulenberg has experimented on pigeons on the action of oxalic acid when breathed. In one of his experiments, .75 grm. of the acid was volatilised into a glass shade, in which a pigeon had been placed; after this had been done five times in two minutes, there was uneasiness, shaking of the head, and cough, with increased mucous secretion of the nasal membrane. On continuing the transmission of the vapour, after eight minutes there was again restlessness, shaking of the head, and cough; after eleven minutes the bird fell and was convulsed. On discontinuing the sublimation, it got up and moved freely, but showed respiratory irritation. On the second day after the experiment, it was observed that the bird's note was hoarse, on the fourth day there was slowness of the heart's action and refusal of food, and on the sixth day the bird was found dead.

684 *Lond. Med. Rep.*, vol. iii. p. 382.

685 *Traité de Toxicologie.*

686 *Edin. Med. and Surg. Journ.*, 1823.

687 *Exper. Wirkungen der Oxalsäure, Virch. Archiv*, Bd. lxxvii. S. 209.

688 *Allg. Med. central Ztg.*, 1877.

689 *Archiv der Pharm.* (3 R.), Bd. xiii. S. 544, 1878.

690 *Treatise on Poisons.*

Examination after death showed slight injection of the cerebral membranes; the cellular tissue in the neighbourhood of the trachea contained in certain places extravasations of blood, varying from the size of a pea to that of a penny; the mucous membrane of the larynx and trachea was swollen and covered with a thick croupous layer; the lungs were partially hepatised, and the pleura thickened; the crop as well as the true intestines still contained some food.[691]

§ 698. **The Effects of Oxalic Acid and Hydropotassic Oxalate on Man.**—The cases of oxalic poisoning have been invariably due to either oxalic acid or hydropotassic oxalate, the neutral sodic or potassic oxalates having hitherto in no instance been taken. The symptoms, and even the locally destructive action of oxalic acid and the acid oxalate, are so similar that neither from clinical nor *post-mortem* signs could they be differentiated by anyone not having a previous knowledge of the case.

The external application of oxalic acid does not appear to cause illness; workmen engaged in trades requiring the constant use of the acid often have the nails white, opaque, and brittle; but no direct injury to health is on record.

A large dose of either causes a local and a remote effect; the local is very similar to that already described as belonging to the mineral acids, i.e., more or less destructive of the mucous membranes with which the acid comes in contact. The remote effects may only be developed after a little; they consist essentially of a profound influence on the nervous system. Though more than 120 cases of oxalic acid poisoning have occurred since Christison wrote his treatise, his graphic description still holds good. "If," says he, "a person immediately after swallowing a solution of a crystalline salt, which tasted purely and strongly acid, is attacked with burning in the throat, then with burning in the stomach, vomiting, particularly of bloody matter, imperceptible pulse, and excessive languor, and dies in half an hour, or still more, in twenty, fifteen, or ten minutes, I do not know any fallacy which can interfere with the conclusion that oxalic acid was the cause of death. No parallel disease begins so abruptly, and terminates so soon; and no other crystalline poison has the same effect." The local action is that of a solvent on the mucous tissues. If from 10 to 30 grms. are swallowed, dissolved in water, there is an immediate sour taste, pain, burning in the stomach, and vomiting. The vomit may be colourless, greenish, or black, and very acid; but there is a considerable variety in the symptoms. The variations may be partly explained by saying that, in one class of cases, the remote or true toxic effects of the poison predominate; in a second, the local and the nervous are equally divided; while in a third, the local effects seem alone to give rise to symptoms.

In a case at Guy's Hospital, in 1842, there was no pain, but vomiting and collapse. In another case which occurred in 1870, a male (aged 48) took 10.4 grms. (162 grains); he had threatening collapse, cold sweats, white and red patches on the tongue and pharynx, difficulty in swallowing, and contracted pupils. Blood was effused from the mouth and anus; on the following day there were convulsions, coma, and death thirty-six hours after taking the poison. In another case, there was rapid loss of consciousness and coma, followed by death in five hours. Death may be very rapid, *e.g.*, in one case (*Med. Times and Gaz.*, 1868) it took place in ten minutes; there was bleeding from the stomach, which doubtless accelerated the fatal result. Orfila has recorded a death almost as rapid from the acid oxalate of potash; a woman took 15 grms.; there was no vomiting, but she suffered from fearful cramps, and death ensued in fifteen minutes. In another case, also recorded by Orfila, there was marked slowing of the pulse, and soporific tendencies. With both oxalic acid and the acid oxalate of potash, certain nervous and other sequelæ are more or less constant, always provided time is given for their development. From the experiments already detailed on animals, one would expect some paresis of the lower extremities, but this has not been observed in man. There is more or less inflammation of the stomach, and often peritonitis; in one case (*Brit. Med. Journal*, 1873) there were cystitis and acute congestion of the kidneys with albuminuria.

In two cases quoted by Taylor, there was a temporary loss or enfeeblement of voice; in one of the two, the aphonia lasted for eight days. In the other, that of a man who had swallowed about 7 grms. (¼ oz.) of oxalic acid, his voice, naturally deep, became in nine hours low and feeble, and continued so for more than a month, during the whole of which time he suffered in addition from numbness and tingling of the legs. As a case of extreme rarity may be mentioned that of a young woman,[692] who took 12 grms. (185 grains) of the acid oxalate of potash, and on the third day died; before death exhibiting delirium so active and intense that it was described as "madness."

§ 699. **Physiological Action.**—Putting on one side the *local* effects of oxalic acid, and regarding only its true toxic effects, there is some difference of opinion as to its action. L. Hermann considers it one of the heart poisons, having seen the frog's heart arrested by subcutaneous doses of sodic oxalate, an observation which is borne out by

[691] *Gewerbe Hygiene*, p. 423.

[692] *Journ. de Chim. Méd.*, 1839, p. 564.

the experiments of Cyon,[693] and not negatived by those of Kobert and Küssner. The poison is believed to act on the extracardial ganglia. Onsum[694] held at one time a peculiar theory of the action of oxalic acid, believing that it precipitated as oxalate of lime in the lung capillaries, causing embolic obstruction; but this view is not now accepted—there are too many obvious objections to it. Kobert and Küssner do not consider oxalic acid a heart poison, but believe that its action is directed to the central nervous system, as attested by sinking of the blood-pressure, the arhythm and retardation of the pulse, the slow breathing, the paralytic symptoms, and the fibrillary muscular contraction; but, with regard to the latter, Locke[695] has observed that a frog's sartorius, immersed in 0.75 sodium oxalate solution, becomes in a few seconds violently active, much more so than in Biederman's normal saline solution. After thirty to forty-five minutes it loses its irritability, which, however, it partially recovers by immersion in 0.6 sodium chloride solution. He thinks this may explain the symptoms of fibrillary muscular contraction observed by Kobert and Küssner, which they ascribe to an action on the central nervous system.

§ 700. **Pathological Changes.**—Kobert and Küssner observed that when oxalate of soda was subcutaneously injected into animals, there was often abscess, and even gangrene, at the seat of the injection. If the poison were injected into the peritoneal cavity, death was so rapid as to leave little time for any coarse lesions to manifest themselves. They were not able to observe a cherry-red colour of the blood, nor did they find oxalate of lime crystals in the lung capillaries; there were often embolic processes in the lung, but nothing typical. They came, therefore, to the conclusion that the state of the kidneys and the urine was the only typical sign. The kidneys were dark, full of blood, but did not show any microscopic hæmorrhages. Twelve hours after taking the poison there is observed in the cortical substance a fine striping corresponding to the canaliculi; in certain cases the whole boundary layer is coloured white. If the poisoning lasts a longer time, the kidneys become less blood-rich, and show the described white striping very beautifully; this change persists several weeks. The cause of this strange appearance is at once revealed by a microscopical examination; it is due to a deposition of oxalate of lime; no crystals are met with in the glomerules. Both by the microscope and by chemical means it may be shown that the content of the kidney in oxalates is large.[696] So far as the tissues generally are concerned, free oxalic acid is not likely to be met with; there is always present sufficient lime to form lime oxalate. The urine was always albuminous and contained a reducing substance, which vanished about the second day after the dose. Hyaline casts and deposits of oxalates in the urine never failed.[697]

§ 701. Observations of the pathological effects of the oxalates on man have been confined to cases of death from the corrosive substances mentioned, and hence the intestinal tract has been profoundly affected.

In the museum of St. Thomas' Hospital is a good example of the effects produced. The case was that of a woman who had taken a large, unknown quantity of oxalic acid, and was brought to the hospital dead. The mucous membrane of the gullet is much corrugated and divided into numerous parallel grooves, these again by little transverse grooves, so that the intersection of the two systems makes a sort of raised pattern. It is noted that in the recent state the mucous membrane could be removed in flakes; in the upper part it was whitish, in the lower slate-coloured. The stomach has a large perforation, but placing the specimen beside another in the same museum which illustrates the effect of the gastric juice, in causing an after-death solution of a portion of the stomach, I was unable to differentiate between the two. The mucous membrane had the same shreddy flocculent appearance, and is soft and pale. The pyloric end is said to have been of a blackish colour, and no lymph was exuded.

§ 702. The pathological changes by the acid oxalate of potash are identical with those of oxalic acid, in both the gullet and stomach being nearly always more or less inflamed or corroded; the inflammation in a few cases has extended right through into the intestinal canal; there are venous hyperæmia, hæmorrhages, and swelling of the mucous membrane of the stomach. The hæmorrhages are often punctiform, but occasionally larger, arranged in rows

---

693 *Virch. Archiv*, Bd. xx. S. 233.

694 Almen afterwards supported Onsum's view; he made a number of microscopical observations, and appears to have been the first who identified oxalate of lime in the kidneys (Upsala, *Läkareförenings förhandl.*, Bd. ii. Hft. iv. S. 265).

695 F. S. Locke, *J. Phys.*, xv. 119; *Journ. Chem. Soc.*, 1893, 480.

696 The important fact of the oxalate-content of kidneys and urine, and the expulsion of casts, was first observed by Mitscherlich in 1854. He noticed in a rabbit, to which had been given 7.5 grms. of oxalic acid, and which had died in thirteen minutes, "*renes paululum magis sanguine replete videbantur, in urina multa corpora inveniebantur, quæ tubulos Bellenianos explese videntur*" (*De acidi acetici, oxalici, tartarici, citrici, formici, et boracici, &c., Berlin*).

697 Rabuteau has discovered by experiment that even the oxalates of iron and copper are decomposed and separated by the kidneys. *Gaz. Méd. de Paris*, 1874.

on the summits of the rugæ; sometimes there is considerable bleeding. In the greater number of cases there is no actual erosion of the stomach, but the inner layer appears abnormally transparent. On examining the mucous membrane under the microscope, Lesser[698] has described it as covered with a layer which strongly reflects light, and is to be considered as caused by a fine precipitate of calcic oxalate. Lesser was unable to find in any case oxalic acid crystals, or those of the acid oxalate of potash. There are many cases of perforation on record, but it is questionable whether they are not all to be regarded as *post-mortem* effects, and not life-changes; at all events, there is little clinical evidence to support the view that these perforations occur during life. In the case (mentioned *ante*) in which death took place by coma, the brain was hyperæmic. The kidneys, as in the case of animals, show the white zone, and are congested, and can be proved by microscopical and chemical means to be rich in oxalates.

§ 703. **Separation of Oxalic Acid from Organic Substances, the Tissues of the Body, &c.**—From what has been stated, no investigation as to the cause of poison, when oxalic acid is suspected, can be considered complete unless the analyst has an opportunity of examining both the urine and the kidneys; for although, in most cases—when the acid itself, or the acid potassic salt has been taken—there may be ample evidence, both chemical and pathological, it is entirely different if a case of poisoning with the neutral sodic salt should occur. In this event, there may be no congested appearance of any portion of the intestinal canal, and the evidence must mainly rest on the urine and kidneys.

Oxalic acid being so widely distributed in the vegetable kingdom, the expert must expect, in any criminal case, to be cross-examined by ingenious counsel as to whether or not it was possible that the acid could have entered the body in a rhubarb-pie, or accidentally through sorrel mixed with greens, &c. To meet these and similar questions it is important to identify, if possible, any green matters found in the stomach. In any case, it must be remembered, that although rhubarb has been eaten for centuries, and every schoolboy has occasionally chewed small portions of sorrel, no poisoning has resulted from these practices. When oxalic acid has been taken into the stomach, it will invariably be found partly in combination with lime, soda, ammonia, &c., and partly free; or if such antidotes as chalk has been administered, it may be wholly combined. Vomiting is nearly always present, and valuable evidence of oxalic acid may be obtained from stains on sheets, carpets, &c. In a recent case of probably suicidal poisoning, the writer found no oxalic acid in the contents of the stomach, but some was detected in the copious vomit which had stained the bed-clothes. The urine also contained a great excess of oxalate of lime—a circumstance of little value taken by itself, but confirmatory with other evidence. If a liquid is strongly acid, oxalic acid may be separated by dialysis from organic matters, and the clear fluid thus obtained precipitated by sulphate of lime, the oxalate of lime being identified by its microscopic form and other characters.

The usual general method for the separation of oxalic acid from organic substances or mixtures is the following:—Extract with boiling water, filter (which in some cases must be difficult or even impossible), and then precipitate with acetate of lead. The lead precipitate may contain, besides oxalate of lead, phosphate, chloride, sulphate, and various organic substances and acids. This is to be decomposed by sulphuretted hydrogen, and on filtering off the sulphide of lead, oxalic acid is to be tested for in the filtrate. This process can only be adopted with advantage in a few cases, and is by no means to be recommended as generally applicable. The best general method, and one which insures the separation of oxalic acid, whether present as a free acid, as an alkaline, or a calcic oxalate, is perhaps the following:—The substance or fluid under examination is digested with hydrochloric acid until a fluid capable of filtration is obtained; the free acid is neutralised by ammonia in very slight excess, and permitted to deposit, and the fluid is then carefully decanted, and the deposit thrown on a filter. The filtrate is added to the decanted fluid, and precipitated with a slight excess of acetate of lime—this precipitate, like the first, being collected on a filter. The first precipitate contains all the oxalic acid which was in combination with lime; the second, all that which was in the free condition. Both precipitates should be washed with acetic acid. The next step is to identify the precipitate which is supposed to be oxalate of lime. The precipitate is washed into a beaker, and dissolved with the aid of heat by adding, drop by drop, pure hydrochloric acid; it is then reprecipitated by ammonia, and allowed to subside completely, which may take some time. The supernatant fluid is decanted, and the precipitate washed by subsidence; it is lastly dried over the water-bath in a tared porcelain dish, and its weight taken. The substance is then identified by testing the dried powder as follows:—

(*a*) It is whitish in colour, and on ignition in a platinum dish leaves a grey carbonate of lime. All other organic salts of lime—viz., citrate, tartrate, &c.—on ignition become coal-black.

(*b*) A portion suspended in water, to which is added some sulphuric acid, destroys the colour of permanganate

[698] Virchow's *Archiv*, Bd. lxxxiii. S. 218, 1881.

of potash—a reaction by which, as is well known, oxalic acid or an oxalate may be conveniently titrated. This reaction is so peculiar to oxalic acid, that there is no substance with which it can be confounded. It is true that uric acid in an acid solution equally decolorises permanganate, but it does so in a different way; the reaction between oxalic acid and permanganate being at first slow, and afterwards rapid, while the reaction with uric acid is just the reverse—at first quick, and towards the end of the process extremely slow.

(*c*) A portion placed in a test-tube, and warmed with concentrated sulphuric acid, develops on warming carbon oxide and carbon dioxide; the presence of the latter is easily shown by adapting a cork and bent tube to the test-tube, and leading the evolved gases through baryta water.

Alexander Gunn[699] has described a new method of both detecting and estimating oxalic acid; it is based on the fact that a small trace of oxalic acid, added to an acid solution of ferrous phosphate, strikes a persistent lemon-yellow colour; the depth of colour being proportionate to the amount of oxalic acid.

The reagents necessary for both quantitative and qualitative testing are as follows:—A standard solution of oxalic acid, of which 100 c.c. equal 1 grm., and a solution of ferrous phosphate, containing about 12.5 per cent. of Fe_32PO_4, with excess of phosphoric acid.

Into each of two Nessler graduated glasses 7.5 c.c. of the ferrous phosphate solution are run and made up to 50 c.c. with distilled water; both solutions should be colourless; 1, 2, or more c.c. of the solution to be tested are then run into one of the Nessler glasses; if oxalic acid be present, a more or less deep tint is produced; this must be imitated by running the standard solution of oxalic acid into the second Nessler cylinder—the calculation is the same as in other colorimetric estimations. It does not appear to be reliable quantitatively, if alum is present; and it is self-evident that the solution to be tested must be fairly free from colour.

§ 704. **Oxalate of Lime in the Urine.**—This well-known urinary sediment occurs chiefly as octahedra, but hour-glass, contracted or dumbbell-like bodies, compound octahedra, and small, flattened, bright discs, not unlike blood discs, are frequently seen. It may be usually identified under the field of the microscope by its insolubility in acetic acid, whilst the ammonio mag. phosphate, as well as the carbonate of lime, are both soluble in that acid. From urates it is distinguished by its insolubility in warm water. A chemical method of separation is as follows:—The deposit is freed by subsidence as much as possible from urine, washed with hot water, and then dissolved in hydrochloric acid and filtered; to the filtrate ammonia is added in excess. The precipitate may contain phosphates of iron, magnesia, lime, and oxalate of lime. On treatment of the precipitate by acetic acid, the phosphates of the alkaline earths (if present) dissolve; the insoluble portion will be either phosphate of iron, or oxalate of lime, or both. On igniting the residue in a platinum dish, any oxalate will be changed to carbonate, and the carbonate of lime may be titrated with d. n. HCl acid and cochineal solution, and from the data thus obtained the oxalate estimated. The iron can be tested qualitatively in the acid solution by ferrocyanide of potassium, or it can be determined by the ordinary methods. If the qualitative detection of oxalate of lime in the deposit is alone required, it is quite sufficient evidence should the portion insoluble in acetic acid, on ignition in a platinum dish, give a residue effervescing on the addition of an acid.

§ 705. **Estimation of Oxalic Acid.**—Oxalic acid is estimated in the free state by direct weighing, or by titration either with alkali or by potassic permanganate, the latter being standardised by oxalic acid. If (as is commonly the case) oxalic acid is precipitated as oxalate of lime, the oxalate may be—

(*a*) Dried at 100° and weighed directly, having the properties already described.

(*b*) Titrated with dilate sulphuric acid and permanganate.

(*c*) Ignited, and the resulting carbonate of lime weighed; or dissolved in standard acid and titrated back—one part of calcic carbonate corresponds to 1.26 part of crystallised oxalic acid, or 0.90 part of $H_2C_2O_4$; similarly, 1 c.c. of standard acid equals .05 of calcic carbonate (or .063 of crystallised oxalic acid).

(*d*) The oxalate may be dissolved in the smallest possible amount of hydrochloric acid, and boiled with ammonio chloride of gold, avoiding exposure to light; every part of gold precipitated corresponds to .961 part of crystallised oxalic acid.

(*e*) The oxalate may be placed in Geissler's carbonic acid apparatus, with peroxide of manganese and diluted sulphuric acid. The weight of the gas which at the end of the operation has escaped, will have a definite relation to that of the oxalate, and if multiplied by 1.4318 will give the amount of crystallised oxalic acid.

[699] *Pharm. Journal*, 1893, 408.

CERTAIN OXALIC BASES—OXALMETHYLINE—OXALPROPYLINE.

§ 706. Hugh Schulz[700] and Mayer have contributed the results of some important researches bearing upon a more exact knowledge of the effects of the oxalic group of poisons, and upon the relation between chemical constitution and physiological effects. They experimented upon *oxalmethyline*, *chloroxalmethyline*, and *oxalpropyline*.

Chloroxalmethyline ($C_6H_5ClN_2$) is a liquid, boiling at 205°, with a weakly narcotic smell. A solution of the hydrochlorate of the base was employed. Subcutaneous injections of .05 grm. into frogs caused narcosis, and both this and the ethylic compound deranged the heart's action, decreasing the number of beats. Thus .05 grm. decreased the number of the beats of the heart of a frog in the course of one and three-quarter hours as follows: 72, 60, 56, 50, 44, 40, 35, 0.

Oxalmethyline produces somewhat similar symptoms, but the nervous system is more affected than in that which contains chlorine.

Oxalpropyline also causes narcosis, and afterwards paralysis of the hinder extremities and slowing of the heart.

The difference between the chlorine-free and the chlorine-containing oxalic bases are summarised as follows:—

	Chlorine-Holding Bases.	Chlorine-Free Bases.
FROGS.	Notable narcosis; no heightened reflex action, muscular cramps, nor spontaneous convulsions.	Narcosis occurs late, and is little pronounced; a notable increase of reflex excitability; more and more muscular paralysis; between times, muscular cramps.
CATS.	Notable narcosis and salivation; no mydriasis; convulsions and paralysis; no change in the respirations.	Great excitement; general shivering, rising to pure clonic convulsions; paralysis of the hind legs; notable mydriasis, jerking, and superficial respiration; weak narcosis.
DOGS.	Notable narcosis; occasional vomiting; the rest as in cats.	Narcosis evident; the rest as in cats.

[700] *Beitrag zur Kenntniss der Wirkung der Oxalbasen auf den Thierkörper. Arch. f. exper. Path. u Pharm.*, 1882.

PART IX. INORGANIC POISONS.

I.—PRECIPITATED FROM A HYDROCHLORIC ACID SOLUTION BY HYDRIC SULPHIDE—PRECIPITATE YELLOW OR ORANGE.[701]

Arsenic—Antimony—Cadmium.

1. ARSENIC.

§ 707. **Metallic Arsenic**, at. wt. 75, specific gravity of solid 5.62 to 5.96, sublimes without fusion in small quantities at 110° (230° F.) *Guy*. It occurs in commerce in whitish-grey, somewhat brittle, crystalline masses, and is obtained by subjecting arsenical pyrites to sublimation in earthen retorts, the arsenic being deposited in suitable receivers on sheet iron. Metallic arsenic is probably not poisonous, but may be changed by the animal fluids into soluble compounds, and then exert toxic effects—volatilised metallic arsenic is easily transformed in the presence of air into arsenious acid, and is therefore intensely poisonous.

§ 708. **Arsenious Anhydride—Arsenious Acid—White Arsenic—Arsenic**, As_2O_3 = 198; specific gravity of vapour, 13.85; specific gravity of opaque variety, 3.699; specific gravity of transparent variety, 3.7385. Composition in 100 parts, As 75.75, O 24.25; therefore one part of metallic arsenic equals 1.32 of As_2O_3. It is entirely volatilised at a temperature of 204.4°.

In analysis it is obtained in brilliant octahedral crystals as a sublimate on discs of glass, or within tubes, the result of heating a film of metallic arsenic with access of air. It is obtained in commerce on a very large scale from the roasting of arsenical pyrites. As thus derived, it is usually in the form of a white cake, the arsenious acid existing in two forms—an amorphous and a crystalline—the cake being generally opaque externally, whilst in the centre it is transparent. According to Kruger, this change from the crystalline to the amorphous condition is dependent upon the absorption of moisture, no alteration taking place in dry air. Both varieties of arsenious anhydride are acid to test-paper.

The solubility of arsenious acid is often a question involving chemical legal matters of great moment. Unfortunately, however, no precisely definite statement can be made on this point, the reason being that the two varieties of arsenic occur in very different proportions in different samples. Both the amorphous and crystalline varieties having very unequal solubilities, every experimenter in succession has given a different series of figures, the only agreement amid the general discrepancy being that arsenic is very sparingly soluble in water.

The statement of Taylor may, however, be accepted as very near the truth, viz., that an ounce of cold water dissolves from half a grain to a grain. According to M. L. A. Buchner,[702] one part of crystalline arsenious acid dissolves after twenty-four hours' digestion in 355 parts of water at 15°; and the amorphous, under the same condition, in 108 of water. A boiling solution of the crystalline acid, left to stand for twenty-four hours, retains one part of acid in 46 of water; a similar solution of the amorphous retains one of arsenic in 30 parts of water, *i.e.*, 100 parts of water dissolve from 2.01 to 3.3 parts of As_2O_3.

Boiling water poured on the powdered substance retains in cooling a grain and a quarter to the ounce; in other words, 100 parts of water retain .10. Lastly, arsenious acid boiled in water for an hour is dissolved in the proportion of 12 grains to the ounce, *i.e.*, 100 parts of water retain 2.5.

K. Chodomisky[703] has investigated the solubility of recrystallised arsenious acid in dilute acids, and his results

---

[701] Fresenius has pointed out that sulphur may mask small quantities of arsenic, antimony, tin, &c., and he recommends that the turbid liquid in which apparently nothing but sulphur has separated should be treated as follows:—A test-tube is half filled with the liquid, and then a couple of c.c. of petroleum ether or of benzene added, the tube closed by the thumb, and the contents well shaken. The sulphur dissolves, and is held in solution by the solvent, which latter forms a clear upper layer. If traces of a metallic sulphide were mixed with the sulphur, thin coloured films are seen at the junction of the two layers, and the sulphides may also coat the tube above the level of the liquid with a slight faintly-coloured pellicle (*Chem. News*, Jan. 4, 1895).

[702] *Bull. de la Société Chem. de Paris*, t. xx. 10, 1873.

[703] *Chem. Centrbl.*, 1889, 569.

are as follows:—100 c.c. of 1.32 per cent. hydrochloric acid dissolves 1.15 grm. As_2O_3 at 18.5°. 100 c.c. of 6 per cent. hydrochloric acid dissolves 1.27 grm. at 18.5°. 100 c.c. of pure hydrochloric acid of the ordinary commercial strength dissolves 1.45 grm. As_2O_3. 100 c.c. of dilute sulphuric acid at 18° dissolves about 0.54 grm.; at 18.5° from 0.65 to 0.72 grm.; and at 80° from 1.09 to 1.19 grm.

§ 709. **Arsine—Arseniuretted Hydrogen**, H_3As.—Mol. weight, 78; vol. weight, 39; specific gravity, 2.702; weight of a litre, 3.4944 grammes; percentage composition, 95.69 As, 4.31 H; volumetric composition, 2 vol. H_3As = half vol. As + 3 vol. H. A colourless inflammable gas, of a fœtid alliaceous odour, coercible into a limpid colourless liquid at a temperature of from -30° to -40°. The products of the combustion of arseniuretted hydrogen are water and arsenious acid; thus, $2H_3As + 6O = 3H_2O + As_2O_3$. If supplied with air in insufficient quantity, if the flame itself be cooled by (for example) a cold porcelain plate, or if the gas pass through a tube any portion of which is heated to redness, the gas is decomposed and the metal separated. Such a decomposition may be compared to the deposit of carbon from ordinary flames, when made to play upon a cooled surface. It may also be decomposed by the electric spark,[704] *e.g.*, if the gas is passed slowly through a narrow tube 0.7 to 0.8 mm. internal diameter, provided with wires 0.5 to 0.6 mm. apart, and a small induction coil used connected with two large Bunsen's cells, then, under these conditions, arsenic as a metal is deposited in the neighbourhood of the sparks. For the decomposition to be complete, the gas should not be delivered at a greater speed than from 10 to 15 c.c. per minute. The gas burns with a blue-white flame, which is very characteristic, and was first observed by Wackenroder. It cannot, however, be properly seen by using the ordinary apparatus of Marsh, for the flame is always coloured from the glass; but if the gas is made to stream through a platinum jet, and then ignited, the characters mentioned are very noteworthy.

Oxygen or air, and arsine, make an explosive mixture. Chlorine decomposes the gas with great energy, combining with the hydrogen, and setting free arsenic as a brown cloud; any excess of chlorine combines with the arsenic as a chloride. Sulphur, submitted to arseniuretted hydrogen, forms sulphuretted hydrogen, whilst first arsenic and then sulphide of arsenic separate. Phosphorus acts in a similar way. Arseniuretted and sulphuretted hydrogen may be evolved at ordinary temperatures without decomposition; at the boiling-point of mercury (350°) they are decomposed, sulphide of arsenic and hydrogen being formed; thus, $3H_2S + 2AsH_3 = As_2S_3 + 6H_2$, a reaction which is of some importance from a practical point of view. Many metals have also the property of decomposing the gas at high temperatures, and setting hydrogen free. Metallic oxides, again, in like manner combine with arsenic, and set water free, *e.g.*, $3CuO + 2H_3As = Cu_3As_2 + 3H_2O$.

Arsine acts on solutions of the noble metals like phosphuretted hydrogen, precipitating the metal and setting free arsenious acid; for example, nitrate of silver is decomposed thus—

$$12AgNO_3 + 2H_3As + 3H_2O = As_2O_3 + 12HNO_3 + 12Ag.$$

Vitali[705] thinks the reaction is in two stages, thus:—

(1) $2AsH_3 + 12AgNO_3 = 2(Ag_3As3AgNO_3) + 6HNO_3$.
(2) $2(Ag_3As,3AgNO_3) + 6H_2O = 6HNO_3 + 6Ag_2 + 2H_3AsO_3$.

This reaction admits of valuable practical application to the estimation of arsenic; for the precipitated silver is perfectly arsenic-free; the excess of nitrate of silver is easily got rid of by a chloride of sodium solution, and the absorption and decomposition of the gas are complete.

In cases of poisoning by arsine, the blood, when examined by the spectroscope (a process the analyst should never omit where it is possible), is of a peculiar inky colour, and the bands between D and C are melted together, and have almost vanished. Such blood, exposed to oxygen remains unaltered.

§ 710. **Arsine in the Arts, &c.**—In the bronzing of brass, in the desilverising of lead by zinc, and subsequent treatment of the silver zinc with hydrochloric acid, in the tinning of sheet iron, and similar processes, either from the use of acids containing arsenic as an impurity, or from the application of arsenic itself, arsine is evolved.

§ 711. **Effects on Animals and Man of Breathing Arsine.**—The most general effect on mammals is to produce jaundice, bloody urine, and bile. In the course of numerous experiments on dogs, Stadelmann[706] found that by

---

[704] N. Klobrikow, *Zeit. Anal. Chem.*, xxix. 129-133.
[705] *L'Orosi*, 1892, 397-411.
[706] *Die Arsenwasserstoff-Vergiftung, Archiv f. exper. Path. u. Pharm.*, Leipzig, 1882.

making them breathe a dose of arsine, which would not be immediately fatal, icterus was always produced under these circumstances, and could be always detected by the appearance of the tissues. The bile is remarkably thickened, and the theory is, that in such cases the jaundice is purely mechanical, the gall-duct being occluded by the inspissated bile. Rabbits experimented upon similarly showed increased biliary secretion, but no jaundice; while it was proved that cats are not so sensitive to arsine as either rabbits or dogs. There are not wanting instances of arsine having been breathed by man—the discoverer of the gas, Gehlen, was in fact the first victim on record. In order to discover a flaw in his apparatus he smelt strongly at the joints, and died in eight days from the effects of the inhalation.

Nine persons, workmen in a factory, were poisoned by arsine being evolved during the treatment by hydrochloric acid of silver-lead containing arsenic. Three of the nine died; their symptoms were briefly as follows:—

(1) H. K., 22 years old; his duty was to pour hydrochloric acid on the metal. Towards mid-day, after this operation, he complained of nausea, giddiness, and *malaise*. In the afternoon he felt an uncommon weight of the limbs, and an oppression in breathing. His fellow-workmen thought that he looked yellow. On going home he lay down and passed into a narcotic sleep. Next morning he went to his work as usual, but was not capable of doing anything; he passed bloody urine several times throughout the day, and fell into a deep sleep, from which he could scarcely be roused. On the third day after the accident, a physician called in found him in a deep sleep, with well-developed jaundice, the temperature moderately high, pulse 100. On the fifth day the jaundice diminished, but it was several months before he could resume his work.

(2) J. T., aged 19, suffered from similar symptoms after five and a half hours' exposure to the gas. He went home, vomited, was jaundiced, and suffered from bloody urine; in six days became convalescent, but could not go to work for many months.

(3) C. E. was very little exposed, but was unwell for a few days.

(4) L. M., 37 years old, was exposed two days to the gas; he vomited, had bloody urine, passed into a narcotic sleep, and died in three days from the date of the first exposure.

(5) J. S., aged 40, was exposed for two days to the gas; the symptoms were similar to No. 4, there was suppression of urine, the catheter drawing blood only, and death in eight days.

(6) M. E., 36 years old; death in three days with similar symptoms.

(7), (8), and (9) suffered like Nos. 1 and 2, and recovered after several months.

The chief *post-mortem* appearance was a dirty green colour of the mucous membrane of the intestines, and congestion of the kidneys. Arsenic was detected in all parts of the body.[707]

Two cases are detailed by Dr. Valette in Tardieu's *Étude*.[708] A mistake occurred in a laboratory, by which a solution of arsenic (instead of sulphuric acid) was poured on zinc to develop hydrogen. Of the two sufferers, the one recovered after an illness of about a week or ten days, the other died at the end of twenty-eight days. The main symptoms were yellowness of skin, vomiting, bloody urine, great depression, slight diarrhœa, headache, and in the fatal case a morbiliform eruption. In a case recorded in the *British Medical Journal*, November 4, 1876, there were none of the usual symptoms of gastric irritation, but loss of memory of recent acts, drowsiness, and giddiness.

§ 712. **The Sulphides of Arsenic.**—Of the sulphides of arsenic, two only, realgar and orpiment, are of any practical importance. *Realgar*, As_2S_2 = 214; specific gravity, 3.356; composition in 100 parts, As 70.01, S 29.91; average composition of commercial product, As 75, S 25. Realgar is found native in ruby-red crystals, and is also prepared artificially by heating together 9 parts of arsenic and 4 of sulphur, or 198 parts of arsenious anhydride with 112 parts of sulphur, $2As_2O_3 + 7S = 2As_2S_2 + 3SO_2$. It is insoluble in water and in hydrochloric acid, but is readily dissolved by potassic disulphide, by nitric acid, and by aqua regia. It is decomposed by caustic potash, leaving undissolved a brown sediment ($As_{12}S$), which contains 96.5 per cent. of arsenic. The dissolved portion is readily converted into arsine by aluminium.

§ 713. **Orpiment, or Arsenic Trisulphide.**—As_2S_3 = 246; specific gravity, 3.48; composition in 100 parts, As 60.98, S 39.02; found native in crystals, presents itself in the laboratory usually as a brilliant yellow amorphous powder, on passing sulphuretted hydrogen through an acid solution of arsenious acid or an arsenite. It is very insoluble in water (about one in a million, *Fresenius*), scarcely soluble in boiling concentrated hydrochloric acid,

[707] Trost, *Vergiftung durch Arsenwasserstoff bei der technischen Gewinnung des Silbers, Vierteljahrsschrift f. gericht. Med.*, xviii. Bd., 2 Heft, S. 6, 1873.

[708] Ambroise Tardieu, *Étude Médico-légale sur l'Empoisonnement*, Obs. xxv. p. 449.

and insoluble generally in dilute acids. Red fuming nitric acid dissolves it, converting it into arsenic and sulphuric acids; ammonia and other alkaline sulphides, the alkalies themselves, alkaline carbonates, bisulphide of potassium, and aqua regia, all dissolve it readily. In the arts it is used as King's yellow. Tanners also formerly employed a mixture of 90 parts of orpiment and 10 of quicklime, under the name of *Rusma*, as a depilatory; but the alkaline sulphides from gas-works are replacing this to a great extent.

§ 714. **Haloid Arsenical Compounds.—The Chloride of Arsenic**, $AsCl_3$ = 181.5; specific gravity liquid, 0° 2.205; boiling-point 134° (273.2°F.), is a heavy, colourless, oily liquid, which has been used as an escharotic in cancerous affections (principally by quacks). In one process of detecting and estimating arsenic, the properties of this substance are utilised. It is immediately decomposed by water into arsenious and hydrochloric acids.

The Iodide of Arsenic (AsI_3) is used occasionally in skin diseases, but is of little interest to the analyst; it is commonly seen in the form of brick-red brilliant flakes.

§ 715. **Arsenic in the Arts.**—The metal is used in various alloys; for example, speculum metal is made of tin, copper, and a little arsenic; white copper is an alloy of copper and arsenic; shot is composed of 1000 parts of lead mixed with 3 of arsenic; the common Britannia metal used for tea-pots, spoons, &c., often contains arsenic; and brass is bronzed with a thin film of arsenic. It was formerly much employed in the manufacture of glass, but is being gradually superseded. It is also now used to some extent in the reduction of indigo blue, and in that of nitro-benzole in the manufacture of aniline.

In cases of suspected poisoning, therefore, and the finding of arsenic in the stomach, or elsewhere, it may be set up as a defence that the arsenic was derived from shot used in the cleansing of bottles, from the bottles themselves, or from metal vessels, such as tea-pots, &c.

The arsenic in all these alloys being extremely insoluble, any solution to a poisonous extent is in the highest degree improbable. It may, however, be necessary to treat the vessels with the fluid or fluids which have been supposed to exert this prejudicial action, and test them for arsenic. The treatment should, of course, be of a severe and exhaustive character, and the fluids should be allowed to stand cold in the vessels for twenty-four hours; then the effect of a gentle heat should be studied, and, lastly, that of boiling temperatures. The analysis of the alloy itself, or of the glass, it would seldom be of value to undertake, for the crushed and finely divided substance is in a condition very different from that of the article when entire, and inferences drawn from such analytical data would be fallacious.

Arsenious anhydride is also used for the preservation of wood, and is thrown occasionally into the holds of vessels in large quantities to prevent vegetable decomposition. In India, again, a solution of arsenic is applied to the walls as a wash, in order to prevent the attacks of insects.

§ 716. **Pharmaceutical, Non-officinal, and other Preparations of Arsenic.**—(1) **Pharmaceutical Preparations.**—The Liquor arsenicalis (Fowler's solution), or solution of arsenic of the pharmacopœia, is composed of:—

Carbonate of Potash,	87 grains (5.64 grms.)
Arsenious Acid,	87 „(5.64 „)
Compound Tincture of Lavender,	5 drachms (17.72 c.c.)

dissolved in 1 pint (567.9 c.c.) of water; every ounce, therefore, contains 4.3 grains of arsenious acid (or 100 c.c. = .9As_2O_3); the strength is therefore nearly 1 per cent.

Liquor Ammonii Arsenitis (not officinal) is made of the same strength, ammonium carbonate being substituted for potassic carbonate.

The *hydrochloric solution of arsenic* is simply arsenious acid dissolved in hydrochloric acid; its strength should be exactly the same as that of Fowler's solution.

A solution of *arseniate of soda*[709] contains the *anhydrous* salt in the proportion of 4 grains to the ounce (.9 in 100 c.c.) of water.

Liquor Arsenii et Hydrargyri Iodidi (Donovan's Solution of Arsenic).—This is not officinal, but is used to some extent in skin diseases; it is a solution of the iodides of mercury and arsenic; strength about 1 per cent. of each of the iodides.

Arseniate of Iron, $Fe_3As_2O_8$, is an amorphous green powder, used to some extent in medicine. It should contain 33.6 per cent. of metallic arsenic.

[709] The formula for arseniate of soda is $Na_2HAsO_47H_2O$, but it sometimes contains more water.

Clemen's Solution.—A solution of the bromide and arseniate of potassium; strength equal to 1 per cent. arsenious acid. Officinal in U.S., France, and Norway.

Pilula Asiatica (not officinal) is composed of arsenious acid, extract of gentian, and black pepper. There is $\frac{1}{12}$th of a grain (5.4 milligrams) of arsenious acid in each pill.

Dr. De Valanguis' Solutio solventes mineralis is composed of 30 grains of As_2O_3 dissolved by 90 minims of HCl in 20 oz. of water; strength = 0.034 per cent. As_2O_3.

(2) **Veterinary Arsenical Medicine.**—Common veterinary preparations containing arsenic are:—A ball for worms, containing in parts—

Calomel,	1.3	per cent.
Arsenious Acid,	1.3	„
Tin Filings,	77.9	„
Venice Turpentine,[710]	19.5	„

A common tonic ball:[711]—

Arsenious Acid,	5 to 10 grains	(.324 to .648 grm.)
Aniseed,	½ oz.	(14 .1744 grms.)
Opium,	30 grains	(1 .94 „)
Treacle,	q. s.	

An arsenical ball, often given by grooms to horses for the purpose of improving their coats, contains in 100 parts:—

Arsenious Acid,	2 .5	per cent.
Pimento,	19.2	„
Extract of Gentian,	78.3	„

Another ball in use is composed of arsenic and verdigris (acetate of copper), of each 8 grains (.518 grm.); cupric sulphate, 20 grains (1.3 grm.); q. s. of linseed meal and treacle.

(3) **Rat and Fly Poisons, &c.**—An arsenical paste sold for rats has the following composition:—

Arsenious Acid,	5 .0	per cent.
Lampblack,	.6	„
Wheat Flour,	46.3	„
Suet,	46.3	„
Oil of Aniseed, a small quantity.		

Another rat poison is composed as follows:—

White Arsenic,	46.8	per cent.
Carbonate of Baryta,	46.8	„
Rose-pink,[712]	5 .8	„
Oil of Aniseed,	.2	„
Oil of Rhodium,	.2	„

Various arsenical preparations are used to kill flies; the active principle of the brown "*papier moure*" is arsenious acid. A dark grey powder, which used to be sold under the name of fly-powder, consisted of metallic arsenic that had been exposed some time to the air.

Fly-water is a strong solution of arsenious acid of uncertain strength, sweetened with sugar, treacle, or honey. Another fly-poison consists of a mixture of arsenious acid, tersulphide of arsenic, treacle, and honey.

(4) **Quack and other Nostrums.**—The analyst may meet with several quack preparations for external use in cancer. A celebrated arsenical paste for this purpose is composed of:—

Arsenious Acid,	8	per cent.

[710] The Venice turpentine is rarely found in ordinary commerce, what is sold under that name consisting of black resin and oil of turpentine.

[711] A similar preparation in common use has the addition of sulphate of zinc.

[712] Alum and carbonate of lead coloured with Brazil and peach woods.

Cinnabar,	70 „
Dragon's Blood,	22 „

Frères Come's Cancer Paste is composed of arsenious acid, 1; charcoal, 1; red mercury sulphide, 4; water, q. s.

The tasteless "*ague drops*" used in the fen countries are simply a solution of arsenite of potash.

Davidson's Cancer Remedy consists, according to Dr. Paris, of equal parts of arsenious acid and powdered hemlock.

In India, arsenic given as a medicine by native practitioners, or administered as a poison, may be found coloured and impure, from having been mixed either with cow's urine, or with the juice of leaves, &c.[713]

Arsenious acid is used by dentists to destroy the nervous pulp of decayed and painful teeth, about the twenty-fifth of a grain (2.5 mgrms.) being placed in the cavity. A common formula is arsenious acid, 2; sulphate of morphine, 1; creasote, q. s. to make a stiff paste. There is no record of any accident having resulted from this practice hitherto; but since the dentist seldom weighs the arsenic, it is not altogether free from danger.

(5) **Pigments, &c.**—*King's yellow* should be As_2S_3, the trisulphide of arsenic or orpiment. It is frequently adulterated with 80 to 90 per cent. of arsenious acid, and in such a case is, of course, more poisonous. King's yellow, if pure, yields to water nothing which gives any arsenical reaction.

A blue pigment, termed *mineral blue*, consists of about equal parts of arsenite of copper and potash, and should contain 38.7 per cent. of metallic arsenic (= to 51.084 As_2O_3H) and 15.6 of copper.

Schweinfurt green (Syn. *Emerald-green*), $(CuAs_2O_4)_3Cu(C_2H_3O_2)_2$ is a cupric arsenite and acetate, and should contain 25 per cent. of copper and 58.4 per cent. of arsenious acid. In analysis, the copper in this compound is readily separated from the arsenic by first oxidising with nitric acid, and then adding to the nitric acid solution ammonia, until the blue colour remains undissolved. At this point ammonium oxalate is added in excess, the solution is first acidified by hydrochloric or nitric acid, and, on standing, the copper separates completely (or almost so) as Oxalate, the arsenic remaining in solution.

Another method is to pass SH_2 to saturation, collect the sulphides on a filter, and, after washing and drying the mixed sulphides, oxidise with fuming nitric acid, evaporate to dryness, and again treat with nitric acid. The residue is fused with soda and potassic nitrate, the fused mass is dissolved in water, acidulated with nitric acid, and the copper is precipitated by potash; the solution is filtered, and in the filtrate the arsenic is precipitated as ammonio-magnesian arseniate or as trisulphide.[714]

Scheele's green ($CuHAsO_3$) is a hydrocupric arsenite, and contains 52.8 per cent. of arsenious anhydride and 33.8 per cent. of copper.

(6) **External Application of Arsenic for Sheep, &c.**—Many of these are simply solutions of arsenic, the solution being made by the farmer. Most of the yellow sheep-dipping compounds of commerce are made up either of impure carbonate of potash, or of soda ash, arsenic, soft soap, and sulphur. The French *bain de Tessier* is composed of:—

Arsenious Acid,	1.00 kgrm.
Ferrous Sulphate,	10.00 „
Peroxide of Iron,	0.40 „
Gentian Powder,	0.20 „

This is to be added to 100 kgrms. of water. Another common application consists of alum and arsenic (10 or 12 to 1), dissolved in two or three hundred parts of water.

(7) **Arsenical Soaps, &c.**—Arsenic is used in preserving the skins of animals. One of the compounds for this purpose, known under the name of *Bécoeur's arsenical soap*, has the following composition:—

Camphor,	3.4 per cent.
Arsenic,	20.2 „
Carbonate of Potash,	56.2 „
Lime,[715]	20.2 „

[713] Chevers, *Med. Jurisprudence for India*, p. 116.

[714] P. Gucci, *Chem. Centrbl.*, 1887, 1528.

[715] The dust from the preserved skins of animals has caused, at least, one case of poisoning. *Ann. d'Hyg. Pub. et de Méd. Lég.*, 2 sér., 1870, t. xxxiii, p. 314.

(8) **Arsenical compounds** used in pyrotechny:—

		Parts.
Blue fires—(1)	Realgar,	2
	Charcoal,	3
	Potassic Chlorate,	5
	Sulphur,	13
	Nitrate of Baryta,	77
(2)	Sulphur,	40.9
	Nitre,	36.8
	Sulphide of Antimony,	12.3
	„ Arsenic,	5
	Charcoal,	5
Green fires—	Metallic Arsenic,	2
	Charcoal,	3
	Chlorate of Potash,	5
	Sulphur,	13
	Nitrate of Baryta,	7
Light green fire—	Charcoal,	1 .75
	Sulphide of Arsenic,	1 .75
	Sulphur,	10.50
	Chlorate of Potash,	23.25
	Nitrate of Baryta,	62.50
White fire—(1)	Arsenious Acid,	.76
	Charcoal,	1 .63
	Sulphide of Antimony,	12.27
	Nitrate of Potash,	36.59
	Sulphur,	48.75
(2)	Realgar,	6 .1
	Sulphur,	21.2
	Nitrate of Potash,	72.7

§ 717. **Statistics.**—During the ten years 1883-92 there were registered in England and Wales 113 deaths from arsenic; of these 57, or about half, were suicidal deaths, and 5 were classed under the head of "murder"; the rest were due to accident. The age and sex distribution of persons dying from accidental or suicidal arsenical poisoning are detailed in the following table:—

DEATHS FROM ARSENIC DURING THE TEN YEARS 1883-1892.

Accident or Negligence.

Ages,	1-5	5-15	15-25	25-65	65 and above	Total
Males,	1	4	3	23	6	37
Females,	4	...	3	4	3	14

Total,	5	4	6	27	9	51

Suicide.

Ages,	15-25	25-65	65 and above	Total
Males,	3	32	2	37
Females,	5	12	3	20
Total,	8	44	5	57

§ 718. **Law Relative to the Sale of Arsenic.**—By the 14th of Vict. c. 12, every person selling arsenic is bound to keep a written record of every particular relative to each transaction, such as the name, abode, and calling of the purchaser, the purpose for which the poison is required, and the quantity sold, &c. These particulars are to be signed also by the purchaser. No person (sec. 2) is allowed to sell arsenic to any one unknown to the seller, unless in the presence of a witness whom the seller is acquainted with. The arsenic sold (sec. 3) is to be mixed with soot or indigo in the proportion of half an ounce of indigo to a pound of arsenic. It, therefore, follows that the coloured substance should not contain more than 70 per cent. of arsenious acid. The Act applies to all the colourless preparations of arsenic: but it is not to affect chemists in making up prescriptions for medical men, or in supplying medical men; nor is it to affect the wholesale dealers in supplying arsenic to retail shops, &c. The penalty for conviction is £20, or less.[716]

§ 719. **Dose.**—The smallest dose of arsenic known to have proved fatal to a human being is .16 grm. (2½ grains). Farriers and grooms are in the habit of giving as much as 1.3 grm. (20 grains) a day to a horse, so that the poisonous dose for this animal must be very large.

The maximum dose for the horned cattle appears to be from .32 to .38 grm. (5 to 6 grains); that for a dog is 16 mgrms. (¼ grain), and even this may, in the smaller kinds, cause illness.

The following may be considered as *dangerous doses* of arsenic:—.13 grm. (2 grains) for an adult; 1.9 grm. (30 grains) for a horse; .64 grm. (10 grains) for a cow; and 32 to 64 mgrms. (½ to 1 grain) for a dog.

§ 720. **Effects of Arsenious Acid on Plants.**—If the root or stem of a plant is immersed in a solution of arsenious acid, the hue of the leaves soon alters in appearance, the green colour becomes of a whitish or brownish hue, and the plant withers; the effect being very similar to that produced by hot water. The toxic action may be traced from below upwards, and analysis will detect minute quantities of arsenic in all portions of the plant.

It has, however, been shown by Gorup-Besanez,[717] that if arsenious acid be mixed with earth, and plants grown in such earth, they only take up infinitesimal quantities of arsenic. Hence, in cases of cattle poisoning, any defence based upon the alleged presence of arsenic in the pasture will be more ingenious than just.

The influence of arsenical fumes as evolved from manufactories upon shrubs and trees is in general insignificant. Pines and firs, five to six years old, have been known to suffer from a disease in which there is a shedding of the leaves, the more tender herbage being at the same time affected. Whatever dangers the practice of steeping corn intended for seed in a solution of arsenious acid, as a preventive of "smut," may possess, it does not appear to influence deleteriously the growth of the future plant.

Superphosphate of manure is frequently rich in arsenic. Dr. Edmund Davy asserts that plants to which such manure is applied take up arsenic in their tissues, and M. Andonard has made a similar statement. Tuson[718] has also undertaken some experiments, which confirm Andonard and Davy's researches. The bearing of this with relation to the detection of arsenic in the stomachs of the herbivora needs no comment.

§ 721. **Effects on Animal Life—Animalcules.**—All infusoria and forms of animalcule-life hitherto observed perish rapidly if a minute quantity of arsenious acid is dissolved in the water in which they exist.

Insects.—The common arsenical fly-papers afford numerous opportunities for observing the action of arsenic

[716] Commercial arsenic is often much adulterated, especially with gypsum, chalk, &c. These are most readily detected by subliming the arsenic. The sublimed arsenic itself may not be entirely pure, sometimes containing arsenical sulphides and antimonious oxide.

[717] *Annal. d. Chemie u. Pharmacie*, Bd. cxxvii., H. 2, 243.

[718] Cooley's *Dictionary*, Art. "Arsenic."

on ordinary flies; within a few minutes (five to ten after taking the poison into their digestive organs) they fall, apparently from paralysis of the wings, and die. Spiders and all insects into which the poison has been introduced exhibit a similar sudden death. It is said that in the neighbourhood of arsenical manufactories there is much destruction among bees and other forms of insect life.

Annelids.—If arsenious acid is applied to the external surface of worms or leeches, the part which it touches perishes first, and life is extinguished successively in the others. If a wound is made first, and the arsenious acid then applied to it, the effects are only intensified and hastened. There is always noticed an augmentation of the excretions; the vermicular movements are at first made more lively, they then become languid, and death is very gradual.

Birds.—The symptoms with birds are somewhat different, and vary according to the form in which the poison is administered, viz., whether as a vapour or in solution. In several experiments made by Eulenberg on pigeons, the birds were secured under glass shades, and exposed to the vapour of metallic arsenic vaporised by heat. It is scarcely necessary to remark that in operating in this way, the poisoning was not by metallic arsenic vapour, but by that of arsenious acid. One of these experiments may be cited:—A pigeon was made to breathe an atmosphere charged with vapour from the volatilisation of metallic arsenic. The bird was immediately restless; in thirty minutes it vomited repeatedly, and the nasal apertures were noticed to be moist; after a little while, the bird, still breathing the arsenious acid atmosphere, was much distressed, shook its head repeatedly, and yawned; in fifty minutes the respiration was laboured, and in fifty-nine minutes there was much vomiting. On removing the bird, after it had been exposed an hour to the vapour (.16 grm. of metallic arsenic having been evaporated in all), it rapidly recovered.

Six days after, the pigeon was again exposed in the same way to the vapour, but this time .56 grm. of metallic arsenic was volatilised. In fifteen minutes there was retching, followed by vomiting. On taking it out after an hour it remained very quiet, ate nothing, and often puffed itself out; the breathing was normal, movements free, but it had unusual thirst. On the second and third day the excretions were frequent and fluid; the cardiac pulsations were slowed, and the bird was disinclined to move. On the fourth day it continued in one place, puffing itself out; towards evening the respirations slowed, the beak gaping at every inspiration. On attempting flight, the wings fluttered and the bird fell on its head. After this it lay on its side, with slow, laboured respiration, the heart-beats scarcely to be felt, and death took place without convulsions, and very quietly. On examining the organs after death, the brain and spinal cord were very bloodless; there were ecchymoses in the lungs; but little else characteristic. The experiment quoted has a direct bearing upon the breathing of arsenical dust; as, for example, that which floats in the air of a room papered with an easily detached arsenical pigment. Other experiments on birds generally have shown that the symptoms produced by arsenious acid in solution, or in the solid form, in a dose insufficient to destroy life, are languor, loss of appetite, and the voidance of large quantities of liquid excreta like verdigris. With fatal doses, the bird remains quiet; there are fluid, sometimes bloody, excretions; spasmodic movements of the pharynx, anti-peristaltic contraction of the œsophagus, vomiting, general trembling of the body, thirst, erection of the feathers, and laboured respiration. The bird becomes very feeble, and the scene mostly closes with insensibility and convulsions.

Mammals, such as cats, dogs, &c., suffer from symptoms fairly identical with those observed in man; but the nervous symptoms (according to P. Hugo) do not predominate, while with rabbits and guinea-pigs, nervous symptoms are more marked and constant.[719] There are vomiting, purging, and often convulsions and paralysis before death. It has been noticed that the muscles after death are in a great state of contraction. The slow poisoning of a dog, according to Lolliot,[720] produced an erythematous eruption in the vicinity of the joints, ears, and other parts of the body; there were conjunctivitis, increased lachrymal secretion, and photophobia; the hair fell off.

§ 722. **Effects of Arsenious Acid on Man.**—The symptoms produced by arsenious acid vary according to the form of the poison—whether solid, vaporous, or soluble—according to the condition of bodily health of the person taking it, and according to the manner in which it is introduced into the animal economy, while they are also in no small degree modified by individual peculiarities of organisation and by habit, as, for instance, in the arsenic-eaters.

Arsenic-Eaters.—In all European countries grooms and horse-dealers are acquainted with the fact that a little arsenic given daily in the corn improves the coat, increases, probably, the assimilation of the food, and renders the horse plump and fat. On the Continent grooms have been known to put a piece of arsenic, the size of a pea, in a little oatmeal, make it into a ball, tie it up in a linen rag, and attach it to the bit; the saliva dissolves, little by little,

[719] *Archiv f. exper. Path. u. Pharmakol*, Leipzig, 1882.
[720] *Étude Physiol. d'Arsène*, Thèse, Paris, 1868.

the poison, while both the gentle irritation and physiological action excite a certain amount of salivation, and the white foam at the mouth, and the champing of the horse, are thought vastly to improve the appearance. Shot, which contains a small quantity of arsenic, have been used for the same purpose, and from half a pound to a pound of small shot has been given to horses. When a horse has been for a long time dosed with arsenic, it seems necessary to continue the practice; if this is not done, the animal rapidly loses his condition. The explanation probably is, that the arsenic stimulates the various cells and glands of the intestinal tract to a superaction, the natural termination of which is an enfeeblement of their secreting power—this especially in the absence of the stimulus. Turning from equine involuntary arsenic-eaters, we find the strange custom of arsenic-eating voluntarily pursued by the races of lower Austria and Styria, especially by those dwelling on the mountains separating Styria from Hungary. In India also (and especially in the Punjaub) the same practice prevails, and here it is often taken as an aphrodisiac. The mountaineers imagine that it increases the respiratory power, nor is there wanting some evidence to show that this is actually the fact, and medicinal doses of arsenic have been in use for some time in cases of asthma and other diseases of the chest. The arsenic-eaters begin with a very small dose, which is continued for several weeks or months, until the system gets accustomed to it. The amount is then slightly augmented until relatively large doses are taken with impunity. In one case[721] it appears that a countryman, in good health, and sixty years of age, took daily 4 grains of arsenious acid, a habit which he had inherited from his father, and which he in turn bequeathed to his son.

The existence of such a custom as arsenic-eating, in its literal sense, has more than once been doubted, but all who have travelled over Styria and other places where the habit prevails have convinced themselves that the facts have not been overstated. For example, Dr. Maclagan, in company with Dr. J. T. Rutter,[722] visited Styria in 1865, and having carefully weighed 5 or 6 grains of arsenic, saw these doses actually swallowed by two men. On collecting their urine, about two hours afterwards, abundant quantitative evidence of its presence was found; but in neither of the men were there the slightest symptoms of poisoning. It is obvious that the existence of such a habit might seriously complicate any inquiry into arsenical poisoning in these regions.

§ 723. **Manner of Introduction of Arsenic.**—Arsenious acid exerts a poisonous action, whether it is taken by the stomach, or introduced into the system by any other channel whatever. The differences in the symptoms produced by external application (as through a wound), and by swallowing arsenious acid in substance or in solution, are not so marked as might be expected. It was probably Hunter who first distinctly recognised the fact that arsenic, even when introduced outwardly by application to an abraded surface, exerts a specific effect on the mucous membrane of the stomach. Brodie[723] states, "Mr. Home informed me that in an experiment made by Mr. Hunter himself, in which arsenic was applied to a wound in a dog, the animal died in twenty-four hours, and the stomach was found to be considerably inflamed. I repeated this experiment several times, taking the precaution of always applying a bandage to prevent the animal licking the wound. The result was that the inflammation of the stomach was commonly more violent and more immediate than when the poison was administered internally, and that it preceded in appearance the inflammation of the wound."

§ 724. **Cases of Poisoning by the External Application of Arsenic.**—A mass-poisoning by the external use of arsenical violet powder to infants occurred in England some years ago. Two deaths from this cause were established by coroners' inquests.[724] Dr. Tidy found the violet powders used in the two cases to have the following composition:—

	1. Per cent.	2. Per cent.
Arsenious Acid,	38.5	38.3
Starch (Potato),	54.8	55.4
Magnesia, &c.	6.7	6.3[725]

[721] Tardieu, *op. cit.*

[722] *Edin. Med. Journ.*, April 1865; *Brit. and For. Med. Chir. Journ.*, Oct. 1865.

[723] *Phil. Trans.*, 1812.

[724] "Gleanings in Toxicology," by C. Meymott Tidy, M.B.—*Lancet*, Aug. 21, 1878.

[725] Two recipes were handed in at the coroner's inquest which pretty fairly represent the composition of ordinary commercial violet powder:—

Although the children were poisoned by absorption through the skin (unless it is allowed that some may have found its way in the form of arsenical dust into the throat, or, what is still more probable, that the infants may from time to time have seized the puff-ball and *sucked* it), the large quantity of .421 grm. (6.5 grains) of arsenious acid was separated in the one case, and .194 grm. (3 grains) in the other. In these cases arose the question which is sure to recur in legal inquiries into poisoning by absorption, viz., whether the poison lying on the surface and folds of the skin could not have been mixed during the *post-mortem* examination with the organs of the body? In these particular cases special care appears to have been taken, and the answer was satisfactory. It is not amiss, however, to call attention to the extreme precaution which such instances necessitate.

A woman, aged 51, had used a solution of arsenious acid to cure the itch; erysipelas of the body, however, followed, and she died after a long illness—one of the symptoms noted being trembling and paresis of the limbs.[726] In a case recorded by Desgranges,[727] a young chambermaid had applied to the unwounded scalp an arsenical ointment for the purpose of destroying vermin. She also suffered from a severe erysipelas, and the hair fell off. Quacks have frequently applied various arsenical pastes to ulcers and cancerous breasts with a fatal result. Instances of this abound; in one, a charlatan applied to a chronic ulcer of the leg an arsenical caustic; the patient showed symptoms of violent poisoning, and died on the sixth day.[728] In another, a lady suffering from some form of tumour of the breast, applied to an unqualified practitioner, who made from fifteen to twenty punctures with a lancet in the swelling, covered a piece of bread with an arsenical compound, and applied the bread thus prepared to the breast. Twelve hours afterwards symptoms of violent gastric irritation commenced; and vomiting and a sanguinolent diarrhœa followed, with death on the fifth day. Arsenic was found in all the organs.[729] Such examples might be multiplied. Arsenic has been in more than one case introduced criminally into the vagina with a fatal result.[730] Foderé, *e.g.*, has recorded the case of a maid-servant who poisoned her mistress by intentionally administering several arsenical enemata.[731] Arsenious acid again has been respired in the form of vapour. One of the best instances of this is recorded by Taylor, and was the subject of a trial at the York Lent Assizes, 1864. The prisoner placed some

---

First Quality, sold at 7s. per gross.

Starch Powder,	28	lbs.
Magnesia,	1 ½	lb.
Orris-root,	1	lb.
Violet Perfume,	1	oz.
Essence of Roses,	5	drops.

Second Quality, sold at 6s. per gross.

Terra Alba (Sulphate of Lime),	14	lbs.
Potato Starch,	21	lbs.
Magnesia,	3	lbs.
Orris-root,	1 ½	lb.
Violet Perfume,	1 ½	oz.
Essence of Roses,	5	drops.

726 Belloc, *Méd. Lég.*, t. iv. p. 124.
727 *Recueil de la Soc. de Méd. de Paris*, t. vi. p. 22, An. vii.; also Tardieu, *Étude Méd. Légale, sur l'Empoisonnement*, Obs. xxvii. p. 457.
728 Mean, *Bibliothèque Méd.*, t. lxxiv., 1821, p. 401.
729 Tardieu, *op. cit.*, Obs. xxix.; Dr. Vernois, *Ann. d'Hyg. et de Méd. Lég.*, t. xxxvi., 1st ser., p. 141, 1846.
730 Ansiaulx, *Clinique Chirurgicale*. Mangor (*Acta. Societ. Reg. Hafniens*, iii. p. 178) gives the case of a man who poisoned his three wives successively with arsenic—the two last by introducing into the vagina a powder composed of flour and arsenic. Another similar case is related by Brisken. Mangor made experiments on mares, showing that when arsenic is applied to the vagina, death may result from inflammation.
731 *Méd. Légale*, iv.

burning pyrites at the doorway of a small room, in which there were eight children, including an infant in the cradle. The other children were removed speedily, but the infant was exposed to the vapour for an hour; it suffered from vomiting and diarrhœa, and died in twenty-four hours. There was slight inflammation of the stomach and intestines, the brain and lungs were congested, and the lining membrane of the trachea of a bright red colour. Arsenic was detected in the stomach, in the lungs, and spleen. The pyrites contained arsenic, and the fatal fumes were in effect composed of sulphurous and arsenious acids.

§ 725. **Arsenic in Wall-Papers.**—It is now an accepted fact that arsenical colours on wall-papers cause illness. The symptoms are those of chronic poisoning, and present nothing distinctive from the effects produced from small doses of arsenic.

Kirschgasser[732] has described the symptoms in detail of twenty-six cases. That arsenic is actually present in patients suffering is often susceptible of proof, by examining skilfully and carefully a considerable volume (from one to two days' collection) of the urine; in most of the cases thus examined arsenic has been discovered. This poisoning is produced, sometimes from the dust, at others from a volatile compound of arsenic, which has the following properties:—It is very volatile (perhaps a gas), it has a strong alliaceous odour, it is not entirely decomposed by a solution of silver nitrate, but is apparently decomposed by a boiling acid solution of potassic permanganate. The author suggests that it may be a compound of CO and As, but this is only a supposition. The existence of this volatile substance has been settled beyond all question by the experiments of Gosio,[733] confirmed by those of Charles Robert Sanger.[734]

This substance appears to be readily enough produced by the action of the common moulds upon organic matter in the presence of small amounts of arsenic; the moulds vary in this property: *Mucor*, *Mucedo*, and *Aspergillum glaucum* react well; on the contrary, *Penicillium glaucum*, *Mucor ramosus*, and several others have either no action, or the action is but slight. One mould, the *Penicillium brevicaule*, has quite a special endowment in forming this peculiar arsenical compound; so much so, that Gosio has proposed its use as a reagent for arsenic, the garlic odour being perceived when the fungus is made to grow in solutions containing organic matter and only traces of arsenic.

§ 726. **Forms of Arsenical Poisoning.**—There are at least four distinct forms of arsenical poisoning, viz., an acute, subacute, a nervous, and a chronic form.

Acute Form.—All those cases in which the inflammatory symptoms are severe from the commencement, and in which the sufferer dies within twenty-four hours, may be called acute. The commencement of the symptoms in these cases is always within the hour; they have been known, indeed, to occur within eight minutes, but the most usual time is from twenty minutes to half an hour. There is an acrid feeling in the throat, with nausea; vomiting soon sets in, the ejected matters being at first composed of the substances eaten; later they may be bilious or even bloody, or composed of a whitish liquid. Diarrhœa follows and accompanies the vomiting, the motions are sometimes like those met with in ordinary diarrhœa and English cholera, and sometimes bloody. There is coldness of the extremities, with great feebleness, and the pulse is small and difficult to feel. The face, at first very pale, takes a bluish tint, the temperature falls still lower; the patient sinks in collapse, and death takes place in from five to twenty hours after the taking of the poison.

There can scarcely be said to be any clinical feature which distinguishes the above description from that of cholera; and supposing that cholera were epidemic, and no suspicious circumstance apparently present, there can be little doubt that a most experienced physician might mistake the cause of the malady, unless surrounding circumstances give some hint or clue to it. In the acute form diarrhœa may be absent, and the patient die, as it were, from "shock." This was probably the cause of death in a case related by Casper,[735] that of Julius Bolle, poisoned by his wife. He took an unknown quantity of arsenic in solution at seven in the morning, and in about three-quarters of an hour afterwards suffered from pain and vomiting, and died in little more than three hours. There were no signs of inflammation in the stomach and intestines, but from the contents of the stomach were separated .0132 grm. of arsenious acid, and .00513 grm. from pieces of the liver, spleen, kidneys, lung, and blood. The dose actually taken is supposed not to have been less than .388 grm. (6 grains).

---

[732] *Vierteljahr. f. gericht Med.*, N. F., ix. 96.

[733] *Azione di alcune Muffe sui Compositi fissi d'Arsenico. Ministero dell'Interno, Laboratori Scientifici della Direzione di Sanita*, Roma, 1892.

[734] "On the Formation of Volatile Compounds of Arsenic from Arsenical Wall-Papers," *American Academy of Arts and Sciences*, vol. xxix.

[735] Case 188 in Casper's *Handbuch*.

§ 727. **The Subacute Form.**—The subacute form is that which is most common; it exhibits some variety of phenomena, and individual cases vary much in the matter of time. The commencement of symptoms is, as in the most acute form, usually within the hour, but exceptions to this rule occur. In a case quoted by Taylor,[736] and recorded by M. Tonnelier, the poison did not cause any marked illness for eight hours; it was found, on *post-mortem* examination, that a cyst had been formed in the stomach which sheathed the arsenic over, and in some degree explained this delay. In another case, again, ten hours elapsed, and this is considered to be the maximum period yet observed. As with the acute form, there is a feeling of nausea, followed by vomiting, which continues although the stomach is quite empty; at first the ejected matter is a watery fluid, but later it may be streaked with blood. The tongue is thickly coated; there is great thirst, but the drinking of any liquid (even of ice-cold water) increases the vomiting. Nearly always pain is felt in the epigastrium, spreading all over the abdomen, and extending to the loin (which is tense and tender on pressure). Deglutition is often painful, and is accompanied by a sort of spasmodic constriction of the pharyngeal muscles. Diarrhœa follows the vomiting, and has the same characters as that previously described; occasionally, however, this feature is absent. In the case recorded by Martineau,[737] a man, aged 25, was seized at 10 A.M. suddenly with vomiting, which persisted all that day and the next, during which time the bowels were obstinately confined. On the second day a purgative was administered, whereupon diarrhœa set in, and continued until his death, which occurred in about two days and sixteen hours from the commencement of the symptoms. This case is also remarkable from the absence of pain or tenderness of the abdomen.

In subacute cases the urine has several times been suppressed, and it is generally scanty and red in colour. Irregularity of the heart's action and feebleness are tolerably constant phenomena. As the end approaches, there is excessive muscular weakness, the face is pale, the eyes hollow; the mucous membranes first, and then the skin, take a bluish tint; the skin itself is covered with perspiration, and there has been noticed a peculiar odour, which has been likened to arsine (arseniuretted hydrogen). The respiration is troubled, convulsive movements of the limbs have been observed, and cramps in the calves of the legs; death follows in a variable time—from twenty-four hours to several days. In certain cases there is a curious remission after violent symptoms, the patient rallies and seems to have recovered; but the appearance is deceptive, for the symptoms recur, and death follows. Recovery may also take place partially from the primary effects, and then inflammatory changes in the stomach, &c., set in, with fever and the ordinary symptoms which are common in all internal inflammation.

A single dose of arsenious acid may cause a prolonged and fatal illness, one of the best known examples being that of the suicide of the Duc de Praslin,[738] who took, with suicidal intent, on Wednesday, August 18, 1847, a dose of arsenious acid. The exact time of the act could not be ascertained, but the first effects appeared at 10 P.M.; there were the usual signs of vomiting, followed on the next day by diarrhœa, fainting, and extreme feebleness of the pulse. On Friday there was a remission of the symptoms, but great coldness of the limbs, intermittency and feebleness of the heart's action, and depression. On Saturday there was slight fever, but no pain or tenderness in the abdomen, vomiting, or diarrhœa; on this day no urine was passed. On the Sunday he complained of a severe constriction of the throat, and deglutition was extremely painful; thirst was extreme, the tongue intensely red, as well as the mucous membrane of the mouth and pharynx, and the patient had a sensation of burning from the mouth to the anus. The abdomen was painful and distended, the heat of the skin was pronounced, the pulse frequent and irregular,—sometimes strong, at others feeble,—the bowels had to be relieved by injections, the urine was in very small quantity; during the night there was no sleep. The duke died at 4.35 A.M. on Tuesday the 24th, the sixth day; intelligence was retained to the last. As the end approached, the respiration became embarrassed, the body extremely cold, and the pulse very frequent.

§ 728. **In the nervous form** the ordinary vomiting and purging are either entirely suppressed, or present in but feeble degree; and under this heading are classed the rare cases in which, in place of the ordinary symptoms, affections of the nervous system predominate. Narcotism, paresis, deepening into paralysis, delirium, and even acute mania, as well as epileptiform convulsions, have all been recorded. In short, the symptoms show so much variety, that an idea of the malady produced in this very rare form can only be obtained by studying the clinical history of cases which have presented this aspect. In a case recorded by Guilbert,[739] a man, thirty-five years of age, had

[736] Taylor's *Principles and Practice of Jurisprudence*, vol. i. p. 251; Flandin, vol. i. p. 535.

[737] Tardieu, *op. cit.*, Obs. xix.

[738] Tardieu, "Relation Médico-Légale de l'Assassinat de la Duchesse de Praslin," *Ann. d'Hyg. Pub. et de Médico-Lég.*, 1847, t. xxxviii. p. 390; also *op. cit.*, Obs. xi.

[739] *Journal de Van der Monde*, 1756, t. iv. p. 353; Tardieu, *op. cit.*, Obs. xiii. p. 430.

swallowed a solution of arsenic, half of which was immediately rejected by vomiting. A little while afterwards his respiration became laborious; the eyes were bathed with tears, which were so acrid as to inflame the eyelids and the cheeks; the muscles of the face were from time to time convulsed; he perspired much, and the perspiration had a fœtid odour; there was some diarrhœa, the urine was suppressed, and from time to time he was delirious. Afterwards the convulsions became general, and the symptoms continued with more or less severity for five days. On the sixth a copious miliary eruption broke out, and the symptoms became less severe. The eruption during fifteen days every now and again reappeared, and at the end of that time the patient was convalescent, but weak, liable to ophthalmia, and had a universal trembling of the limbs.

In one of Brodie's[740] experiments on rabbits, 7 grains of arsenious acid were inserted in a wound in the back; the effect of which was to paralyse the hind legs. In other experiments on animals, paralysis of the hind legs has been frequently noticed, but paralysis certainly is rare in man; in the case, however, recorded by Barrier,[741] of the five men who took by mistake a solution of arsenious acid, one of them was found stretched on the ground with the inferior extremities paralysed.

In a case of "mass" poisoning reported by Dr. Coqueret,[742] three persons ate by mistake an unknown quantity of arsenious acid—two of them only suffered slightly, but the third severely, vomiting occurring almost immediately, and continuing with frequency until the end of the fourth day. Two hours after swallowing the poison, the patient took the hydrated oxide of iron as an antidote. On the sixth day there was stupor and a semi-delirious state, with an eruption of a pustular character compared to that of the small-pox. These symptoms continued more or less until the fifteenth day, when they diminished, and ultimately the patient recovered. In a case related by Tardieu,[743] in which a person died on the eleventh day from the effects of the poison, towards the end, as a specially marked symptom, there was noted hyperæsthesia of the inferior extremities, so that the least touch was painful.

§ 729. **Absence of Symptoms.**—In a few cases there have been a remarkable absence of symptoms, and this both in man and animals. Seven horses were fed with oats accidentally mixed with arseniate of soda. The first succumbed three hours after taking the poison, without having presented any symptom whatever; he fell suddenly, and in a short time expired.[744] It is related by Orfila,[745] that a woman, aged 27, expired in about twelve hours from a large dose of arsenious acid; there were the usual *post-mortem* appearances, but in life no sign of pain, no vomiting, and but little thirst.

§ 730. **Slow Poisoning.**—Slow poisoning has been caused accidentally by arsenical wall-paper, in the manufacture of arsenical pigments, by the admixture of small quantities of arsenic with salt or other condiments, and repeated small doses have been used for criminally producing a fatal illness intended to simulate disease from natural causes. The illness produced by small intermittent doses may closely resemble in miniature, as it were, those produced by large amounts; but, on the other hand, they may be different and scarcely to be described otherwise than as a general condition of ill-health and *malaise*. In such cases there is loss of appetite, feebleness, and not unfrequently a slight yellowness of the skin. A fairly constant effect seen, when a solution of arsenious acid is given continuously for a long time, is an inflammation of the conjunctivæ, as well as of the nasal mucous membrane—the patient complains of "always having a cold." This inflammatory action also affects the pharynx, and may extend to the air-passages, and even to the lung-tissue. At the same time there is often seen an exanthem, which has received a specific name—"*eczema arsenicale*." Salivation is present, the gums are sore, at times lacerated. In chronic poisoning by arsenic, nervous symptoms are almost constant, and exhibit great variety; there may be numbness, or the opposite condition, hyperæsthesia, in the extremities. In certain cases fainting, paresis, paralysis, and sometimes convulsions occur; towards the end a sort of hectic fever supervenes, and the patient dies of exhaustion.

§ 731. **The Maybrick Case.**[746]—The Maybrick case may be considered an example of poisoning extending over a considerable period of time:—Mr. James Maybrick, a Liverpool cotton-broker, aged 49, married Florence Elizabeth, an American lady, aged 21. They had two children. The marriage proved an unhappy one. Some two years before his death in May 1889 they had occupied two separate rooms. Seven weeks before the husband's death,

[740] "The Action of Poisons," *Phil. Trans.*, 1812.

[741] *Journ. de Médecine*, 1783, p. 353; Tardieu, *op. cit.*, Obs. xiv. p. 431.

[742] *Journ. de Connaiss. Méd. Chirurg.*, 1839, p. 155; Tardieu, *op. cit.*, Obs. xv. p. 482.

[743] *Op. cit.*, Obs. xvii. p. 434.

[744] Bouley (Jeune), *Ann. d'Hyg. et de Médico-Lég.*, 1834, t. xii. p. 393.

[745] Tome i. Obs. iv. p. 314.

[746] "The Maybrick Trial and Arsenical Poisoning," by Thos. Stevenson, M.D., *Guy's Hosp. Rep.*, 1889.

Mrs. Maybrick went to London on a false pretext, and lived for some days at an hotel, ostensibly the wife of another man. Two days after her return, Mr. and Mrs. Maybrick attended the Grand National race meeting, and there a serious quarrel arose between them respecting the man with whom she had cohabited in London; they returned from the race, each separately, and she slept apart. Next day an apparent reconciliation took place through the intervention of Dr. Fuller, the family medical attendant.

On or about April 12-19th, 1889, Mrs. Maybrick purchased arsenical fly-papers. On April 13-20th Mr. Maybrick visited London, and consulted Dr. Fuller for dyspepsia, who prescribed nux vomica, acids, and mild remedies (but no arsenic); in one bottle of medicine, ostensibly made according to Dr. Fuller's prescription, arsenic was subsequently found.

Up to Saturday, April 27th, Mr. Maybrick was in his usual health; he was then sick, numbed, and in pain, and had cramps; he told his clerk he had been an hour in the water-closet, but whether for diarrhœa or constipation does not appear; he ascribed the symptoms to an overdose of Fuller's medicine. About this date fly-papers were found by the servants soaking in Mrs. Maybrick's bedroom in a sponge-basin, carefully covered up. On the 29th she again purchased two dozen fly-papers from another chemist. On April 28th Mr. Maybrick was sick and ill; at 11 A.M. Dr. R. Humphreys was called in; Mr. Maybrick complained of a peculiar sensation about his heart, and said he was in dread of paralysis. He attributed his illness to a strong cup of tea taken before breakfast. On the following day he was better, and on the 30th still improving. On May 1st and 2nd Mr. Maybrick went to his office and lunched, both days, off revalenta food, prepared at home and warmed at his office in a new saucepan purchased for the occasion; on one of these days the lunch was forgotten, and was sent to Mr. Maybrick by his wife; and on one of the two days, it is not clear which, Mr. Maybrick complained that his lunch did not agree with him, and he attributed it to inferior sherry put into his food.

In a jug found at the office, and in which food had been taken there, a trace of the food still remained after Mr. Maybrick's death, and arsenic was found therein.

On May 3rd the last fatal illness set in. It is uncertain what food he had after breakfast; he went to the office, and returned home between 5 and 6 P.M. He had been seen by Dr. Humphreys in the morning, and appeared then not quite so well; he found him at midnight suffering from what he thought was severe sciatica; the patient said he had been sick from revalenta. On May 4th he was continually sick, nothing could be retained on the stomach, but the sciatic pain was gone; on May 5th the vomiting continued, the patient complained of the sensation of a hair sticking in the throat, and of a filthy taste in the mouth. The throat and fauces were only slightly reddened, the tongue was furred.

On May 6th there was less vomiting, but otherwise the condition was the same, and Fowler's solution ordered, but only a quantity equal to $^1/_{300}$ grain was actually taken.

May 7th the condition was improved, but there was no increase of power. Dr. W. Carter was called in consultation. The vomiting was passing away, and diarrhœa commencing. The throat was red, dry, and glazed; there were incessant attempts to cough up an imaginary hair. No cramps, no pain in the stomach or intestines, nor conjunctivitis. On this day the first direct evidence of diarrhœa is recorded, the medical men actually seeing a loose motion. The result of the consultation was that Mr. Maybrick must have taken some irritant in his food or drink.

On the 8th a professional nurse took charge. During the 8th and 9th severe tenesmus set in with diarrhœa, and blood was observed in the fæces. Now arsenic was suspected, the urine was examined by Dr. Humphreys, and a rough analysis was made of some Neaves' food which the patient had been taking.

The patient died on the 10th, at 8.30 P.M.

The *post-mortem* appearances were as follows:—

The tongue was dark, the top of the gullet slightly red, but otherwise healthy, save at the lower end, where the mucous membrane was gelatinous, and was dotted over with black dots, like frogs' spawn.

There was a small shallow ulcer in the mucous membrane of the larynx at the back of the epiglottis. The free margin of the epiglottis was rough and eroded; and on the posterior aspect of the ericoid cartilage there were two small red patches. In the stomach were from 5-6 ozs. of brownish fluid. At the cardiac end there was a large vermilion-red patch, interspersed here and there with small dark ecchymoses (spoken of by Dr. Humphreys as a flea-bitten appearance); to this followed a non-inflamed space, and near the pyloric orifice, and extending 2 inches from it, was another red inflamed portion of mucous membrane. In the small intestine the mucous membrane was red and inflamed, from 3 inches below the pylorus to about 3 feet downwards. About 18 or 20 feet lower down, *i.e.*, a little below the ileo-cæcal valve, the mucous membrane was again inflamed to a lesser extent over a space of about 2 feet; the lower end of the rectum was also red and inflamed. No arsenic was found in the stomach or its contents, or in the spleen. Arsenic was present in the liver, in the intestines, and in the kidneys. The quantity separated altogether amounted to over 0.1 grain. The liver weighed 48 ozs., and from 12 ozs. of the liver 0.076 grain of arsenic, reckoned as As_2O_3, was separated.

The whole course of the symptoms and the *post-mortem* examination showed that the deceased died from an irritant poison; and from the fact of a small quantity of arsenic having been found in the body, there can be little doubt but that the poison was arsenic. The symptoms were somewhat anomalous, but not more so than in other recorded cases of undoubted arsenical poisoning. The facts that tended to connect the accused with the death were as follows:—On the night of either May 9th or the 10th Mrs. Maybrick was observed to remove from the table an opened bottle of Valentine's meat juice, and take it into an inner dressing-room, and then replace it—the acts being surreptitious. In replacing it, she was observed to take it either from the pocket of her dressing-gown or from an inner pocket. The lining of this pocket was found to be impregnated with As_2O_3. The juice was found to contain 0.5 grain As_2O_3, and the liquid was of lower gravity than commercial juice; it had probably, therefore, been diluted.

The following is a list of things containing arsenic:—

1. Mrs. Maybrick's dressing-gown.
2. „ apron.
3. A handkerchief wrapped around a bottle.
4. Packet of arsenic "for cats." (Arsenious acid mixed with charcoal.) Tumbler containing milk, with handkerchief soaking in it; at least 20 grains of As_2O_3 in the tumbler mixed with charcoal.
5. A portion of a handkerchief.
6. A bottle containing a strong solution of arsenious acid and several grains of undissolved arsenious acid.
7. A bottle containing from 15-20 grains of solid arsenic and a few drops of solution.
8. A saturated solution of arsenious acid and some solid arsenious acid.
9. Valentine's meat juice.
10. Price's glycerin; ⅔ grain in the whole bottle.
11. A bottle containing 0.1 grain of arsenious acid.
12. A bottle from Mr. Maybrick's office containing a few drops of medicine prescribed by Dr. Fuller (decidedly arsenical).
13. Jug from the office with remains of food.
14. Sediment from trap of w.c. and lavatory drain containing As_2O_3.

Mrs. Maybrick was convicted, but afterwards the sentence was commuted to penal servitude for life.

§ 732. **Post-mortem Appearances in Animals.**—P. Hugo[747] has made some minute researches as to the pathological appearances met with in animals. His experiments were made on seven dogs, eight guinea-pigs, five rabbits, two pigeons, and five cats—all poisoned by arsenious acid. According to Hugo, so far as these animals were concerned, changes were more constant in the intestine than in the stomach.

Stomach.—Changes in the mucous membrane were especially noticed in the great curvature and towards the pylorus; the pylorus itself, and a part of the cardiac portion, remained unchanged. The mucous membrane in dogs and cats was red, with a tinge of blue—in many cases the redness was in streaks, with injection of the capillaries. The stomach of plant-eaters was less altered, and a microscopical examination of the mucous tissues did not show any fatty change.

The Intestines.—In dogs and cats changes were evident; in rabbits and guinea-pigs they were not so marked, but the intestines of the last were extremely tender and brittle, very moist, and filled with a slimy, serous, grey-white fluid; nevertheless, the changes in all these animals appear to be of essentially the same nature. The most striking effect is the shedding of a pseudo-membrane; in quite recent cases there is a layer of from 1 to 1½ mm. wide of a transparent, frog-spawn-like jelly streaking the intestine. In later stages it becomes thicker, while occasionally it resembles a diphtheritic exudation. The mucous membrane itself is deep purple-red, showing up by the side of the pseudo-membrane. With regard to the villi, the epithelial layer is detached, and the capillary network filled with blood and enlarged.

The Liver.—Hugo met only occasionally with fatty degeneration of the liver, but there was marked steatosis of the epithelium of the gall-bladder of dogs. A fact not prominently noticed before, is (at all events, in dogs) a serous transudation into the pleural sac and acute œdema of the lungs; the exudation may be excessive, so that more than 100 c.c. of serous fluid can be obtained from the thorax; there is also usually much fluid in the pericardium. In

[747] *Beiträge zur Pathologie der acuten Arsenikvergiftung., Archiv für exper. Pathol. u. Pharmakol.*, Leipzig, 1882.

two of Hugo's experiments there was fluid in the cerebral ventricles; and in all there was increased moisture of the brain substance with injection of the capillary vessels, especially of the pia.

§ 733. **Post-mortem Appearances.**—A remarkable preservation of the body is commonly, but not constantly, observed. When it does occur it may have great significance, particularly when the body is placed under conditions in which it might be expected to decompose rapidly. In the celebrated Continental case of the apothecary Speichert (1876), Speichert's wife was exhumed eleven months after death. The coffin stood partly in water, the corpse was mummified. The organs contained arsenic, the churchyard earth no arsenic. R. Koch was unable to explain the preservation of the body, under these conditions, in no other way than from the effect of arsenic; and this circumstance, with others, was an important element which led to the conviction of Speichert.

When arsenious acid is swallowed in substance or solution, the most marked change is that in the mucous membrane of the stomach and intestines; and, even when the poison has been absorbed by the skin, or taken in any other way, there may be a very pronounced inflammatory action. On the other hand, this is occasionally absent. Orfila[748] relates a case in which a man died in thirteen hours after having taken 12 grms. of arsenious acid:—"The mucous membrane of the stomach presented in its whole extent no trace of inflammation, no redness, and no alteration of texture." Many other similar cases are on record; and, according to Harvey's statistics, in 197 cases, 36 (about 18.2 per cent.) presented no lesion of the stomach.

The usual changes produced by arsenious acid may be studied in the museums of the London hospitals. In Guy's Hospital Museum there are three preparations. In preparation 1798^{32} is seen a large stomach with the mucous membrane at certain points abraded, and at the great curvature the whole coats are thinned; it is also somewhat congested. In preparation 1798^{64} is a portion of coagulated lymph, from the stomach of a lad, aged 14, who had taken accidentally a piece of cheese charged with arsenious acid, prepared for the purpose of destroying rats. He lived twenty-eight hours, and presented the ordinary symptoms. The lymph has a membranous appearance, and the rugæ of the stomach are impressed upon it. It is said when recent to have presented numerous bright bloody spots, although there was no visible breach of substance on the surface of the stomach. The mucous membrane of the stomach is stated to have been injected, and there was also diffuse injection of the duodenum. Preparation 1798^{80} is the stomach of a person who survived thirteen hours after taking a fatal dose of arsenious acid; and in the same museum there is a wax model of the appearances which the fresh preparation exhibited, showing a large oval patch coated with mucus and the poison. The stomach was intensely inflamed, the cæcum injected. The rest of the intestine was healthy.

In the museum of University College there are two preparations, one[749] exhibiting intense swelling and congestion of the gastric mucous membrane, which is of a perfectly vermilion colour. Another preparation (No. 2868) shows the effect of a small dose of arsenic on the stomach; there are spots of arborescent extravasation, and slight congestion of the summits of the rugæ, but in other respects it is normal. There is also a cast of Peyer's patches from the same case, showing great prominence of the glands, with some injection of the intestinal mucous membrane.

In St. Thomas' Hospital there is an interesting preparation (No. 8) showing the gastric mucous membrane dotted all over with minute ulcers, none of which have an inflammatory zone.[750] I have not, however, seen in any museum a preparation of the curious emphysematous condition of the mucous membrane, which has more than once been met with. For example, in a case related by Tardieu,[751] Schwann, a labourer, died from the effects of arsenic in thirty-six hours. The autopsy showed that the mucous membrane of the stomach and small intestine was covered with a pasty coating, and was elevated in nearly its whole extent by bullæ filled with gas, forming true emphysematous swellings which encroached upon the diameter of the intestine. There was neither redness nor ulceration, but the mucous membrane was softened.

The author saw, many years ago, at Barnard Castle, an autopsy made on a gentleman who died from arsenic. In this case the mucous membrane of the stomach presented a peculiar appearance, being raised here and there by little blebs, and very slightly reddened.

---

[748] Tome i. Obs. v.

[749] This preparation at the time of my visit had no number.

[750] In a case related by Orfila, t. i. Obs. xv., death resulted from the outward application of arsenic; the mucous membrane of the stomach was natural in colour, but there were four ulcers, one of which was 50 centimetres in diameter.

[751] *Op. cit.*, Obs. i. p. 468.

§ 734. The inflammatory and other changes rarely affect the gullet. Brodie[752] never observed inflammation of the œsophagus as an effect of arsenic; but, when arsenic is swallowed in the solid state, as in the suicide of Soufflard, graphically described by Orfila,[753] it may be affected. In Soufflard's case there was a vivid injection of the pharynx and gullet.

In many instances, when the arsenic has been taken in the solid form, the crystals with mucus and other matters adhere to the lining membrane. I have seen in the stomach of a horse, poisoned by an ounce of arsenic, an exquisite example of this. The inflammatory changes may be recognised many months after death owing to the antiseptic properties of arsenic; nevertheless, great caution is necessary in giving an opinion, for there is often a remarkable redness induced by putrefactive changes in healthy stomachs. Casper,[754] on this point, very justly observes:—"If Orfila quotes a case from Lepelletier, in which the inflammatory redness of the mucous membrane of the stomach was to be recognised after nine months' interment, and if Taylor cites two cases in which it was observed nineteen and twenty-one months after death respectively, this is in contradiction of all that I, on my part, have seen in the very numerous exhumed corpses examined by me in relation to the gradual progress of putrefaction and of saponification, and I cannot help here suspecting a confusion with the putrefactive imbibition redness of the mucous membrane."

If examined microscopically, the liver and kidneys show no change, save a fatty degeneration and infiltration of the epithelial cells. In the muscular substance of the heart, under the endocardium, there is almost constantly noticed ecchymosis. In the most acute cases, in which a cholera-like diarrhœa has exhausted the sufferer, the blood may be thickened from loss of its aqueous constituents, and the whole of the organs will present that singularly dry appearance found in all cases in which there has been a copious draining away of the body fluids. In the narcotic form of arsenical poisoning, the vessels of the brain have been noted as congested, but this congestion is neither marked nor pathognomonic. Among the rare pathological changes may be classed glossitis, in which the whole tongue has swollen, and is found so large as almost to fill the mouth. This has been explained, in one case, as caused by solid arsenious acid having been left a little time in the mouth before swallowing it. On the other hand, it has also been observed when the poison has been absorbed from a cutaneous application. When arsenic has been introduced into the vagina, the ordinary traces of inflammatory action have been seen, and, even without direct contact, an inflammation of the male and female sexual organs has been recorded, extending so far as gangrene. As a rule, putrefaction is remarkably retarded, and is especially slow in those organs which contain arsenic; so that, if the poison has been swallowed, the stomach will retain its form, and, even to a certain extent, its natural appearance, for an indefinite period. In corpses long buried of persons dying from arsenical poisoning, the ordinary process of decay gives place to a saponification, and such bodies present a striking contrast to others buried in the same graveyard. This retardation of putrefaction is what might, *à priori*, be expected, for arsenic has been long in use as a preservative of organic tissues.

§ 735. **Physiological Action of Arsenic.**—The older view with regard to the essential action of arsenic was, without doubt, that the effects were mainly local, and that death ensued from the corrosive action on the stomach and other tissues—a view which is in its entirety no longer accepted; nevertheless, it is perfectly true that arsenic has a corrosive local action; it will raise blisters on the skin, will inflame the tongue or mucous membranes with which it comes in contact; and, in those rapid cases in which extensive lesions have been found in the alimentary canal, it can hardly be denied that instances of death have occurred more from the local than the constitutional action. In the vast majority of cases, however, there is certainly insufficient local action to account for death, and we must refer the lethal result to a more profound and intimate effect on the nervous centres. The curious fact, that, when arsenic is absorbed from a cutaneous surface or from a wound, the mucous membrane of the stomach inflames, is explained by the absorption of the arsenic into the blood and its separation by the mucous membrane, in its passage exerting an irritant action. The diarrhœa and hyperæmia of the internal abdominal organs have been referred to a paralysis of the splanchnic nerves, but Esser considers them due to an irritation of the ganglia in the intestinal walls. Binz has advanced a new and original theory as to the action of arsenious acid; he considers that the protoplasm of the cells of many tissues possess the power of oxidising arsenious acid to arsenic acid, and this arsenic acid is again, by the same agency, reduced to arsenious acid, in this way, by the alternate oxidation and reduction of the arsenious acid, the cells are decomposed, and a fatty degeneration takes place. Thus arsenic causes fatty

[752] *Phil. Trans.*, 1812.

[753] T. i. p. 319.

[754] *Handbuch*, vol. ii. p. 420.

changes in the liver, kidney, and other cells by a process analogous to the action of phosphorus. T. Araki[755] also considers that both arsenic and phosphorus lessen oxidation, and points out that lactic acid appears in the urine when either of these poisons are taken, such acid being the result of insufficient oxidation. A notable diminution of arterial pressure has been observed. In an experiment by Hugo[756] .03 grm. of As_2O_3 was injected intravenously, the normal arterial pressure being 178 mm. Ten minutes after injection the pressure sank to 47 mm.; in sixteen minutes it again rose to 127 mm. Accumulative action of arsenic does not occur. Hebra has given, in skin diseases, during many months, a total quantity of 12 grms. without evil result.

§ 736. **Elimination of Arsenic.**—Arsenic is separated especially by the urine,[757] then through the bile, and by the perspiration. The eruption often observed on the skin has been referred to the local action of small quantities of arsenic in this way eliminated. It is found in the urine first after from five to six hours, but the elimination from a single dose is not finished till a period of from five to eight days; it has often been looked for twelve days after taking it, but very seldom found. According to Vitali, the arsenic in the urine is not free, but probably displaces phosphorus in phospho-glyceric acid; possibly it may also replace phosphorus in lecithin.

§ 737. **Antidote and Treatment.**—In any case in which there is opportunity for *immediate* treatment, ferric hydrate should be administered as an antidote. Ferric hydrate converts the soluble arsenious acid into the insoluble ferric arseniate, the ferric oxide being reduced to ferrous oxide. It is necessary to use ferric hydrate recently prepared, for if dried it changes into an oxyhydrate, or even if kept under water the same change occurs, so that (according to the experiments of Messrs. T. & H. Smith) after four months the power of the moist mass is reduced to one-half, and after five months to one-fourth.

It is obvious that ferric hydrate is not in the true sense of the word an antidote, for it will only act when it comes in contact with the arsenious acid; and, when once the poison has been removed from the stomach by absorption into the tissues, the administration of the hydrate is absolutely useless. Ferric hydrate may be readily prepared by adding strong ammonia to the solution or tincture of ferric chloride, found in every medical man's surgery and in every chemist's shop, care being taken to add no caustic excess of ammonia; the liquid need not be filtered, but should be at once administered. With regard to other methods of medical treatment, they are simply those suggested by the symptoms and well-known effects of the poison. When absorbed, the drinking of water in excess cannot but assist its elimination by the kidneys.

§ 738. **Detection of Arsenic.**—The analyst may have to identify arsenic in substance, in solution, in alloys, in wall-papers, in earth, and in various animal, fatty, resinous, or other organic matters.

Arsenious Acid in Substance.—The general characters of arsenious acid have been already described, and are themselves so marked as to be unmistakable. The following are the most conclusive tests:—

(1) A small fragment placed in the subliming cell, and heated to about the temperature of 137.7° (286° F.), at once sublimes in the form of an amorphous powder, if the upper glass disc is cool; but if heated (as it should be) to nearly the same temperature as the lower, characteristic crystals are obtained, remarkable for their brilliancy and permanency, and almost always distinct and separate. The prevailing form is the regular octahedron, but the rhombic dodecahedron, the rectangular prism, superimposed crystals, half crystals, deep triangular plates like tetrahedra, and irregular and confused forms, all occasionally occur.

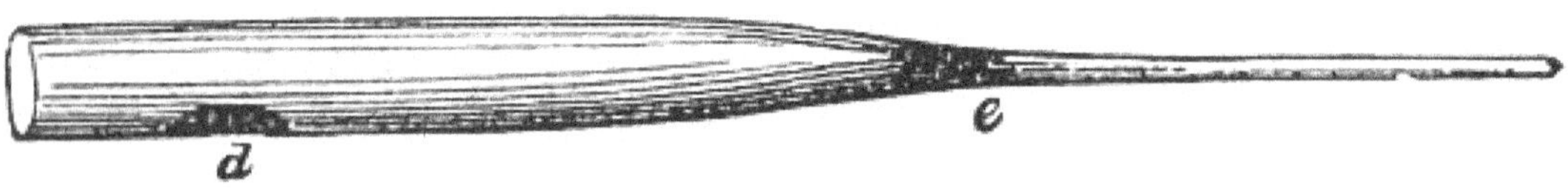

(2) A beautiful and well-known test is that of Berzelius:—A small hard-glass tube is taken, and the closed end drawn out to the size of a knitting needle. Within the extreme point of this fine part is placed the fragment (which may be no more than a milligramme) and a splinter of charcoal, fine enough to enter freely the narrow part, as

755 *Zeit. physiol. Chem.*, xvii. 311-339.

756 *Op. cit.*

757 An old experiment of Orfila's has some practical bearings, and may be cited here. A dog was treated by .12 grm. of arsenious acid, and supplied plentifully with liquid to drink; his urine, analysed from time to time during ten days, gave abundant evidences of arsenic. On killing the animal by hanging on the tenth day, no arsenic could be detected in any of the organs of the body; it had been, as it were, washed out.

shown in the figure. The portion of the tube containing the charcoal (*e*) is first heated until it glows, and then the extreme end; if arsenic is present, a mirror-like coating is easily obtained in the broader portion of the tube (*d*). That this coating is really arsenical can be established by the behaviour of metallic crusts of arsenic towards solvents. The portion of the tube containing the crust may also be broken up, put in a very short, wide test-tube (the mouth of which is occupied by a circle of thin microscopic glass) and heated, when the arsenic will sublime on to the glass disc, partly as a metal and partly as crystalline arsenious acid.

(3) Arsenious acid, itself inodorous, when heated on coal, after mixing it with moist oxalate of potash, evolves a peculiar garlic-like odour. To this test oxide of antimony adulterated with arsenic will respond, if there is only a thousandth part present. Simply projecting arsenious acid on either red-hot charcoal or iron produces the same odour.

(4) A little bit of arsenious acid, heated in a matrass with two or three times its weight of acetate of potash, evolves the unsupportable odour of kakodyl.

Arsenites and Arseniates, mixed with oxalate of soda and heated in a matrass, afford distinct mirrors, especially the arsenites of the earths and silver; those of copper and iron are rather less distinct.

Sulphides of Arsenic are reduced by any of the processes described below.

In Solution.—An acid solution of arsenious acid gives, when treated with SH_2, a canary-yellow precipitate, soluble in ammonia, carbonate of ammonia, and bisulphite of potash, and also a metallic sublimate when heated in a tube with the reducing agents in the manner described below. By these properties the sulphide is distinguished and, indeed, separated from antimony, tin, and cadmium.

The sulphides of tin and cadmium are certainly also yellow, but the latter is quite insoluble in ammonia, while the former gives no metallic sublimate when heated with reducing substances.

The sulphide of antimony, again, is orange, and quite insoluble in potassic bisulphite, and scarcely dissolves in ammonia.

A small piece of sodium amalgam placed in a test-tube or flask containing an arsenic-holding liquid, or the liquid made alkaline with soda or potash and a little bit of aluminium added, produces in a short time arsine, which will blacken a piece of paper, soaked in nitrate of silver, and inserted in the mouth of the flask. This is certainly the most convenient test for arsenic. No antimoniuretted hydrogen (*stibine*) is given off from an alkaline solution and no SH_2.

Marsh's Original Test for Arsenic consisted in evolving nascent hydrogen by zinc and sulphuric acid, and then adding the liquid to be tested. The apparatus for Marsh's test, in its simplest form, consists of a flask provided with a cork conveying two tubes, one a funnel reaching nearly to the bottom of the flask; the other, a delivery tube, which is of some length, is provided with a chloride of calcium bulb,[758] and towards the end is turned up at right angles, the end being narrowed. By evolving hydrogen from zinc and sulphuric acid, and then adding portions of the liquid through the funnel, arseniuretted hydrogen in a dry state is driven along the leading tube, can be ignited on its issue, and on depressing a piece of cold porcelain, a dark metallic spot of arsenic is obtained.[759] Or, if any portion of the tube be made red-hot, the metal is deposited in the same way as a ring. The apparatus admits of much complication and variety. One of the most useful additions is, perhaps, the interposition of a small gasometer. This consists of a cylindrical glass vessel with entrance and exit tubes, open at the bottom, immersed in water in a larger vessel, and counterpoised by weights and rollers, exactly like the large gasometers used at gasworks; the exit tube must have a stop-cock, and the gas must pass over calcic chloride in order to dry it thoroughly.

M. Blondlot has observed[760] that if pure zinc, a weak solution of arsenious acid, and a sulphuric acid containing nitric acid or nitrous compounds, be mixed together, the arsenic passes into a solid hydrate, which is deposited on the surface of the zinc; this is, however, prevented by the addition of a little stannous chloride dissolved in hydrochloric acid.

The precautions to be observed in Marsh's test are:—

---

[758] Otto recommends the first half of the drying tube connected with the development flask to be filled with caustic potash, the latter half with chloride of calcium (*Ausmittelung der Gifte*). Dragendorff approves of this, but remarks that it should be used when arsenic alone is searched for, since caustic potash decomposes stibine. The potash fixes SH_2, and prevents the formation of chloride of arsenic; on the other hand, it absorbs some little AsH_3.

[759] For identification of arsenical films, see below.

[760] Blondlot, "Transformation de l'arsenic en hydrure solide par l'hydrogène aissant sous l'influence des composés nitreux."—*Jour. de Pharm. et de Chim.*, 3e sér., t. xliv. p. 486.

(1) Absolute freedom of the reagents used from arsenic, antimony,[761] and other impurities.
(2) The sulphuric acid should be diluted with five times its weight of water, and if freshly prepared should be cooled before use. Strong acid must not be employed.[762]
(3) The fluid to be tested should be poured in little by little.
(4) Nitrous compounds, nitric acid, hydrochloric acid, chlorides, are all more or less prejudicial.
(5) The gas should come off regularly in not too strong a stream, nor out of too small an opening.
(6) The gas should pass through the red-hot tube at least one hour, if no stain is at once detected.
(7) Towards the end of the operation, a solution of stannous chloride in hydrochloric acid is to be added to the contents of the flask. This addition precipitates any arsenic present in a finely divided state, in which it is readily attacked by nascent hydrogen.[763]

The characteristics of the metallic stains which may occur either on glass or porcelain in the use of Marsh's test, may be noted as under:—

Mirror or Crust of Arsenic	Mirror or Crust of Antimony
Is deposited at a little distance from the flame.	Is deposited close to the flame, and on both sides of it, and is therefore notched.
An arsenical stain is in two portions, the one brownish, the other a glittering black.	The stain is tolerably homogeneous, and usually has a tin-like lustre.
On heating, it is rapidly volatilised as arsenious acid.	Volatilisation very slow; no crystalline sublimate obtainable.
On transmission of a stream of SH_2, whilst immediately behind the stain a gentle heat is applied, the arsenic is changed to yellow sulphide;[764] if dry ClH is now transmitted, the arsenical sulphide is unchanged.	The same process applied in the case of antimony produces the orange or black sulphide; and on passing dry ClH, chloride of antimony volatilises without the application of heat.
Chloride of lime dissolves the arsenic completely.	Antimony not affected.
Protochloride of tin has no action on metallic arsenic.	Dissolves slowly but completely the antimony stain.
The arsenic stain, dissolved in *aqua regia*, or ClH and chlorate of potash, and then treated with tartaric acid, ammonia, and magnesia mixture, gives a precipitate of ammonia magnesian arseniate.[765]	No precipitate with antimony.

761 With regard to purity of reagents, Sonnenschein states that he has once found chlorate of potash contaminated with arsenic.—Sonnenschein, *Gericht. Chemie*, p. 139.

762 M. A. Gautier uses sulphuric acid diluted with five times its weight of water; when the hydrogen has displaced the air, he adds to the arsenical matter 45 grms. of this acid and 5 grms. of pure sulphuric acid.—*Bull. de la Société Chim. de Paris*, 1875, t. xxiv.

763 F. W. Schmidt, *Zeit. anorg. Chem.*, i. 353-359.

764 It is desirable to dissolve away the free sulphur often deposited with the arsenical sulphide by bisulphide of carbon.

765 Schönbein has proposed ozone as an oxidiser of arsenical stains. The substance containing the stain, together with a piece of moist phosphorus, is placed under a shade, and left there for some time; the oxidisation product is, of course, coloured yellow by SH_2 if it is arsenious acid, orange if antimony. The vapour of iodine colours metallic arsenic pale yellow, and later a brownish hue; on exposure to the air it loses its colour. Iodine, on the other hand, gives with antimony a carmelite brown, changing to orange.

An arsenical ring may be also treated as follows:—Precipitated zinc sulphide is made into a paste with a little water, and introduced into the end of the tube; the same end is then plunged into dilute sulphuric acid, and the ring heated, when the arsenical sulphide will be produced.

The mirror or crust of arsenic is usually described and weighed as being composed of the pure metal, but J. W. Rettgers has investigated the matter, and the following is an abstract of his results:—

There is no amorphous form of arsenic, the variety generally thus called being crystalline. Two modifications can be distinguished: the one being a hexagonal silver-white variety possessed of metallic lustre, specifically heavier and less volatile than the second kind, which is black in colour, crystallises apparently in the regular system, and constitutes the true arsenic mirror. The former modification corresponds to red hexagonal phosphorus (red phosphorus having been recently proved by the author to be crystalline), and the latter to yellow phosphorus, which crystallises in the regular system. Both modifications of arsenic are perfectly opaque; deposits which are yellow or brown, and more or less transparent, consist of the suboxide and hydride, As_2O and AsH. The brown spot on porcelain produced by contact with a flame of arseniuretted hydrogen is not a thin film of As, but one of the brown solid hydride AsH, formed by the decomposition of AsH_3. This view is confirmed by the fact that arsenic sublimed in an indifferent gas (*e.g.*, CO_2) is deposited in one or other of the modifications described above, the brown transparent product being obtained only in the presence of H or O. Moreover, pure arsenic is insoluble in all solvents, whereas the film on porcelain (AsH) is soluble in many solvents, including hydrocarbons of the benzene series (*e.g.*, xylene), warm methylene iodide, and hot caustic potash.

Hence quantitative results from weighing arsenical mirrors can never be accurate, because the mirrors consist of mixtures of hydride and suboxide.

Reinsch's Test.—A piece of bright copper foil, boiled in an acid liquid containing either arsenic or antimony, or both, becomes coated with a dark deposit of antimony or arsenic, as the case may be. The arsenical stain, according to Lippert, is a true alloy, consisting of 1 arsenic to 5 copper.[766] Properly applied, the copper will withdraw every trace of arsenic or antimony from a solution. Dr. John Clark[767] has lately introduced some improvements in Reinsch's process. His experiments have been directed to the means of proving the presence of arsenic or antimony in the stain on the copper with greater certainty, and at the same time estimating the amount when they occur together.

The material to be tested is boiled gently in a porcelain vessel with dilute hydrochloric acid and a small strip of copper about 1 inch long by ¼ inch broad, till the absence of arsenic or antimony has been ascertained, or a coating has been produced. When the coating is decided, the piece of copper is taken out, washed first with water, then with a little alcohol to get rid of fatty matter, and finally with water. It is then placed in a mixture of dilute caustic potash and peroxide of hydrogen, and allowed to digest in the cold. At the same time a second piece of copper is introduced into the material which has given a deposit on the first piece, the washings of the first piece being added, and the boiling continued.

The treatment of the first piece of copper by caustic potash and peroxide of hydrogen dissolves any antimony or arsenic and restores the copper to its original brightness; when this is accomplished, the second piece of copper is taken out and replaced by the first, and this second piece, if stained, is digested with potash, peroxide of hydrogen, and washed as in the former case. The process is repeated until the slips of copper cease to be stained in the slightest degree—until, in short, the whole arsenic or antimony has been withdrawn.

The alkaline liquid contains the arsenic, as arsenate of potassium; the antimony, if present, as antimonate; and the solution is also contaminated by a little hydrated copper oxide; this latter separates on boiling, and can be filtered off, and the filtrate is boiled down to a small bulk. The liquid is washed into a small distillation-flask with strong hydrochloric acid, ferrous chloride is added, the flask, fitted with a safety tube, is connected with a condenser, and the arsenic distilled into water. To obtain the last traces of arsenic it may be necessary to distil it twice in this way, adding, each time, fresh strong acid and distilling to dryness. The distillate is then tested for arsenic by adding an equal bulk of saturated SH_2 water. The sulphide of arsenic may be dealt with as described below.

The residue in the flask is now tested for antimony by saturating with SH_2; should antimony be present, the precipitate by SH_2 will probably be dark coloured, because of a small quantity of copper. The precipitate is collected, dissolved in dilute caustic soda, boiled, filtered to remove copper sulphide, the filtrate acidified by hydrochloric acid, and sulphuretted hydrogen water added. If antimony was present, this time the precipitate will be of an orange colour, and may be dealt with as described below.

The test experiments with regard to this combined process appear satisfactory.

---

[766] *Journ. f. pract. Chem.*, xiii. 168.

[767] *Journ. Chem. Soc.*, June 1893, 886.

§ 739. **Arsenic in Glycerin.**—Arsenic has been frequently found in commercial glycerin, the quantity varying from 0.1 to 1 mgrm. in 100 c.c. The best method to detect the presence of arsenic in glycerin is as follows:—A mixture of 5 c.c. of hydrochloric acid (1 : 7) and 1 grm. of pure zinc is placed in a long test-tube, the mouth of which is covered with a disc of filter-paper previously moistened with one or two drops of mercuric chloride solution, and dried. If arsenic is present, a yellow stain is produced upon the filter-paper within fifteen minutes, and it subsequently becomes darker.[768]

§ 740. **Arsenic in Organic Matters.**—Orfila and the older school of chemists took the greatest care, in searching for arsenic, to destroy the last trace of organic matter. Orfila's practice was to chop up the substance and make it into a paste with 400 to 700 grms. of water; to this .010 grm. KHO in alcohol was added, and .020 grm. of potassic nitrate. The substances were heated up to from 80° to 90° for some time, until they were pretty well dissolved; the organic matter was then burnt off in a Hessian crucible heated to redness, on which small quantities of the matters were placed at a time. When the whole had thus been submitted to red heat, the melted mass was run into an almost red-hot porcelain basin, and allowed to cool. Afterwards, it was again heated with concentrated sulphuric acid, until all nitric and nitrous fumes were dissipated; on dissolving and filtering in water, the liquid was introduced into a Marsh's apparatus. Orfila never seems to have failed in detecting arsenic by this process. For an organ like the liver, he considered that 100 grms. of potash and 86 of strong sulphuric acid were necessary in order to destroy the organic matters.

The liability of the various reagents used to impurity, and the probability of loss in these operations, have tended to discredit destruction of the organic matter by a red heat, and chemists generally have preferred to oxidise animal matters by a moist process. The organic substance is divided finely and digested with dilute hydrochloric acid, and from time to time crystals of potassic chlorate are thrown in until all the fluid is very thin and capable of passing through a filter. The filtrate must now be submitted to the prolonged action of sulphuretted hydrogen,[769] and the sulphide of arsenic separated from free sulphur by dissolving in sodic sulphide. After filtering, the arsenic sulphide may be again thrown down by the addition of hydrochloric acid, collected on a filter, and still further purified by solution in ammonic carbonate; once more precipitated by hydrochloric acid, and lastly identified by conversion into magnesia pyro-arseniate (see below). The above process is a general and safe way of detecting arsenic in almost any organic tissue, but the author prefers the distillation process described below.

From ordinary pills, quack extracts, and similar preparations, drying, powdering, and exhaustion with boiling dilute HCl, will remove the whole of the arsenic, if in a soluble state.

Oils and matters consisting almost entirely of fat, suspected of containing arsenic, are gently heated, and allowed to deposit any insoluble matter they may contain; the oil is then decanted, and, if necessary, filtered from any deposit; saponified by alcoholic potash, the soap decomposed by HCl, the fatty acids separated, and the arsenic looked for both in the first deposit and in the solution, now fairly free from fat, and easy to treat.

In searching for arsenic in the fluids or tissues of the body, the analyst is generally at the mercy of the pathologist, and sometimes the work of the chemist leads to a negative result, solely from not having the proper organ sent to him.[770]

Brodie long ago stated that when arsenious acid had been given in solution to any animal capable of vomiting, no arsenic could be detected in the stomach; this statement is too absolute, but in the majority of cases true.

In all cases the chemist should have portions of the brain, spinal cord, liver, kidneys, lungs, and muscular tissue, as well as the stomach and its contents.

According to the experiments of Scolosuboff,[771] arsenic is generally greatest in the marrow, then in the brain, next in the liver, and least in the muscles, and the following may be taken as a fairly accurate statement of the relative proportion in which arsenic is likely to be found in the body, 100 grms. being taken of each:—

Muscles,	1
Liver,	10.8

[768] "Arsenic in Glycerin," by Dr. H. B. H. Paul and A. J. Cownley, *Pharm. Journ.*, Feb. 24, 1894.

[769] The SH_2 should be washed by passing it through two or more washing bottles supplied with warm dilute HCl—a few samples of sulphide of iron give off an arseniferous gas, so that this precaution is necessary.

[770] For example, in cases of poisoning by external application, more than once merely the empty stomach and a piece of intestine have been forwarded to the writer.

[771] *Bull. Soc. Chim.* (2), xxiv. p. 124.

Brain,	36.5
Spinal Marrow,	37.3

But Ludwig's[772] experiments and conclusions are entirely opposed to this, since both in acute and chronic cases he found as follows (per cent. As_2O_3):—

Brain,	.0002
Liver,	.001
Kidney,	.0004
Muscle,	.00025

So that he detected in the liver five times more than in the brain. M. P. Hamberg has also confirmed the fact, that more is found in the liver and kidneys than in the nervous tissues.

Chittenden[773] found in a body the following quantities of arsenic estimated as arsenious acid:—

	Grain.
Stomach and gullet,	0.158
Intestines,	0.314
Liver,	0.218
Kidney,	0.029
Lungs and spleen,	0.172
Heart,	0.112
Brain,	0.075
Diaphragm,	0.010

The whole arsenic present was estimated as equal to 3.1 grains of arsenious acid, viz., 2.628 grains absorbed, and 0.472 unabsorbed; of the absorbed portion 8.3 per cent. was found in the liver.

With regard to the preliminary treatment of the stomach and fluids submitted to the analyst, the careful noting of appearances, the decantation, washing, and examination[774] (microscopical and chemical) of any deposit, are precautions so obviously dictated by common sense, that they need only be alluded to in passing. Of some considerable moment is the question which may be put to the analyst in court, in reference to the possible entrance of arsenic into the living body, by accidental and, so to speak, *subtle* means. Such are the inhaling of the fumes from the burning of arsenical candles,[775] and of emanations from papers (see above),[776] as well as the possible entrance of arsenic into the body after death from various sources, such as arsenical earth, &c.[777]

§ 741. **Imbibition of Arsenic after Death.**—The arguments which are likely to be used, in favour of a corpse having become arsenical may be gathered from a case related by Sonnenschein:—Certain bodies were exhumed in two churchyards; the evidence went to show that they had been poisoned by arsenic, and this substance was actually

[772] *Ueber die Verhaltung des Arsens im thierischen Organismus nach Einverleibung von Arseniger Säure. Med. Jahrbuch*, 1880.

[773] *American Chemical Journal*, v. 8.

[774] From some observations of Fresenius in a recent number of the *Zeitschrift f. anal. Chem.*, it would seem necessary to test all glass vessels used; for it is difficult at present to purchase arsenic-free glass.

[775] See a case of poisoning (non-fatal) of a lady by the use of arsenical candles, *Med. Times and Gazette*, vol. iii., 1876, p. 367.

[776] To solve this question, it has been at times considered necessary to analyse an extraordinary number of things. In the "affaire Danval" (*Journ. d'Hygiène*, 2e sér., No. 108, July 1878), more than sixty different articles, comprising drugs, drinks, perfumes, bed-curtains, wall-paper, and other matters, were submitted to the experts.

[777] The following important case is related by Sonnenschein:—

Nicholas Nobel and his wife, Jerome, were buried two metres from each other in the churchyard at Spinal, the earth of which notoriously contained arsenic. A suspicion of poisoning arose. The bodies were exhumed, and arsenic was found in the stomach and intestines of Nobel, but not the slightest trace in the corpse of the wife. The remains of the bodies were reinterred, and after six months, on a fresh suspicion of poisoning arising, again exhumed. The corpse of the woman had been put naked in the moist earth during a heavy shower, but this time also no arsenic was detected in it.

found in the bodies, while at the same time it was discovered to exist also in traces in the earth of the churchyard. The theory for the defence was, that although the arsenic in the earth was in an insoluble state, yet that it might combine with lime as an arsenite of lime; this arsenite would become soluble by the action of carbonic acid set free by vegetation, and filter down to the corpse. Sonnenschein suspended a quantity of this earth in water, and passed CO_2 through it for twelve hours; on filtering, the liquid gave no evidence of arsenic. A similar result was obtained when an artificial mixture of 1 grm. of arsenious acid and 1 pound of earth were submitted to the same process.

The fact would appear to stand thus: oxide of iron in ordinary earth retains arsenic, and requires treatment with a concentrated acid to dissolve it. It therefore follows that, if a defence of arsenical earth is likely to be set up, and the analyst finds that by mere extraction of the tissues by *water* he can detect arsenic, the defence is in all probability unsound. The expert should, of course, deal with this question on its merits, and without prejudice. According to Eulenberg,[778] in arsenical earth—if, after having been crushed and washed, it lies for some time exposed to the disintegrating action of the air—soluble arsenical salts are formed, which may find their way into brooks and supplies of drinking water. We may infer that it is hardly probable (except under very peculiar circumstances) for a corpse to be contaminated internally with an estimable quantity of arsenic from the traces of arsenic met with in a few churchyards.

It occasionally happens that an exhumation is ordered a very long time after death, when no organs or parts (save the bones) are to be distinguished. In the case of a man long dead, the widow confessing that she had administered poison, the bones were analysed by Sonnenschein, and a small quantity of arsenic found. Conièrbe and Orfila have both asserted that arsenic is a normal constituent of the bones—a statement which has been repeatedly disproved. Sonnenschein relates:[779]—"I procured from a churchyard of this place (Berlin) the remnants of the body of a person killed twenty-five years previously, and investigated several others in a similar way, without finding the least trace of arsenic. Similar experiments in great number were repeated in my laboratory, but in no case was arsenic recognised." The opinion of the expert, should he find arsenic in the bones, must be formed from the amount discovered, and other circumstances.

A difficult case on which to form an opinion is one recorded by William P. Mason,[780] as follows:—

The deceased, a farmer, bachelor, sixty-five years of age, and in good health, was taken violently sick shortly after breakfast, with vomiting and distress in the stomach. Although a physician was summoned, the symptoms increased in severity, and a little after midnight death ensued. The funeral took place three days later. Certain very damaging pieces of circumstantial evidence having been collected, the housekeeper was arrested on the charge of murder, it having been shown, among other things, that on the day preceding the death she had purchased an ounce of white arsenic.

Thirty-five days after death (from March 20 to April 25) the body was exhumed, and found in a state of remarkable preservation, and free from cadaveric smell. The stomach presented evidences of inflammation.

Portions sent for analysis were the stomach, portion of intestine, portion of liver, one kidney, and the heart. Arsenic was found in all these parts. White octahedral crystals were found in the contents of the stomach, which on separation gave arsenical reaction.

The arsenic found was:—

Stomach and intestine,	0.2376	grm.
Liver and kidney,	0.0032	„
Heart,	0.0007	„
Total as metallic arsenic,	0.2415	„

The amount of arsenic recovered and produced in court was in quantity sufficient to produce death. Some time after the analytical report was made to the coroner, it was learned that an embalming fluid, highly arsenical in character, had been used upon the body by the undertaker at the time of preparation for burial. No injection of this embalming fluid was practised, but cloths wrung out in the fluid were laid upon the face and chest, and were kept constantly wet therewith during a period of many hours. In all about two quarts of embalming fluid were so used. Its composition appeared to be a strongly acidified solution of sodium arsenite and zinc sulphate. Only the arsenic and zinc were determined quantitatively, and they were found to be, zinc (metallic), 1.978 per cent., and arsenic

[778] *Gewerbe Hygiene*, p. 234.

[779] *Gerichtl. Chem.*, p. 212.

[780] *Chem. News*, Feb. 23, 1894.

(metallic), 1.365 per cent. by weight. An amount of this fluid measuring 15.7 c.c. would thus contain a weight of arsenic equal to that actually recovered from the body.

Extended medical testimony was offered by the prosecution, tending to show that, under the given circumstances, no fluid of any kind could have reached the stomach through the nose or mouth after death, thus anticipating what the defence afterwards claimed, that the undertaker was responsible for the arsenic discovered in the remains.

In order to gather further light upon the possibility of cadaveric imbibition of embalming fluid through the unbroken skin, test was made for zinc in the heart and stomach, and distinct traces of the metal were found in each instance. That at least a portion of the arsenic found in the body was due to *post-mortem* causes was thus distinctly proven. A weighed portion (62 grms.) of the stomach and contents was then most carefully analysed quantitatively for both zinc and arsenic with the following results:—Arsenic, 0.0648 grm., and zinc, 0.0079 grm. Bearing in mind the relative quantities of the two metals in the embalming fluid, it will be seen that the arsenic found in the 62 grms. of the stomach was nearly twelve times larger than it should have been to have balanced the zinc which was also present. This fact, together with the discovery of crystals of white arsenic in the stomach, constituted the case for the prosecution, so far as the chemical evidence was concerned.

The defence made an unsuccessful effort to show that the crystals of the tri-oxide originated from the spontaneous evaporation of the embalming fluid. The prosecution met this point by proving that such fluid had been abundantly experimented upon by exposure to a very low temperature during an interval of several months, and also by spontaneous evaporation with a view of testing that very question, and that the results had in every case been negative. Special importance was given these experiments, because of the well-known separation of octahedral crystals during the spontaneous evaporation of a hydrochloric acid solution of the white oxide, it having also appeared that, in the manufacture of the embalming fluid, the arsenic was used as white arsenic.

A very strong point was finally raised for the defence by the inability of the expert on the side of the prosecution to state positively whether or not an embalming fluid of the above composition would diffuse as a whole through dead tissue, or its several parts would be imbibed at different rates of speed, the zinc portion becoming arrested by albuminoid material and being therefore outstripped by the arsenic, or *vice versa*. The prisoner was ultimately acquitted.

In a case which occurred in the Western States of America, there was good reason for believing that arsenic had been introduced into the corpse of a man *after* his decease. With regard to the imbibition of arsenic thus introduced, Orfila[781] says:—"I have often introduced into the stomach (as well as the rectum) of the corpses of men and dogs 2 to 3 grms. of arsenious acid, dissolved in from 400 to 500 grms. of water, and have examined the different viscera at the end of eight, ten, or twenty days. Constantly I have recognised the effects of cadaveric imbibition. Sections of the liver or other organs which touch the digestive canal, carefully cut and analysed, furnished arsenic, which could not be obtained sensibly (or not at all) from sections which had not been in contact with this canal. If the corpse remained long on the back after arsenious acid had been introduced into the stomach, I could obtain this metal from the left half of the diaphragm and from the inferior lobe of the left lung, whilst I did not obtain it from other portions of the diaphragm nor from the right lung." Dr. Reece has also made some experiments on the imbibition of arsenic after death. He injected solutions of arsenious acid into the stomach of various warm-blooded animals, and found at various periods arsenic, not alone in the intestinal canal, but also in the spleen, liver, and kidneys.

§ 742. **Analysis of Wall-Paper for Arsenic.**—The separation of arsenic from paper admits of great variety of manipulation. A quick special method is as follows:—The paper is saturated with chlorate of potash solution, dried, set on fire in a suitable plate, and instantly covered with a bell-glass. The ash is collected, pulverised, and exhausted with cold water, which has previously thoroughly cleansed the plate and bell-glass; the arsenic in combination with the potash is dissolved, whilst oxides of chromium, copper, aluminium, tin, and lead remain in the insoluble portion.[782]

Fresenius and Hintz[783] have elaborated a method for the examination of wall-papers, fabrics, yarns, and similar substances, which, provided the reagents are pure, is accurate and easy. Twenty-five grms. of the substance are placed in a half-litre distilling flask or retort, and 250 c.c. of HCl, specific gravity 1.19, added; after digestion for

[781] *Op. cit.*, t. i. p. 309.
[782] Kapferschlaeger: *Rev. Universelle des Mines*, 1876.
[783] *Zeit. anal. Chem.*, xxvii. 179-182.

an hour, 5 c.c. of a saturated solution of ferrous chloride are added, and the liquid slowly distilled until frothing stops any farther distillation. A further quantity of 100 c.c. HCl is then added, and distilled over. The receiver, in each case, contains water, and must be kept cool. The united distillates are diluted to 800 c.c. and saturated with SH_2. The arsenious sulphide is collected on an asbestos filter. After partial washing, it is heated with bromine in HCl of 1.9 specific gravity, and the solution again distilled with ferrous chloride. The distillate, on now being treated with SH_2, gives arsenious sulphide free from organic matter.

§ 743. **Estimation of Arsenic.**—Most of the methods for the quantitative determination of arsenic are also excellent tests for its presence. It may be regarded, indeed, as an axiom in legal chemistry, that the precise amount of every substance detected, if it can be weighed or estimated by any process whatever, should be accurately stated. Indefinite expressions, such as "a small quantity was found," "traces were detected," &c., are most objectionable. The more perfect of the methods of evolving arsenic can be made quantitative. For example, the galvanic process introduced by Bloxam may be utilised as follows:—A fractional part of the arsenical solution is taken for the experiment; the bottom of a narrow-necked bottle of about 100 c.c. capacity is removed, and replaced by a piece of vegetable parchment. The neck of the bottle carries a cork, which is pierced by (1) a platinum wire, which is attached to a platinum electrode; (2) a short tube, bent at right angles, and connected by piping with a longer tube, which has also a rectangular bend, and dips into a solution of silver nitrate; (3) an ordinary funnel-tube, reaching nearly to the bottom. The bottle is placed in a beaker of such a size as to leave a small interval between the two, and the whole apparatus stands in a large vessel of cold water. Dilute sulphuric acid is now put into the bottle, and also into the beaker, so that the fluid reaches exactly the same level in each. The positive platinum electrode of a battery of six of Grove's cells, or other efficient combination, is immersed in the liquid outside the bottle, connection with the negative plate is established, and hydrogen very soon comes off, and passes over into the nitrate of silver solution. When all the air is expelled, a portion of the rectangular tube is heated to redness, and if there is no stain nor any reduction of the silver, the acid is pure. If the gas is passed for a long time into the silver solution, the silver will be reduced to some extent by the hydrogen, although arsenic-free;[784] so that it is better to rely upon the metallic ring or stain, which is certain to be formed on heating a portion of the tube red-hot, and keeping it at that temperature for *at least ten minutes*. The liquid is then passed through the funnel in successive portions; if arsenic is present, there will be a decided metallic ring on heating the tube as before, and if antimony is present, there will also be a stain; the distinctions between these stains have been described earlier.

The tube is kept red-hot until the stain is very distinct; then the source of heat is removed, and the gas allowed to bubble through the argentic nitrate solution, which it decomposes, as before detailed. This process is continued until, on placing the delivery tube in a sample of clear nitrate of silver solution, there is no darkening of colour. In certain cases this may take a long time, but the apparatus, once set to work, requires little superintendence. At the conclusion, the whole of the arsenic is separated,—part is in the silver solution as arsenious acid, part in the tube as a ring of metallic arsenic. The portion of the tube containing the metallic arsenic should be cut off with a file and weighed, the arsenic then removed and re-weighed; the loss is the metal approximately. Or, the weight of the film may be estimated by having a set of similar deposits of known weight or quantities, in tubes exactly corresponding to those used in the analysis, and comparing or matching them.

The arsenious acid in the nitrate of silver may be dealt with in several ways. The equation given shows clearly that pure arsine, passed into nitrate of silver solution, decomposes it in such a manner that, if either the silver deposited or the free acid is estimated, the quantity of arsenic can from such data be deduced. In operating on organic liquids, ammonia and other products may be given off, rendering either of the indirect processes inadvisable. A very convenient method, applicable in many cases, is to throw out the silver by hydrochloric acid, alkalise the filtrate by bicarbonate of soda, and titrate with iodine solution. The latter is made by dissolving exactly 12.7 grms. of pure dry iodine by the aid of 18 grms. of potassic iodide in one litre of water, observing that the solution must take place in the cold, without the application of heat. The principle of the titration is, that arsenious acid, in the presence of water and free alkali, is converted into arsenic acid—

$$As_2O_3 + 4I + 2Na_2O = As_2O_5 + 4NaI.$$

The end of the reaction is known by adding a little starch-paste to the solution; as soon as a blue colour appears, the process is finished.

Another convenient way by which (in very dilute solutions of arsenious acid) the arsenic may be determined,

[784] Nitrate of silver solution is reduced by H_2, CH_3, PH_3, and SbH_3; hence it is absolutely necessary in any qualitative examination to prove that arsenious acid has actually been produced in the silver solution.

is a colorimetric method, which depends on the fact that sulphuretted hydrogen, when arsenious acid is present in small quantity, produces no precipitate at first, but a yellow colour, proportionate to the amount of arsenic present. The silver solution containing arsenious acid is freed from silver by hydrochloric acid; a measured quantity of saturated SH_2 water is added to a fractional and, if necessary, diluted portion, in a Nessler cylinder or colorimetric apparatus, and the colour produced exactly imitated, by the aid of a dilute solution of arsenious acid, added from a burette to a similar quantity of SH_2 water in another cylinder, the fluid being acidified with HCl.

§ 744. **Destruction of the Organic Matter by Nitric Acid, and Subsequent Reduction of the Arsenic Acid to Arsine (Arseniuretted Hydrogen), and final Estimation as Metallic Arsenic.**—This process, which is essentially a combination of several, has been much improved in its details by R. H. Chittenden and H. H. Donaldson.[785] 100 grms. of the suspected matters, cut up into small pieces, are heated in a porcelain dish of suitable size, stirred by means of a glass rod with 23 c.c. of pure concentrated nitric acid, and heated up to from 150° to 160°. When the matters assume a yellow or orange colour, the bath is removed from the source of heat, and 3 c.c. of pure concentrated sulphuric acid added, and the mixture stirred, when the mass becomes brown, swells up, and evolves dense nitrous and other fumes. The vessel is again heated to 180°, and while hot 8 c.c. of pure concentrated nitric acid are added, drop by drop, with continual stirring. After this addition, it is heated to 200° for fifteen minutes, and the result on cooling is a hard carbonaceous residue wholly free from nitric acid. The arsenic is in this way oxidised into arsenic acid, which is easily soluble in water. The contents of the dish are, therefore, perfectly extracted by boiling water, the aqueous extract filtered, and evaporated to dryness. The next process is to obtain the arsenic in a metallic state:—

The flask, a Bunsen's wash-bottle of 200 c.c. capacity, is provided with a small separating funnel of 65 c.c. capacity, with glass stop-cock. This is a very material aid to the obtaining of a slow and even evolution of gas, an important desideratum when all loss is to be avoided; for with only a funnel tube, every time a small portion of fluid is added, a sudden rush of gas takes place, with probably a small, but still more or less appreciable, loss. But the separating funnel, filled with the acid mixture, can be so arranged as to give a constant and regular supply of fluid at the rate of two or three drops per minute, more or less. The gas generated is dried by a calcic chloride tube, and then passes through a tube of hard glass, heated to a red heat by a miniature furnace of three Bunsen lamps with spread burners, so that a continuous flame of 6 inches is obtained, and with a proper length of cooled tube not a trace of arsenic passes by. The glass tube where heated is wound with a strip of wire gauze, both ends being supported upon the edges of the lamp frame, so that the tube does not sink down when heated. The small furnace is provided with two appropriate side pieces of sheet metal, so that a steady flame is always obtained. When the quantity of arsenic is very small, the tube is naturally so placed that the mirror is deposited in the narrow portion; but when the arsenic is present to the extent of 0.005 grm., the tube should be 6 mm. in inner diameter, and so arranged that fully 2 inches of this large tube are between the flame and the narrow portion. When the quantity of arsenic is less, the tube can naturally be smaller.

Acids of different strengths are made as follows:—

Acid No. 1.

545 c.c. pure conc. H_2SO_4.
5000 c.c. H_2O.

Acid No. 2.

109 c.c. pure conc. H_2SO_4.
1640 c.c. Acid No. 1.

Acid No. 3.

218 c.c. pure conc. H_2SO_4.
1640 c.c. Acid No. 1.

[785] *American Chem. Journ.*, vol. ii., No. 4; *Chem. News*, Jan. 1881, p. 21.

Acid No. 4.

530 c.c. pure conc. H_2SO_4.
1248 c.c. H_2O.

25 to 35 grms. of granulated zinc, previously alloyed with a small quantity of platinum, are placed in the generator, and everything being in position, the apparatus is filled with hydrogen by the use of a small quantity of acid No. 2. After a sufficient time has elapsed, the gas is lighted at the jet, and the glass tube heated to a bright redness.

The arsenical solution in concentrated form is mixed with 45 c.c. of acid No. 2, and the mixture passed into the separating funnel, from which it is allowed to flow into the generator at such a rate that the entire fluid is introduced in one hour or one and a half; 40 c.c. of acid No. 3 are then added and allowed to flow slowly into the generator, and, lastly, 45 c.c. of acid No. 4. The amount of time required will vary with the amount of arsenic: 2 to 3 mgrms. of arsenic will require about two to three hours for the entire decomposition, while 4 to 5 mgrms. will need perhaps three to four hours. Where the amount of arsenic is small, only 25 grms. of zinc are needed, and but 45 c.c. of acid No. 2, 30 c.c. of acid No. 3, and 30 c.c. of acid No. 4; but when 4 to 5 mgrms. of arsenic are present, it is better to take the first mentioned quantities of zinc and acids.

The arsenic being thus collected as a large or small mirror of metal, the tube is cut at a safe distance from the mirror, so that a tube of perhaps 2 to 6 grms. weight is obtained. This is carefully weighed, and then the arsenic removed by simple heating; or, if the arsenic is to be saved (as in a toxicological case), dissolved out with strong nitric acid. The tube is then cleaned, dried, and again weighed, the difference giving the weight of metallic arsenic, from which, by a simple calculation, the amount of arsenious oxide can be obtained. Some test results are given as follows; they were obtained by introducing definite quantities of arsenious oxide in the form of a solution mixed with 45 c.c. of No. 2 acid, &c.:—

Quantity of Arsenic introduced.	Wt. of Metallic Arsenic found.	Theoretical Wt. of Metallic Arsenic.
0.005 grm. As_2O_3	0.00373	0.00378
0.005 „ „	0.00370	0.00378
0.004 „ „	0.00300	0.00303
0.002 „ „	0.00151	0.00151

Sanger estimates and tests for minute quantities of arsenic by the Marsh-Berzelius process, and uses a generator of hydrogen; that is to say, the hydrogen is evolved in the ordinary way from zinc and sulphuric acid, and the issuing gas dried by calcic chloride; but into this flask is also delivered from another flask, charged with sulphuric acid and zinc, pure hydrogen, so that into the second flask, little by little, may be added the solution to be tested; and, owing to the generating flask, the gas may be made to give a uniform current, and at the end of the operation all arsine swept out. To estimate the quantities of arsenic in the gas, the reduction tube is heated, and a mirror or mirrors obtained, and compared with a set of standard mirrors. The standard mirrors are made as follows:—One grm. of arsenious oxide, purified by repeated sublimation, is dissolved with the aid of a little sodic bicarbonate, and, after acidification with dilute sulphuric acid, made up to 1 litre. This standard solution contains 1 mgrm. of As_2O_3 in every c.c., and is used to make a second standard solution, containing 0.01 mgrm., to every c.c., by diluting 10 c.c. to a litre. Of this last solution, 1 c.c., 2 c.c., 3 c.c., and so on, are measured and introduced into the reduction flask, and the standard mirrors obtained. It is recommended, for obvious reasons, to make more than one standard for each quantity, for the appearance of the mirrors from the same amount of arsenic varies. The tubes are hermetically sealed, and, when not in use, kept in the dark.

This process is convenient for small amounts of arsenic; but, as stated before, the results are given as metallic arsenic, whereas the films appear never to be composed of pure metallic arsenic, but a mixture of hydride and suboxide. Test experiments give, however, fair results.[786]

§ 745. **Arsine Developed from an Alkaline Solution.**—Fleitmann discovered in 1851 that arsenic, mixed with finely divided zinc, and excess of soda or potash added, evolved arsine; but no stibine was evolved under the same conditions. In 1873 J. W. Gatehouse suggested the use of aluminium and sodic hydrate as a modification of

[786] *Proc. American Academy of Arts and Sciences*, vol. xxvi.

Fleitmann's test, for the purpose of distinguishing between arsenic and antimony; and this is now the usual process adopted. The hydrogen comes off regularly even in the cold, but it is best to apply a little heat. This test will evolve arsine from arsenious acid, and also from arsenic trisulphide; but it is not available for the detection of arsenic, when the arsenic is in the form of arsenic acid. According to Clark,[787] it is not adapted for quantitative purposes, because, owing to the formation of solid hydride, about one-fifth remains behind.

E. W. Davy, in 1876, proposed the use of sodium amalgam for the generation of arsine; on the whole, it is, however, not so convenient as the aluminium process.

The liquid to be tested is made strongly alkaline with pure sodic or potassic hydrate placed in a flask connected with a tube dipping into a 4 per cent. solution of silver nitrate, a few pieces of sheet aluminium added, and the flask gently heated; any arsine present will reduce the silver. The silver solution thus blackened may be treated in the manner described.

§ 746. **Precipitation as Tersulphide.**—Despite the advantages of some of the processes described, which are (to a certain extent) easy and accurate, not a few chemists still prefer the old method of precipitation with hydric sulphide SH_2, because, although tedious, it has stood the test of experience. If this be used, it is well in most cases to pass sulphurous anhydride through the liquid until it smells strongly of the gas, for by this means any arsenic acid present is reduced, the sulphurous anhydride is quickly got rid of by a current of carbonic anhydride, and then the liquid is saturated with hydric sulphide. In the ordinary way, much time is often wasted in saturating the liquid with this gas. Those, however, who have large laboratories, and daily employ hydric sulphide, possess (or should possess) a water saturated with the gas under pressure; such a liquid, added in equal volume to an arsenical solution, is able to convert the whole of the arsenic into sulphide in a very few minutes. Those who do not possess this hydric sulphide water can saturate in an hour the liquid to be tested, by passing the gas in under pressure.[788] A convenient method is to evolve SH_2 from sulphide of antimony and ClH; the gas passes first into a wash-bottle, and then into a strong flask containing the solution under trial. This flask is furnished with a safety-valve, proportioned to the strength of the apparatus; the two tubes dipping into the wash-bottle and the last flask are provided with Bunsen's valves, which only allow the gas to pass in one direction. The hydric sulphide is then driven over by heat, and when sufficient gas has in this way passed into the liquid, the flame is withdrawn, and the apparatus allowed to stand for some hours, the valves preventing any backward flow of the liquid or gas. When the precipitate has settled to the bottom, the supernatant fluid is carefully passed through a filter, and the precipitate washed by decantation in the flask, without transference to the filter, if it can be avoided.

The impure sulphide is washed with water, then with alcohol, then with carbon disulphide, then, after having got rid of the lead, again with alcohol, and finally with water; it is then dissolved in ammonia, the ammonia solution filtered, and the filtrate evaporated to dryness on a sand-bath, at a somewhat high temperature; in this way it is freed from sulphur and, to a great extent, from organic matter; after weighing, it may be purified or identified by some of the following methods:—

(*a*) **Solution in Ammonia and Estimation by Iodine.**[789]—The filter is pierced, the sulphide washed into a flask by ammonia water (which need not be concentrated), and dissolved by warming, filtered from any insoluble matter, and estimated by iodine and starch.

(*b*) **Oxidation of the Sulphide and Precipitation as Ammonia Magnesian Arseniate, or Magnesia Pyro-Arseniate.**—The tersulphide, as before, is dissolved in ammonia (not omitting the filter-paper, which should be soaked in this reagent), the solution filtered, and evaporated to dryness. The dry residue is now oxidised by fuming nitric acid, taking care to protect the dish with a large watch-glass (or other cover) during the first violent action; the dish is then heated in the water-bath until all the sulphur has disappeared, and only a small bulk of the liquid remains; it is then diluted and precipitated by "magnesia mixture."[790] The fluid must stand for several hours, and, if

[787] *Journ. Chem. Soc.*, 1893, 884.

[788] Hydric sulphide gas has been liquefied, and is now an article of commerce, being sold in iron bottles.

[789] P. Champion and H. Pellett, *Bull. Soc. Chim.* (2), xxvj. pp. 541-544.

[790] Magnesia Mixture:—

Sulphate of magnesia,	1
Chloride of ammonium,	1
Solution of ammonia,	4
Water,	8

Dissolve; then allow to stand for several days; finally filter, and keep for use.

the arsenic is to be determined as the usual ammoniacal salt, it must be passed through a weighed filter, and washed with a little ammoniacal water (1 : 3). The solubility of the precipitate is considerable, and for every 16 c.c. of the filtrate (not the washings) 1 mgrm. must be allowed. The precipitate, dried at 100°, $2(NH_4MgAsO_4)H_2O$, represents 39.47 per cent. metallic arsenic.

The solubility of the magnesium arseniate itself, and the general dislike which chemists have to weighing in such hygroscopic material as a filter, are, perhaps, the main reasons for the variation of this old method, which has lately come into notice. Rose proposed some time ago the conversion of the double salt into the pyro-arseniate—a method condemned by Fresenius and Parnell, but examined and pronounced a practicable and accurate process by Remol, Rammelsberg, Thorpe, Fuller, Wittstein, Emerson, Macivor, Wood, and Brauner. The modification of Rose's process, recommended by Wood,[791] and still further improved by Brauner,[792] may be accepted.

The precipitation is effected by magnesia mixture, with the addition of half its bulk of alcohol. The solution is allowed to stand for several hours, until it is possible to decant the clear liquid from the precipitate; the latter is now dissolved in ClH, reprecipitated as before, thrown on a small filter, and washed with a mixture of one volume of ammonia, two volumes of alcohol, and three of water.

The precipitate is now dried, and transferred as completely as possible from the filter into a small porcelain crucible, included in a larger one made of platinum, moistened with nitric acid, covered and heated at first gently, lastly to a bright redness; the filter is then treated similarly, and the crucible with its contents weighed. Pyro-arseniate of arsenic ($Mg_2As_2O_7$) contains 48.29 per cent. of metallic arsenic.

(*c*) **Conversion of the Trisulphide of Arsenic into the Arsenomolybdate of Ammonia.**—The purified sulphide is oxidised by nitric acid, the acid solution is rendered alkaline by ammonia, and then precipitated by a molybdenum solution, made as follows:—100 grms. of molybdic acid are dissolved in 150 c.c. of ordinary ammonia and 80 of water; this solution is poured drop by drop into 500 c.c. of pure nitric acid and 300 c.c. of water; it is allowed to settle, and, if necessary, filtered. The molybdic solution must be mixed in excess with the liquid under treatment, the temperature raised to 70° or 80°, and nitric acid added in excess until a yellow coloration appears; the liquid is then passed through a tared filter, and dried at 100°. It contains 5.1 per cent. of arsenic acid [3.3 As].[793]

(*d*) **Conversion of the Sulphide into Metallic Arsenic.**—If there should be any doubt as to the nature of the precipitated substances, the very best way of resolving this doubt is to reduce the sulphide to metal; the easiest method of proving this is to dissolve in potash and obtain arsine by the action of aluminium; or if it is desired to evolve arsine from an acid solution with zinc in the usual way, then by dissolving a slight excess of zinc oxide in potash or soda, and dissolving in this the arsenic sulphide; the zinc combines with all the sulphur, and converts the sulpharsenite into arsenite; the zinc sulphide is filtered off, and the filtrate acidified and introduced into Marsh's apparatus. The original process of Fresenius was to mix the sulphide with carbonate of soda and cyanide of potassium, and place the mixture in the wide part of a tube of hard German glass, drawn out at one end to a capillary fineness. Carbonic anhydride, properly dried, was passed through the tube, and the portion containing the mixture heated to redness; in this way the arsenical sulphide was reduced, and the metal condensed in the capillary portion, where the smallest quantity could be recognised. A more elaborate and accurate process, based on the same principles, has been advocated by Mohr.[794]

A convenient quantity of carbonate of soda is added to the sulphide, and the whole mixed with a very little water, and gently warmed. The yellow precipitate is very soon dissolved, and then the whole is evaporated carefully, until it is in a granular, somewhat moist, adhesive state. It is now transferred to a glass tube, open at top and bottom, but the top widened into a funnel; this tube is firmly held perpendicularly on a glass plate, and the prepared sulphide hammered into a compact cylinder by the aid of a glass rod, which just fits the tube. The cylinder is now dried over a flame, until no more moisture is to be detected, and then transferred into a glass tube 4 or 5 inches long, and with one end drawn to a point (the weight of this tube should be first accurately taken). The tube is connected with the following series:—(1) A chloride of calcium tube; (2) a small bottle containing nitrate of silver solution; (3) a hydrogen-generating bottle containing zinc and sulphuric acid. The hydrogen goes through the argentic nitrate solution, leaving behind any sulphur and arsenic it may contain; it is then dried by chloride of calcium, and streams in a pure dry state over the cylinder of prepared sulphide (no error with regard to impurities in the gas is likely to

[791] *Zeitschrift für anal. Chem.*, vol. xiv. p. 356.
[792] *Ibid.*, xvj. pp. 57, 58.
[793] Champion and Pellett, *Bull. Soc. Chim.*, Jan. 7, 1877.
[794] Mohr's *Toxicologie*, p. 57.

occur; but in rigid inquiries it is advisable to heat a portion of the tube, previous to the insertion of the cylinder, for some time, in order to prove the absence of any external arsenical source); when it is certain that pure hydrogen, unmixed with air, is being evolved, the portion of the tube in which the cylinder rests is heated slowly to redness, and the metallic arsenic sublimes at a little distance from the source of heat. Loss is inevitable if the tube is too short, or the stream of hydrogen too powerful.

The tube after the operation is divided, the portion soiled by the soda thoroughly cleansed, and then both parts weighed; the difference between the weight of the empty tube and the tube + arsenic gives the metallic arsenic. This is the process as recommended by Mohr; it may, however, be pointed out that the glass tube itself loses weight when any portion of it is kept red-hot for some little time; and, therefore, unless the crust is required in the original tube, it is better to divide it, carefully weigh the arsenical portion, remove the crust, and then re-weigh. The method is not perfectly accurate. The mirror is not pure metallic arsenic, and if the white alkaline residue be examined, arsenic will be detected in it, the reason being that the arsenical sulphide generally contains pentasulphide of arsenic as well as free sulphur. Now the pentasulphide does not give up metallic arsenic when treated as before detailed; nor, indeed, does the trisulphide, if mixed with much sulphur, yield an arsenical crust. It is, therefore, of great moment to free the precipitate as much as possible from sulphur, before attempting the reduction.

The development of a reducing gas from a special and somewhat complicated apparatus is not absolutely necessary. The whole process of reduction, from beginning to end, may take place in a single tube by any of the following processes:—(1) The sulphide is mixed with oxalate of soda (a salt which contains no water of crystallisation), and the dry mixture is transferred to a suitable tube, sealed at one end. An arsenical mirror is readily obtained, and, if the heat is continued long enough, no arsenic remains behind—an excellent and easy method, in which the reducing gas is carbonic oxide, in an atmosphere of carbonic anhydride. (2) The sulphide is oxidised by *aqua regia*, and the solution evaporated to complete dryness. The residue is then dissolved in a few drops of water, with the addition of some largish grains of good wood charcoal (which absorb most of the solution), and the whole carefully dried. The mass is now transferred to a tube closed at one end, a little charcoal added in the form of an upper layer, and heat applied first to this upper layer, so as to replace the air with CO_2, and then to bring the whole tube gradually to redness from above downwards. In this case also the whole of the arsenic sublimes as a metallic mirror.

There are various other modifications, but the above are trustworthy, and quite sufficient. Brugelmann's method of determining arsenic, elsewhere described, would appear to possess some advantages, and to promise well; but the writer has had no personal experience of it with regard to arsenic.

§ 747. **Conversion of Arsenic into Arsenious Chloride** ($AsCl_3$).—This process, first employed by Schneider and Fyfe, and afterwards modified by Taylor, differs from all the preceding, since an attempt is made to separate by one operation volatile metallic chlorides, and to destroy the organic matter, and thus obtain two liquids—one a distillate—tolerably clear and free from solid particles, whilst the mass in the retort retains such metals as copper, and is in every way easy to deal with.

Schneider and Fyfe employed sulphuric acid and common salt; but Taylor recommends hydrochloric acid, which is in every respect preferable. As recommended by Taylor, all matters, organic or otherwise, are to be completely desiccated before their introduction into a retort, and on these dried substances sufficient pure hydrochloric acid poured, and the distillation pushed to dryness. Every one is well aware how tedious is the attempt to dry perfectly the organs of the body (such as liver, &c.) at any temperature low enough to ensure against volatilisation of such a substance as, *e.g.*, calomel. This drying has, therefore, been the great stumbling-block which has prevented the general application of the process. It will be found, however, that drying in the ordinary way is by no means necessary. The writer cuts up the solid organ (such as liver, brain, &c.) with scissors into small pieces, and transfers them to a retort fitted by an air-tight joint to a Liebig condenser; the condenser in its turn being connected with a flask by a tube passing through an india-rubber stopper dipping into a little water. Another tube from the same flask is connected with india-rubber piping, which is connected with a water-pump, the fall tube of which terminates in the basement of a house over a gully. The distillation is now carried on to carbonisation; on cooling, a second quantity of hydrochloric acid is added, and the last fraction of the distillate examined for arsenic. If any is found, a third distillation is necessary. At the termination of the operation the retort is washed with water, the solution filtered, and this solution and the distillate are each separately examined for arsenic. If properly performed, however, the second distillation brings over the whole of the arsenical chloride,[795] and none will be found in the retort. With the above arrangement there can be no odour, nor is there any loss of substance. In the distillate the arsenic can hardly be in the form of arsenious chloride, but rather arsenious acid and hydrochloric acid; for the chloride easily splits up in the presence of water into these substances. It is best to convert it into the trisulphide. Taylor[796] recommends evolving arsine in the usual way, and passing the arsine (AsH_3) into solution of silver nitrate, finally estimating it as an arseniate of silver. Objections with regard to the impurity of reagents should be met by blank experiments. Kaiser[797] has proposed and practised a modification of this method, which essentially consists in the use of sulphuric acid and sodic chloride (as in Schneider and Fyfe's original process), and in passing the distillate first into a flask containing a crystal or two of potassium chlorate, and thence into an absorption bulb; in the latter most of the arsenic is found in the form of arsenic acid, the chloride having been oxidised in its passage. The apparatus is, however, complicated in this way without a corresponding advantage.[798] Lastly, E. Fischer[799] has shown that it is a considerable advantage to add from 10 to 20 c.c. of a saturated solution of ferrous chloride before distilling with HCl. In this way all the arsenic, whether as arsenic or arsenious acids, is easily converted into chloride.

2. ANTIMONY.

§ 748. **Metallic Antimony.**—Atomic weight, 120.3 (R. Schneider), 120.14 (Cook[800]); specific gravity, 6.715; fusing-point about 621° (1150° F.). In the course of analysis, metallic antimony may be seen as a black powder thrown down from solutions; as a film deposited on copper or platinum; and, lastly, as a ring on the inside of a tube from the decomposition of stibine. At a bright red-heat it is volatilised slowly, even when hydrogen is passed over it; chlorine, bromine, and iodine combine with it directly. It may be boiled in concentrated ClH without solution; but *aqua regia*, sulphides of potassium and sodium readily dissolve it. The distinction between thin films of this metal and of arsenic on copper and glass are pointed out earlier. It is chiefly used in the arts for purposes of alloy, and enters to a small extent into the composition of fireworks.

§ 749. **Antimonious Sulphide.**—Sulphide of antimony = 336; composition in 100 parts, Sb 71.76, S 28.24. The commercial article, known under the name of black antimony, is the native sulphide, freed from silicious matter by fusion, and afterwards pulverised. It is a crystalline metallic-looking powder, of a steel-grey colour, and is often much contaminated with iron, lead, copper, and arsenic.

The amorphous sulphide (as obtained by saturating a solution of tartar emetic with SH_2) is an orange-red powder, soluble in potash and in ammonic, sodic, and potassic sulphides; and dissolving also in concentrated hydrochloric acid with evolution of SH_2. It is insoluble in water and dilute acid, scarcely dissolves in carbonate of ammonia, and is quite insoluble in potassic bisulphite. If ignited gently in a stream of carbonic acid gas, the weight remains constant. To render it anhydrous, a heat of 200° is required.

The recognition of arsenic in the commercial sulphide is most easily effected by placing 2 grms. or more in a suitable retort (with condenser), adding hydrochloric acid, and distilling. The chloride of arsenic passes over before the chloride of antimony; and by not raising the heat too high, very little antimony will come over, even if the distillation be carried almost to dryness. The arsenic is detected in the distillate by the ordinary methods.

Several lamentable accidents have happened through mistaking the sulphide of antimony for oxide of manganese, and using it with potassic chlorate for the production of oxygen. The addition of a drop of hydrochloric acid, it is scarcely necessary to say, will distinguish between the two.

Antimony is frequently estimated as sulphide. An amorphous tersulphide of mercury, containing a small admixture of antimonious oxide and sulphide of potassium, is known under the name of *Kermes mineral*, and has lately been employed in the vulcanising of india-rubber. Prepared in this way, the latter may be used for various

[795] Dragendorff asserts to the contrary; but we may quote the authority of Taylor, who has made several experiments, in which he obtained all the arsenic as chloride. The writer has performed the process many times, each time carefully testing the mass in the retort for arsenic; but the result proved that it had entirely passed over.

[796] *Principles of Medical Jurisprudence*, vol. i. p. 267.

[797] *Zeitschr. f. anal. Chem.*, xiv. pp. 250-281.

[798] Selmi (*Atti dell. Accademia dei Lincei*, Fasc. ii., 1879) proposed a modification of Schneider's process. The substances are treated with hot, pure sulphuric acid, and at the same time the liquid is traversed by a stream of hydrochloric acid gas. The resulting distillate is tested for arsenic by Marsh's process. Selmi states that, operating in this way, he has detected $^1/_{400}$ of a mgrm. of As_2O_3 in 100 grms. of animal matter.

[799] *Scheidung u. Bestimmung d. Arsens*; Liebig's *Annalen d. Chemie*, Bd. ccvii. p. 182.

[800] *Ann. Phys. Chem.* (2), v. pp. 255-281.

purposes, and thus become a source of danger. It behoves the analyst, therefore, in searching for antimony, to take special care not to use any india-rubber fittings which might contain the preparation.

A *pentasulphide of antimony* (from the decomposition of Schleppe's salt [$Na_3Sb_6S_4 + 9H_2O$], when heated with an acid) is used in calico-printing.

§ 750. **Tartarated Antimony, Tartrate of Potash and Antimony, or Tartar Emetic**, is, in a medico-legal sense, the most important of the antimonial salts. Its formula is $KSbC_4H_4O_7H_2O$, and 100 parts, theoretically, should contain 35.2 per cent. of metallic antimony. The B.P. gives a method of estimation of tartar emetic not free from error, and Professor Dunstan has proposed the following:—Dissolve 0.3 grm. of tartar emetic in 80 c.c. of water, add to this 10 c.c. of a 5 per cent. solution of sodium bicarbonate, and immediately titrate with a decinormal solution of iodine, using starch as an indicator. One c.c. of $^{n}/_{10}$ iodine = 0.0166 grm. tartar emetic; therefore, if pure, the quantity used by 0.3 grm. should be 18 c.c. Tartar emetic occurs in commerce in colourless, transparent, rhombic, octahedral crystals, slightly efflorescing in dry air.

A crystal, placed in the subliming cell, decrepitates at 193.3° (380° F.), sublimes at 248.8° (480° F.) very slowly and scantily, and chars at a still higher temperature, 287.7° (550° F.). On evaporating a few drops of a solution of tartar emetic, and examining the residue by the microscope, the crystals are either tetrahedra, cubes, or branched figures. 100 parts of cold water dissolve 5 of tartar emetic, whilst the same quantity of boiling water dissolves ten times as much, viz., 50. The watery solution decomposes readily with the formation of algæ; it gives no precipitate with ferrocyanide of potassium, chloride of barium, or nitrate of silver, unless concentrated.

§ 751. **Metantimonic Acid**, so familiar to the practical chemist from its insoluble sodium salt, is technically applied in the painting of glass, porcelain, and enamels; and in an impure condition, as antimony ash, to the glazing of earthenware.

§ 752. **Pharmaceutical, Veterinary, and Quack Preparations of Antimony.**[801]

(1) **Pharmaceutical Preparations**:—

Oxide of Antimony (Sb_2O_3) is a white powder, fusible at a low red heat, and soluble without effervescence in hydrochloric acid, the solution responding to the ordinary tests for antimony. Arsenic may be present in it as an impurity; the readiest means of detection is to throw small portions at a time on glowing charcoal, when very small quantities of arsenic will, under such conditions, emit the peculiar odour. Carbonate of lime appears also to have been found in the oxide of commerce.

Antimonial Powder is composed of one part of oxide of antimony and two parts of phosphate of lime; in other words, it ought to give 33.3 per cent. of Sb_2O_3.

Tartar Emetic itself has been already described. The preparations used in medicine are—

The Wine of Antimony (Vinum antimoniale), which is a solution of tartar emetic in sherry wine, and should contain 2 grains of the salt in each ounce of the wine (0.45 grm. in 100 c.c.).

Antimony Ointment (Unguentum antimonii tartarati) is a mechanical mixture of tartar emetic and lard, or simple ointment;[802] strength 20 per cent. There is no recorded case of conviction for the adulteration of tartar emetic; cream of tartar is the only probable addition. In such a case the mixture is less soluble than tartar emetic itself, and on adding a small quantity of carbonate of soda to a boiling solution of the suspected salt, the precipitated oxide at first thrown down, becomes redissolved.

Solution of Chloride of Antimony is a solution of the terchloride in hydrochloric acid; it is a heavy liquid of a yellowish-red colour, powerfully escharotic; its specific gravity is 1.47; on dilution with water, the whitish-yellow oxychloride of antimony is precipitated. One drachm (3.549 c.c.) mixed with 4 ounces (112 c.c.) of a solution of tartaric acid (.25 : 4) gives a precipitate with SH_2, which weighs *at least* 22 grains (1.425 grm.). This liquid is used on very rare occasions as an outward application by medical men; farriers sometimes employ it in the foot-rot of sheep.

Purified Black Antimony (Antimonium nigrum purificatum) is the purified native sulphide Sb_2S_3; it should be absolutely free from arsenic.

Sulphurated Antimony (Antimonium sulphuratum) is a mixture of sulphide of antimony, Sb_2S_3, with a small and variable amount of oxide, Sb_2O_3. The P.B. states that 60 grains (3.888 grms.) dissolved in ClH, and poured into

[801] The history of antimony as a drug is curious. Its use was prohibited in France in 1566, because it was considered poisonous, one Besnier being actually expelled from the faculty for transgressing the law on this point. The edict was repealed in 1650; but in 1668 there was a fresh enactment, confining its use to the doctors of the faculty.

[802] Simple ointment is composed of white wax 2, lard 3, almond oil 3 parts.

water, should give a white precipitate of oxychloride of antimony, which (properly washed and dried) weighs about 53 grains (3.444 grms.). The officinal compound pill of subchloride of mercury (*Pilula hydrargyri subchloridi composita*) contains 1 grain (.0648 grm.) of sulphurated antimony in every 5 grains (.324 grm.), *i.e.*, 20 per cent.

(2) **Patent and Quack Pills**:—

Dr. J. Johnson's Pills.—From the formula each pill should contain:—

	Grains.		Grms.
Compound Extract of Colocynth,	2 .5	=	.162
Calomel,	.62	=	.039
Tartar Emetic,	.04	=	.002
Oil of Cassia,	.12	=	.007
	3 .28	=	.210

The oil of cassia can be extracted by petroleum ether; the calomel sublimed and identified by the methods given in the article on "Mercury"; the antimony deposited in the metallic state on platinum or tin; and the colocynth extracted by dissolving in water, acidifying, and shaking up with chloroform. On evaporating the chloroform the residue should taste extremely bitter; dissolved in sulphuric acid it changes to a red colour, and dissolved in Fröhde's reagent to a cherry-red. It should also have the ordinary reactions of a glucoside.

Mitchell's Pills contain in each pill:—

	Grains.		Grms.
Aloes,	1 .1	=	.070
Rhubarb,	1 .6	=	.103
Calomel,	.16	=	.010
Tartar Emetic,	.05	=	.003
	2 .91	=	.186

The mineral substances in this are easy of detection by the methods already given; the aloes by the formation of chrysammic acid, and the rhubarb by its microscopical characters.

Dixon's Pills probably contain the following in each pill:—

	Grains.		Grms.
Compound Extract of Colocynth,	2 .0	=	.1296
Rhubarb,	1 .0	=	.0648
Tartar Emetic,	.06	=	.0038
	3 .06	=	.1982

(3) **Antimonial Medicines, chiefly Veterinary**:[803]—

Liver of Antimony is a preparation formerly much used by farriers. It is a mixture of antimonious oxide, sulphide of potassium, carbonate of potassium, and undecomposed trisulphide of antimony (and may also contain sulphate of potassium), all in very undetermined proportions. When deprived of the soluble potash salts, it becomes the *washed saffron of antimony* of the old pharmacists. A receipt for a grease-ball, in a modern veterinary work, gives, with liver of antimony, cream of tartar and guaiacum as ingredients.

Hind's Sweating-ball is composed of 60 grains (3.888 grms.) of tartar emetic and an equal portion of assafœtida, made up into a ball with liquorice-powder and syrup. The assafœtida will be readily detected by the odour, and the antimony by the methods already recommended.

Ethiops of Antimony, very rarely used now, is the mechanical mixture of the sulphides of antimony and

[803] There has long prevailed an idea (the truth of which is doubtful) that antimony given to animals improves their condition; thus, the *Encyclop. Brit.*, 5th ed., art. "Antimony":—"A horse that is lean and scrubby, and not to be fatted by any means, will become fat on taking a dose of antimony every morning for two months together. A boar fed for brawn, and having an ounce of antimony given him every morning, will become fat a fortnight sooner than others put into the stye at the same time, and fed in the same manner, but without the antimony." Probably the writer means by the term *antimony* the impure sulphide. To this may be added the undoubted fact, that in Brunswick the breeders of fat geese add a small quantity of antimonious oxide to the food, as a traditional custom.

mercury—proportions, 3 of the former to 2 of the latter.

The Flowers of Antimony is an impure oxysulphide of antimony, with variable proportions of trioxide and undecomposed trisulphide.

Diaphoretic Antimony (calcined antimony) is simply antimoniate of potash.

Glass of Antimony is a mixture of sulphide and oxide of antimony, contaminated with a small quantity of silica and iron.

A quack pill, by name, **Ward's Red Pill**, is said to contain glass of antimony and dragon's blood.

Antimonial Compounds used in Pyrotechny:—

Blue Fire:—

Antimonious sulphide,	1
Sulphur,	2
Nitre,	6

This composition is used for the blue or Bengal signal-light at sea. Bisulphide of carbon and water are solvents which will easily separate the powder into its three constituents.

Crimson Fire:—

Potassic Chlorate,	17.25
Alder or Willow Charcoal,	4.5
Sulphur,	18.
Nitrate of Strontia,	55.
Antimonious Sulphide,	5.5

The spectroscope will readily detect strontia and potassium, and the analysis presents no difficulty. In addition to these a very great number of other pyrotechnical preparations contain antimony.

§ 753. **Alloys.**—Antimony is much used in alloys. The ancient *Pocula emetica*, or everlasting emetic cups, were made of antimony, and with wine standing in them for a day or two, they acquired emetic properties. The principal antimonial alloys are Britannia and type metal, the composition of which is as follows:—

		Tin, per cent.	Copper, per cent.	Antimony, per cent.
Britannia Metal,	Best,	92.0	1.8	6.2
	Common,	92.1	2.0	5.9
	For Castings,	92.9	1.8	5.3
	For Lamps,	94.0	1.3	4.7

		Tea Lead, per cent.	Antimony, per cent.	Block Tin, per cent.
Type Metal, -	(1.)	75	20	5
	(2.)	70	25	5
Metal for Stereotype,		84.2	13.5	2.3

There is also antimony in brass, concave mirrors, bell-metal, &c.

§ 754. **Pigments.**—Cassella and Naples yellow are principally composed of the antimoniate of lead.

Antimony Yellow is a mixture of antimoniate of lead with basic chloride of lead.

§ 755. **Dose.**—A medicinal dose of a soluble antimonial salt should not exceed 97.2 mgrms. (1½ grain). With circumstances favouring its action, a dose of 129.6 mgrms. (2 grains) has proved fatal;[804] but this is quite exceptional, and few medical men would consider so small a quantity dangerous for a healthy adult, especially since most posological tables prescribe tartar emetic as an emetic in doses from 64.8 to 194.4 mgrms. (1 to 3 grains). The smallest dose which has killed a child appears to be 48.5 mgrms. (¾ grain).[805] The dose of tartar emetic for horses and cattle is very large, as much as 5.832 grms. (90 grains) being often given to a horse in his gruel three times a

[804] Taylor, Guy's Hosp. Reports, Oct. 1857.

[805] Op. cit.

day. 3.8 grms. (60 grains) are considered a full, but not an excessive, dose for cattle; .38 grm. (6 grains) is used as an emetic for pigs, and half this quantity for dogs.

§ 756. **Effects of Tartar Emetic and of Antimony Oxide on Animals.**—Large doses of tartar emetic act on the warm-blooded animals as on man; whether the poison is taken by the mouth, or injected subcutaneously, all animals able to vomit[806] do so. The heart's action, at first quickened, is afterwards slowed, weakened, and lastly paralysed. This action is noticed in cold as well as in warm-blooded animals. It is to be ascribed to a direct action on the heart; for if the brain and spinal cord of the frog be destroyed—or even if a solution of the salt be applied direct to the frog's heart separated from the body—the effect is the same. The weak action of the heart, of course, causes the blood-pressure to diminish, and the heart stops in diastole. The voluntary muscles of the body are also weakened; the breathing is affected, partly from the action on the muscles. The temperature of the body is depressed (according to F. A. Falck's researches) from 4.4° to 6.2°.

The effect of small doses given repeatedly to animals has been several times investigated. Dr. Nevin[807] experimented upon eleven rabbits, giving them tartar emetic four times a day in doses of 32.4 mgrms. (½ grain), 64.8 mgrms. (1 grain), and 129.6 mgrms. (2 grains). Five died, the first after four, the last after seventeen days; three were killed after one, three, and four days respectively, two after an interval of fourteen days, and one thirty-one days after taking the last dose. There was no vomiting; diarrhœa was present in about half the number; one of the rabbits, being with young, aborted. The chief symptoms were general dulness, loss of appetite, and in a few days great emaciation. Four of the five that died were convulsed before death, and several of the animals exhibited ulcers of the mucous membrane of the mouth, in places with which the powder had come in contact. Caillol and Livon have also studied the action of small doses of the white oxide of antimony given in milk to cats. A cat took in this way in 109 days .628 grm. The animal passed gradually into a cachectic state, diarrhœa supervened, and it died miserably thin and exhausted.

§ 757. **Effects of Tartar Emetic on Man.**[808]—The analogy between the symptoms produced by arsenic and antimony is striking, and in some acute cases of poisoning by tartar emetic, there is but little (if any) clinical difference. If the dose of tartar emetic is very large, there may be complete absence of vomiting, or only a single evacuation of the stomach. Thus, in a case mentioned by Taylor, in which a veterinary surgeon swallowed by mistake 13 grms. (200 grains) of tartar emetic, vomiting after fifteen minutes could only be induced by tickling the throat. So, again, in the case reported by Mr. Freer, a man, aged 28, took 7.77 grms. (120 grains) of tartar emetic by mistake for Epsom salts; he vomited only once; half an hour after taking the poison he had violent pain in the stomach and abdomen, and spasmodic contraction of the abdomen and arms; the fingers were firmly contracted, the muscles quite rigid, and there was involuntary aqueous purging. After six hours, during which he was treated with green tea, brandy, and decoction of oak-bark, he began to recover, but suffered for many nights from profuse perspirations.

With more moderate and yet large doses, nausea and vomiting are very prominent symptoms, and are seldom delayed more than half an hour. The regular course of symptoms may therefore be summed up thus:—A metallic

---

[806] L. Hermann (*Lehrbuch der experimentellen Toxicologie*) remarks that the vomiting must be considered as a reflex action from the inflammatory excitement of the digestive apparatus, especially of the stomach. It is witnessed if the poison is administered subcutaneously or injected into the brain. Indeed, it is established that (at least, so far as the muscles are concerned) the co-ordinated movements producing vomiting are caused by excitement of the medulla oblongata. Giannussi and others found that after section between the first and third vertebræ of dogs, and subsequent administration of tartar emetic, no vomiting took place; and Grimm's researches seem to show that the suspected *vomit-centre* is identical with the respiratory centre, so that the vomiting movement is only an abnormal respiratory movement. L. Hermann, however, considers the theory that when tartar emetic is introduced into the vessels the *vomit-centre* is directly excited, erroneous, for (1) in introducing it by the veins much larger doses are required to excite vomiting than by the stomach; and (2), after subcutaneous injection of the salt, antimony is found in the first vomit. His explanation, therefore, is that antimony is excreted by the intestinal tract, and in its passage excites this action. Majendie's well-known experiment—demonstrating that, after extirpation of the stomach, vomiting movements were noticed—is not considered opposed to this view.

[807] Lever, *Med. Chir. Journ.*, No. 1.

[808] Antimony occasionally finds its way into articles of food through obscure channels. Dr. Page has recorded the fact of antimonial lozenges having been sold openly by an itinerant vendor of confectionery. Each lozenge contained nearly a quarter of a grain (.16 mgrms.), and they caused well-marked symptoms of poisoning in the case of a servant and two children. How the antimony got in was unknown. In this case it appears to have existed not as tartar emetic, but as an insoluble oxide, for it would not dialyse in aqueous solution.—"On a remarkable instance of Poisoning by means of Lozenges containing Antimony," by David Page, M.D., Medical Officer of Health, *Lancet*, vol. i., 1879, p. 699.

taste in the mouth, repeated vomitings, which are sometimes bloody, great faintness and depression, pains in the abdomen and stomach, and diarrhœa, which may be involuntary. If the case is to terminate fatally, the urine is suppressed, the temperature falls, the face becomes cyanotic, delirium and convulsions supervene, and death occurs in from two to six days. Antimony, like arsenic, often produces a pustular eruption. Solitary cases deviate more or less from the course described, *i.e.*, severe cramps affecting all the muscles, hæmorrhage from the stomach, kidney, or bowel, and death from collapse in a few hours, have all been noticed. In a case recorded by Mr. Morley,[809] a surgeon's daughter, aged 18, took by mistake an unknown quantity of antimonial wine; she soon felt sleepy and powerless, and suffered from the usual symptoms in combination with tetanic spasms of the legs. She afterwards had enteritis for three weeks, and on recovery her hair fell off. Orfila relates a curious case of intense spasm of the gullet from a large dose of tartar emetic.

§ 758. **Chronic Antimonial Poisoning.**—The cases of Palmer and J. P. Cook, M. Mullen, Freeman, Winslow, Pritchard, and the remarkable Bravo case have, in late years, given the subject of chronic antimonial poisoning a considerable prominence. In the trials referred to, it was shown that medical men might easily mistake the effects of small doses of antimony given at intervals for the action of disease—the symptoms being great nausea, followed by vomiting, chronic diarrhœa, alternating with constipation, small frequent pulse, loss of voice, great muscular weakness, depression, with coldness of the skin and a clammy perspiration. In the case of Mrs. Pritchard,[810] her face was flushed, and her manner so excited as to give an ordinary observer the idea that she had been drinking; and with the usual symptoms of vomiting and purging, she suffered from cramps in the hands. Dr. Pritchard tried to make it appear that she was suffering from typhoid fever, which the symptoms in a few respects only resembled.

According to Eulenberg, workmen, exposed for a long period to the vapour of the oxide of antimony, suffer pain in the bladder and a burning sensation in the urethra, and continued inhalation even leads to impotence and wasting of the testicles.[811]

§ 759. **Post-mortem Appearances.**—The effect of large doses of tartar emetic is mainly concentrated upon the gastro-intestinal mucous membrane. There is an example in the museum of University College Hospital of the changes which resulted from the administration of tartar emetic in the treatment of pneumonia. These are ascribed in the catalogue, in part to the local action of the medicine, and in part to the extreme prostration of the patient. In the preparation (No. 1052) the mucous membrane over the fore border of the epiglottis and adjacent part of the pharynx has been destroyed by sloughing; the ulceration extends into the upper part of the œsophagus. About an inch below its commencement, the mucous membrane has been entirely removed by sloughing and ulceration, the circular muscular fibres being exposed. Above the upper limit of this ulcer, the mucous membrane presents several oval, elongated, and ulcerated areas, occupied by strips of mucous membrane which have sloughed. In other places, irregular portions of the mucous membrane, of a dull ashen-gray colour, have undergone sloughing; the edges of the sloughing portion are of colours varying from brown to black.

It is seldom that so much change is seen in the gullet and pharynx as this museum preparation exhibits; but redness, swelling, and the general signs of inflammation are seldom absent from the stomach and some parts of the intestines. On the lining membrane of the mouth, ulcers and pustules have been observed.

In Dr. Nevin's experiments on the chronic poisoning of rabbits already referred to, the *post-mortem* appearances consisted in congestion of the liver in all the rabbits; in nearly all there was vivid redness of the stomach; in two cases there was ulceration; in some, cartilaginous hardness of the pylorus; while, in others, the small intestines presented patches of inflammation. In two of the rabbits the solitary glands throughout the intestines were prominent, yellow in colour, and loaded with antimony. The colon and rectum were healthy, the kidneys congested; the lungs were in most congested, in some actually inflamed, or hepatised and gorged with blood. Bloody extravasations in the chest and abdomen were frequent.

Saikowsky,[812] in feeding animals daily with antimony, found invariably in the course of fourteen to nineteen days fatty degeneration of the liver, and sometimes of the kidney and heart. In the experiment of Caillol and Livon also all the organs were pale, the liver had undergone fatty degeneration, and the lung had its alveoli filled with large degenerated cells, consisting almost entirely of fat. The mesenteric glands also formed large caseous masses,

---

[809] *Brit. Med. Journ.*, Oct. 14, p. 70.

[810] *Edin. Med. Journ.*, 1865.

[811] In the first operations of finishing printers' types, the workmen inhale a metallic dust, which gives rise to effects similar to lead colic; and probably in this case the lead is more active than the associated antimony.

[812] Virchow's *Arch. f. path. Anat.*, Bd. xxv.; also, *Centralblatt f. Med. Wissen.*, No. 23, 1865.

yellowish-white in colour, which, under the microscope, were seen to be composed of fatty cells, so that there is a complete analogy between the action of arsenic and antimony on the body tissues.

§ 760. **Elimination of Antimony.**—Antimony is mainly eliminated by the urine. In 1840, Orfila showed to the *Académie de Médecine* metallic antimony, which he had extracted from a patient who had taken .12 grm. of tartar emetic in twenty-four hours. He also obtained antimony from an old woman, aged 80, who twelve hours before had taken .6 grm. (9¼ grains)—a large dose, which had neither produced vomiting nor purging. In Dr. Kevin's experiments on rabbits, antimony was discovered in the urine after the twelfth dose, and even in the urine of an animal twenty-one days after the administration of the poison had been suspended.

§ 761. **Antidotes for Tartar Emetic.**—Any infusion containing tannin or allied astringent principles, such as decoctions of tea, oak-bark, &c., may be given with advantage in cases of recent poisoning by tartar emetic, for any of the salt which has been expelled by vomiting may in this way be decomposed and rendered harmless. The treatment of acute poisoning which has proved most successful, has been the encouraging of vomiting by tickling the fauces, giving strong green tea and stimulants. (See Appendix.)

§ 762. **Effects of Chloride or Butter of Antimony.**—Only a few cases of poisoning by butter of antimony are on record: its action, generally speaking, on the tissues is like that of an acid, but there has been considerable variety in the symptoms. Five cases are recorded by Taylor; three of the number recovered after taking respectively doses of 7.7 grms. (2 drachms) and 15.5 grms. (4 drachms), and two died after taking from 56.6 to 113 grms. (2 to 4 ounces). In one of these cases the symptoms were more like those of a narcotic poison, in the other fatal case there was abundant vomiting with purging. The autopsy in the first case showed a black appearance from the mouth to the jejunum, as if the parts had been charred, and extensive destruction of the mucous membrane. In the other case there were similar changes in the stomach and the upper part of the intestines, but neither the lips nor the lower end of the gullet were eroded. In a case recorded by Mr. Barrington Cooke,[813] a farmer's wife, aged 40, of unsound mind, managed to elude the watchfulness of her friends, and swallowed an unknown quantity of antimony chloride about 1.30 P.M. Shortly afterwards she vomited several times, and had diarrhœa; at 2.30 a medical man found her lying on her back insensible, and very livid in the face and neck. She was retching, and emitting from her mouth a frothy mucous fluid, mixed with ejected matter of a grumous colour; the breathing was laboured and spasmodic; the pulse could not be felt, and the body was cold and clammy. She expired at 3.30, about one hour and a half from the commencement of symptoms, and probably within two hours from the taking of the poison. The autopsy showed no corrugation of the tongue or inner surface of the lining membrane of the mouth, and no appearance of the action of a corrosive upon the lips, fauces, or mucous membrane of the œsophagus. The whole of the mucous membrane of the stomach was intensely congested, of a dark and almost black colour, the rest of the viscera were healthy. Chemical analysis separated antimony equivalent to nearly a grm. (15 grains) of the chloride, with a small quantity of arsenic, from the contents of the stomach.

§ 763. **Detection of Antimony in Organic Matters.**—In acute poisoning by tartar emetic it is not impossible to find a mere trace only in the stomach, the greater part having been expelled by vomiting, which nearly always occurs early, so that the most certain method is, where possible, to analyse the ejected matters. If it should be suspected that a living person is being slowly poisoned by antimony, it must be remembered that the poison is mainly excreted by the kidneys, and the urine should afford some indication. The readiest way to test is to collect a considerable quantity of the urine (if necessary, two or three days' excretion), concentrate by evaporation, acidify, and then transfer the liquid to a platinum dish, in which is placed a slip of zinc. The whole of the antimony is in time deposited on the platinum dish, and being thus concentrated, may be subsequently identified in any way thought fit.

Organic liquids are boiled with hydrochloric acid; organic solids are extracted with the same acid in the manner described; or, if the distillation process given earlier be employed, the antimony may be found partly in the distillate, and partly in the retort. In any case, antimony in solution may be readily detected in a variety of ways—one of the most convenient being to concentrate on tin or platinum, to dissolve out the antimonial film by sulphide of ammonium, and thus produce the very characteristic orange sulphide.

If a slip of pure tinfoil be suspended for six hours in a solution, which should not contain more than one-tenth of its bulk of ClH, and exhibit no stain or deposit, it is certain that antimony cannot be present. It may also

[813] *Lancet*, May 19, 1883.

conveniently be deposited on a platinum dish,[814] by filling the same with the liquid properly acidulated, and inserting a rod of zinc; the metallic antimony can afterwards be washed, dried, and weighed.

Reinsch's and Marsh's tests have been already described, and require no further notice. There is, however, a very beautiful and delicate means of detecting antimony, which should not be omitted. It is based upon the action of stibine (SbH_3) on sulphur.[815] When this gas is passed over sulphur, it is decomposed according to equation, $2SbH_3 + 6S = Sb_2S_3 + 3SH_2$, the action taking place slowly in diffused daylight, but very rapidly in sunshine. An ordinary flask for the evolution of hydrogen (either by galvanic processes or from zinc and sulphuric acid), with its funnel and drying-tubes, is connected with a narrow tube having a few fragments of sulphur, kept in place by plugs of cotton wool. The whole apparatus is placed in sunshine; if no orange colour is produced when the hydrogen has been passing for some time, the liquid to be tested is poured in gradually through the funnel, and if antimony should be present, the sulphur acquires a deep orange colour. This is distinct even when so small a quantity as .0001 grain has been added through the funnel. The sulphide of antimony thus mixed with sulphur can, if it is thought necessary, be freed from the sulphur by repeated exhaustion with bisulphide of carbon. The stibine does not, however, represent all the antimony introduced, a very large proportion remaining in the evolution flask;[816] hence it cannot be employed for quantitative purposes. Moreover, the test can, of course, only be conveniently applied on sunny days, and is, therefore, in England more adapted for summer.[817] Often, however, as mentioned elsewhere, when the analyst has no clue whatever to the nature of the poison, it is convenient to pass SH_2 in the liquid to saturation.[818] In such a case, if antimony is present (either alone or in combination with other sulphides), it remains on the filter, and must be separated and identified as follows:—The sulphides are first treated with a solution of carbonate of ammonia, which will dissolve arsenic, if present, and next saturated *in situ* with pure sulphide of sodium, which will dissolve out sulphide of antimony, if present. The sulphide of antimony will present the chemical characters already described, more particularly—

(1) It will evolve SH_2 when treated with HCl, and at the same time pass into solution.[819]

(2) The solution evaporated to get rid of free HCl gives with water a thick cheesy precipitate of basic chloride of antimony. This may be seen if only a drop or two of the solution be taken and tested in a watch-glass.

(3) If tartaric acid be added to the solution, this precipitation does not occur.

(4) The solution from (3) gives an orange precipitate with SH_2.

Such a substance can only be sulphide of antimony. With regard to (2), bismuth would act similarly, but under the circumstances could not be present, for the sulphide of bismuth is insoluble in sodic sulphide.

§ 764. **Quantitative Estimation.**—The quantitative estimation of antimony is best made by some volumetric process, *e.g.*, the sulphide can be dissolved in HCl, some tartrate of soda added, and then carbonate of soda to weak alkaline reaction. The strength of the solution of tartarised antimony thus obtained can now be estimated by a decinormal solution of iodine, the end reaction being indicated by the previous addition of a little starch solution, or by a solution of permanganate of potash, either of which should be standardised by the aid of a solution of tartar emetic of known strength.

3. CADMIUM.

§ 765. **Cadmium**, Cd = 112; specific gravity, 8.6 to 8.69; fusing-point, 227.8° (442° F.); boiling-point, 860° (1580° F.).—Cadmium in analysis is seldom separated as a metal, but is estimated either as oxide or sulphide.

§ 766. **Cadmium Oxide**, CdO = 128—cadmium, 87.5 per cent.; oxygen, 12.5 per cent.—is a yellowish or

---

[814] According to Fresenius (*Zeitschr. f. anal. Chem.*, i. 445), a solution which contains $^1/_{10000}$ of its weight of antimony, treated in this way, gives in two minutes a brown stain, and in ten a very notable and strong dark brown film. When in the proportion of 1 to 20,000, the reaction begins to be certain after a quarter of an hour; with greater dilution it requires longer time, 1 to 40,000 giving a doubtful reaction, and 1 to 50,000 not responding at all to this test.

[815] See Ernest Jones on "Stibine," *Journ. Chem. Soc.*, vol. i., 1876.

[816] Rieckter, *Jahresbericht*, 1865, p. 255.

[817] The action of salts of cæsium with chloride of antimony might be used as a test for the latter. A salt of cæsium gives a white precipitate with chloride of antimony in concentrated ClH; it contains 30.531 per cent. of antimony, and corresponds to the formula $SbCl_3CsCl$. Chloride of tin acts similarly.—E. Godeffroy, *Berichte der deutschen Chem. Gesellschaft*, Berlin, 1874.

[818] The solution must not be too acid.

[819] By adding chloride of tin to a solution of chloride of antimony in sufficient quantity, and passing SO_2 through the liquid, the whole of the antimony can be thrown down as sulphide, whilst the tin remains in solution. Thus,—

$$9SnCl_2 + 2SbCl_3 + 3SO_2 + 12ClH = Sb_2S_3 + 9SnCl_4 + 6OH_2.$$

—Federow, *Zeitschrift für Chemie*, 1869, p. 16.

reddish-brown powder, non-volatile even at a white heat; insoluble in water, but dissolving in acids. Ignited on charcoal, it is reduced to metal, which volatilises, and is then deposited again as oxide, giving to the coal a distinct coat of an orange-yellow colour in very thin layers; in thicker layers, brown.

§ 767. **Cadmium Sulphide**, CdS = 144—Cd, 77.7 per cent.; S, 22.3 per cent.—known as a mineral termed Greenockite. When prepared in the wet way, it is a lemon-yellow powder, which cannot be ignited in hydrogen without loss, and is insoluble in water, dilute acids, alkalies, alkaline sulphides, sulphate of soda, and cyanide of potassium. The solution must not contain too much hydrochloric acid, for the sulphide is readily soluble with separation of sulphur in concentrated hydrochloric acid. It may be dried in the ordinary way at 100° without suffering any decomposition.

§ 768. **Medicinal Preparations.**—*The Iodide of Cadmium* (CdI_2) occurs in white, flat, micaceous crystals, melting at about 215.5° (419.9° F.), and at a dull red heat giving off violet vapour. In solution, the salt gives the reactions of iodine and cadmium. The ointment of iodide of cadmium (*Unguentum cadmii iodidi*) contains the iodide in the proportion of 62 grains to the ounce, or 14 per cent.

Cadmium Sulphate is officinal in the Belgian, Portuguese, and French pharmacopœias.

§ 769. **Cadmium in the Arts, &c.**—Cadmium is used in various alloys. The sulphide is found as a colouring ingredient in certain toilet soaps, and it is much valued by artists as a pigment. The iodide of cadmium is employed in photography, and an amalgam of metallic cadmium to some extent in dentistry.

§ 770. **Fatal Dose of Cadmium.**—Although no deaths from the use of cadmium appear to have as yet occurred, its use in photography, &c., may lead to accidents. There can be no question about the poisonous action of cadmium, for Marmé,[820] in his experiments on it with animals, observed giddiness, vomiting, syncope, difficulty in respiration, loss of consciousness, and cramps. The amount necessary to destroy life can only be gathered from the experiments on animals. A strong hound died after the injection of .03 grm. (.462 grain) subcutaneously of a salt of cadmium; rabbits are poisoned if from 19.4 to 38.8 mgrms. (.3 to .6 grain) are introduced into the stomach. A watery solution of .5 grm. (7.5 grains) of the bromide administered to a pigeon caused instant death, without convulsion; the same dose of the chloride killed a second pigeon in six minutes; .25 grm. (3.85 grains) of sulphite of cadmium administered to a pigeon excited vomiting, and after two hours diarrhœa; it died in eight days. Another pigeon died from a similar dose in fourteen days, and cadmium, on analysis, was separated from the liver. From the above cases it would seem probable that 4 grms. (61.7 grains) would be a *dangerous* dose of a soluble salt of cadmium for an adult, and that in a case of chronic poisoning it would most probably be found in the liver.

§ 771. **Separation and Detection of Cadmium.**—If cadmium be in solution, and the solution is not too acid, on the addition of SH_2 there is precipitated a yellow sulphide, which is distinguished from antimony and arsenical sulphides by its insolubility in ammonia and alkaline sulphides. Should all three sulphides be on the filter (an occurrence which will seldom, perhaps never, happen), the sulphide of arsenic can be dissolved out by ammonia, the antimony by sulphide of sodium, leaving the sulphide of cadmium as the residue.[821]

The further tests of the sulphide are:—

(1) It dissolves in dilute nitric acid to a colourless fluid, with separation of sulphur.

(2) The solution, filtered and freed from excess of nitric acid by evaporation, gives with a solution of ammonic carbonate a white precipitate of carbonate of cadmium insoluble in excess. This distinguishes it from zinc, which gives a similar white precipitate, but is soluble in the excess of the precipitant.

(3) The carbonate thus obtained, heated on platinum foil, is changed into the brown-red non-volatile oxide.

(4) The oxide behaves on charcoal as already detailed.

(5) A metallic portion can be obtained by melting the oxide with cyanide of potassium; it is between zinc and tin in brilliancy, and makes a mark on paper like lead, but not so readily. There are many other tests, but the above are conclusive.

If cadmium in any case be specially searched for in the organs or tissues, the latter should be boiled with nitric acid. The acid solution is filtered, saturated with caustic potash, evaporated to dryness, and ignited; the residue is dissolved in dilute hydrochloric acid, and treated after filtration with SH_2. Cadmium may also be estimated volumetrically by digesting the sulphide in a stoppered flask with ferric chloride and hydrochloric acid; the resulting ferrous compound is titrated with permanganate, each c.c. of a d.n. solution of permanganate = .0056 grm. of cadmium.

---

[820] *Zeitschr. f. rationelle Med.*, vol. xxix. p. 1, 1867.

[821] It is unnecessary to state that absence of sulphur is presupposed.

II.—PRECIPITATED BY HYDRIC SULPHIDE IN HYDROCHLORIC ACID SOLUTION—BLACK. Lead—Copper—Bismuth—Silver—Mercury.

1. LEAD.

§ 772. **Lead**, Pb = 207.—Lead is a well-known bluish-white, soft metal; fusing-point, 325°; specific gravity, 11.36.

Oxides of Lead.—The two oxides of lead necessary to notice here briefly are—litharge and minium.

Litharge, or Oxide of Lead, PbO = 223; specific gravity, 9.2 to 9.5—Pb 92.82 per cent., O 7.18—is either in crystalline scales, a fused mass, or a powder, varying in colour (according to its mode of preparation) from yellow to reddish-yellow or orange. When prepared below the temperature of fusion it is called "*massicot*." It may be fused without alteration in weight; in a state of fusion it dissolves silicic acid and silicates of the earths. It must not be fused in platinum vessels.

Minium, or Red Lead, 2PbO, PbO_2; specific gravity, 9.08, is a compound of protoxide of lead with the dioxide. It is of a brilliant red colour, much used in the arts, and especially in the preparation of flint-glass.

§ 773. **Sulphide of Lead**, PbS = 239; Pb, 86.61 per cent., S, 13.39 per cent., occurring in the usual way, is a black precipitate insoluble in water, dilute acids, alkalies, and alkaline sulphides. It dissolves in strong nitric acid with separation of sulphur, and in strong hydrochloric acid, with evolution of SH_2. Fuming nitric acid does not separate sulphur, but converts the sulphide into sulphate.

§ 774. **Sulphate of Lead**, $PbSO_4$ = 303; specific gravity, 6.3; PbO, 73.61 per cent., SO_3, 26.39 per cent., when produced artificially is a heavy white powder, of great insolubility in water, 22,800 parts of cold water dissolving only one of lead sulphate; and if the water contains sulphuric acid, no less than 36,500 parts of water are required. The salts of ammonia (especially the acetate and tartrate) dissolve the sulphate, and it is also soluble in hyposulphite of soda. The sulphate can be readily changed into the carbonate of lead, by boiling it with solutions of the alkaline carbonates. The sulphate of lead, fused with cyanide of potassium, yields metallic lead; it may be also reduced on charcoal, and alone it may be fused without decomposition, provided reducing gases are excluded.

§ 775. **Acetate of Lead**, **Sugar of Lead**, $Pb(C_2H_3O_2)_2 3OH_2$ = 379, is found in commerce in white, spongy masses composed of acicular crystals. It may, however, be obtained in flat four-sided prisms. It has a sweet metallic taste, is soluble in water, and responds to the usual tests for lead. The P.B. directs that 38 grains dissolved in water require, for complete precipitation, 200 grain measures of the volumetric solution of oxalic acid, corresponding to 22.3 grains of oxide of lead.

§ 776. **Chloride of Lead**, $PbCl_2$ = 278; specific gravity, 5.8; Pb, 74.48 per cent., Cl, 25.52 per cent., is in the form of brilliant crystalline needles. It is very insoluble in cold water containing hydrochloric or nitric acids. According to Bischof, 1635 parts of water containing nitric acid dissolve one part only of chloride of lead. It is insoluble in absolute alcohol, and sparingly in alcohol of 70 to 80 per cent. It fuses below red heat without losing weight; at higher temperatures it may be decomposed.

Carbonate of Lead.—The commercial carbonate of lead (according to the exhaustive researches of Wigner and Harland[822]) is composed of a mixture of neutral carbonate of lead and hydrate of lead, the best mixture being 25 per cent. of hydrate, corresponding to an actual percentage of 12.3 per cent. carbonic acid. The nearer the mixture approximates to this composition the better the paint; whilst samples containing as much as 16.33 per cent., or as little as 10.39 per cent., of CO_2 are practically useless.

§ 777. **Preparations of Lead used in Medicine, the Arts, &c.**

(1) **Pharmaceutical**:—

Lead Plaster (*Emplastrum plumbi*) is simply a lead soap, in which the lead is combined with oleic and margaric acids, and contains some mechanically included glycerin.

Lead Iodide, PbI_2, is contained in the *Emplastrum plumbi iodidi* to the extent of 10 per cent., and in the *Unguentum plumbi iodidi* to the extent of about 12.5 per cent.

Acetate of Lead is contained in a pill, a suppository, and an ointment. The pill (*Pilula plumbi cum opio*) contains 75 per cent. of lead acetate, and 12.5 per cent. of opium, the rest confection of roses. The suppository (*Suppositoria plumbi composita*) contains 20 per cent. of acetate of lead, and 6.6 per cent. of opium, mixed with oil

[822] "On the Composition of Commercial Samples of White Lead," by G. W. Wigner and R. H. Harland.—*Analyst*, 1877, p. 208.

of theobroma. The ointment (*Unguentum plumbi acetatis*) contains 20.6 per cent. of lead acetate, mixed with benzoated lard.

The solution of subacetate of lead (*Liquor plumbi subacetatis*) is the subacetate, $Pb(C_2H_3O_2)_2PbO$, dissolved in water; it contains nearly 27 per cent. of subacetate.

A dilute solution of the stronger, under the name of *Liquor plumbi subacetatis dilutus*, and commonly called Goulard water, is prepared by mixing 1 part (by volume) of the solution and 1 part of spirit, and 78 parts of distilled water; the strength is equal to 1.25 per cent.

There is an ointment, called the *Compound Ointment of subacetate of lead*, which contains the subacetate in about the proportion of 2 per cent. of the oxide, the other constituents being camphor, white wax, and almond oil.

Carbonate of Lead.—The ointment (*Unguentum plumbi carbonatis*) should contain about 12.5 per cent. of the carbonate, and the rest simple ointment.

(2) **Quack Nostrums, &c.**:—

The quack medicines composed of lead are not very numerous.

Liebert's **Cosmetique Infaillible** is said to have for its basis nitrate of lead.

One of "**Ali Ahmed's Treasures of the Desert**," viz., the antiseptic malagma, is a plaster made up of lead plaster 37.5 per cent., frankincense 25 per cent., salad oil 25 per cent., beeswax 12.5 per cent.

Lewis' Silver Cream contains white precipitate and a salt of lead.

Goulard's Balsam is made by triturating acetate of lead with hot oil of turpentine.

There are various ointments in use made up of litharge. Some herbalists in the country (from cases that have come under the writer's own knowledge) apply to cancerous ulcers, &c., a liniment of linseed and other common oils mixed with litharge and acetate of lead.

Acetate of lead may also be found as a constituent of various eye-waters.

(3) **Preparations of Lead used in the Arts, &c.**:—

Ledoyen's Disinfecting Fluid has for its basis nitrate of lead.

In various hair-dyes the following are all used:—Litharge, lime, and starch; lime and carbonate of lead; lime and acetate of lead; litharge, lime, and potassic bicarbonate. The detection of lead in the hair thus treated is extremely easy; it may be dissolved out by dilute nitric acid.

Lead Pigments.—The principal pigments of lead are white, yellow, and red.

White Pigments:—

White Lead, **Flake White Ceruse**, **Mineral White**, are so many different names for the carbonate of lead already described.

Newcastle White is white lead made with molasses vinegar.

Nottingham White.—White lead made with alegar (sour ale), often, however, replaced by permanent white, *i.e.*, sulphate of baryta.

Miniature Painters' White, **White Precipitate of Lead**, is simply lead sulphate.

Pattison's White is an oxychloride of lead, $PbCl_2PbO$.

Yellow Pigments:—

Chrome Yellow may be a fairly pure chromate of lead, or it may be mixed with sulphates of lead, barium, and calcium. The pigment known as "Cologne yellow" consists of 25 parts of lead chromate, 15 of lead sulphate, and 60 of calcic sulphate. The easiest method of analysing chrome yellow is to extract with boiling hydrochloric acid in the presence of alcohol, which dissolves the chromium as chloride, and leaves undissolved chloride of lead, sulphate of lead, and other substances insoluble in ClH. Every grain of chromate of lead should yield 0.24 grain of oxide of chromium, and 0.4 grain of chloride of lead.

Turner's Yellow, **Cassella Yellow**, **Patent Yellow**, is an oxychloride of lead ($PbCl_27PbO$) extremely fusible.

Dutch Pink sometimes contains white lead.

Red Pigments:—

Chrome Red is a bichromate of lead.

Red Lead or **Minium** is the red oxide of lead.

Orange Red is an oxide prepared by calcining the carbonate.

The chief preparations of lead which may be met with in the arts, in addition to the oxides and the carbonate, are—

The **Nitrate of Lead**, much used in calico-printing.

The **Pyrolignite of Lead**, which is an impure acetate used in dyeing; and

The **Sulphate of Lead** is a by-product in the preparation of acetate of aluminium for dyeing.

The alloys containing lead are extremely numerous; but, according to the experiments of Knapp,[823] the small quantity of lead in those used for household purposes has no hygienic importance.

§ 778. **Statistics of Lead-Poisoning.**—In the ten years, 1883 to 1892, no less than 1043 persons died from the effects of lead; of these, 3 only were suicidal, the remaining 1040 were mainly from the manufacture of white lead or from the use of lead in the arts or from the accidental contamination of food or drink.

The following table shows in what manner the 1040 were distributed as to age and sex:—

DEATHS FROM LEAD-POISONING IN ENGLAND AND WALES DURING THE TEN YEARS 1883-1892.

Ages,	0-1	1-5	5-15	15-25	25-65	65 and above	Total
Males,	...	4	14	44	733	36	831
Females,	3	5	...	68	129	4	209
Total,	3	9	14	112	862	40	1040

§ 779. **Lead as a Poison.**—All the compounds of lead are said to be poisonous; but this statement cannot be regarded as entirely correct, for the sulphocyanide has been proved by experiment not to be so,[824] and the sulphide is also probably inactive. In the treatment of cases of lead-poisoning, the flowers of sulphur given internally appear to be successful.[825]

Lead-poisoning, either in its obscure form (producing uric acid in the blood, and, as a consequence, indigestion and other evils), or in the acute form (as lead colic and various nervous affections), is most frequent among those who are habitually exposed to the influence of the metal in its different preparations, viz., workers of lead, house-painters, artists, gilders, workers of arsenic, workers of gold, calico-printers, colourists, type-founders, type-setters, shot-founders, potters, faience makers, braziers, and many others.[826] In white-lead factories so large a number of the employés suffer from poisoning that it has excited more than once the attention of the Government.[827]

Lead, again, has been found by the analyst in most of the ordinary foods, such as flour, bread, beer, cider, wines, spirits, tea, vinegar, sugar, confectionery, &c., as well as in numerous drugs, especially those manufactured by the

---

[823] *Dingl. Polytech. Journ.*, vol. ccxx. pp. 446-453.

[824] Eulenberg, *Gewerbe Hygiene*, p. 712.

[825] Mohr's *Toxicologie*, p. 78.

[826] The attention which the use of lead in the arts has always excited is evident from the fact that one of the oldest works on Trade Hygiene (by Stockhausen) is entitled, *De lithargyrii fumo noxio, morbifico ejusque metallico frequentiori morbo vulgo dicto hüttenkatze*, Gaslar, 1556.

[827] A departmental committee, appointed to inquire into the white lead and allied industries, in a report presented to the Home Secretary stated:—

"8. (*a*) It is known that if lead (in any form), even in what may be called infinitesimal quantities, gains entrance into the system for a lengthened period, by such channels as the stomach, by swallowing lead dust in the saliva, or through the medium of food and drink; by the respiratory organs, as by the inhalation of dust; or through the skin; there is developed a series of symptoms, the most frequent of which is colic. Nearly all the individuals engaged in factories where lead or its compounds are manipulated look pale, and it is this bloodlessness and the presence of a blue line along the margin of the gums, close to the teeth, that herald the other symptoms of plumbism. (*b*) A form of paralysis known as wrist-drop or lead-palsy occasionally affects the hands of the operatives. There is, in addition, a form of acute lead-poisoning, most frequently met with in young girls from 18 to 24 years of age, which is suddenly developed and is extremely fatal. In it the first complaint is headache, followed sooner or later by convulsions and unconsciousness. Death often terminates such a case within three days. In some cases of recovery from convulsions total blindness remains.

"9. There has been considerable doubt as to the channels by which the poison enters the system. The committee have taken much evidence on this subject, and have arrived at the conclusion (*a*) that carbonate of lead may be absorbed through the pores of the skin, and that the chance of this is much increased during perspiration and where there is any friction between the skin and the clothing; (*b*) that minute portions of lead are carried by the hands, under and round the nails, &c., on to the food, and so into the stomach; (*c*) but that the most usual manner is by the inhalation of lead dust. Some of this becomes dissolved in the alkaline secretions of the mouth, and is swallowed by the saliva, thus finding its way to the stomach. Other particles of dust are carried to the lungs, where they are rendered soluble and absorbed by the blood."—*Report of Chief Inspector of Factories for 1893.*

aid of sulphuric acid (the latter nearly always containing lead), and those salts or chemical products which (like citric and tartaric acids) are crystallised in leaden pans. Hence it follows that in almost everything eaten or drunk the analyst, as a matter of routine, tests for lead. The channels through which it may enter into the system are, however, so perfectly familiar to practical chemists, that a few *unusual* instances of lead-poisoning only need be quoted here.

A cabman suffered from lead colic, traced to his taking the first glass of beer every morning at a certain public-house; the beer standing in the pipes all night, as proved by analysis, was strongly impregnated with lead.[828]

The employment of red lead for repairing the joints of steam pipes has before now caused poisonous symptoms from volatilisation of lead.[829] The use of old painted wood in a baker's oven, and subsequent adherence of the oxide of lead to the outside of the loaves, has caused the illness of sixty-six people.[830]

Seven persons became affected with lead-poisoning through horse-hair coloured with lead.[831]

The manufacture of *American overland cloth* creates a white-lead dust, which has caused serious symptoms among the workmen (*Dr. G. Johnson*). The cleaning of pewter pots,[832] the handling of vulcanised rubber,[833] the wrapping up of various foods in tinfoil,[834] and the fingering of lead counters covered with brine by fishmongers, have all caused accidents in men.

The lead in glass, though in the form of an insoluble silicate, is said to have been dissolved by vinegar and other acid fluids to a dangerous extent. This, however, is hardly well established.[835]

§ 780. **Effects of Lead Compounds on Animals.**—Orfila and the older school of toxicologists made a number of experiments on the action of sugar of lead and other compounds, but they are of little value for elucidating the physiological or toxic action of lead, because they were, for the most part, made under unnatural conditions, the gullet being ligatured to avoid expulsion of the salt by vomiting. Harnack, in order to avoid the local and corrosive effects of sugar of lead, used an organic compound, viz., plumbic triethyl acetate, which has no local action. Frogs exhibited symptoms after subcutaneous doses of from 2 to 3 mgrms., rabbits after 40 mgrms.; there was increased peristaltic action of the intestines, with spasmodic contraction rising to colic, very often diarrhœa, and death followed through heart paralysis. Dogs given the ethyl compound exhibited nervous symptoms like chorea. Gusserno[836] has also made experiments on animals as to the effects of lead, using lead phosphate, and giving from 1.2 grm. to a rabbit and a dog daily. Rosenstein[837] and Heubel[838] used small doses of acetate, the latter giving dogs daily from .2 to .5 grm. The results arrived at by Gusserno were, mainly, that the animals became emaciated, shivered, and had some paralysis of the hinder extremities; while Rosenstein observed towards the end epileptiform convulsions, and Heubel alone saw, in a few of his cases, colic. A considerable number of cattle have been poisoned from time to time with lead, and one instance of this fell under my own observation. A pasture had been manured with refuse from a plumber's yard, and pieces of paint were in this way strewn about the field in every direction; a herd of fifteen young cattle were placed in the field, and in two or three days they all, without exception, began rapidly to lose condition, and to show peculiar symptoms—diarrhœa, loss of appetite; in two, blindness, the retina presenting an appearance not unlike that seen in Bright's disease; in three, a sort of delirium. Four died, and showed on *post-mortem* examination granular conditions of the kidneys, which was the most striking change observable. In the fatal cases, paralysis of the hind extremities, coma, and convulsions preceded death. In another case[839] seven cows and a bull died from eating lead paint; the symptoms were loss of appetite, obstinate constipation, suspension of rumination, dry muffle, quick breathing, and coma. In other cases a marked symptom has been paralysis. Cattle[840] have also several times been poisoned from eating grass which has been splashed by the spray from bullets, as in

[828] *Chem. News.*
[829] Eulenberg, *Op. cit.*, p. 708.
[830] *Annales d'Hygiène.*
[831] Hitzig, *Studien über Bleivergiftung.*
[832] *Med. Gazette*, xlviij. 1047.
[833] *Pharm. Journ.*, 1870, p. 426.
[834] Taylor, *Prin. Med. Jurisprud.*, i.
[835] See *Aerztl. Intelligenzbl. f. Baiern*, Jahrg., 1869; *Buchner's Rep. Pharm.*, Bd. xix. p. 1; *Med. Centrbl.*, Jahrg., 1869, p. 40.
[836] Virchow's *Archiv. f. path. Anat.*, vol. xxi. p. 443.
[837] *Ib.*, vol. xxxix. pp. 1 and 74.
[838] *Pathogenese u. Symptome der chronischen Bleivergiftung*, Berlin, 1871.
[839] See a paper by Professor Tuson, *Veterinarian*, vol. xxxviii., 1861.
[840] *Ib.*; also Taylor, *Op. cit.*

pastures in the vicinity of rifle butts; here we must allow that the intestinal juices have dissolved the metal, and transformed it into compounds capable of being taken into the system.

§ 781. **Effects of Lead Compounds on Man—Acute Poisoning.**—Acute poisoning by preparations of lead is not common, and, when it does occur, is seldom fatal. With regard to the common acetate, it would seem that a large single dose is less likely to destroy life than smaller quantities given in divided doses for a considerable period. The symptoms produced by a considerable dose of sugar of lead usually commence within a few minutes; there is immediately a metallic taste, with burning, and a sensation of great dryness in the mouth and throat; vomiting, which occurs usually within fifteen minutes, is in very rare cases delayed from one to two hours. The retching and vomiting are very obstinate, and continue for a long time; the matters thrown up are sometimes streaked with blood; there is pain in the abdomen of a colicky character—a pain relieved by pressure. The bowels are, as a rule, constipated, but occasionally relaxed. The stools at a later date are black from the presence of lead sulphide. The urine, as a rule, is diminished. The breath has a foul odour, and the tongue is coated; the skin is dry, and the pulse small and frequent. The full development of the toxic action is completed by the appearance of various nervous phenomena—headache, shooting pains in the limbs, cramps in the legs, and local numbness. All the symptoms enumerated are not present in each case; the most constant are the vomiting and the colic. If the sufferer is to die, death occurs about the second or third day. If the patient recovers, convalescence may be much retarded, as shown in the case of two girls,[841] who had each swallowed an ounce of lead acetate by mistake, and who suffered even after the lapse of a year from pain and tenderness in the stomach and sickness.

There are "mass-poisonings" by acetate of lead on record, which afford considerable insight into the varying action of this salt on different individuals. A case (*e.g.*) occurred at Stourbridge in 1840,[842] in which no less than 500 people were poisoned by thirty pounds of lead acetate being accidentally mixed with eighty sacks of flour at a miller's. The symptoms commenced after a few days; constriction of the throat, cramping and twisting pains round the umbilicus, rigidity of the abdominal muscles, dragging pains at the loins, cramps and paralysis of the lower extremities. There was obstinate constipation; the urine was scanty and of a deep red colour, and the secretions were generally arrested; the pulse was slow and feeble; the countenance depressed, often livid; and the gums showed the usual blue line. The temperature of the skin was low. In only a few cases was there sickness, and in these it soon ceased. It is curious that not one of the 500 cases proved fatal, although some of the victims were extremely ill, and their condition alarming. It was specially observed that, after apparent convalescence, the symptoms, without any obvious cause, suddenly returned, and this even in a more aggravated form. Remittance of this kind is of medico-legal import; it might, for example, be wrongly inferred that a fresh dose had been taken. In the 500 cases there were no inflammatory symptoms; complete recovery took some time. On examining the bread the poison was found so unequally distributed that no idea could be formed as to the actual amount taken.

There is also recorded[843] an outbreak of lead-poisoning among 150 men of the 7th Infantry at Tione, in the Southern Tyrol. One case proved fatal, forty-five required treatment in hospital. The symptoms were pallor, a blue line in the gums, metallic taste in the mouth, a peculiar odour of the breath, a loaded tongue with a bluish tint, obstinate constipation with loss of appetite whilst all complained, in addition, of dragging of the limbs and of the muscles of the chest, and difficulty of breathing. In the severer cases there were tetanic spasms, muscular tremors, and anæsthesia of the fingers and toes. The pulse and temperature were normal, save in a few cases in which there were fever and sweats at night. *In none was there colic*, but the constipation was obstinate. In two of the worst cases there was strangury. Acute cases occur occasionally from poisoning by *the carbonate of lead*. Dr. Snow recorded an instance (in 1844) of a child who had eaten a piece as big as a marble, ground up with oil. For three days the child suffered from pain in the abdomen and vomiting, and died ninety hours after taking the poison. In another case, in which a young man took from 19 to 20 grms. of lead carbonate in mistake for chalk as a remedy for heartburn, the symptoms of vomiting, pain in the stomach, &c., commenced after a few hours; but, under treatment with magnesic sulphate, he recovered.

The chromate of lead is still more poisonous (see Art. "Chromium").

§ 782. **Chronic Poisoning by Lead.**—Chronic poisoning by lead—often caused by strange and unsuspected channels, more frequently an incident, nay, almost a necessity, of certain trades, and occasionally induced by a cunning criminal for the purpose of simulating natural disease—is of great toxicological and hygienic importance.

---

[841] Prov. *Med. Journal*, 1846.

[842] Recorded by Mr. Bancks, *Lancet*, May 5, 1849, p. 478.

[843] Königschmied, *Centralbl. Allg. für Gesundheitspflege*, 2 Jahrg., Heft 1.

In the white-lead trade it is, as might be expected, most frequently witnessed; but also in all occupations which involve the daily use of lead in almost any shape. The chief signs of chronic poisoning are those of general ill-health; the digestion is disturbed, the appetite lessened, the bowels obstinately confined, the skin assumes a peculiar yellowish hue, and sometimes the sufferer is jaundiced. The gums show a black line from two to three lines in breadth, which microscopical examination and chemical tests alike show to be composed of sulphide of lead; occasionally the teeth turn black.[844] The pulse is slow, and all secretions are diminished. Pregnant women have a tendency to abort. There are also special symptoms, one of the most prominent of which is often lead colic.

In 142 cases of lead-poisoning, treated between 1852 and 1862 at the Jacob's Hospital, Leipzig, forty-four patients (or about 31 per cent.) suffered from colic. Arthralgia—that is, pains in the joints—is also very common; it seldom occurs alone, but in combination with other symptoms. Thus, in seventy-five cases of lead-arthralgia treated at Jacob's Hospital, in only seven were pain in the joints without other complications, fifty-six being accompanied by colic, five by paralysis, and seven by other affections of the nervous system. The total percentage of cases of lead-poisoning, in which arthralgia occurs, varies from 32 to 57 per cent.

Paralysis, in some form or other, Tanqueril[845] found in 5 to 8 per cent. of the cases, and noticed that it occurred as early as the third day after working in lead. The muscles affected are usually those of the upper extremity, then the legs, and still more rarely the muscles of the trunk. It is only exceptionally that the paralysis extends over an entire limb; it more usually affects a muscular group, or even a single muscle. Its common seat is the extensors of the hand and fingers; hence the expression "dropped-wrist," for the hands droop, and occasionally the triceps and the deltoid are affected. The paralysis is usually symmetrical on both sides. Although the extensors are affected most, the flexors nearly always participate, and a careful investigation will show that they are weakened. If the paralysis continues, there is a wasting and degeneration of the muscle, but this is seen in paralysis from any cause. The muscular affection may cause deformities in the hands, shoulders, &c. Anæsthesia of portions of the skin is generally present in a greater or less degree. A complete analgesia affecting the whole body has been noticed to such an extent that there was absolute insensibility to burns or punctures; but it is usually confined to the right half of the body, and is especially intense in the right hand and wrist.

§ 783. The older writers recognised the toxic effect of lead on the nervous system. Thus Dioscorides speaks of delirium produced by lead, Aretaeus of epilepsy, and Paul of Ægina refers to it as a factor of epilepsy and convulsions. But in 1830, Tanqueril first definitely described the production of a mental disease, which he called "*lead encephalopathy*." This he divided into four forms—(1) a delirious form; (2) a comatose; (3) a convulsive; and (4) a combined form, comprising the delirious, convulsive, and comatose. Dr. Henry Rayner,[846] and a few other English alienists, have directed their attention to this question; and, according to Dr. Rayner's researches, the number of male patients admitted into Hanwell Asylum, engaged in trades such as plumbing, painting, and the like, is larger in proportion to the number admitted from other trades than it should be, compared with the proportion of the various trades in the county of Middlesex, as ascertained from the census. Putting aside coarse lead-poisoning, which may occasionally produce acute mania, the insanity produced by prolonged minute lead intoxications possesses some peculiar features. It develops slowly, and in nearly all cases there are illusions of the senses, of hearing, taste, or smell, and especially of sight. Thus, in one of Dr. Rayner's cases the patient saw round him "wind-bags blown out to look like men," apparitions which made remarks to him, and generally worried him. Besides this form, there is also another which closely resembles general paralysis, and, in the absence of the history, might be mistaken for it.

§ 784. The degenerative influence on the organ of sight is shown in six of Dr. Robertson's patients, whose insanity was ascribed to lead—four of the six were either totally or partially blind.

The amaurosis has been known to come on suddenly, and after a very brief exposure to lead, *e.g.*, a man, thirty-four years of age, after working for three days in a white-lead factory, was seized with intense ciliary neuralgia, had

[844] The black line soon develops; Masazza has seen it in a dog, exposed to the influence of lead, in so short a period as three days (*Riforma med.*, 1889, Nos. 248-257, 1).

[845] Tanqueril des Planches, *Traité des Maladies de Plomb*, Paris, 1839. Tanqueril's monograph is a classical work full of information.

[846] See an important paper, "Insanity from Lead-Poisoning," by Drs. H. Rayner, Robertson, Savage, and Atkins, *Journ. of Mental Science*, vol. xxvi. p. 222; also a paper by Dr. Barton, *Allgemeine Zeitschrift für Psychiatrie*, Bd. xxxvij. H. 4, p. 9.

pains in his limbs and symptoms of lead-poisoning, and the right eye became amaurotic.[847] This form of impairment or loss of vision is different from the *Retinitis albuminurica*,[848] which may also be produced as a secondary effect of the poison; the kidneys in such cases being profoundly affected. The kind of diseased kidney produced by lead is the granular contracted kidney.

Eulenberg speaks of the sexual functions being weakened, leading to more or less impotence.

Lewy,[849] in 1186 patients suffering from lead-poisoning, has found caries or necrosis in twenty-two cases, or about 1.8 per cent.; fifteen were carious affections of the upper jaw, four of the fore-arm, two of the thigh, and one of the rib and sternum. Epilepsy and epileptiform convulsions occur in a few cases; it is very possible that the epilepsy may be a result of the uræmic poisoning induced by diseased kidneys.

Five cases of fatal poisoning occurred between 1884-6 among the employés of a certain white-lead factory in the east of London. The cases presented the following common characters. They were all adult women, aged from 18 to 33, and they had worked at the factory for short periods, from three to twelve months. They all exhibited mild symptoms of plumbism, such as a blue line round the gums, and more or less ill-defined indisposition; paralyses were absent. They were all in their usual state of health within a few hours or days preceding death. Death was unexpected, mostly sudden. In four cases it was preceded by epileptic fits and coma; but in the fifth case no convulsions were noted, although they may have occurred in the night.

The author[850] had an opportunity of investigating by chemical means the distribution of lead in the fourth and fifth cases in the liver, kidney, and brain.

In the fourth case, from 402 grms. of liver 24.26 mgrms. of lead sulphate were separated. The right kidney (weighing 81 grms.) yielded 5.42 mgrms. of lead sulphate. The brain was dehydrated with alcohol, and then treated with ether, hot alcohol, and chloroform until an albuminoid residue remained; lead was extracted from each of these portions, viz., the alcohol used for dehydration, the ethereal and chloroform extracts, and the albuminoid residue, as follows:—

	Mgrms. of Lead Sulphate.
Soluble in cold alcohol,	1.11
Soluble in ether and chloroform and hot alcohol,	25.47
Albuminoid residue,	7.76
	34.34

In the fifth case, the brain was examined more in detail, and the lead present estimated in the following solutions and substances:—

1. Alcohol used for dehydration. This may be called "the watery extract," for, after the brain has remained in strong alcohol for some weeks, the result is that the alcohol contains much water and substances extracted with water.
2. White matter—(*a*) from cerebrum; (*b*) from cerebellum.
3. Kephalin—(*a*) from cerebrum; (*b*) from cerebellum.
4. Ether extract, kephalin-free—(*a*) from cerebrum; (*b*) from cerebellum.
5. Substances soluble in cold alcohol—(*a*) from cerebrum; (*b*) from cerebellum.
6. The albuminoid residue—(*a*) from cerebrum; (*b*) from cerebellum.

The general results were as follows:—

	Cerebrum, 460.8 grms. Mgrms. of $PbSO_4$.	Cerebellum, 156.2 grms. Mgrms. of $PbSO_4$
White matter freed from kephalin by ether,	0.0	5.0
Kephalin,	1.5	6.0

[847] Samelsohn, *Monatsbl. f. Augenheilk.*, vol. xi. p. 246, 1873. See also a case of lead amaurosis, described by Mr. W. Holder, *Pharm. Journ.*, Oct. 14, 1876.

[848] Ran, *Arch. f. Ophthal.*, vol. i. (2), p. 205, 1858, and Schmidt's *Jahrbuch*, Bd. cxxxiii. p. 116; Bd. cxliii. p. 67.

[849] *Die Berufskrank. d. Bleiarbeiter*, Wien, 1873, S. 61.

[850] "The Distribution of Lead in the Brains of two Lead Factory Operatives," *Journ. of Mental Science*, Jan. 1888.

Ether extract, kephalin-free,	0.0	0.0
Substances soluble in cold alcohol,	0.0	0.0
Albuminoid residue,	40.0	6.0
	41.5	17.0

The aqueous extract contained 1.5 mgrm. of lead sulphate. In neither of the cases did the pathologist ascertain the total weight of the brain, but, presuming that the weight was an average weight, and that the lead in the remainder of the brain was similarly distributed, the amount of lead calculated as sulphate would amount to 117 mgrms. From these results it appears to the author probable that lead forms a substitution compound with some of the organic brain matters. This view would explain the absence of changes apparent to the eye found in so many of the fatal cases of lead encephalopathy.

§ 785. Lead taken for a long time causes the blood to be impregnated with uric acid. In 136 cases of undoubted gout, 18 per cent. of the patients were found to follow lead occupations, and presented signs of lead impregnation.[851]

Ellenberger and Hofmeister[852] found that, with chronic poisoning of sheep with lead, excretion of hippuric acid ceased, and the output of uric acid was diminished. This may be explained by the formation of glycocol being arrested.

§ 786. There are some facts on record which would seem to countenance the belief that disease, primarily caused by an inorganic body like lead, may be transmitted. M. Paul (*e.g.*) has related the history of the offspring (thirty-two in number) of seven men, who were suffering from lead-poisoning—eleven were prematurely born and one still-born; of the remaining twenty, eight died in the first year, four in the second, and five in the third year, so that of the whole thirty-two, only three survived three years.

The influence of the poison on pregnant women is, indeed, very deleterious. M. Paul noted that in four women who were habitually exposed to the influence of lead, and had fifteen pregnancies, ten terminated by abortion, two by premature confinement, three went the full term, but one of the three children was born dead, a second only lived twenty-four hours; so that, out of the whole fifteen, one only lived fully. In another observation of M. Paul's, five women had two natural confinements before being exposed to lead. After exposure, the history of the thirty-six pregnancies of these women is as follows:—there were twenty-six abortions (from two to five months), one premature confinement, two infants born dead, and five born alive, four of whom died in the first year.

Chronic poisoning may be nearly always accounted for by the inhaling of lead dust, or by the actual swallowing of some form of lead; but, if we are to accept the fact narrated by the late Dr. Taylor, viz., that he himself had an attack of lead colic from sitting in a room for a few hours daily, in which there was a large canvas covered with white lead and drying oil, and one or two other similar cases,[853] we must allow that there is some subtle volatile organic compound of lead evolved. In the present state of our knowledge, it seems more reasonable to account for such cases by the suggestion that lead has entered the system by an unsuspected channel.

In 1882, a very interesting case occurred at Keighley, in which a mechanic, aged 42, died from the supposed effects of lead-poisoning, induced from drinking the town water, which was proved by Mr. Allen to contain about $\frac{3}{5}$ of a grain of lead per gallon. For six months he had been out of health, and a week before his death he suffered from colic, vomiting, constipation, and a blue line round the gums, and occasional epileptiform seizures. After death the kidneys were found granular, and the heart somewhat enlarged. The viscera were submitted to Mr. Allen for analysis; no lead was found in the heart or brain, a slight, non-estimable trace in the kidneys, and about a grain was separated from the liver and spleen. Dr. Tidy, who was called in as an expert, gave a very guarded opinion, rather against the theory of direct lead-poisoning; and the verdict returned by the jury was to the effect that the deceased died from granular kidney, accelerated by lead-poisoning. Murder by the administration of doses of sugar of lead is rare, but such a case has occurred.

At the Central Criminal Court, in December 1882, Louisa Jane Taylor was indicted for poisoning Mary Ann Tregillis at Plumstead, and convicted. From the evidence it appeared that the prisoner, who was thirty-six years of

[851] "On Lead Impregnation in Relation to Gout," by Dyce Duckworth, M.D., *St. Barth. Hosp. Reports*, vol. xvii., 1881.

[852] *Arch. f. wiss. u. pract. Thierheilk.*, Bd. x., 1884.

[853] The gate-keeper of a graveyard at Bordeaux continually used the remnants of crosses, covered with lead paint, to replenish his fire; the chimney smoked; gradually paralysis of the extensors of the right wrist developed itself, and he suffered from colic and other signs of lead-poisoning.—Marmisse, *Gaz. des Hôpit.*, No. 25, 1866.

age, came to reside with Mr. and Mrs. Tregillis, an aged couple of eighty-five and eighty-one years respectively. The prisoner was proved to have purchased at different times an ounce and half an ounce of sugar of lead, and to have added a white powder to the medicine of Mrs. Tregillis. The illness of the latter extended from about August 23 to October 23—a period of two months. It is difficult to say when the first dose could have been given, but it was probably some time between August 13 and 23, while the administration, without doubt, ceased on or before October 6, for on that date different nursing arrangements were made. The symptoms observed were nausea, vomiting, pain in the pit of the stomach, burning in the throat, very dark teeth, a blue line round the gums, and slight jaundice. There was great muscular weakness, with trembling of the hands, and a week before death there was paralysis of the right side.

Lead was discovered in most of the viscera, which were in great part normal, but the kidneys were wasted, and the mucous membrane blackened. The actual quantity of lead recovered by analysis was small, viz., 16.2 mgrms. ($^1/_4$ grain) from the liver; from 8 ounces of brain, 3.2 mgrms. ($^1/_{20}$ grain); from half of the stomach, 16.2 mgrms. ($^1/_4$ grain); and from the spleen, the kidneys, and the lungs, small quantities. It is, therefore, probable that, if the whole body had been operated upon, the yield would have been more than .15 grm. (a little over 2 grains); but then, it must be remembered that the deceased lived, at least, seventeen days after the last dose.

§ 787. **Post-mortem Appearances.**—In acute cases of poisoning by the acetate, there may sometimes be found a slight inflammatory appearance of the mucous membrane of the stomach and intestines. Orfila considered that streaks of white points adherent to the mucous membrane were pathognomonic; but there have been several cases in which only negative or doubtful signs of inflammatory or other action have presented themselves. A general contraction of the intestines has often been noticed, and is of considerable significance when present; so also is a grey-black mucous membrane caused by deposited lead sulphide. Loen found in dogs and guinea-pigs, poisoned by lead, local inflammation areas in the lungs, liver, and kidneys; but in no case fatty degeneration of the epithelial cells of the liver, kidneys, or intestines. As a rule, no unabsorbed poison will be found in the stomach; the case related by Christison, in which a person died on the third day after taking at a single dose some large quantity of acetate of lead; and at the autopsy a fluid was obtained from the stomach, which had a sweet metallic taste, on evaporation smelt of acetic acid, and from which metallic lead was obtained—is so very extraordinary in every respect, that its entire accuracy is to be questioned. In death from chronic lead-poisoning, there is but little that can be called diagnostic; a granular condition of the kidneys, and all the pathological changes dependent on such a condition, are most frequently seen. If the patient has suffered from colic, a constriction of portions of the intestine has been noticed; also, in cases in which there has been long-standing paralysis of groups of muscles, these muscles are wasted, and possibly degenerated. In instances, again, in which lead has induced gout, the pathological changes dependent upon gout will be prominent. The blue line around the gums, and sometimes a coloration by sulphide of lead of portions of the intestines, may help a proper interpretation of the appearances seen after death; but all who have given any attention to the subject will agree that, simply from pathological evidence, it is impossible to diagnose chronic lead-poisoning.

§ 788. **Physiological Action of Lead.**—The action of lead is still obscure, but it is considered to have an effect mainly on the nervous centres. The paralysed muscles respond to the direct current, but not to the induced, leading to the suspicion that the intramuscular terminations of the nerves are paralysed, but that the muscular substance itself is unattacked. On the other hand, the restriction of the action to groups of muscles supports the theory of central action.

The lead colic is due to a true spasmodic constriction of the bowel, the exciting cause of which lies in the walls of the bowel itself; the relief given by pressure is explained by the pressure causing an anæmia of the intestinal walls, and thus lessening their sensibility. The slowing of the pulse produced by small doses is explained as due to a stimulation of the inhibitory nerves; and, lastly, many nervous phenomena, such as epilepsy, &c., are in part due to imperfect elimination of the urinary excreta, causing similar conditions to those observed in uræmia.

§ 789. **Elimination of Lead.**—When a large dose of acetate or carbonate is taken, part is transformed into more or less insoluble compounds—some organic, others inorganic; so that a great portion is not absorbed into the body at all, but passes into the intestines, where, meeting with hydric sulphide, part is changed into sulphide, colouring the alvine evacuations black. Some of the lead which is absorbed is excreted by the kidneys, but the search often yields only traces. Thudichum[854] states that in fourteen cases of lead-poisoning, in two only was obtained a weighable quantity from a day's urine; in the remaining twelve lead was detected, but only by the brownish colour

[854] *Pathology of the Urine*, p. 550.

produced in an acid solution of the ash by hydric sulphide.

The elimination of lead by the kidneys is favoured by certain medicines, such, for example, as potassic iodide. Annuschat found in dogs poisoned by lead from 3.8 to 4.1 mgrms. in 100 c.c. of urine; but, after doses of potassic iodide, the content of lead rose to 6.9 and even to 14 mgrms. Lead appears to be eliminated by the skin, being taken up by the epithelial cells, and minute, insoluble particles coming away with these cells. If a person who has taken small doses of lead for a time be placed in a sulphur water-bath, or have his skin moistened with a 5 per cent. solution of sodium sulphide, the upper layer of the epidermis is coloured dark; but the perspiration excited by pilocarpin or other agency contains no lead.

§ 790. **Fatal Dose**—(*a.*) **Sugar of Lead.**—It may almost be said that it is impossible to destroy human life with any single dose likely to be taken or administered. In three cases an ounce (28.3 grms.) has been taken without fatal result. Although it must be allowed that repeated moderate doses, extending over some time, are more dangerous to health and life than a single large dose, yet there seems to be in some individuals a great tolerance of lead. Christison has given .18 grm. in divided doses daily for a long time without any bad effect, save the production of a slight colic. Swieten has also given daily 3.9 grms. (60 grains) in ten days without observing toxic effects. That, in other cases, less than a grain per gallon of some lead compound dissolved in drinking-water, or in some way introduced into the economy, causes serious illness, is most inexplicable.

(*b.*) **The Basic Acetate** in solution is more poisonous apparently than the acetate—60 c.c. (1½ drms.) have caused serious symptoms.

(*c.*) **The Carbonate of Lead.**—Doses of anything like 28 grms. (an ounce) would probably be very dangerous to an adult; the only case of death on record is that of a child who took some unknown quantity, probably, from the description of the size of the lump, about 10 grms. (2½ drms.).

§ 791. **Antidotes and Treatment.**—Soluble sulphates (especially magnesic sulphate) have been given largely in both acute and chronic cases; in the acute, it stands to reason that it is well to ensure the presence of plenty of sulphates in the stomach and intestines, in order to form the sparingly soluble lead sulphate, should any residue remain; but to expect this double decomposition to go on in the blood and tissues is not based upon sound observation. The chronic lead-poisoning is best treated by removal from the source of mischief, the administration of large quantities of distilled water, and medicinal doses of potassic iodide.

§ 792. **Localisation of Lead.**—In a dog, which was killed by chronic lead-poisoning, Heubel found in the bones 0.18 to 0.27 per 1000 of lead; in the kidneys, 0.17 to 0.20; liver, 0.10 to 0.33; spinal cord, 0.06 to 0.11; brain, 0.04 to 0.05; muscles, 0.02 to 0.04; in the intestines traces, 0.01 to 0.02; in the spleen, the blood, and the bile, he also only found traces. Ellenberger and Hofmeister found in the kidneys of the sheep, 0.44 to 0.47; liver, 0.36 to 0.65; pancreas, 0.54; salivary glands, 0.42; bile, 0.11 to 0.40; bones, 0.32; fæces, 0.22; spleen, 0.14; central nervous system, 0.07 to 0.18; blood, 0.05 to 0.12; flesh, 0.05 to 0.08; urine, 0.06 to 0.08; and in the unstriped muscles and the lungs, 0.03 per 1000 of lead.

Without going so far as to say that lead is a natural constituent of the body, it is certain that it may be frequently met with in persons who have been apparently perfectly healthy, and quite free from all symptoms of lead-poisoning. Legrip found in the liver and spleen of a healthy person, 5.4 mgrms. of lead oxide in every kilogram; Oidtmann, in the liver of a man fifty-six years of age, 1 mgrm. of lead oxide per kilogram, and in the spleen 3 mgrms. per kilogram. Hence, the analyst, in searching for poison, must be very careful in his conclusions. Grave and serious errors may also arise from complications; suppose, *e.g.*, that a deceased person previous to death had partaken of game, and inadvertently swallowed a shot—if the analyst had not carefully searched the contents of the stomach for *solid* bodies, but merely treated them at once with acid solvents, he would naturally get very decided lead reactions, and would possibly conclude, and give evidence to the effect, that a poisonous soluble salt of lead had been administered shortly before death.

§ 793. **Detection and Estimation of Lead.**—A great number of fluids (such as beer, wines, vinegar, water, &c.), if they contain anything like the amount of one-tenth of a milligramme in 100 c.c., will give a very marked dark colour with SH_2. It is, however, usually safest in the first place to concentrate the liquid, to add an acid, and deposit the lead on platinum, in the way to be shortly described. Nearly all the lead from oils and fatty matter may be dissolved out by shaking up the fat with dilute nitric acid; if necessary, the fat should previously be melted.

If (in the usual course of routine research) a hydrochloric acid solution is obtained from the treatment or destruction of organic substances by that agent, and lead sulphide (mixed possibly with other sulphides) is filtered off, any arsenical sulphide may first be extracted from the filter by ammonia, and any antimonious sulphide by sodic sulphide; then the sulphide may be extracted by warm hydrochloric acid, which will leave undissolved such sulphides as those of copper and mercury. On diluting the liquid, and filtration at a boiling temperature, crystals of lead chloride will be deposited on cooling.

If, however, organic matters are *specially* searched for lead, hydrochloric acid is not the best solvent, but nitric should always be preferred; and, if there is reason to think that the lead exists in the form of sulphate, then the proper solvent is either the acetate or the tartrate of ammonia; but, in either case, the solution should contain an excess of ammonia. It must, however, be remembered that organic matters retain lead with great tenacity, and that in all cases where it can with any convenience be effected, the substances should be not only carbonised, but burnt to an ash; for Boucher has shown[855] that carbon retains lead, and that the lead in carbon resists to a considerable extent the action of solvents.

In the case of sulphate of lead, which may be always produced in an ash from organic substances by previous treatment with sufficient sulphuric acid, a very excellent method of identification is to convert it into sugar of lead. To do this, it is merely necessary to boil it with carbonate of ammonia, which changes it into carbonate of lead; treatment with acetic acid will now give the acetate; the solution may (if the lead is in very small quantity) be concentrated in a watch-glass, a drop evaporated to dryness on a circle of thin microscopic glass, and the crystals examined by the microscope; the same film next exposed to the fumes of SH_2, which will blacken it; and lastly, the solution (which should be sweet) tasted. A crystalline substance, possessing a sweet taste, and blackening when exposed to SH_2, can, under the circumstances, be no other substance than acetate of lead.

If the analyst does not care for this method, there is room for choice. Lead in solution can be converted into sulphide; in this case it is, however, absolutely necessary that there should be no great excess of acid, since as little as 2.5 per cent. of free hydrochloric acid will prevent all the lead going down. On obtaining the sulphide, the latter, as already described, can be converted into chloride by hydrochloric acid, and the crystalline chloride is extremely characteristic.

From the solution of the chloride the metal may be obtained in a solid state by inserting a piece of zinc in the solution contained in a crucible; the lead will be deposited gradually, and can be then collected, washed, and finally fused into a little globule on charcoal. A lead bead flattens easily when hit with a hammer, and makes a mark on paper. Solutions of the chloride also give a heavy precipitate of lead sulphate, when treated with a solution of sodic sulphate.

When lead is in very minute quantity, an electrolytic method is generally preferable; the lead is precipitated on platinum by using exactly the same apparatus as in Bloxam's test, described earlier; the liquid to be tested being placed in the inner cell, the lead film may now be identified, dissolved in nitric acid, and estimated by a colorimetric process. For the estimation of the minute fractions of a grain by a colour method, it is merely necessary to have a very dilute solution of acetate of lead, to add a known volume of SH_2 water to the liquid to be tested in a Nessler cylinder, noting the colour, and add to another a known quantity of the standard lead solution and the same quantity of SH_2 as was added to the first.

The process has an advantage which is great, viz., that it either detects copper, or proves its absence at the same time; and there are few cases in which the analyst does not look for copper as well as for lead. Lead, if in sufficient quantity, may be most conveniently estimated as oxide, sulphate, or chloride; the chief properties of these substances have been already described.

§ 794. **The Detection of Lead in Tartaric Acid, in Lemonade, and Aërated Waters.**—To detect lead in tartaric acid a convenient method is to burn it to an ash, digest in a little strong sulphuric acid, and then add either sodic chloride or a drop of HCl; lead, if present, is precipitated as chloride, giving a pearly opalescence. Lemonades often contain minute quantities of iron and copper as well as lead. Neither copper nor iron are precipitated by ammonium sulphide in presence of potassic cyanide. On the other hand, the sulphide of lead is not soluble in the alkaline cyanides. Hence a liquid which, on the addition of potassium cyanide and then ammonium sulphide, becomes dark coloured, or from which a precipitate separates, contains lead.[856]

2. COPPER.

§ 795. **Copper**, Cu = 63.5; specific gravity, from 8.921 to 8.952; fusing-point, 1091° (1996° F.). Copper in analysis occurs either as a film or coating on such metals as platinum, iron, &c., or in a state of fine division; or, finally, as a bead. In thin films, copper has a yellowish or a yellowish-red colour; it dissolves readily in nitric, slowly in hydrochloric acid. If air be excluded, hydrochloric acid fails to dissolve copper, and the same remark applies to

[855] *Ann. d'Hygiène*, t. xli.

[856] F. L. Teed, *Analyst*, xvii. 142-143.

ammonia; but, if there be free access of air, ammonia also acts as a slow solvent. Metallic copper in a fine state of division can be fused at a white heat to a bright bluish-green globule, which, on cooling, is covered with black oxide.

§ 796. **Cupric Oxide** (CuO = 79.5; specific gravity, 6.5, composition in 100 parts, Cu 79.85, O 20.15) is a brownish-black powder, which remains in the absence of reducing gases unaltered at a red heat. It is nearly insoluble in water, but soluble in ClH, NO_3H, &c.; it is hygroscopic, and, as every one who has made a combustion knows, is readily reduced by ignition with charcoal in the presence of reducing gases.

§ 797. **Cupric Sulphide**, CuS = 95.5, produced in the wet way, is a brownish powder so insoluble in water that, according to Fresenius, 950,000 parts of water are required to dissolve one part. It is not quite insoluble in ClH, and dissolves readily in nitric acid with separation of sulphur. By ignition in a stream of H it may be converted into the subsulphide of copper. It must always be washed by SH_2 water.

§ 798. **Solubility of Copper in Water and Various Fluids.**—The solubility of copper in water and saline solutions has been very carefully studied by Carnelley.[857] Distilled water exerts some solvent action, the amount varying, as might be expected, according to the time of exposure, the amount of surface exposed, the quantity of water acting upon the copper, &c. It would appear that, under favourable circumstances, 100 c.c. of distilled water may dissolve .3 mgrm. of copper (.2 grain per gallon).

With regard to salts, those of ammonium exert a solvent action on copper more decided than that of any others known. With the others, however, the nature of the base exerts little influence, the action of the salt depending chiefly on the nature of its acid radical. Thus, beginning with the least effective, the following is the order of dissolving strength:—Nitrates, sulphates, carbonates, and chlorides. It will then at once be evident that a water, contaminated by sewage, and therefore containing plenty of ammonia and chlorides, might exert a very considerable solvent action on copper.

Almost all the oils and fats, as well as syrups, dissolve small quantities of copper; hence its frequent presence in articles of food cooked or prepared in copper vessels. In the very elaborate and careful experiments of Mr. W. Thompson,[858] the only oils which took up no copper, when digested on copper foil, were English neats'-foot oil, tallow oil, one sample of olive oil, palm-nut oil, common tallow oil, and white oil, which was protected from the air by a thick coating of oxidised oil on its surface.

The formation of copper compounds with the fatty acids takes place so readily that Jeannel[859] has proposed the green colouring of fats by copper as a test for the presence of copper; and Bottger[860] recommends a copper holding brandy to be shaken up with olive oil to free it from copper.

Lehmann has made some useful researches on the amount of copper taken up by fats under different conditions. 100 c.c. of strongly rancid fat dissolved in fourteen days 8.7 mgrms. of copper; but when heated to 160° for one hour, and then allowed to stand, a similar amount was found. Some rancid butter was rubbed into a brass bowl of 90 c.c. capacity, and then allowed to stand for twenty-four hours; the butter became of a blue-green colour. Into this dish, thus partially attacked by fatty acids, 50 c.c. of rancid butter was poured in a melted condition, and allowed to stand for twenty-four hours. The amount taken up was found to be equal to 10 mgrms. of copper for every 100 c.c. of fluid butter.

Hilger found a fatty soup, which had stood twelve hours in a clean copper vessel, to contain 0.163 per cent. copper. According to Tschirch, the easiest fatty salt to form is the oleate, hydrated copper oxide dissolving in oleic acid with great ease, and even copper oxide dissolving to some extent; the palmitate and the stearate are not so readily produced; hence the amount of copper dissolved is greater in the case of olive oil and butter (both rich in oleic acids) than in the case of the firmer animal fats. Acid solutions, such as clarets, acetic acid, vinegars, and so forth, as might be expected, dissolve more or less copper. The amount likely to be dissolved in practice has been investigated by Lehmann. He steeped 600 square metres of copper sheeting or brass sheeting in vessels holding 2 litres of acid claret; the sheets were in some of the experiments wholly immersed, in others partly so. More copper was dissolved by the wine when the copper was partly immersed than when it was wholly immersed; and more copper was dissolved from brass sheeting than from pure copper sheeting. With a sheet of copper, partly immersed, claret may contain as much as 56 mgrms. per litre. Lehmann also investigated the amount of copper, as acetate,

[857] *Journ. Chem. Soc.*, 1876, vol. ii. p. 4.
[858] "Action of Fatty Oils on Metallic Copper," *Chem. News*, vol. xxxiv. pp. 176, 200, 313.
[859] *L'Union pharmac.*, xvii. 81.
[860] *Arch. de Pharm.*, 1853, cxxvi. 67.

which could be dissolved in wine before the taste betrayed its presence: with 50 mgrms. per litre no copper taste; with 100 mgrms. there was a weak after taste; with 150 mgrms. it was scarcely drinkable, and there was a strong after taste; with 200 mgrms. per litre it was quite undrinkable, and the colour was changed to bluish-green. Vinegar, acting under the most favourable circumstances on sheet brass or copper, dissolved, in seven days, 195 mgrms. of copper per litre from the copper sheet, 195 from the brass sheet.

Lehmann discusses the amount of copper which may be taken at a meal under the circumstance that everything eaten or drank has been artificially coppered, but none "coppered" to the extent by which the presence of the metal could be betrayed by the taste; and the following is, he thinks, possible:—

300 c.c. of soup boiled in a copper vessel,	20 mgrms. Cu.
1 litre of wine which has been standing in a copper vessel,	50 „
50 c.c. vinegar which has been kept in a copper vessel,	10 „
50 grms. of fat which has been used for frying in a copper vessel,	5 „
200 grms. of strongly coppered peas,	50 „
500 grms. of strongly coppered bread,	60 „

The total only amounts to 195 mgrms. of copper, which only slightly exceeds a high medicinal dose. The metal is tasted more easily in liquids, such as wine, than in bread; bread may be coppered so that at a meal a person might eat 200 mgrms. of a copper compound without tasting it.

It is pretty well accepted that cooking in clean bright copper vessels will not contaminate any ordinary food sufficiently to be injurious to health.

§ 799. **Copper in the Vegetable and Animal Kingdom and in Foods.**—Copper is widely distributed in the vegetable kingdom, and is a constant constituent of the chief foods we consume; the following quantities, for example, have been separated from the chief cereals:—

Wheat,	5 .2 to 10.8 mgrms.	per kilo.
Rye,	5 mgrms.	„
Oats,	8 .5 „	„
Barley,	11.8 „	„
Rice,	1 .6 „	„
Bread,	1 .5 to 4.4 mgrms.	„

It has also been found in vermicelli (2-10 mgrms. per kilo.), groats (1.6-3 mgrms. per kilo.), potatoes (1.8 mgrm. per kilo.), beans (2-11 mgrms. per kilo.). In similar small quantities it has also been found in carrots, chicory, spinach, hazel-nuts, blackberries, peaches, pears, figs, plums, tamarinds, black pepper, and many other fruits and spices. The most common food which has a high copper content is cocoa, which contains from 12 mgrms. to 29 mgrms. per kilo., the highest amount of copper being in the outer husk; copper has also been found in many supplies of drinking water, in aërated waters, in brandies, wines, and many drugs.

It has been calculated that the ordinary daily food of an average man contains the following:—

	Copper.
900 grms. bread,	0.45 mgrm.
260 grms. meat,	0.25 „
200 grms. fruit and vegetables,	0.25 „
	0.95 mgrm.

That is to say, that, neglecting altogether foods artificially contaminated with copper, each of us eats daily about 1 mgrm. of copper (0.015 grain).

In the animal kingdom it is a constant and natural constituent of the blood of the cephalopods, crustacea, and gasteropods, and is nearly always present in the liver and kidneys of domestic animals, as well as in men. Dr. Dupré[861] found .035 to .029 grain (1.8 to 2 mgrms.) in human livers, or about 1 part in 500,000. Bergeron and L. L'Hôte's researches on fourteen bodies, specially examined for copper, fully substantiate those of Dr. Dupré; in twelve the copper was found in quantities of from .7 to 1.5 mgrm.; in the remaining two the amount of copper was

[861] *Analyst*, No. 13, 1877.

very minute, and was not estimated.[862] Copper is also found normally in the kidneys, and Dupré[863] detected in human kidneys about 1 in 100,000 parts; it is also found in the bile, and in minute traces in the blood.[864]

In the kidneys and livers of the ruminants copper may always be found, a sheep's liver containing about 1 part in 20,000.[865] Church found copper in the feathers of the wings of the turaco; melopsitt in the feathers of a parroquet (*Melopsittacus undulatus*).[866] In these cases the copper enters into the composition of the colouring matter to which the name of "turacin" has been given. Turacin contains 7 per cent. of copper, and gives to analysis numbers which agree with the formula of $C_{82}H_{81}Cu_2N_9O_{32}$.

Copper has been discovered in aërated waters, its presence being due to the use of copper cylinders, the tin lining of which had been rendered defective by corrosion.[867]

Accidents may also occur from the use of copper boilers. Mr. W. Thompson found in one case[868] no less than 3.575 grains in a gallon (51 mgrms. per litre) in water drawn from a kitchen boiler.

At Roubaix, in France, sulphide of copper had been deposited on the roof, as a consequence of the use of copper flues; the sulphide was changed into sulphate by the action of the air, and washed by the rain into the water-tank.[869]

That preserved vegetables are made of a bright and attractive green colour by impregnation with copper, from the deliberate use of copper vessels for this purpose, is a fact long known. Green peas especially have been coloured in this way, and a number of convictions for this offence have taken place in England.

§ 800. **The "Coppering" of Vegetables.**—The fact that green vegetables, such as peas, beans, cucumbers, and so forth, preserve their green colour, if boiled in copper vessels, has long been known. In this "coppering" the French have been more active than the English traders; the French operate in two different ways. One method is, to dip from 60 to 70 litres of the green vegetables in 100 litres of 0.3 to 0.7 per cent. of copper sulphate, to leave them there for from five to fifteen minutes, then to remove them, wash and sterilise in an autoclave. A second method is to put the vegetables into a copper vessel, the wall of which is connected with the negative pole of an electric current, the positive pole dips in a solution of salt in the same vessel, the current is allowed to pass for three minutes, and the vegetables are afterwards sterilised. Fruits are simply allowed to stand with water in copper vessels, the natural acidity of the juice dissolving sufficient copper.

The amount of copper taken up in this way is appreciable, but yet not so much as might be expected; the prosecutions for selling "coppered" peas in England have been based upon quantities varying from 1 to 3 grains per lb.; the highest published amount of copper found in peas artificially coloured is 0.27 per kilo., or 18.9 grains per lb.

The reason why vegetables preserve their green colour longer when treated with a copper salt has been proved by Tschirch[870] to be owing to the formation of a phyllocyanate of copper.

Phyllocyanic acid is a derivative of chlorophyll, and allied to it in composition; the formula of $C_{24}H_{28}N_2O_4$ has been ascribed to it. Under the action of acids generally, mineral or organic, chlorophyll splits up into this acid and other compounds. Copper phyllocyanate, $(C_{24}H_{27}N_2O_4)_2Cu$, contains 8.55 per cent. of copper; it forms black lamellæ, dissolving easily in strong alcohol and chloroform, but insoluble in water; it is a little soluble in ether, insoluble in petroleum ether, and dissolved neither by dilute acetic acid, nor by dilute nor concentrated hydrochloric acid. The compound dissolves in caustic alkali on warming. In alcohol it forms a beautiful non-fluorescent solution. A solution of 1 : 100,000 is still coloured strongly green.

This solution, in a stratum of 25 mm. thick, gives four absorption bands when submitted to spectroscopic observation, and Tschirch has worked out a process of estimation of the amount of copper phyllocyanate based upon the disappearance of these bands on dilution.

Green substances, so carefully treated that they only contain phyllocyanate of copper, would yield but small quantities of copper, and probably they would not be injurious to health; but the coppering is usually more extensive,

862 *Compt. Rendus*, vol. lxxx. p. 268.

863 *Op. cit.*

864 Hoppe-Seyler, *Handbuch der physiologisch. Analyse*, p. 415.

865 Dupré, *op. cit.*

866 *Chem. News*, xxviij. 212.

867 "On the Presence of Lead and Copper in Aërated Waters," by Dr. James Milne, *Chem. News*, xxxi. p. 77.

868 *Chem. News*, xxxi. No. 801.

869 Author's *Dictionary of Hygiène*, p. 167.

870 *Das Kupfer*, Stuttgart, 1893.

and copper leguminate and other compounds are formed; for the vegetables, when exhausted by alcohol, give a residue which, successively exhausted by water, by soda-lye, and lastly by hydrochloric acid, parts with copper into the three solvents mentioned.

It might be argued that, from the insoluble character of the phyllocyanate of copper, and especially seeing that it does not dissolve in strong hydrochloric acid, that it would be perfectly innocuous; but Tschirch has proved that, whether the tartrate of copper (dissolving easily in water), or copper oxide (not dissolving at all in water, but soluble in hydrochloric acid), or phyllocyanate of copper (insoluble both in water and in hydrochloric acid) be used, the physiological effect is the same.

Copper may be found in spirits, owing to the use of copper condensers, a remark which applies also to the essential oils, such as *oleum cajepute*, *menthæ*, &c.[871] In France, it has been added fraudulently to absinthe, to improve its colour.[872] Green sweetmeats, green toys, green papers, have all been found to contain definite compounds of copper to a dangerous extent.

§ 801. **Preparations of Copper used in Medicine and the Arts.**

(1) **Medicinal Preparations**:—

Sulphate of Copper, **Cupri Sulphas**, $CuSO_45H_2O$.—This well-known salt is soluble in water at ordinary temperature, 3 parts of water dissolving 1 of the sulphate; but boiling water dissolves double its weight; 1 part of copper sulphate dissolves in 2½ of glycerin; it reddens litmus, and is slightly efflorescent; its solution responds to all the usual tests for copper and sulphuric acid. A watery solution of the salt to which twice its volume of a solution of chlorine has been added, gives, when treated with ammonia in excess, a clear sapphire-blue solution, leaving nothing undissolved, and thus showing the absence of iron. Besides iron, sulphate of copper has been found to contain zincic sulphate.

Nitrate of Copper, $Cu(NO_3)_23H_2O$, is officinal; it is very soluble.

Cuprum Aluminatum.—A preparation, called cuprum aluminatum (*Pierre divine*), is in use in France and Germany, chiefly as an external wash. It is composed of 16 parts cupric sulphate, 16 potassic nitrate, 16 alum, fused in a crucible, a little camphor being afterwards added.

Regular and irregular medical practitioners, veterinary surgeons, farriers, and grooms, all use sulphate of copper (bluestone) as an application to wounds. Copper as an *internal* remedy is not in favour either with quacks or vendors of patent medicines. The writer has not yet found any patent pill or liquid containing it.

(2) **Copper in the Arts.**—Copper is used very extensively in the arts; it enters into the composition of a number of alloys, is one of the chief constituents of the common bronzing powders, is contained in many of the lilac and purple fires of the pyrotechnist, and in a great variety of pigments. The last-mentioned, being of special importance, will be briefly described:—

Pigments:—

Schweinfurt and Scheele's Green[873] are respectively the aceto-arsenite and the arsenite of copper (see article "Arsenic").

Brighton Green is a mixture of impure acetate of copper and chalk.

Brunswick Green, originally a crude chloride of copper, is now generally a mixture of carbonate of copper and chalk or alumina.

Mountain Green, or **Mineral Green**, is the native green carbonate of copper, either with or without a little orpiment.

Neuwieder Green is either the same as mountain green, or Schweinfurt green mixed with gypsum or sulphate of baryta.

Green Verditer is a mixture of oxide and carbonate of copper with chalk.

Verdigris is an acetate of copper, or a mixture of acetates. Its formula is usually represented as $(C_2H_3O_2)CuO$. It is much used in the arts, and to some extent as an external application in medicine. Its most frequent impurities or adulterations are chalk and sulphate of copper.

§ 802. **Dose—Medicinal Dose of Copper.**—Since sulphate of copper is practically the only salt administered

[871] According to Eulenberg (*Gewerbe Hygiene*, p. 716), *Oleum cajepute*, *Menth. pip.*, *Melissæ*, *Tanaceti*, &c., are almost always contaminated with copper.

[872] Tardieu, *Étude Méd. Lég. sur l'Empoisonnement.*

[873] The synonyms for Schweinfurt green are extremely numerous:—Mitic green, Viennic green, imperial green, emerald green, are the principal terms in actual use.

internally, the dose is generally expressed as so many grains of sulphate. This salt is given in quantities of from .016 to .129 grm. (¼ to 2 grains) as an astringent or tonic; as an emetic, from .324 to .648 grm. (5 to 10 grains).

The sulphate of copper is given to horses and cattle in such large doses as from 30 up to 120 grains (1.9 to 7.7 grms.); to sheep, from 1.3 to 2.6 grms. (20 to 40 grains); rabbits, .0648 to .1296 grm. (1 to 2 grains).

§ 803. **Effects of Soluble Copper Salts on Animals.**—Harnack has made some experiments on animals with an alkaline tartrate of copper, which has no local action, nor does it precipitate albumin. ½ to ¾ mgrm. of copper oxide in this form, administered subcutaneously, was fatal to frogs, .05 grm. to rabbits, .4 grm. to dogs. The direct excitability of the voluntary muscles was gradually extinguished, and death took place from heart paralysis. Vomiting was only noticed when the poison was administered by the stomach.[874] The temperature of animals poisoned by copper, sinks, according to the researches of F. A. Falck, many degrees. These observations are in agreement with the effects of copper salts on man, and with the experiments of Orfila, Blake, C. Ph. Falck, and others.

Roger[875] experimented on the effect of copper leguminate which was administered subcutaneously; he found gradual increasing paralysis of the motor spinal tracts, which finally destroyed life by paralysis of the breathing centre. The heart beat after the breathing had stopped. The irritability and contractility of the muscles of frogs were lost, while sensibility remained. He also found that, if the copper was injected into the intestinal vessels, the dose had to be doubled in order to destroy life; this is, doubtless, because the liver, as it were, strained the copper off and excreted it through the bile. Roger was unable to destroy life by large doses of copper given by the mouth, for then vomiting supervened and the poison in great part was removed.

Bernatzic[876] considers that the poisonous properties of copper are similar to those of zinc and silver. He says: "Silver, copper, and zinc are, in their medicinal application, so much allied that, with regard to their action, they graduate one into the other and show only minor differences; copper, which is a little the more poisonous of the three so far as its remote action is concerned, stands between the other two. If taken, in not too small a quantity, for a long time, the functional activity of the muscular and nervous systems is influenced injuriously, the development of the animal cells is inhibited, the number of the red blood corpuscles decreased, and therefore the oxidising process and metabolism are likewise diminished, leading ultimately to a condition of marked cachexia. . . . From a toxic point of view, the three metals named also stand near each other, and their compounds differ from other metals injurious to the organism in this, that they do not produce notable changes of the tissues or coarse functional disturbances leading to death as other poisonous metals, and therefore are not to be considered poisons in the same sense as lead, mercury, arsenic, antimony, phosphorus are considered poisons; for, on stopping the entry of the poison, any injurious effect is completely recovered from and the functions again become normal."

Lehmann[877] has also experimented on the effects of copper; his experiments were made on both animals and men. He found that small quantities were more thoroughly absorbed than medium or large doses; the method of separation appeared to be different in different animals—thus, the chief copper-excreting organ in dogs is the liver; in rabbits, the intestine; and in man, the kidneys. Of 3 mgrms. of copper taken by a man in three days, 1 mgrm., or a third, was recovered from the urine. Lehmann experimented on 6 rabbits, 4 cats, and 1 dog. During the first few days the animals were given 10 to 30 mgrms. of copper, in the form of a salt, in their food; then the dose was raised to 50 mgrms. or even to 100 mgrms., and the experiment continued for from two to four months; in one case, six months. The sulphate, acetate, chloride, oleate, butyrate, and lactate were all tried, but no essential difference in action discovered. Apart from slight vomiting, and in a few cases, as shown by *post-mortem*, a slight catarrh of the stomach, the animals remained well. A few increased in weight. Nervous symptoms, cramps, convulsions, diarrhœa, or the reverse, were not observed. The analysis of the organs showed considerable copper absorption; the liver of the cats gave a mean amount of 12 mgrms. of copper, and in the other organs there was more copper than is found in cases of acute poisoning.

Lehmann has also made experiments upon himself and his pupils on the effect of the sulphate and the acetate when taken for a long time:—

---

[874] On the other hand, Brunton and West have observed vomiting produced in animals after injection of copper peptone into the jugular vein.—*Barth. Hosp. Rep.*, 1877, xii.

[875] *Revue de Médecine*, 1877, xii.

[876] *Encycloped. d. ges. Heilkunde*, xi. S. 429.

[877] *Münch. med. Wochenschrift*, 1891, Nr. 35 u. 36.

One of the experimenters took	for 50	days 10	mgrms. daily Cu as sulphate.
,, ,, ,,	then for 30 ,,	20 ,,	,,
Another took	for 3 days	5	mgrms. as acetate.
,,	then for 10 days	10 ,,	,,
,,	,, 1 day	15 ,,	,,
,,	,, 19 days	20 ,,	,,
,,	,, 18 days	30 ,,	,,

None of these daily doses had the least effect.

Five farther experiments showed that 75 to 127 mgrms. of copper in peas and beans, divided in two meals, could be taken daily without effect; but if 127 mgrms. were taken at one meal in 200 grms. of peas, then, after a few hours, there might be vomiting; and Lehmann concludes that doses of copper in food of about 100 mgrms. may produce some transient derangement in health, such as sickness, a nasty taste in the mouth, and a general feeling of discomfort, but nothing more; some slight colicky pains and one or two loose motions are also possible, but were not observed in Lehmann's experiments.

§ 804. **Toxic Dose of Copper Salts.**—This is a difficult question, because copper salts generally act as an emetic, and therefore very large doses have been taken without any great injury. In fact, it may be laid down that a medium dose taken daily for a considerable time is far more likely to injure health, or to destroy life, than a big dose taken at once. In Tschirch's[878] careful experiments on animals, he found 10 mgrm. doses of CuO given daily to rabbits, the weight of which varied from 1200 to 1650 grms., caused injury to health, that is, about 3.5 mgrms. per kilo. If man is susceptible in the same proportion, then daily doses of 227.5 mgrms. (or about 3½ grains) would cause serious poisonous symptoms; although double or treble that quantity might in a single dose be swallowed and, if thrown up speedily, no great harm result. 120 grms. of sulphate of copper have been swallowed, and yet the patient recovered after an illness of two weeks.[879] Lewin[880] mentions the case of an adult who recovered after ten days' illness, although the dose was 15 grms.; there is also on record the case of a child, four and a half years old, who recovered after a dose of 16.5 grms. (a little over half an ounce). On the other hand, 7.7 grms. have been with difficulty recovered from.[881] A woman died in seventy-two hours after taking 27 grms. (7 drms.) of copper sulphate mixed with 11.6 grms. (3 drms.) of iron sulphide; 56.6 grms. (2 ozs.) of copper acetate have caused death in three days; 14.2 grms. (0.5 oz.) in sixty hours.[882]

§ 805. **Cases of Acute Poisoning.**—Acute poisoning by salts of copper is rare; in the ten years ending 1892, there were registered in England 8 deaths from this cause—3 suicidal (2 males, 1 female) and 5 accidental (4 males, 1 female). The symptoms produced by the sulphate of copper are those of a powerful irritant poison: there is immediate and violent vomiting; the vomited matters are of a greenish colour—a green distinguished from bile by the colour changing to blue on the addition of ammonia. There is pain in the stomach, and in a little time affections of the nervous system, as shown by spasms, cramps, paralysis, and even tetanus. Jaundice is a frequent symptom, if life is prolonged sufficiently to admit of its occurrence.

One of the best examples of acute poisoning by copper sulphate is recorded by Maschka.[883] A youth, sixteen years old, took an unknown large dose of powdered copper sulphate, mixed with water. Half an hour afterwards there was violent vomiting, and he was taken to the hospital. There was thirst, retching, constriction in the throat, a coppery taste in the mouth, and pain in the epigastrium, which was painful on pressure. The vomit was of a blue colour, and small undissolved crystals of copper sulphate were obtained from it. The patient was pale, the edges of the lips and the angles of the mouth were coloured blue, the surface of the tongue had also a blue tint, the temperature was depressed, the extremities cold, nails cyanotic, and the pulse small and quick. Several loose greenish-yellow evacuations were passed; there was no blood. The urine was scanty, but contained neither blood nor albumen. During the night the patient was very restless; the next morning he had violent headache, pain in the epigastrium, burning

[878] *Das Kupfer*, Stuttgart, 1893.

[879] Referred to by Bernatzic, on the authority of Ketli, in *Encycl. d. ges. Heilkunde*, xi. S. 433.

[880] *Toxicologie*, S. 133.

[881] D Taylor, *op. cit.*

[882] Sonnenschein, *op. cit.*

[883] *Wiener med. Wochenschr.*, 1871, Nro. 26, p. 628.

in the mouth and gullet, but no vomiting. The urine was scanty, contained blood, albumen, and colouring matter from the bile. On the fourth day there was marked jaundice. The mucous membrane was very pale, the temperature low, pulse frequent, and great weakness, cardiac oppression, and restlessness were experienced. There were diarrhœa and tenesmus, the motions being streaked with blood; the urine also contained much blood. The liver was enlarged. The patient died in a state of collapse on the seventh day.

In 1836 a girl, sixteen months old, was given bluestone to play with, and ate an unknown quantity; a quarter of an hour afterwards the child was violently sick, vomiting a bluish-green liquid containing some pieces of sulphate of copper. Death took place in four hours, without convulsions, and without diarrhœa.

§ 806. **Subacetate of Copper, Subchloride, and Carbonate**, all act very similarly to the sulphate when given in large doses.

§ 807. **Post-mortem Appearances.**—In Maschka's case, the chief changes noted were in the liver, kidneys, and stomach. The substance of the liver was friable and fatty; in the gall-bladder there were but a few drops of dark tenacious bile. The kidneys were swollen, the cortical substance coloured yellow, the pyramids compressed and pale brown. In the mucous membrane of the stomach there was an excoriation the size of a shilling, in which the epithelium was changed into a dirty brown mass, easily detached, laying bare the muscular substance beneath, but otherwise normal.

In a case of poisoning by verdigris (subacetate of copper) recorded by Orfila,[884] the stomach was so much inflamed and thickened that towards the pyloric end the opening into the intestine was almost obliterated. The small intestines throughout were inflamed, and perforation had taken place, so that part of the green liquid had escaped into the abdomen. The large intestines were distended in some parts, contracted in others, and there was ulceration of the rectum. In other cases a striking discoloration of the mucous membrane, being changed by the contact of the salt to a dirty bluish-green, has been noticed, and, when present, will afford valuable indications.

§ 808. **Chronic Poisoning by Copper.**—Symptoms have arisen among workers in copper or its salts, and also from the use of food accidentally contaminated by copper, which lend support to the existence of chronic poisoning. In the symptoms there is a very great resemblance to those produced by lead. There is a green line on the margin of the gums. Dr. Clapton[885] found the line very distinct in a sailor and two working coppersmiths, and the two men were also seen by Dr. Taylor. Cases of chronic poisoning among coppersmiths have also been treated by Dr. Cameron,[886] but this symptom was not noticed. Corrigan speaks of the line round the gums, but describes it as purple-red. Among workers in copper, Lancereaux[887] has seen a black coloration of the mucous membrane of the digestive canal; its chemical characters appear to agree with those of carbon.

Metallic copper itself is not poisonous. A Mr. Charles Reed has published a letter in the *Chemical News* of Jan. 12, 1894, stating that he was, when a boy, wounded in the shin by a copper percussion-cap, and the cap remained in the tissues; it was removed from the shin after a sojourn thereof some twelve years; about the year 1873 he noticed that whenever a piece of clean iron or steel came in contact with his perspiration it was at once covered with a bright coating of copper, and this continued until the percussion-cap was removed. Presuming the truth of this, it shows conclusively that metallic copper deposited in the tissues is in itself not poisonous, and farther, that one method of elimination is by the skin. The experiments already cited throw doubt as to whether repeated small doses of copper taken for a long time produce in a scientific sense chronic poisoning; those which apparently support the view that there is such a thing as chronic poisoning by copper, have been produced by copper mixed with other metals; and there is the possibility that these cases are really due to lead or arsenic, and not to copper. The great use of late years of solutions of copper sulphate as a dressing to plants, for the purpose of preventing the ravages of various parasites, has provided, so far as animals are concerned, much material for the judgment of this question. Sheep have been fed with vines which have been treated with copper sulphate, oxen and pigs have consumed for a long time grass treated with a 3 per cent. of copper sulphate, without the least health disturbance. Mach[888] has fed cows with green food coppered up to 200 mgrms. of copper sulphate, without observing the slightest bad effect, for long periods of

[884] *Toxicologie*, vol. i. p. 787 (5th ed.).

[885] *Med. Times and Gazette*, June 1868, p. 658.

[886] *Med. Times and Gazette*, 1870, vol. i. p. 581.

[887] *Atlas of Pathological Anatomy.*

[888] Mach, *Bericht über die Ergebnisse der im Jahre 1886 ausgeführten Versuche zur Bekämpfung der Peronospora*, St. Michele, Tyrol.

time; and Tschirch[889] summarises the evidence as to chronic poisoning as follows:—"So it appears the contention that there is no chronic poisoning in men or animals is at present uncontradicted; it is farther to be considered proved that the small amounts of copper naturally in food, or carefully introduced into food, are not injurious to the health of those that take such food, because the liver, kidneys, and other organs excrete the copper through the urine and bile, and prevent a pernicious accumulation." At the same time, Tschirch does not consider the question is definitely settled; the experiments should, he thinks, have been continued not for months, but for years, to obtain a trustworthy judgment.

It may also be remarked that, if we are to rely upon the separation of copper by the kidneys and the liver, those organs are presumed to be in a healthy state, which is not the case with a percentage of the population; to persons whose liver or kidneys are unsound, even the small amounts of copper found in "coppered" peas may act as a poison, and the experiments previously detailed throw no light upon the action of copper under such circumstances.

§ 809. **Detection and Estimation of Copper.**—Copper may occur either in the routine process of precipitating by SH_2, or it may, as is generally the case, be searched for specially. If copper is looked for in a precipitate produced by SH_2, it is taken for granted that the precipitate has first been treated successively by carbonate of ammonia, sulphide of sodium, and hydrochloric acid; in other words, arsenic, antimony, and lead have been removed. The moist precipitate is now treated with warm nitric acid, which dissolves out copper sulphide with separation of sulphur; if there is sufficient copper, the fluid shows a blue colour, which of itself is an indication of copper being present. The further tests are—(1) Ammonia gives a deeper blue; (2) ferrocyanide of potash a brown-red colour or precipitate; (3) a few drops mixed with a solution of tartrate of soda, alkalised with sodic hydrate, and boiled with a crystal or two of grape-sugar, gives quickly a red precipitate of oxide of copper; (4) a needle or a clean iron wire, or any simple galvanic combination, immersed in, or acting on, the liquid, soon becomes coated with the very characteristic reddish metallic film. Various other tests might be mentioned, but the above are ample.

Special Examinations for Copper.

(1) **In Water and Liquids generally.**—The liquid may be concentrated, and the copper separated by electrolysis. A simple method is to place the liquid in a large platinum dish, and insert a piece of zinc, adding a sufficient quantity of ClH to dissolve the zinc entirely; the copper is found as an adherent film on the inner surface of the dish. It is neater, however, and more accurate, to connect the platinum dish with the negative plate of a battery, suspending in the liquid the positive electrode. The modifications of this method are numerous; some chemists use (especially for small quantities of copper) two small platinum electrodes, either of foil or of wire, and on obtaining the film, weigh the electrode, then dissolve the copper off by nitric acid, and re-weigh. Such solid substances as peas are conveniently mashed up into a paste with water and ClH; an aliquot part is carefully weighed and put in a platinum dish, connected, as before described, with a battery; at the end of from twelve to twenty-four hours all the copper is deposited, and the dish with its film dried and weighed. The weight of the clean dish, *minus* the coppered dish, of course equals the copper. Fat and oils are best thoroughly washed with hot acid water, which will, if properly performed, extract all the copper. By the use of separating funnels and wet filters, the fat or oil can be separated from the watery liquid.

A galvanic test has been proposed, which is certainly very delicate, $^1/_{100}$ of a mgrm. in solution being recognised with facility. A zinc platinum couple is made with two wires; on leaving this in an acid liquid containing a mere trace of copper, after several hours the platinum will be found discoloured. If the discoloration is from copper, on exposing the wire to hydrobromic acid fumes (easily produced from the action of potassic bromide and sulphuric acid) and bromine, the wire will become of a violet colour. This colour is easily recognised by rubbing the wire on a piece of porcelain.[890]

(2) **Animal Matters**, such as the liver, brain, spinal cord, &c., are best entirely burnt to an ash, and the copper looked for in the latter.[891] The same remark applies to bread and substances consisting almost entirely of starchy matters. Any injurious quantity of copper can, however, be extracted with hydrochloric acid and water; and, although this method of extraction is not quite so accurate, it is quicker.

§ 810. **Volumetric Processes for the Estimation of Copper.**—A number of volumetric processes have been

[889] *Op. cit.*

[890] *Chem. News*, Nov. 30, 1877.

[891] In exhumation of long buried bodies, it may be necessary to know the composition of the soil. Sonnenschein mentions a skull, now in the museum at Madrid, which was dug out of an old Roman mine, and is quite green from copper compounds.—Sonnenschein's *Handbuch*, p. 83.

devised for the estimation of copper, but for the purposes of this work it is unnecessary to detail them. When copper is in too small a quantity to be weighed, it may then be estimated by a colorimetric process.

One of the best of these is based upon the brown colour which ferrocyanide of potash produces in very dilute solutions of copper. A standard copper solution is obtained by dissolving sulphate of copper in a litre of water, so that each c.c. contains 0.1 mgrm. Cu, and a solution of ferrocyanide of potash in water is prepared, strength 4 per cent. It is also convenient to have a solution of nitrate of ammonia, which is found to render the reaction much more delicate.

The further details are on the well-known lines of colorimetric estimations.

3. BISMUTH.

§ 811. **Bismuth**, Bi = 210; sp. gr., 9.799; fusing-point, 264° (507.2° F.).—Bismuth, as obtained in the course of analysis, is either a black metallic powder or an extremely brittle bead of a reddish-white colour. The compounds which it will be necessary to briefly notice are the peroxide and tersulphide.

§ 812. **The peroxide of bismuth**, Bi_2O_3 = 468; sp. gr., 8.211; Bi, 89.64 per cent., O, 10.36 per cent., as prepared by igniting the carbonate or nitrate, is a pale lemon coloured powder, which can be fused without loss of weight, but is reduced on charcoal, or in a stream of carbon dioxide, to the metallic state. It is also reduced by fusion with potassic cyanide or by ignition with ammonium chloride.

§ 813. **The Sulphide of Bismuth**, Bi_2S_3 = 516; Bi, 81.25 per cent., S, 18.75 per cent., occurs, in the course of analysis, as a brownish-black or quite black precipitate, insoluble in water, dilute acids, alkalies, alkaline sulphides, sulphate of soda, and cyanide of potassium, but dissolving in moderately concentrated nitric acid with separation of sulphur. It continually increases in weight when dried in the ordinary way, and is completely reduced when fused with cyanide of potassium.

§ 814. **Preparations of Bismuth used in Medicine and the Arts.**

(1) **Pharmaceutical Preparations**:—

Bismuthi Subnitras, $BiONO_3.H_2O$.—A heavy white powder, insoluble in water, and responding to the usual tests for bismuth and nitric acid. The formula should yield 77 per cent. of bismuth oxide. Commercial preparations, however, vary from 79 to 82 per cent.

Bismuth Lozenges (Trochisci bismuthi) are composed of subnitrate of bismuth, magnesia carbonate, precipitated lime carbonate, sugar, and gum, mixed with rose water. Each lozenge should contain 0.13 grm. (2 grains) of subnitrate of bismuth.

Solution of Citrate of Bismuth and Ammonia (Liquor Bismuthi et Ammoniæ citratis), a colourless neutral or slightly alkaline fluid, sp. gr. 1.07, responding to the tests for bismuth and ammonia. As an impurity lead may be present, citric acid being so frequently contaminated with lead. Carbonate of bismuth (*Bismuthi carbonas*), $(Bi_2O_2CO_3)_2H_2O$ is a fine white powder answering to the tests for carbon dioxide and bismuth; it should yield 89.1 per cent. of bismuth oxide.

A Nitrate of Bismuth, $Bi(NO_3)_3$, an oleate of bismuth, an oxide of bismuth, a subgallate of bismuth (*dermatol*), and a subiodide of bismuth are also used in medicine.

(2) **Bismuth in the Arts.**[892]

The chief use of bismuth is in alloys and solders. The Chromate is employed in calico-printing, and the subnitrate as a paint under the name of pearl-white.

The salts of bismuth also occur in washes for the hair, and pearl-white is used as a cosmetic, but only to a small extent.

§ 815. **Medicinal Doses of Bismuth.**—The subnitrate and carbonate are prescribed in doses from .0648 to 1.296 grm. (1 to 20 grains); the valerianate, from .1296 to .648 grm. (2 to 10 grains); and the solution, from 1.7 c.c. to 5.2 c.c. (½ drachm to 1½ drachm).

§ 816. **Toxic Effects of Bismuth.**—From the researches of Meyer and Steinfeld[893] on animals, it appears that if birds or mammals are poisoned with bismuth salts introduced subcutaneously, or by direct injection, into the veins, death follows in from twenty-four to forty-eight hours, the fatal issue being preceded by convulsions; after death, the colon is intensely blackened, and it may be ulcerated, while the small intestines and the stomach are

[892] Bismuth is contained in all copper coinage—from the Bactrian coins to our own; in all cupreous ores, except the carbonates, and in nearly all specimens of commercial copper.—Field, *Chem. News*, xxxvi. 261.

[893] L. Feder-Meyer, *Rossbach's pharmak. Unters.*, iii., 1882, No. 23; Steinfeld, *Wirkung des Wismut. Inaug. Diss.*, Dorpat, 1884; *Arch. exp. P.*, Bd. xx. 1886.

healthy. If, however, sulphur preparations are given by the mouth, there is then blackening of the stomach, and there may also be ulcers. Meyer is of the opinion that SH_2 precipitates bismuth in the parenchyma, and the particles occluding the capillaries thus cause small local necroses; that which escapes precipitation is mainly excreted by the kidneys. Poisonous symptoms in man have been known to occur from the treatment of wounds with bismuth preparations;[894] the symptoms have been somewhat similar to mercurial poisoning; there have been noticed stomatitis with salivation, loosening of the teeth, a black colour of the mucous membrane of the mouth and ulceration, also catarrh of the intestines, and the inflammatory condition of the kidneys usual when that organ has to excrete metallic substances not natural to the body, the "metallniere," or metal kidney, of the German writers. One case is recorded of death in nine days of an adult after taking 7.7 grms. (2 drms.) of bismuth subnitrate. The recorded symptoms were a metallic taste in the mouth, pain in the throat, vomiting, purging, coldness of the surface, and spasms of the arms and legs. A *post-mortem* examination showed inflammatory changes in the gullet, windpipe, and throughout the intestinal canal. Recovery has, however, taken place from a single dose three times the amount mentioned. It is possible that the fatal case was due to impure bismuth.

§ 817. **Extraction and Detection of Bismuth in Animal Matters.**—Bismuth appears to be excreted principally by the bowels as sulphide of bismuth; but it has also been detected in the urine, spleen, and liver; and Lubinsky has found it in the saliva and in the epithelium of the mouth of persons taking one of its preparations. Without denying the possibility of its existing in a soluble state in the saliva, its presence in the mouth may, under such circumstances, be ascribed to the lodgment of particles of subnitrate or subcarbonate of bismuth in the interstices of the teeth, &c. It will then be evident that, if a person is supposed to have been poisoned by a large dose of bismuth, and the analyst fail to find it in the stomach, the contents of the bowels should be next examined.

The extraction of bismuth must be undertaken by nitric acid, and boiling for at least two hours may be necessary to dissolve it out from the tissues. Such organs as the liver and spleen are boiled in a finely divided state with a litre of dilute nitric acid (strength, 5 per cent.), for the time mentioned, filtered, and the filtrate evaporated to dryness; the remainder is then carbonised by strong nitric acid; and, finally, the charcoal is boiled with equal parts of nitric acid and water, and the whole evaporated to dryness. By this method every trace of bismuth is extracted. The dry residue may now be brought into solution, and tested for bismuth. The best solvent for the nitrate of bismuth is dilute nitric acid 50 per cent.; the dry residue is therefore dissolved in 100 or 200 c.c. of the acid, and fractional parts taken for examination:—

(1) The solution, poured into a large volume of warm distilled water, gives a crystalline precipitate of subnitrate of bismuth. The only metal giving a similar reaction is antimony, and this is excluded by the method employed.

(2) The filtered fluid gives on addition of sodic chloride a precipitate of oxychloride. This, again, is distinguished from oxychloride of antimony by its insolubility in tartaric acid.

(3) Any bismuth precipitate, fused with soda on charcoal, gives a brittle bead of bismuth; the coal is coated whilst warm a dark orange-yellow, on cooling citron-yellow.

(4) The bead may be identified by powdering it, placing it in a short subliming tube, and passing over it dry chlorine. The powder first turns black, then melts to an amber-yellow fluid, and finally, by prolonged heating, sublimes as terchloride of bismuth.

(5) A very delicate test proposed by Abel and Field, in 1862,[895] specially for the detection of bismuth in copper (but by no means confined to mineral analysis), utilises the fact that, if iodide of lead be precipitated from a fluid containing the least trace of bismuth, instead of the yellow iodide the scales assume a dark orange to a crimson tint. A solution of nitrate of lead is used; to the nitric acid solution ammonia and carbonate of ammonia added; the precipitate washed, and dissolved in acetic acid; and, finally, excess of iodide of potassium added. It is said that thus so small a quantity as .00025 grm. may be detected in copper with the greatest ease, the iodide of lead becoming dark orange; .001 grain imparts a reddish-brown tinge, and .01 grain a crimson.

(6) A solution of a bismuth salt, which must contain no free HCl, when treated with 10 parts of water, 2 of potassium iodide, and 1 part of cinchonine, gives a red orange precipitate of cinchonine iod.-bismuth.[896]

(7) Van Kobell's test, as modified by Hutchings,[897] and proposed more especially for the detection of bismuth in minerals, is capable of being applied to any solid compound suspected of containing the metal:—A mixture of

894 *B. Med. Journal*, 1887, i. 749.

895 *Journ. Chem. Soc.*, 1862, vol. xiv. p. 290; *Chem. News*, vol. xxxvi. p. 261.

896 E. Légar, *Bull. de la Soc. Chim.*, vol. iv., 1888, 91.

897 *Chem. News*, vol. xxxvi. p. 249.

precipitated and purified cuprous iodide, with an equal volume of flowers of sulphur, is prepared, and 2 parts of this mixture are made into a paste with 1 part of the substance, and heated on a slip of charcoal on an aluminium support by the blowpipe flame. If bismuth be present, the red bismuth iodide will sublime, and on clean aluminium is easily distinguishable.

There are many other tests, but the above are sufficient.

§ 818. **Estimation of Bismuth.**—The estimation of bismuth, when in any quantity easily weighed, is, perhaps, best accomplished by fusing the sulphide, oxide, or other compound of bismuth, in a porcelain crucible with cyanide of potassium; the bismuth is reduced to the metallic state, the cyanide can be dissolved out, and the metallic powder washed (first with water, lastly with spirit), dried, and weighed.

Mr. Pattison Muir has shown[898] that bismuth may be separated from iron, aluminium, chromium, and manganese, by adding ammonia to the acid solutions of these metals.

This observation admits of many applications, and may be usefully taken advantage of in the separation of bismuth from the nitric acid solution of such animal matters as liver, &c. The acid liquid is partially neutralised by ammonia, and, on diluting with warm water containing a little sodium or ammonium chloride, the whole of the bismuth is precipitated as oxychloride, which may be collected, and fused with cyanide of potassium, as above.

If the bismuth precipitate is in small quantity, or if a number of estimations of bismuth are to be made, it is most convenient to use a volumetric process. In the case first mentioned, the oxychloride could be dissolved in nitric acid, sodium acetate added in excess, and sufficient acetic acid to dissolve any precipitate which has been produced, and then titrated by the following method, which we also owe to Mr. Pattison Muir:—

Estimation of Bismuth by Potassium Dichromate.[899]—A solution of recrystallised potassium dichromate (strength, 1 per cent.) is prepared. A known weight of pure bismuthous oxide (Bi_2O_3) is dissolved in excess of nitric acid, and a solution of sodium acetate is added to this liquid until a copious white precipitate is thrown down; acetic acid is then added in quantity sufficient to dissolve the precipitate completely, and to insure that, when the liquid is made up with water to a fixed volume, no precipitate shall be formed. A certain volume of this liquid is withdrawn by means of a pipette, placed in a beaker, and heated to boiling; the potassium dichromate is then gradually run in from a burette, the liquid being boiled between each addition of the solution, until a drop of the supernatant liquid gives a faint reddish-brown coloration when spotted with silver nitrate on a white slab.

Another very generally applicable volumetric method for bismuth has been proposed by Mr. Muir.[900] This depends on the fact (observed by Sonchay and Leussen),[901] that normal bismuth oxalate splits up on boiling into a basic oxalate of the composition $Bi_2O_32C_2O_3 + OH_2$, but slightly soluble in nitric acid. The process is performed by precipitating the bismuth by excess of oxalic acid, dissolving the precipitate (first purified from free oxalic acid) in dilute hydrochloric acid, and lastly, titrating by permanganate. The absence of free hydrochloric acid before precipitating must be insured.

4. SILVER.

§ 819. **Silver** = 108; specific gravity, 10.5; fusing-point, 1023° (1873° F.).—Silver, as separated in analysis, is either a very white, glittering, metallic bead, or a dull grey powder. It does not lose weight on ignition, and is soluble in dilute nitric acid.

§ 820. **Chloride of Silver**, $AgCl$ = 143.5; specific gravity, 5.552; Ag, 75.27 per cent., Cl, 24.73 per cent., is a dense, white, curdy precipitate, when produced in the wet way. It is very insoluble in water, dilute nitric acid, and dilute sulphuric acid; in many warm solutions (especially aqueous solutions of the chlorides generally), the alkaline and alkaline-earthy nitrates, and tartaric acid solutions, the silver is dissolved to an appreciable extent, but deposited again on diluting and cooling. The complete solvents of chloride of silver are—ammonia, cyanide of potassium, and hyposulphite of soda. Chloride of silver cannot be fused at a high heat without some slight loss by volatilisation; on coal in the R.F., it fuses very easily to a globule. It can with soda be reduced to metal, and can also readily be reduced by ignition in a current of hydrogen, carbon oxide, or carburetted hydrogen gas.

§ 821. **Sulphide of Silver**, Ag_2S = 248; specific gravity, 7.2; Ag, 87.1 per cent., S, 12.9 per cent., when prepared in the wet way, is a black precipitate, insoluble in water, dilute acids, and alkaline sulphides. If ignited in hydrogen it may be reduced to the metallic state; it is soluble in nitric acid, with separation of sulphur.

[898] Pattison Muir on "Certain Bismuth Compounds," *Journ. Chem. Soc.*, p. 7, 1876.

[899] Pattison Muir on "Certain Bismuth Compounds," *Journ. Chem. Soc.*, vol. i. p. 659, 1879.

[900] *Ibid.*, 1877.

[901] *Ann. Chem. Pharm.*, vol. cv. p. 245.

§ 822. **Preparations of Silver used in Medicine and the Arts.**

(1) **Medicinal Preparations:**—

Nitrate of Silver, $AgNO_3$; Ag, 63.51 per cent., N_2O_5, 36.49 per cent. This salt is either sold crystallised in colourless rhombic prisms, or in the form of small white pencils or sticks. It gives the reactions for silver and nitric acid, and stains the skin black. 100 parts, dissolved in distilled water, should give, with hydrochloric acid, a precipitate which, when washed and dried, weighs 83.4 parts. The silver is, however, far more quickly estimated by the blowpipe than in the wet way. One grm. fused in a cavity on charcoal should give a little globule of metallic silver, weighing about .6351 grm. The chief adulterations of this substance are copper, lead, and nitrate of potash. If all the silver is precipitated by hydrochloric acid, carefully filtered off, and the filtrate evaporated to dryness, any residue will denote adulteration or impurity.

Argenti Oxidum, Oxide of Silver, $Ag_2O = 232$; Ag, 93.19 per cent.—A dark olive-brown powder, soluble in ammonia and nitric acid. By ignition it readily yields metallic silver. The P.B. directs that 29 grains of the oxide should yield 27 of metallic silver.

Nitrate of Silver and Potash (Argentum nitricum cum kali nitrico), $AgNO_3 + KNO_3$.—This preparation is in most of the pharmacopœias, Austrian, German, Danish, Swedish, Russian, Swiss, and the British; it is directed by the B.P. to be composed of 1 part of silver nitrate and 1 part of potassic nitrate fused together. A "toughened silver nitrate" is made by fusing together potassic nitrate 5, silver nitrate 95. Mild caustic points are used by oculists by fusing 1 of silver nitrate with 2, 3, 3½, and 4 parts of potassic nitrate.

(2) **Silver in the Arts.**—The uses of the metal in coinage, articles for domestic purposes, for ornament, &c., are too well known to require enumeration. The only forms in which silver is likely to give rise to accident are the salts used in medicine, photography, in the dyeing of hair, and in the manufacture of marking inks.

Hair-dyes.—About one-half of the hair-dyes in use are made with nitrate of silver. The following are only a few of the recipes:—

Aqua Orientalis.—Grain silver 2 drms., nitric acid 1 oz., steel filings 4 drms., distilled water 1½ oz.—the whole finally made up to 3½ fluid ozs., and filtered.

Argentan Tincture.—Nitrate of silver 1 drachm, rose water 1 fluid oz., sufficient nitrate of copper to impart a greenish tint.

Eau d'Afrique.—Two solutions—one of nitrate of silver, the other of potash, containing ammonium sulphide.

The photographer uses various salts of silver, the chief of which are—the nitrate, iodide, bromide, cyanide, and chloride of silver.

Marking Inks.—Some of the more important recipes for marking ink are as follows:—

Nitrate of silver 1.0 part, hot distilled water 3.6 parts, mucilage, previously rubbed with sap-green, 1.0 part. With this is sold a "pounce," or preparation consisting of a coloured solution of sodic carbonate. Another preparation is very similar, but with the addition of ammonia and some colouring matter, such as indigo, syrup of buckthorn, or sap-green. A third is made with tartaric acid and nitrate of silver, dissolved in ammonia solution, and coloured.

Redwood's Ink consists of equal parts of nitrate of silver and potassic bitartrate, dissolved in ammonia, with the addition of archil green and sugar; according to the formula, 100 parts should equal 16.6 of silver nitrate.

Soubeiran's Ink is composed of cupric nitrate 3, argentic nitrate 8, sodic carbonate 4, and the whole made up to 100 parts, in solution of ammonia. In one of Mr. Reade's inks, besides silver, an ammoniacal solution of a salt of gold is used.

§ 823. **Medicinal Dose of Silver Compounds.**—The nitrate and the oxide of silver are given in doses from .0162 to .1296 grm. (¼ grain to 2 grains). Anything like .1944 to .2592 grm. (3 or 4 grains) would be considered a large, if not a dangerous dose; but nothing definite is known as to what would be a *poisonous* dose.

§ 824. **Effects of Nitrate of Silver on Animals.**—Nitrate of silver is changed into chloride by the animal fluids, and also forms a compound with albumen. Silver chloride and silver albumenate are both somewhat soluble in solutions containing chlorides of the alkalies, which explains how a metallic salt, so very insoluble in water, can be absorbed by the blood.

The action of soluble salts of silver on animals has been several times investigated. There appears to be some difference between its effects on warm and cold-blooded animals. In frogs there is quickly an exaltation of the functions of the spinal cord, tetanic convulsions appear, similar to those induced by strychnine; later, there is disturbance of the respiration and cessation of voluntary motion.

The first symptoms with dogs and cats are vomiting and diarrhœa; muscular weakness, paralysis, disturbance of the respiration, and weak clonic convulsions follow. Rouget, as well as Curci, considers that the action of silver is directed to the central nervous system; there is first excitement, and then follows paralysis of the centres of respiration and movement. Death occurs through central asphyxia. According to the researches of F. A. Falck, subcutaneous injections of silver nitrate into rabbits cause a fall of temperature of 6.7° to 17.6°, the last being the greatest fall which, in his numerous researches on the effect of poisons on temperature, he has seen.

Chronic poisoning, according to the experiments of Bogoslowsky on animals, produces emaciation, fatty degeneration of the liver, kidneys, and also of the muscles—a statement confirmed by others.

§ 825. **Toxic Effects of Silver Nitrate in Man**—(1) **Acute Poisoning.**—This is very rare. Orfila relates an attempt at suicide; but most of the cases have been accidental, and of these, in recent times, about five are recorded, mostly children. The accident is usually due to the application of the solid nitrate to the throat, as an escharotic, the stick breaking or becoming detached, and being immediately swallowed; such an accident is related by Scattergood.[902] A piece of silver nitrate ¾ inch long, slipped down the throat of a child, aged fifteen months—vomiting immediately occurred, followed by convulsions and diarrhœa; chloride of sodium was administered, but the child died in six hours. In other cases paralysis and an unconscious state has been observed.

(2) **Chronic Poisoning.**—Salts of silver taken for a long period cause a peculiar and indelible colour of the skin, the body becomes of a greyish-blue to black colour, it begins first around the nails and fingers, then patches of a similar hue appear in different parts of the body, and gradually coalesce, being most marked in those parts exposed to the light. The colour is not confined to the outer skin, but is also seen in the mucous membranes. There is also a slight inflammation of the gums, and a violet line around their edge. Ginpon observed this line after two months' treatment of a patient by silver nitrate; the whole quantity taken being 3.9 grms. (about 60 grains). The peculiar colour of the skin is only seen after large dose; after 8 grms. taken in divided doses Chaillon could not observe any change, but after 15 grms. had been taken it was evident. So also Riemer has recorded a case, in which, after a year's use of silver nitrate (total quantity 17.4 grms.) a greyish-black colour of the face was produced, and, when nearly double the quantity had been taken, the colour had invaded the whole body.

§ 826. **Post-mortem Appearances.**—In the acute case recorded by Scattergood, the mucous membranes of the gullet, of the great curvature of the stomach, and parts of the duodenum and jejunum were eroded, and particles of curd-like silver chloride adhered to the mucous membrane.

In the case recorded by Riemer of the long-continued use of silver nitrate, the serous and mucous membranes were coloured dark; the choroid plexus was of a blue-black; the endocardium, the valves of the heart, and the aorta pale to dark grey, as well as the rest of the vessels; the colouring was confined to the intima. The liver and kidney also showed similar pigmentation. The pigment (probably metallic silver) was in the form of very fine grains, and, as regards the skin, was situate under the *rete Malpighia* in the upper layer of the corium, and also in the deeper connective tissue and in the sweat glands. Liouville has also found the kidneys of a woman similarly pigmented, who took silver nitrate daily for 270 days, in all about 7 grms., five years before her death.

§ 827. **Detection and Estimation of Silver.**—The examination of the solid salts of silver usually met with (viz., the nitrate, bromide, iodide, cyanide, and chloride) is most speedy by the dry method on charcoal; in this way in less than 120 seconds any practical chemist could identify each compound. The nitrate, bromide, iodide, and cyanide, all, if ignited on charcoal, yield buttons of metallic silver—deflagration, bromine vapours, iodine vapours, and cyanogen vapours being the respective phenomena observed. Chloride of silver fuses to a pearl-grey, brown, or black globule on charcoal, according to its purity; but is only in the R.F. gradually reduced to metal. With soda, or fused in hydrogen or coal gas, the reduction is rapid enough.

Nitrate of Silver in solution might be identified by a very large number of tests, since it forms so many insoluble salts. In practice one is, however, satisfied with three tests, viz.: (1) A curdy precipitate of chloride, on the addition of hydrochloric acid or alkaline chlorides, soluble only in ammonia, cyanide of potassium, or hyposulphite of soda; (2) a yellow precipitate, but little soluble in ammonia, on the addition of iodide of potassium; and (3) a blood-red precipitate on the addition of chromate of potash.

The separation of silver from the contents of the stomach is best ensured by treating it with cyanide of potassium; for, unless a very large quantity of silver nitrate has been taken, it is tolerably certain that the whole of it has passed into chloride, and will, therefore, not be attacked easily by acids. The contents of the stomach, then, or the tissues themselves, are placed in a flask and warmed for some time with cyanide of potassium, first, if necessary, adding ammonia. The fluid is separated from the solid matters by subsidence (for an alkaline fluid of this kind will scarcely filter), and then decomposed by hydrochloric acid in excess. The flask containing this fluid is put

902 *Brit. Med. Journal*, May 1871.

on one side in a warm place, and the clear fluid decanted from the insoluble chloride. The latter is now collected on a filter, well washed with hot water, and then dried and reduced on charcoal; or it may be put in a little porcelain crucible with a rod of zinc and a few drops of hydrochloric acid. The silver is soon deposited, and must be washed with water, then with sulphuric acid. By the aid of a wash-bottle the particles of silver are now collected on a small filter, again washed, and on the moist mass a crystal of nitrate of potash and a little carbonate of soda laid. The whole is then dried, and all the filter cut away, save the small portion containing the silver. This small portion is now heated on charcoal until a little button of pure silver is obtained, which may first be weighed, then dissolved in nitric acid, and tested by the methods detailed.

In a similar way hair, suspected of being dyed with silver, can be treated with chlorine gas, and the chloride dissolved in potassic cyanide.

Spots on linen, and, generally, very small quantities of silver, may be detected by a simple galvanic process:—The substance is treated with solution of cyanide of potassium, and submitted to a weak galvanic current, using for the negative plate a slip of copper, for the positive, platinum; the silver is deposited on the former.

5. MERCURY.

§ 828. **Mercury**, Hg = 200; specific gravity, 13.596; boiling-point, 350° (662° F.); it becomes solid at -39.4 (-39 F.). This well known and familiar fluid metal evaporates and sublimes to a minute extent at all temperatures above 5°.

When precipitated or deposited in a finely divided state, the metal can be united into a single globule only if it is fairly pure; very slight *fatty* impurities especially will prevent the union. It is insoluble in hydrochloric acid, soluble to a slight extent in dilute cold sulphuric acid, and completely soluble in concentrated sulphuric and in nitric acids. It combines directly with chlorine, bromine, and iodine, which, in presence of free alkali, readily dissolve it. It is unalterable at 100°, and, when exposed to a high temperature, sublimes unchanged.

Mercurous Chloride (Calomel, HgCl = 235.5; specific gravity, 7.178; subliming temperature, 111.6°; Hg, 84.94 per cent., Cl, 15.06 per cent.), when prepared in the wet way is a heavy white powder, absolutely insoluble in cold, but decomposed by boiling water. It may be converted into the mercuric chloride by chlorine water and aqua regia. Chloride of ammonium, potassium, and sodium, all decompose calomel into metallic mercury and mercuric chloride. It is easily reduced to metal in a tube with soda, potash, or burnt magnesia.

§ 829. **Sulphide of Mercury** (HgS, Hg, 86.21 per cent., S, 13.79 per cent.) is a black powder, dissolving in nitromuriatic acid, but very insoluble in other acids or in water. It is also insoluble in alkaline sulphides, with the exception of potassic sulphide.

§ 830. **Medicinal Preparations of Mercury.**—Mercury in the liquid state has been occasionally administered in constipation; its internal use is now (or ought to be) obsolete. Gmelin has found samples contaminated with metallic bismuth—a metal which only slightly diminishes the fluidity of mercury; the impurity may be detected by shaking the mercury in air, and thus oxidising the bismuth. Mercury may also contain various mechanical impurities, which are detected by forcing the metal by means of a vacuum pump through any dense filtering substance. Tin and zinc may be dissolved out by hydrochloric acid, and all fixed impurities (such as lead and bismuth) are at once discovered on subliming the metal.

Mercury and Chalk (Hydrargyrum cum creta).—Mercury, 33.33 per cent.; chalk, 66.67.

Blue Pill (Pilula hydrargyri).—Mercury in a finely divided state, mixed with confection of roses and liquorice root; the mercury should be in the proportion of 33.33 per cent.[903]

[903] The chemical composition of blue pill varies according to its age. Harold Senier has made a careful series of analyses, with the following result (*Pharm. Journ.*, Feb. 5, 1876):—

	Age.	Metallic Mercury.	Mercuric Oxide.	Mercurous Oxide.	Ash.	Organic Matter.
1	18 hours,	32 .49	none.	a trace.	1 .20	66 .31
2	3 weeks,	32 .26	.09	.25	1 .20	66 .20
3	3 months,	32 .60	.24	.62	1 .18	66 .36
4	3 „	31 .15	.44	1 .60	1 .12	65 .69
5	6 „	32 .44	.50	.80	1 .70	64 .56
6	14 „	29 .86	.98	2 .60	1 .20	65 .36
7	19 „	31 .59	.50	2 .50	1 .00	64 .41

Mercury Plaster (Emplastrum hydrargyri).—Made with mercury, olive oil, sulphur, and lead plaster; it should contain Hg, 33 per cent.; sulphur, 18 per cent.

Ammoniac and Mercury Plaster (Emplastrum ammoniaci cum hydrargyro).—Gum, ammonia, mercury, olive oil, and sulphur; it should contain 20 per cent. of Hg, and .1 per cent. of sulphur.

Mercurial Ointment (Unguentum hydrargyri).—Mercury mixed with lard and suet, the strength should be nearly 50 per cent. mercury; commercial samples often contain as little as 38 per cent.

Compound Mercury Ointment (Unguentum hydrargyri compositum).—Made with ointment of mercury, yellow wax, olive oil, and camphor; it should contain 22.2 per cent. Hg.

Liniment of Mercury (Linimentum hydrargyri) is made of mercurial ointment, solution of ammonia, and liniment of camphor; it contains about 16½ per cent. of mercury.

Mercurial Suppositories (Suppositoria hydrargyri).—Composed of ointment of mercury and oil of theobroma. Each suppository should weigh 15 grains and contain ⅓ of its weight of mercurial ointment.

Acetate of Mercury (Mercurous acetate) is not contained in the B.P., but is officinal on the Continent. It is a salt occurring in white micaceous scales, soluble in 133 parts of cold water, giving the reactions of acetic acid and mercury, and very readily decomposed.

Mercuric Ethyl Chloride (Hydrargyrum æthylo-chloratum) is used as a medicine on the Continent. It occurs in white, glittering, crystalline scales, which take on pressure a metallic appearance, and possess a peculiar ethereal odour; it is but little soluble in water and ether, with difficulty in cold alcohol, but copiously soluble on boiling, and depositing crystals on cooling. It sublimes at about 40° without residue; on quick heating it burns with a weak flame, developing a vapour of metallic taste and unpleasant odour. It gives no precipitate with silver nitrate, nor with albumen.

Corrosive Sublimate (Mercuric chloride), $HgCl_2 = 271$; Hg, 73.8 per cent., Cl, 26.1 per cent.—In commerce this salt occurs in transparent, heavy, colourless masses, which have a crystalline fracture; if placed in the subliming cell described earlier, it sublimes at about 82.2° (180° F.), and melts at higher temperatures. The sublimate is generally in groups of plates drawn to a point at both ends, in crystalline needles, or in octahedra with a rectangular base. It dissolves in 16 parts of cold water and about 3 of boiling, and is very soluble in solutions of the alkaline chlorides; it dissolves also in ether, and can be, to a great extent, withdrawn from aqueous solutions by this agent. Alcohol dissolves nearly one-third its weight of the salt, and its own weight when boiling. It combines with albumen; gives, when in solution, a precipitate of mercuric oxide when tested with solution of potash; a white precipitate with ammonia; a scarlet with iodide of potassium; and a black precipitate of finely divided mercury with protochloride of tin. If a crystal (when placed in the subliming cell) gives a crystalline sublimate at about the temperature mentioned, and this sublimate becomes of a red colour when treated with a droplet of iodide of potassium, it can be no other substance than corrosive sublimate.

Solution of Perchloride of Mercury (Liquor hydrargyri perchloridi) is simply 10 grains of perchloride of mercury and chloride of ammonium in a pint of water; 100 c.c. therefore should contain 114 mgrms. corrosive sublimate.

Yellow Mercurial Lotion (Lotio hydrargyri flava).—Perchloride of mercury, 18 grains, mixed with 10 ounces of solution of lime.

Calomel[904] **(Hydrargyri subchloridum).**—The properties of calomel have been already described. It sometimes contains as an impurity corrosive sublimate, which may be dissolved out by ether. Carbonate of lead, sulphate, and carbonate of baryta, gum, and starch, are the usual adulterants mentioned. If on the application of heat calomel entirely sublimes, it must be free from the substances enumerated.

Oleate of Mercury (Hydrargyri oleatum) is composed of 1 part of yellow oxide and 9 parts of oleic acid.

Black Mercurial Lotion (Lotio hydrargyri nigra).—Calomel, 30 grains, mixed with 10 fluid ounces of lime-water.

Compound Pill of Subchloride of Mercury.—Calomel and sulphurated antimony, each 1 ounce, guiac resin 2 ounces, castor-oil 1 fluid ounce. One grain (.0648 grm.) of calomel, and the same quantity of antimony sulphide,

8	2 years,	28 .40	1 .80	4 .22	2 .10	63 .48
9	(?)	30 .23	1 .06	3 .24	1 .05	64 .44

[904] It would appear that in America a cosmetic is in use, consisting of calomel mixed into a paste with water.—*Vide* "A Dangerous Cosmetic," by C. H. Piesse, *Analyst* (25), 1878, p. 241.

are contained in every 5 grains (324 mgrms.) of the pill mass, *i.e.*, calomel 20 per cent.

Ointment of Subchloride of Mercury (Unguentum hydrargyri subchloridi).—Calomel mixed with benzoated lard; strength about 1 : 6½.

White Precipitate (Hydrargyrum ammoniatum, NH_2HgCl).—A white, heavy powder, subliming by heat without residue, and insoluble in water, alcohol, and ether. With soda, it yields a metallic sublimate. When boiled with potash, ammonia is evolved, the yellow oxide of mercury formed, and chloride of potassium passes into solution. It should contain 79.5 per cent. of mercury.

The fusible white precipitate of the pharmacopœia of the Netherlands does not appear to be of constant composition, varying between 69.4 to 65.6 per cent. of mercury.[905] It melts on heating, and leaves as a residue chloride of sodium.

Commercial white precipitate is frequently adulterated; Barnes has found carbonates of lead and lime, the latter to the extent of nearly 2 per cent.[906] Calomel, according to Nickles,[907] has been substituted for white precipitate, but this was several years ago. The methods for detection are obvious.

Ointment of Ammoniated Mercury (Unguentum hydrargyri ammoniati).—1 part of ammoniated mercury mixed with 9 parts of simple ointment.

Red Iodide of Mercury (Hydrargyrum iodidum rubrum, HgI_2).—A crystalline powder of a scarlet colour, becoming yellow on gentle heating. It is very insoluble in water, one part requiring from 6000 to 7000 parts; soluble in 130 parts of cold, 150 of hot alcohol; and dissolving freely in ether, or in aqueous solution of iodide of potassium.

Ointment of Red Iodide of Mercury (Unguentum hydrargyri iodidi rubri).—16 grains of the substance mixed with an ounce of simple ointment.

Green Iodide of Mercury (Hydrargyri iodidum viride, HgI).—A dingy, greenish-yellow powder, darkening on exposure to light, and easily decomposed into the red iodide.

Red Oxide of Mercury (Hydrargyri oxidum rubrum), HgO = 216; Hg, 92.12 per cent.; specific gravity, 11 to 11.3; small, red, shining, crystalline scales, very insoluble in water, requiring about 20,000 parts; entirely soluble in hydrochloric acid. By a heat below redness it may be volatilised, and at the same time decomposed into mercury and oxygen. Its principal impurity is nitric acid, readily detected by the usual tests, or by heating in a test-tube, when, if nitric acid is present, orange vapours will be evolved. Fixed red powders (such as brick-dust and minium) are detected by being left as a residue, after the application of heat sufficient to volatilise the mercury. An ointment (strength 1 : 8) is officinal.

Sulphate of Mercury.—A white crystalline powder, decomposed by water into the very insoluble basic salt of mercury, known as *Turbith mineral*, $HgSO_42HgO$.

Turbith, or Turpeth, Mineral is contained in the French pharmacopœia, $HgSO_42HgO$; Hg, 82.4 per cent.; specific gravity, 8.319. It requires for solution 2000 parts of cold, and 600 of boiling water; but dissolves with tolerable ease in hydrochloric acid.

The Sulphide of Mercury, known in commerce under the name of *Ethiops mineral*, is officinal in France, the Netherlands, and Germany. Its properties have been already described. The German and Dutch pharmacopœias require in it 50, the French only 33⅓ per cent. of metallic mercury.

Hahnemann's Soluble Mercury (Hydrargyrum solubile Hahnemanni) is officinal in the Dutch pharmacopœia. As found in commerce it contains metallic mercury, nitric acid, and ammonia. The mercury should be in the proportion of 86.33 per cent., the ammonia 2.44 per cent.

Crystallised Nitrate of Mercury (Hydrargyrum nitricum oxidulatum) is officinal in the pharmacopœias of Germany, Switzerland, and France. The salt is in white crystals, giving the reactions of nitric acid and mercury, decomposed by the addition of water, but fully soluble in water, if first moistened with nitric acid. The formula of the neutral salt is $Hg2NO_3HgO2H_2O$, which requires 69.4 per cent. of mercury. An acid solution of mercuric nitrate is officinal.

An Ointment of Nitrate of Mercury (Unguentum hydrargyri nitratis) (often called citrine ointment) is contained in the B.P.; it is made with 4 parts of mercury, nitric acid 12, lard 15, olive oil, 32; the strength is about 1 in 15½.

A Chloride of Mercury and Quinine exists in commerce, prepared by mixing 1 part of corrosive sublimate in

---

905 Hirsch, *Die Prüfung der Arzeneimittel*.

906 *Proceed. Brit. Pharm. Conf.*, 1867, p. 10.

907 *Journ. Pharm. et Chim.*, le Série, 1858, vol. viij. p. 399.

solution with 3 parts of quinine chloride, evaporating, and crystallising.

Cyanide of Mercury, HgCy, is contained in the French pharmacopœia. It occurs in small, colourless, prismatic crystals, easily soluble in water. If to the solution chloride of tin be added, a black precipitate of reduced metal and stannous oxide is thrown down, and the odour of prussic acid is developed.

Mercuric Sulphide (Sulphide of Mercury, Cinnabar, Vermilion) is officinal in Germany, the Netherlands, and France; HgS = 232; specific gravity, solid, 8.2; Hg, 86.21 per cent., O, 13.79 per cent. For medicinal purposes it is made artificially. It is a beautiful red powder, insoluble in all alkaline and all acid liquids, with the exception of aqua regia. The solution gives the reactions of a sulphide and mercury. On heating, it must burn away entirely without residue; adulterations or impurities are—minium, lead, copper, and other metals. The detection of minium is conveniently executed in the dry way. Pure cinnabar, when heated in a matrass, gives a black sublimate, which becomes red on friction. If minium is present, sulphide of lead remains as a residue, and may be recognised on coal; the same remark applies to sulphide of antimony. If it be desired to take the percentage of mercury in cinnabar, equal parts of oxalate and cyanide of potassium should be well mixed with the cinnabar, and heated in the bent tube described below; by this means the whole of the metallic mercury is readily obtained.[908]

§ 831. **Mercury in the Arts.**—The use of mercury in the arts is so extensive, that any one in analytical practice is almost certain occasionally to meet with cases of accidental poisoning, either from the vapour[909] or some of its combinations.

Quicksilver is used in the extraction of gold, the silvering of mirrors, the construction of barometers, and various scientific instruments and appliances; also for the preservation of insects, and occasionally for their destruction.[910] An alloy with zinc and cadmium is employed by dentists for stopping teeth; but there is no evidence that it has been at all injurious, the mercury, probably, being in too powerful a state of combination to be attacked by the fluids in the mouth.[911] Cinnabar has also been employed to give a red colour to confections, and it may be found in tapers, cigarette papers, and other coloured articles. The nitrate of mercury in solution finds application in the colouring of horn, in the etching of metals, in the colouring of the finer sorts of wool, and in the hat manufacture.

The sulphocyanide of mercury gives, when burnt, a most abundant ash, a fact utilised in the toy known as Pharaoh's serpent; the products of combustion are mercurial vapours and sulphurous anhydride. That the substance itself is poisonous, is evident from the following experiment:—.5 grm. was given to a pigeon without immediate result; but ten hours afterwards it was indisposed, refused its food, and in forty hours died without convulsions.[912]

§ 832. The more Common Patent and Quack Medicines containing Mercury.

Mordant's Norton's Drops.—This patent medicine is a mixture of the tincture of gentian and ginger, holding in solution a little bichloride of mercury, and coloured with cochineal.

Solomon's Anti-impetigines is a solution of bichloride of mercury, flavoured and coloured.

Poor Man's Friend.—An ointment of nitrate of mercury.

Brown's Lozenges.—Each lozenge contains ½ grain of calomel, and 3½ grains of resinous extract of jalap; the rest is white sugar and tragacanth.

Ching's Worm Lozenges.—Each lozenge contains 1 grain of calomel; the rest white sugar and tragacanth, with saffron as a colouring matter.

Storey's Worm Cakes.—Each cake 2 grains of calomel, 2 grains of cinnabar, 6 grains of jalap, 5 grains of ginger, and the remainder sugar and water.

Wright's Pearl Ointment is said to be made up of 8 ozs. of white precipitate rubbed to a cream in 1 pint of Goulard's extract, and to the mixture is added 7 lbs. of white wax and 10 lbs. of olive oil.

---

[908] Dr. Sutro has published a case (quoted by Taylor), in which the vapour of vermilion, applied externally, produced poisonous symptoms; yet, according to Polak, the Persians inhale it medicinally, smoking it with tobacco, catechu, mucilage, &c., the only bad effect being an occasional stomatitis.—Eulenberg, *Gewerbe Hygiene*, p. 741.

[909] A singular case is cited by Tardieu (*Étude méd.-légal sur l'Empoisonnement*), in which a man, supposing he had some minerals containing gold, attempted the extraction by amalgamation with mercury. He used a portable furnace (for the purpose of volatilising the mercury) in a small room, and his wife, who assisted him, suffered from a very well-marked stomatitis and mercurial eruption.

[910] Forty-three persons were salivated from fumigating rooms with mercury for the purpose of destroying bugs (Sonnenschein's *Handbuch*, p. 96).

[911] More danger is to be apprehended from the vulcanised rubber for artificial teeth; and, according to Dr. Taylor, accidents have occurred from the use of such supports or plates.

[912] Eulenberg, *Op. cit.*, p. 472.

Keyser's Pills.—The receipt for these pills is—red oxide of mercury 1½ oz., distilled vinegar (dilute acetic acid) 1 pint; dissolve, add to the resulting solution manna 2 lbs., and triturate for a long time before the fire, until a proper consistence is attained; lastly, divide the mass into pills of 1½ grain each.

Mitchell's Pills.—Each pill contains aloes .8 grain, rhubarb 1.6 grain, calomel .16 grain, tartar emetic .05 grain.

Many **Antibilious Pills** will be found to contain calomel, a few mercury in a finely divided state.

§ 833. **Mercury in Veterinary Medicine.**—Farmers and farriers use the ointment (*blue ointment*) to a dangerous extent, as a dressing for the fly, and wholesale poisoning of sheep has been in several instances the consequence.[913] Ethiops mineral and Turpeth mineral are given to dogs when affected by the distemper, worms, or the mange. Mercury, however, is not very frequently given to cattle by veterinary surgeons, ruminants generally appearing rather susceptible to its poisonous effects.

§ 834. **Medicinal and Fatal Dose—Horses.**—Cinnabar 14.2 grms, (½ oz.), calomel 14.2 grms. (½ oz.) or more, corrosive sublimate .13 to .38 grm. (2 to 6 grains), and as much as 1.3 grm. (20 grains) have been given in farcy.

Cattle.—Mercury with chalk 3.8 to 11.6 grms. (1 to 3 drms.), calomel 3.8 to 7.7 grms. (1 to 2 drms.) for worms; .65 to 1.3 grm. (10 to 20 grains) as an alterative; Ethiops mineral, 7.7 to 15.5 grms. (2 to 4 drms.).

Dogs.—Ethiops or Turpeth mineral .13 to 1.3 grm. (2 to 20 grains), according to the size.

Fowls.—Mercury and chalk are given in fractions of a grain.

Hogs are also treated with mercury and chalk; the dose usually given does not exceed .32 grm. (5 grains).

It may be remarked that many of the doses quoted appear very large; the writer cannot but consider that 20 grains of corrosive sublimate administered to a horse would be more likely to kill the animal than to cure the disease.

Man.—Corrosive sublimate has been fatal in a dose so small as .19 grm. (3 grains); white precipitate has caused dangerous symptoms in doses of from 1.9 to 2.6 grm. (30 to 40 grains); the cyanide of mercury has killed a person in a dose of .64 grm. (10 grains)—*Christison*; and Turpeth mineral has proved fatal in doses of 2.6 grms. (40 grains).

Other preparations of mercury have also been fatal, but a doubt has existed as to the precise quantity. Sometimes, also, there is probably a chemical change in the substance, so that it is impossible to state the fatal dose. For example, it is well known that calomel, under the influence of alkaline chlorides, can be converted into the bichloride—a fact which probably explains the extensive corrosive lesions that have been found after death from large doses of calomel.

§ 835. **Poisoning by Mercury—Statistics.**—In the Registrar-General's death returns for the ten years ending 1892, it appears that in England the deaths from mercurial poisoning[914] were 40 males, 19 females; of these, 16 males and 18 females were cases of suicide, the remainder were referred to accident.

The effects of the different compounds of mercury may be divided into two groups, viz., (1) Those caused by the finely divided metal and the non-corrosive compounds; (2) the effects caused by the corrosive compounds.

§ 836. (1) Effects of Mercurial Vapour, and of the Non-Corrosive Compounds of Mercury.

(*a*) **Vegetable Life.**—Priestly and Boussingault have shown that plants under a glass shade in which mercury is exposed in a saucer, first exhibit black spots on the leaves; ultimately, the latter blacken entirely, and the plants die.

(*b*) **Animal Life.**—Mercury in the form of vapour is fatal to animal life, but it is only so by repeated and intense application. Eulenberg[915] placed a rabbit under a large glass shade, and for four days exposed it daily for two hours to the volatilisation of 2 grms. of mercury on warm sand; on the sixth and seventh day 1.5 grm. was volatilised. On the fifteenth day there was no apparent change in the aspect of the animal; 5 grms. of mercury were then heated in a retort, and the vapour blown in at intervals of ten minutes. Fourteen days afterwards the gums were reddened and swollen, and the appetite lost; the conjunctivæ were also somewhat inflamed. The following day these symptoms disappeared, and the animal remained well.

In another experiment 20 grms. of mercury were volatilised, and a rabbit exposed to the vapour under a small glass shade. The following day the conjunctivæ were moist and reddened; two days afterwards 10 grms. of mercury were volatilised in the same way; and in two days' interval other 10 grms. were volatilised in three-quarters of an hour. There was no striking change noticeable in the condition of the animal, but within forty-eight hours it was

[913] Twenty-five tons of blue ointment are said to have been sold to farmers by a druggist in Boston, Lincolnshire, in the course of a single year.—Taylor's *Medical Jurisprudence*, vol. i. p. 279.

[914] The deaths are registered under the term "*Mercury*," but the majority are poisonings by "*Corrosive Sublimate*."

[915] *Op. cit.*, p. 728.

found dead. The cause of death proved to be an extravasation of blood at the base of the brain. The bronchia were reddened throughout, and the lungs congested. Mercury, as with man, is also readily absorbed by the broken or unbroken skin; hence thousands of sheep have been poisoned by the excessive and ignorant external application of mercurial ointment as a remedy against the attacks of parasites. The sheep become emaciated, refuse food, and seem to be in pain, breathing with short quick gasps.

In experiments on rabbits, dogs, and warm-blooded animals generally, salivation and stomatitis are found to occur as regularly as in man; so also in animals and man, paralytic and other nervous affections have been recorded.

§ 837. (*c*) **Effects on Man.**—In 1810[916] an extraordinary accident produced, perhaps, the largest wholesale poisoning by mercurial vapour on record. The account of this is as follows:—H.M.S. "Triumph," of seventy-four guns, arrived in the harbour of Cadiz in the month of February 1810; and in the following March, a Spanish vessel, laden with mercury for the South American mines, having been driven on shore in a gale, was wrecked. The "Triumph" saved by her boats 130 tons of the mercury, and this was stowed on board. The mercury was first confined in bladders, the bladders again were enclosed in small barrels, and the barrels in boxes. The heat of the weather, however, was at this time considerable; and the bladders, having been wetted in the removal from the wreck, soon rotted, and mercury, to the amount of several tons, was speedily diffused as vapour through the ship, mixing more or less with the bread and the other provisions. In three weeks 200 men were affected with ptyalism, ulceration of the mouth, partial paralysis, and, in many instances, with diarrhœa. The "Triumph" was now ordered to Gibraltar, the provisions were removed, and efforts were made to cleanse the vessel. On restowing the hold, every man so employed was salivated. The effects noted were not confined to the officers and ship's company, for almost all the stock died from the fumes—mice, cats, a dog, and even a canary bird shared the same fate, though the food of the latter was kept in a bottle closely corked up. The vapour was very deleterious to those having any tendency to pulmonic affections. Three men, who had never complained before they were saturated with mercury, died of phthisis; one, who had not had any pulmonic complaint, was left behind at Gibraltar, where his illness developed into a confirmed phthisis. Two died from gangrene of the cheeks and tongue. A woman, confined to bed with a fractured limb, lost two of her teeth; and many exfoliations of the jaw took place.

Accidents from the vapour of mercury, quite independently of its applications in the arts, have also occurred, some of them under curious circumstances. Witness, again, a case mentioned by Seidel,[917] in which a female, on the advice of an old woman, inhaled for some affection or other 2.5 grms. of mercury poured on red-hot coals, and died in ten days with all the symptoms of mercurial poisoning.

The metal taken in bulk into the stomach has been considered non-poisonous, and, probably, when perfectly pure, it is so; we have, however, the case of a girl who swallowed 4½ ozs. by weight of the liquid metal, for the purpose of procuring abortion—this it did not effect; but, in a few days, she suffered from a trembling and shaking of the body and loss of muscular power. These symptoms continued for two months, but there was no salivation and no blue marks on the gums. This case is a rare one, and a pound or more has been taken without injury.

§ 838. **Absorption of Mercury by the Skin.**—Mercury in a finely divided form, rubbed into the skin, is absorbed, and all the effects of mercurialism result. This method of administering mercury for medicinal purposes has long been in use, but, when the inunction is excessive, death may occur. Thus, Leiblinger records a case in which three persons were found dead in bed; the day before they had rubbed into the body, for the purpose of curing the itch, a salve containing 270 grms. of mercury finely divided.

It is difficult to say in what proportion workers in mercury, such as water-gilders, &c., suffer. According to Hirt, not only do 1.5 to 2.1 per cent. of the workmen employed in smelting mercury ores suffer acutely, but as high a proportion as 8.7 per cent. are slightly affected.

§ 839. **Symptoms of Poisoning by Mercury Vapour.**—The symptoms of poisoning by mercury vapour, or by the finely divided metal, are the same as those which arise from the corrosive salts, with the exception of the local action. In mild cases there is pallor, languor, and sore mouth (from slightly inflamed gums), fœtid breath, and disorder of the digestive organs. If the action is more intense, there is an inflammation of the gums and, indeed, of the whole mouth, and salivation, which is sometimes so profuse that as much as two gallons of saliva have been secreted daily. The saliva is alkaline, has a bad odour, and its specific gravity in the early stages is increased, but ultimately becomes normal; the gums are raised into slight swellings, which gradually enlarge and coalesce. The

[916] "An Account of the Effect of Mercurial Vapours on the Crew of His Majesty's Ship 'Triumph,' in the year 1810."—*Phil. Trans.*, 113, 1823.
[917] Maschka's *Handbuch*, Bd. ii. 295.

teeth that are already carious, decay more rapidly; they become loose, and some may be shed; the inflammatory action may extend to the jaw, and necrosis of portions of the bone is no unusual occurrence. On recovery, the cheeks sometimes form adhesions with the gums, and cicatrices always mark the loss of substance which such an affection entails. With the stomatitis there are disturbances of the gastro-intestinal tract—nausea and vomiting, pain in the stomach, and diarrhœa alternating with constipation. Conjunctivitis is very common, both in man and animals, from exposure to mercury vapours. The further action of the metal is shown in its profound effects on the nervous system. The patient is changed in his disposition, he is excitable, nervous, or torpid; there are sleeplessness and bad dreams, at the same time headache, noises in the ears, giddiness, faintings, &c.

§ 840. **Mercurial Tremor.**—Mercurial tremor[918] may follow, or accompany the above state, or it may be the chief and most prominent effect. It specially affects the arms, partly withdrawing the muscles from the control of the will, so that a person affected with mercurial tremor is incapacitated for following any occupation, especially those requiring a delicate and steady touch. In cases seriously affected, the tremor spreads gradually to the feet and legs, and finally the whole body may be invaded. The patient is no longer master of his muscles—the muscular system is in anarchy, each muscle aimlessly contracting and relaxing independently of the rest—the movement of the legs becomes uncertain, the speech stuttering, the facial expressions are even distorted into grimaces, and the sufferer sinks into a piteous state of helplessness. The convulsive movements generally cease during sleep. The tremors are accompanied by interference with the functions of other organs: the respiration is weakened and difficult; dyspnœa, or an asthmatic condition, results; the pulse is small and slow; paresis, deepening into paralysis of the extremities, or of a group of muscles, follows; and, lastly, if the condition is not alleviated, the patient becomes much emaciated and sinks from exhaustion. Pregnant women are liable to abortion, and the living infants of women suffering from tremor have also exhibited tremor of the limbs.

In the case of the "mass poisoning" on board the "Triumph," it has been mentioned that several of the sailors became consumptive, and the same effect has been noticed among all workers in the metal; it is now, indeed, an accepted fact that the cachexia induced by mercurialismus produces a weak habit of body specially liable to the tuberculous infection.

The course of the poisoning is generally more rapid when it has resulted from the taking of mercury internally as a medicine than when inhaled by workers in the metal, *e.g.*, a patient suffering from mercurial tremor shown to the Medical Society by Mr. Spencer Watson in 1872, had resisted for seven years the influence of the fumes of mercury; and then succumbed, exhibiting the usual symptoms. Idiosyncrasy plays a considerable *rôle*; some persons (and especially those whose kidneys are diseased) bear small doses of mercury ill, and are readily salivated or affected; this is evidently due to imperfect elimination.

§ 841. **Mercuric Methide**, $Hg(CH_3)_2$.—This compound is obtained by the action of methyl iodide on sodium amalgam in the presence of acetic ether. It is a dense, stable liquid, of highly poisonous properties. In 1865, mercuric methide, in course of preparation in a London laboratory, caused two cases of very serious slow poisoning.[919] One was that of a German, aged 30, who was engaged in preparing this compound for three months, and during this time his sight and hearing became impaired; he was very weak, his gums were sore, and he was ultimately admitted into St. Bartholomew's Hospital, February 3rd, 1865. His urine was found to be albuminous, and his mental faculties very torpid. On the 9th he became noisy, and had to be put under mechanical restraint. On the 10th he was semi-comatose, but there was no paralysis; his breath was very offensive, his pupils dilated; at intervals he raised himself and uttered incoherent howls. There was neither sensation nor motion in the left leg, which was extended rigidly; the knee and the foot were turned slightly inward. On the 14th he died insensible.

The only appearance of note seen at the autopsy was a congestion of the grey matter in the brain; the kidneys and liver were also congested, and there were ecchymoses in the kidneys.

The second case—a young man, aged 23, working in the same laboratory—was admitted into the hospital, March 28th, 1865. In the previous January he had been exposed to the vapour of mercuric methide for about a fortnight; during the illness of the other assistant he felt ill and weak, and complained of soreness of the gums and

---

[918] A case of mercurial tremor (in *Bericht. des K. K. Allgem. Krankenhauses zu Wien im Jahre 1872*, Wien, 1873) is interesting, as showing the influence of pregnancy. A woman, twenty years of age, employed in making barometers, had, in 1869, mercurial tremor and salivation. During a three months' pregnancy the tremor ceased, but again appeared after she had aborted. She again became pregnant, and the tremor ceased until after her confinement in November 1871. The tremor was so violent that the patient could not walk; she also had stomatitis; but ultimately, by treatment with galvanism and other remedies, she recovered.

[919] *St. Barth. Hosp. Reports*, vol. i., 1866, p. 141.

looseness of the teeth. He had also dimness of vision, pain and redness of the eyes, giddiness, nausea and vomiting, the ejected matters being greenish and watery. At the beginning of March his sight and taste became imperfect—all things tasted alike; his tongue was numb and his gums sore, he was also salivated slightly. A week before admission he lost his hearing, and first his hands and then his feet became numb; on admission his breath was very offensive, his pupils dilated; the sight impaired; he was very deaf, and his powers of speech, taste, and smell were deficient. There was anæsthesia of the body, and the movement of the limbs was sluggish and difficult. He continued in the hospital for nearly a month, with but little change. On April 24th, it was noticed that he was getting thinner and slightly jaundiced; he moved his arms aimlessly in an idiotic manner, and passed his urine involuntarily. On April 27th he was more restless, and even violent, shrieking out and making a loud, incoherent noise, or laughing foolishly; he passed his motions and urine beneath him. On July 7th he was in a similar state—perfectly idiotic. He died on April 7th, 1866, about a year and three months from his first exposure to the vapour; the immediate cause of death was pneumonia. The *post-mortem* appearances of the brain and membranes differed little from the normal state; the grey matter was pink, but otherwise healthy; there was a considerable amount of cerebro-spinal fluid; the arachnoid along the longitudinal fissure was thickened; the total weight of the brain with medulla was 41 ozs. The stomach was of enormous size; the pyramids of the kidneys were congested, as was also the small intestine; the lungs showed the usual signs of pneumonia.[920]

§ 842. **Effects of the Corrosive Salts of Mercury.**—The type of the corrosive salts is mercuric chloride, or corrosive sublimate—a compound which acts violently when administered, either externally or internally, in large doses.[921] If the poison has been swallowed, the symptoms come on almost immediately, and always within the first half hour; the whole duration also is rapid. In 36 cases collected by F. A. Falck, 11 died on the first or second day, and 11 on the fifth day; so that 61 per cent. died in five days—the remainder lived from six to twenty-six days. The shortest fatal case on record is one communicated to Dr. Taylor by Mr. Welch; in this instance the man died from an unknown quantity within half an hour.

In the very act of swallowing, a strong metallic taste and a painful sensation of constriction in the throat are experienced. There is a burning heat in the throat extending downwards to the stomach. All the mucous membranes with which the solution comes in contact are attacked, shrivelled, and whitened; so that, on looking into the mouth, the appearance has been described as similar to that produced by the recent application of silver nitrate. The local changes may be so intense as to cause œdema of the glottis, and death through asphyxia. In a few minutes violent pain is felt in the stomach; so much so, that the sufferer is drawn together, and is in a fainting condition; but there are rare cases in which pain has been absent. There are nausea and vomiting, the ejected matters being often streaked with blood; after the vomiting there is purging; here also the motions are frequently bloody.[922] The temperature of the body sinks, the respiration is difficult, and the pulse small, frequent, and irregular. The urine is generally scanty, and sometimes completely suppressed.[923] Sometimes there is profuse hæmorrhage from the bowel, stomach, or other mucous membrane, and such cases are accompanied by a considerable diminution of temperature. In a case recorded by Lœwy,[924] after a loss of blood by vomiting and diarrhœa, the temperature sank to 33.4°. The patient dies in a state of collapse, or insensibility, and death is often preceded by convulsions.

§ 843. Two remarkable cases of death from the external use of corrosive sublimate are recorded by Anderseck. An ointment, containing corrosive sublimate, was rubbed into the skin of two girls, servants, in order to cure the itch. The one, during the inunction, complained of a burning of the skin; the other also, a little while after, suffered in the same way. During the night the skin of each swelled, reddened, and became acutely painful. There were thirst and vomiting, but no diarrhœa, On the following day there was an eruption of blebs or little blisters. On the third day they had diarrhœa, tenesmus, fever, and diminution of the renal secretion; on the fourth day, fœtid breath,

[920] *St. Barth. Hosp. Reports*, vol. ii. p. 211.

[921] The effects on animals are similar to those on man. Richard Mead gave a dog with bread 3.8 grms. (60 grains) of corrosive sublimate:—"Within a quarter of an hour he fell into terrible convulsions, casting up frequently a viscid frothy mucus, every time more and more bloody, till, tired and spent with this hard service, he lay down quietly, as it were, to sleep, but died the next morning."

[922] The mixture of blood with the evacuations is more constantly observed in poisoning by corrosive sublimate than in poisoning by arsenic, copper, or lead.

[923] In a case recorded by Dr. Wegeler (Casper's *Wochenschrift*, January 10, 1846, p. 30), a youth, aged 17, swallowed 11.6 grms. (3 drachms) of the poison. No pain was experienced on pressure of the abdomen; he died on the sixth day, and during the last three days of life no urine was secreted.

[924] *Vierteljahrsschr. für ger. Med.*, 1864, vol. i. p. 187.

stomatitis, hyperæsthesia of the body, and a feeling of "pins and needles" in the hands and feet were noted. The first girl died in the middle of the fifth day, fully conscious; the other died on the sixth. So also Taylor[925] gives the case of a girl, aged 9, who died from the effects of an alcoholic solution of corrosive sublimate (strength, 80 grains to the oz.) applied to the scalp as a remedy for ringworm. The same author[926] further quotes the case of two brothers who died—the one on the fifth, the other on the eleventh day—from the effects of absorbing corrosive sublimate through the unbroken skin.

§ 844. **The Nitrates of Mercury** are poisons, but little (if at all) inferior in corrosive action to mercuric chloride. Death has resulted from both the external and internal use. Application of the nitrate as an escharotic to the *os uteri*, in one case,[927] produced all the symptoms of mercurial poisoning, but the woman recovered; in another case,[928] its use as a liniment caused death.

§ 845. When taken internally, the symptoms are scarcely different from those produced by corrosive sublimate. It seems an unlikely vehicle for criminal poisoning, yet, in the case of *Reg.* v. *E. Smith* (Leicester Summer Assizes, 1857), a girl was proved to have put a solution of nitrate of mercury in some chamomile tea, which had been prescribed for the prosecutrix. The nauseous taste prevented a fatal dose being taken; but the symptoms were serious.

§ 846. **Mercuric Cyanide** acts in a manner very similar to that of corrosive sublimate, 1.3 grm. (about 20 grains) in one case,[929] and in another[930] half the quantity, having destroyed life.

§ 847. **White Precipitate** (ammoniated mercury), as a poison, is weak. Out of fourteen cases collected by Taylor, two only proved fatal; one of these formed the subject of a trial for murder, *Reg.* v. *Moore* (Lewes Lent Assizes, 1860). The effects produced are vomiting, purging, &c., as in corrosive sublimate.[931] Other preparations of mercury, such as the red iodide, the persulphide, and even calomel,[932] have all a more or less intense poisonous action, and have caused serious symptoms and death.

§ 848. **Treatment of Acute and Chronic Poisoning.**—In acute poisoning, vomiting usually throws off some of the poison, if it has been swallowed; and the best treatment seems to be, to give copious albuminous drinks, such, for example, as the whites of eggs in water, milk, and the like. The vomiting may be encouraged by subcutaneous injections of apomorphine. The after-treatment should be directed to eliminating the poison, which is most safely effected by very copious drinks of distilled water (see "Appendix").

The treatment of slow poisoning is mainly symptomatic; medicinal doses of zinc phosphide seem to have done good in mercurial tremors. Potassic iodide is also supposed to assist the elimination of mercury.

§ 849. **Post-mortem Appearances.**—The pathological effects seen after chronic poisoning are too various to be distinctive. In the museum of the Royal College of Surgeons there is (No. 2559) the portion of a colon derived from a lady aged 74.[933] This lady had been accustomed for forty-three years to take a grain of calomel every night; for many years she did not suffer in health, but ultimately she became emaciated and cachectic, with anasarca and albuminuria. The kidneys were found to be granular, and the mucous membrane of a great part of the intestine of a remarkable black colour, mottled with patches of a lighter hue, presenting somewhat the appearance of a toad's back. From the portion of colon preserved mercury was readily obtained by means of Reinsch's test. The black deposit is in the submucosa, and it is, without doubt, mercurial, and probably mercury sulphide. In acute poisoning (especially by the corrosive salts) the changes are great and striking. After rapid death from corrosive sublimate, the escharotic whitening of the mouth, throat, and gullet, already described, will be seen. The mucous membrane right throughout, from mouth to anus, is more or less affected and destroyed, according to the dose and concentration of the poison. The usual appearances in the stomach are those of intense congestion, with ecchymoses, and portions of it may be destroyed. Sometimes the coats are very much blackened; this is probably due to a coating of sulphide of mercury.

In St. George's Hospital Museum (Ser. ix. 43, y. 337) there is a stomach, rather large, with thickened mucous

---

[925] *Op. cit.*

[926] *Poisons*, 1848, p. 394.

[927] *Med. Gazette*, vol. 45, p. 1025.

[928] *Edin. Monthly Journal*, 1864, p. 167.

[929] Orfila, i. p. 735.

[930] Christison, p. 427.

[931] See Dr. Th. Stevenson, "Poisoning by White Precipitate," *Guy's Hospital Reports*, vol. xix. p. 415.

[932] Seidel quotes a case from Hasselt, in which a father, for the purpose of obtaining insurance money, killed his child by calomel.

[933] *Path. Soc. Trans.*, xviii. 111.

coats, and having on the mucous surface a series of parallel black, or black-brown lines of deposit; it was derived from a patient who died from taking corrosive sublimate. With the severe changes mentioned, perforation is rare.[934] In the intestines there are found hyperæmia, extravasations, loosening of the mucous membrane, and other changes. The action is particularly intense about the cæcum and sigmoid flexure; in one case,[935] indeed, there was little inflammatory redness of the stomach or of the greater portion of the intestine, but the whole surface of the cæcum was of a deep black-red colour, and there were patches of sloughing in the coats. The kidneys are often swollen, congested, or inflamed; changes in the respiratory organs are not constantly seen, but in a majority of the cases there have been redness and swelling of the larynx, trachea, and bronchi, and sometimes hepatisation of smaller or larger portions of the lung.

In St. George's Hospital Museum, there are (from a patient dying in the hospital) preparations which well illustrate what pathological changes may be expected in any case surviving for a few days. The patient was Francis L——, aged 45, admitted to the hospital, February 27, 1842. He took a quantity of corrosive sublimate spread on bread and butter, was immediately sick, and was unable to take as much as he had intended. The stomach-pump and other remedies were used. On the following day his mouth was sore, and on March 1st his vision was dim; his mouth was drawn over to the right side, and he lost power over the left eyelid, but he had no pain; he passed some blood from the bowel. On the 2nd he passed much blood, and was salivated; still no pain. On March 4, on the evening of the sixth day, he expired; he was drowsy during the last day, and passed watery evacuations.

Prep. 14a, Ser. ix., shows the pharynx, œsophagus, and tongue; there is ulceration of the tonsils, and fibrinous exudation on the gullet. The stomach (43b, 199) shows a large dark slough, three inches from the cardiac extremity; the margin surrounding the slough is thickened, ulcerated, and irregular in shape, the submucous tissue, to some extent, being also thickened; there is fibrine in the ileum, pharynx, and part of the larynx. The action extended to the whole intestine, the rectum in prep. 145a, 36, is seen to be thickened, and has numerous patches of effused fibrine.

It is a curious fact that the external application of corrosive sublimate causes inflammatory changes in the alimentary canal of nearly the same intensity as if the poison had been swallowed. Thus, in the case of the two girls mentioned *ante*, there was found an intense inflammation of the stomach and intestines, the mucous tissues being scarlet-red, swollen, and with numerous extravasations.

§ 850. The effects of the nitrate of mercury are similar to the preceding; in the few cases which have been recorded, there has been intense redness, and inflammation of the stomach and intestines, with patches of ecchymosis. White precipitate, cyanide of mercury, mercuric iodide, and mercurous sulphide (turpeth-mineral) have all caused inflammation, more or less intense, of the intestinal tract.

§ 851. **Elimination of Mercury.**—The question of the channels by which mercury is eliminated is of the first importance. It would appear certain that it can exist in the body for some time in an inactive state, and then, from some change, be carried into the circulation and show its effects.[936] Voit considers that mercury combines with the albuminous bodies, separating upon their oxidation, and then becoming free and active.[937]

Ullmann[938] found most mercury in the following order:—Kidneys, liver, spleen, a small quantity in the stomach, no mercury in the small intestine, but some in the large intestine; small weighable quantities in the heart and skeletal muscles, also in the lungs; but no mercury, when the dose was small, in brain, the salivary glands, abdominal glands, thyroid glands, the bile, or the bones.

The main channel by which absorbed mercury passes out of the body is the kidneys, whilst mercurial compounds of small solubility are in great part excreted by the bowel. A. Bynssen,[939] after experimenting with mercuric chloride (giving .015 to .15 grm., with a little morphine hydrochlorate), came to the conclusion that it could be detected in the urine about two hours, and in the saliva about four hours, after its administration; he considered that the elimination was finished in twenty-four hours.

[934] There is only one case of perforation on record.

[935] *Lancet*, 1845, p. 700.

[936] Tuson gave a mare, first, 4 grains, and afterwards 5 grains of corrosive sublimate twice a day; at the end of fourteen days, in a pint of urine no mercury was detected, but at the end of three weeks it was found.

[937] *Voit, Physiol. chem. Unters.*, Augsburg, 1857.

[938] *Chem. Centr.*, 1892, ii. 941.

[939] *Journal de l'Anat. et de Physiol.*, 1872, No. 5, p. 500. On the separation of mercury by the urine, see also Salkowsky in Virchow's *Archiv*, 1866.

From the body of a hound that, in the course of thirty-one days, took 2.789 grms. of calomel (2.368 Hg) in eighty-seven doses, about 94 per cent. of the substance was recovered on analysis:—

		Mercurous Sulphide. Grms.
In the	fæces,	2.1175
„	urine,	0.0550
„	brain, heart, lungs, spleen, pancreas, kidneys, scrotum, and penis,	0.0090
„	liver,	0.0140
„	muscles,	0.0114
		2.2069

This equals 1.9 of metallic mercury.[940] Thus, of the whole 2.2 grms. of mercuric sulphide separated, over 95 per cent. was obtained from the fæces.

This case is of considerable interest, for there are recorded in toxicological treatises a few cases of undoubted mercurial poisoning in which no poison had been detected, although there was ample evidence that it had been administered by the mouth. In such cases, it is probable that the whole length of the intestinal canal had not been examined, and the analysis failed from this cause. When (as not unfrequently happens) the mercurial poison has entered by the skin, it is evident that the most likely localities are the urine, the liver, and the kidneys.[941]

In a case related by Vidal,[942] the *Liquor Bellostii* (or solution of mercuric nitrate) was ordered by mistake instead of a liniment. Although externally applied, it caused salivation, profuse diarrhœa, and death in nine days. The whole of the intestinal tract was found inflamed with extravasations, and mercury detected in the liver.

In any case of external application, if death ensues directly from the poison, evidence of its presence will probably be found; but too much stress must not be laid upon the detection of mercury, for, as Dr. Taylor says, "Nothing is more common than to discover traces of mercury in the stomach, bowels, liver, kidneys, or other organs of a dead body."[943]

§ 852. **Tests for Mercury.**—Mercury, in combination and in the solid form, is most readily detected by mixing the substance intimately with dry anhydrous sodic carbonate, transferring the mixture to a glass tube, sealed at one end, and applying heat. If mercury be present, a ring of minute globules condenses in the cool part of the tube. If the quantity of mercury is likely to be very minute, it is best to modify the process by using a subliming cell, and thus obtain the sublimate on a circle of thin glass in a convenient form for microscopical examination. If there is any doubt whether the globules are those of mercury or not, this may be resolved by putting a fragment of iodine on the lower disc of the subliming cell, and then completing it by the disc which contains the sublimate (of course, the supposed mercurial surface must be undermost); on placing the cell in a warm, light place, after a time the scarlet iodide is formed, and the identification is complete. Similarly, a glass tube containing an ill-defined metallic ring of mercury can be sealed or corked up with a crystal of iodine, and, after a few hours, the yellow iodide, changing to scarlet, will become apparent. There are few (if any) tests of greater delicacy than this.

Mercury in solution can be withdrawn by acidulating the liquid, and then inserting either simply a piece of gold foil, gold wire, or bright copper foil; or else, by a galvanic arrangement, such as iron wire wound round a gold coin, or gold foil attached to a rod of zinc; or, lastly, by the aid of gold or copper electrodes in connection with a battery. By any of these methods, mercury is obtained in the metallic state, and the metal with its film can be placed in a subliming cell, and globules deposited and identified, as before described.

The **Precipitating Reagents** for mercury are numerous: a solution of stannous chloride, heated with a solution of mercury, or any combination, whether soluble or insoluble, reduces it to the metallic state.

Mercurous Salts in solution yield, with potash, soda, or lime, a black precipitate of mercurous oxide. **Mercuric Salts**, a bright yellow precipitate of mercuric oxide.

---

[940] Riederer, in Buchner's *Neues Repert. f. Pharm.*, Bd. xvii. 3, 257, 1868.

[941] A woman died from the effects of a corrosive sublimate lotion applied by a quack to a wound in her leg. The writer found no poison in the stomach, but separated a milligramme of metallic mercury from the liver; the urine and intestines were not sent.

[942] *Gaz. des Hôp.*, Juillet 1864.

[943] Taylor, *Medical Jurisprudence*, i. p. 288.

Mercurous Salts yield black precipitates, with sulphides of ammonium and hydrogen. **Mercuric Salts** give a similar reaction, but, with sulphuretted hydrogen, first a whitish precipitate, passing slowly through red to black.

Mercurous Salts, with solutions of the chlorides, give a white precipitate of calomel; the **Mercuric Salts** yield no precipitate under similar circumstances. **Mercurous Salts**, treated with iodide of potassium, give a green mercurous iodide; **Mercuric**, a scarlet.

§ 853. **The Detection of Mercury in Organic Substances and Fluids.**—Ludwig's process, previously described, is found in practice the best. Fluids, such as urine, must be evaporated to dryness, and then treated with hydrochloric acid. Such organs as the liver are cut up and boiled in 20 per cent. HCl. Distinct evidence of mercury in the liver has been obtained on a piece of copper gauze, in a case where a child had been given 2 grains of calomel before death. "Four ounces of the liver were treated with hydrochloric acid and water, and a small piece of pure copper placed in the acid liquid while warm, and kept there for about forty-eight hours. It acquired a slight silvery lustre, and globules of mercury were obtained from it by sublimation."

To detect the cyanide of mercury may require special treatment, and Vitali[944] recommends the following process:—The fluid is acidified with tartaric acid and neutralised by freshly precipitated $CaCO_3$; a slight excess of hydric sulphide is added, and the flask allowed to rest for twenty-four hours in the cold. Then a further quantity of SH_2 is added, and a current of hydrogen passed through the liquid; the effluent gas is first made to bubble through a solution of bismuth nitrate in dilute nitric acid (for the purpose of absorbing SH_2), and then through aqueous potash (to absorb HCl); in the first flask the analyst will separate and identify mercury sulphide, while in the last flask there will be potassic cyanide, which will respond to the usual tests.

In those cases where no special search is made for mercury, but an acid (hydrochloric) solution is treated with sulphuretted hydrogen, mercury is indicated by the presence of a black precipitate, which does not dissolve in warm nitric acid.

The further treatment of the black sulphide may be undertaken in two ways:—

(1) It is collected on a porcelain dish, with the addition of a little nitric acid, and evaporated to dryness in order to destroy organic matter. Hydrochloric and a few drops of nitric acid are next added; the action is aided by a gentle heat, the solution finally evaporated to dryness on the water-bath, and the residue taken up by warm distilled water. The solution is that of a persalt of mercury, and the mercury can be separated by electrolysis, or indicated by the tests already detailed.

(2) The other method, and the most satisfactory, is to mix the sulphide while moist with dry carbonate of soda, make it into a pellet which will easily enter a reducing or subliming tube, dry it carefully, and obtain a sublimate of metallic mercury.

A neat method of recognising mercury when deposited as a film on copper has been proposed by E. Brugnatelli:[945] the copper, after being washed, is transferred to a glass vessel, and a porcelain lid, on which a drop of gold chloride solution has been placed, adjusted over the dish. The whole is heated by a water-bath. The mercury vapour reduces the gold chloride, and gold is deposited as a bluish-violet stain; $^1/_{10}$ mgrm. mercury may by this test be identified.

Of special methods for the separation and detection of mercury, Ludwig's[946] is, without a doubt, the best when organic matters have to be dealt with; the finely divided solid substances are boiled for some hours with hydrochloric acid, strength 20 per cent.; then the liquid is cooled to 60°, and potassic chlorate added in half gramme quantities until the dark liquid becomes clear; the liquid is cooled and filtered, and the substances on the filter washed with water. To the filtrate 5 grms. of zinc dust are added, and the liquid is violently shaken from time to time; a second portion is afterwards added, and also vigorously shaken. After some hours the clear liquid is separated from the zinc and the zinc washed, first with water, then with a little soda solution, and finally, again with water. The zinc is now collected on a glass-wool filter, treated with absolute alcohol to remove water, and dried by suction in a stream of air. The zinc is put into a combustion-tube, the tube being drawn out into a thin capillary extremity, and a combustion made, the mercury collecting at the capillary part. It is a necessary refinement, should the zinc be contaminated with a trace of organic matter, to pack the combustion-tube as follows:—First, the zinc dust on which any mercury present has been deposited, then a plug of asbestos; next, some cupric oxide; and lastly, some pure zinc dust. Bondzynski[947]

[944] *L'Orosi*, xii. 181-196.
[945] *Gazzetta*, xix. 418-422.
[946] *Zeit. f. physiolog. Chemie*, 1882, i. 495; *Chem. Centrblt.*, 1892, ii. 941.
[947] *Zeit. f. anal. Chem.*, xxxii. 302-305.

prefers to use copper rather than zinc; for he says that zinc so frequently contains cadmium, which latter metal also gives a mirror, so that, unless the mercury is afterwards identified by turning it into an iodide, error may be caused.

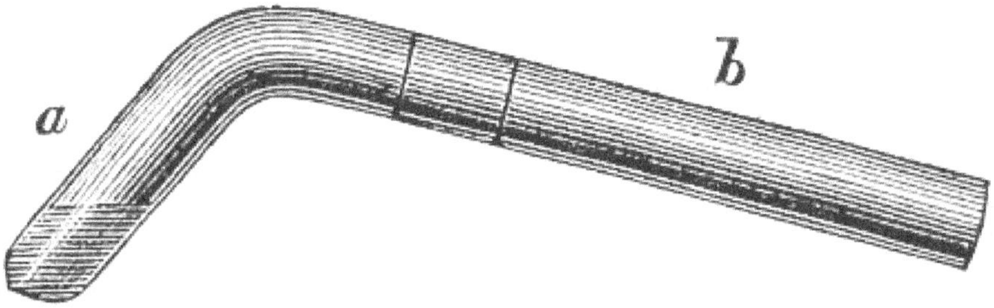

§ 854. **Estimation of Mercury.**—All pharmaceutical substances containing mercury, as well as the sulphide prepared in the wet way, and minerals, are best dealt with by obtaining and weighing the metal in the solid state. The assay is very simple and easy when carried out on the method that was first, perhaps, proposed by Domeyko. A glass tube (which should not be too thin), closed at one end, is bent, as shown in the figure, the diameter should be about three lines, the length from 7 to 8 inches, the shorter arm not exceeding 2 inches. The powdered substance is mixed with two or three times its weight of litharge, and introduced into the tube at *a*. The portion of the tube containing the mercury is at first heated gently, but finally brought to a temperature sufficient to fuse the substance and soften the glass. The mercury collects in an annular film at *b* in the cooler limb, and may now, with a little management of the lamp, be concentrated in a well-defined ring; the portion of the tube containing this ring is cut off, weighed, then cleansed from mercury, and reweighed. Many of the pharmaceutical preparations do not require litharge, which is specially adapted for ores, and heating with sodic carbonate (in great excess) will suffice. Mercury mixed with organic matter must be first separated as described, by copper or gold, the silvered foil rolled up, dried, introduced into the bent tube, and simply heated without admixture with any substance; the weight may be obtained either by weighing the foil before and after the operation, or as above.

§ 855. **Volumetric Processes for the Estimation of Mercury.**—When a great number of mercurial preparations are to be examined, a volumetric process is extremely convenient. There are several of these processes, some adapted more particularly for mercuric, and others for mercurous compounds. For mercuric, the method of Personne[948] is the best. The conversion of the various forms of mercury into corrosive sublimate may be effected by evaporation with aqua regia, care being taken that the bath shall not be at a boiling temperature, or there will be a slight loss.

Personne prefers to heat with caustic soda or potash, and then pass chlorine gas into the mixture; the excess of chlorine is expelled by boiling, mercuric chloride in presence of an alkaline chloride not being volatilised at 100°. The standard solutions required for this process are:—

(1) 33.2 grms. of potassic iodide in 1 litre of water, 1 c.c. = 0.01 grm. Hg, or 0.01355 grm. $HgCl_2$.

(2) A solution of mercuric chloride containing 13.55 grms. to the litre, 1 c.c. = 0.1 grm. Hg.

The process is founded on the fact that, if a solution of mercuric chloride be added to one of potassic iodide, in the proportion of one of the former to four of the latter, mercuric iodide is formed, and immediately dissolved, until the balance is overstepped, when the red colour is developed; the final reaction is very sharp, and with solutions properly made is very accurate. The mercuric solution must always be added to the alkaline iodide; a reversal of the process does not answer. It therefore follows that the solution to be tested must be made up to a definite bulk, and added to a known quantity of the potassic iodide until the red colour appears.

Mercurous Salts may be titrated with great accuracy by a decinormal solution of sodic chloride. This is added to the cold solution in very slight excess, the calomel filtered off, the filtrate neutralised by pure carbonate of soda, and the amount of sodic chloride still unused found by titration with nitrate of silver, the end reaction being indicated by chromate of potash. Several other volumetric processes are fully described in works treating upon this branch of analysis.

[948] *Comptes Rendus*, lvi. 68; Sutton's *Vol. Anal.*, 177.

III.—PRECIPITATED BY HYDRIC SULPHIDE FROM A NEUTRAL SOLUTION.
Zinc—Nickel—Cobalt.

1. ZINC.

§ 856. **Zinc**—At. wt., 65; specific gravity, 6.8 to 7.1; fusing-point, 412° (773° F.)—is a hard, bluish-white, brittle metal, with a crystalline fracture. Between 100° and 150° it becomes ductile, and may be easily wrought, but at a little higher temperature it again becomes brittle, and at a bright red heat it fuses, and then volatilises, the fumes taking fire when exposed to the air. In analysis, zinc occurs either as a metallic deposit on a platinum foil or dish, or as a brittle bead, obtained by reducing a zinc compound with soda on charcoal.

The salts of zinc to be briefly described here are the carbonate, the oxide, and the sulphide,—all of which are likely to occur in the separation and estimation of zinc, and the sulphate and chloride,—salts more especially found in commerce, and causing accidents from time to time.

§ 857. **Carbonate of Zinc**, in the native form of calamine, contains, as is well known, 64.8 per cent. of oxide of zinc; but the carbonate obtained in the course of an analysis by precipitating the neutral hot solution of a soluble salt of zinc by carbonate of potash or soda, is carbonate of zinc *plus* a variable quantity of hydrated oxide of zinc. Unless the precipitation takes place at a boiling temperature, the carbonic anhydride retains a portion of the oxide of zinc in solution. By ignition of the carbonate, oxide of zinc results.

§ 858. **Oxide of Zinc** (ZnO = 81; specific gravity, 5.612; Zn, 80.24, O, 19.76) is a white powder when cool, yellow when hot. If mixed with sufficient powdered sulphur, and ignited in a stream of hydrogen, the sulphide is produced; if ignited in the pure state in a rapid stream of hydrogen gas, metallic zinc is obtained; but, if it is only a feeble current, the oxide of zinc becomes crystalline, a portion only being reduced.

§ 859. **Sulphide of Zinc** (ZnS = 97; specific gravity, 4.1; Zn, 67.01, S, 32.99).—The sulphide obtained by treating a neutral solution of a soluble salt of zinc by hydric sulphide is hydrated sulphide, insoluble in water, caustic alkalies, and alkaline sulphides, but dissolving completely in nitric or in hydrochloric acid. When dry, it is a white powder, and if ignited contains some oxide of zinc. The anhydrous sulphide is produced by mixing the precipitated sulphide with sulphur, and igniting in a crucible in a stream of hydrogen gas.

Pharmaceutical Preparations.—The officinal compounds of zinc used in medicine are the *acetate*, *carbonate*, *chloride*, *oxide*, *sulphate*, *sulphocarbolate*, and *valerianate*.

Sulphate of Zinc ($ZnSO_4 7H_2O$ 161 + 126; specific gravity, crystals, 1.931).—This salt is officinal in all the pharmacopœias, is used in calico-printing, and is commonly known as *white vitriol*. By varying the temperature at which the crystals are allowed to be formed, it may be obtained with 6, 5, 2, or 1 atoms of water. The commercial sulphate is in crystals exactly similar to those of Epsom salts; it is slightly efflorescent, and gives the reactions of zinc and sulphuric acid.

§ 860. **Chloride of Zinc** is obtained by dissolving zinc in hydrochloric acid, or by direct union of zinc and chlorine. Chloride of zinc is the only constituent in the well-known "Burnett's disinfectant fluid." A solution of chloride of zinc may be heated until it becomes water-free; when this takes place it still remains fluid, and makes a convenient bath, for warmth may be applied to it above 370° without its emitting fumes to inconvenience; at a red heat it distils. A concentrated solution of zinco-ammonic chloride ($2H_4NClZnCl_2$) is used for the purpose of removing the film of oxide from various metals preparatory to soldering.

§ 861. **Zinc in the Arts.**—The use of zinc as a metal in sheeting cisterns, articles for domestic use, alloys, &c., is well known; oxide of zinc enters largely into the composition of india-rubber. Sulphide of zinc has been employed as a substitute for white lead, and may possibly supersede it. Zinc white is further employed as a pigment, and, mixed with albumen, is an agent in calico-printing; it is also used in the decoloration of glass, in the polishing of optical glasses, and in the manufacture of artificial meerschaum pipes.[949]

Chromate of Zinc ($ZnCrO_4$) is used in calico-printing, and there is also in commerce a basic chromate known as *zinc yellow*. Zinc green, or Rinman's green, is a beautiful innocuous colour, formed by igniting a mixture of dry zincic and cobaltous carbonates.

The use of zinc vessels in the preparation of foods may occasionally bring the metal under the notice of the analyst. When exposed to a moist atmosphere, zinc becomes covered with a thin film of oxide, perfectly insoluble in ordinary water; but, if the water should be charged with common salt, a considerable quantity may be dissolved.

[949] Artificial meerschaum pipes are composed of zinc white, magnesia usta, and caseine ammonium.

It may generally be laid down as a rule that the solvent power of water on zinc has a direct relation to the chlorides present, whilst carbonate of lime greatly diminishes this solubility.[950]

Milk may become contaminated by zinc; for, it is a matter of common knowledge, that milk contained in zinc vessels does not readily turn sour. This may be explained by the zinc oxide combining with the lactic acid, and forming the sparingly soluble lactate of zinc $2(C_3H_5O_3)Zn + 3H_2O$, thus withdrawing the lactic acid as fast as it is formed, preventing the coagulation of the casein. With regard to this important practical subject, MM. Payne and Chevallier made several experiments on the action of brandy, wine, vinegar, olive oil, soup, milk, &c., and proved that zinc is acted on by all these, and especially by alcoholic, acetic, and saline liquids. M. Schaufféle has repeated these experiments, and determined the amount of zinc dissolved in fifteen days by different liquids from a galvanised iron as well as a zinc vessel.

The amount found was as follows:—

	The liquid from the zinc vessel, grms. per litre.		The liquid from the galvanised iron vessel, grms. per litre.	
Brandy,	0	.95	0	.70
Wine,	3	.95	4	.10
Orange-flower water,	0	.50	0	.75
Vinegar,	31	.75	60	.75
Fatty soup,	0	.46	1	.00
Weak soup,	0	.86	1	.76
Milk,	5	.13	7	.00
Salt water,	1	.75	0	.40
Seltzer water,	0	.35	0	.30
Distilled water,	traces.		traces.	
Ordinary water,	traces.		traces.	
Olive oil,	none.		none.	

§ 862. **Effects of Zinc, as shown by Experiments on Animals.**—Harnack, in experiments with sodium-zinc oxide pyrophosphate, has shown that the essential action of zinc salts is to paralyse the muscles of the body and the heart, and, by thus affecting the circulation and respiration, to cause death; these main results have been fully confirmed by Blake, Letheby, and C. Ph. Falck. For rabbits the lethal dose is .08 to .09 grm. of zinc oxide, or about .04 per kilogrm. The temperature during acute poisoning sinks notably—according to F. A. Falck's researches on rabbits, from about 7.3° to 13.0°. Zinc is eliminated mainly by the urine, and has been recognised in that fluid four to five days after the last dose. It has also been separated in small quantity from the milk and the bile.

§ 863. **Effects of Zinc Compounds on Man—(a) Zinc Oxide.**—The poisonous action of zinc oxide is so weak that it is almost doubtful whether it should be considered a poison. Dr. Marcett has given a pound (453.6 grms.) during a month in divided doses without injury to a patient afflicted with epilepsy; and the workmen in zinc manufactories cover themselves from head to foot with the dust without very apparent bad effects. It is not, however, always innocuous, for Popoff has recorded it as the cause of headache, pain in the head, cramps in the calves of the legs, nausea, vomiting, and diarrhœa; and he also obtained zinc from the urine of those suffering in this manner.[951] Again, a pharmacy student[952] filled a laboratory with oxide of zinc vapour, and suffered from well-marked and even serious poisonous symptoms, consisting of pain in the head, vomiting, and a short fever. It must be remembered that, as the ordinary zinc of commerce is seldom free from arsenic, and some samples contain gallium, the presence of these metals may possibly have a part in the production of the symptoms described.

[950] Ziurek, indeed, found in a litre of water contained in a zinc cistern no less than 1.0104 grm. of zinc, and the same water showed only 0.074 grm. of common salt to the litre.—*Vierteljahrsschr. für gericht. Medicin*, 1867, Bd. 6, p. 356.

[951] The so-called "zinc fever" has only been noticed in the founding of brass; it is always preceded by well-marked shivering, the other symptoms being similar to those described.

[952] Rust's *Magazin*, Bd. xxi. § 563.

§ 864. **(b) Sulphate of Zinc.**—Sulphate of zinc has been very frequently taken by accident or design, but death from it is rare. The infrequency of fatal result is due, not to any inactivity of the salt, but rather to its being almost always expelled by vomiting, which is so constant and regular an effect, that in doses of 1.3 grm. (20 grains), sulphate of zinc is often relied upon in poisoning from other substances to quickly expel the contents of the stomach. In a case reported by Dr. Gibb, an adult female swallowed 4.33 grms. (67 grains), but no vomiting occurred, and it had to be induced by other emetics; this case is unique. It is difficult to say what would be a fatal dose of zinc sulphate, but the serious symptoms caused by 28 grms. (1 oz.) in the case of a groom in the service of Dr. Mackenzie, leads to the view that, although not fatal in that particular instance, it might be in others. The man took it in mistake for Epsom salts: a few minutes after he was violently sick and purged, and was excessively prostrated, so that he had to be carried to his home; the following day he had cramps in the legs, and felt weak, but was otherwise well.

In a criminal case related by Tardieu and Roussin, a large dose of zinc sulphate, put into soup, caused the death of an adult woman of sixty years of age in about thirty hours.[953] The symptoms were violent purging and vomiting, leading to collapse. From half of the soup a quantity of zinc oxide, equal to 1.6 grm. of zinc sulphate, was separated. Zinc was also found in the stomach, liver, intestines, and spleen—(see also a case of criminal poisoning recorded by Chevallier).[954]

§ 865. **(c) Zinc Chloride.**—Chloride of zinc is a powerful poison, which may kill by its primary or secondary effects; its local action as a caustic is mainly to be ascribed to its intense affinity for water, dehydrating any tissue with which it comes in contact. The common use of disinfecting fluids containing zinc chloride, such as Burnett's fluid, leads to more accidents in England than in any other European country. Of twenty-six cases of poisoning by this agent, twenty-four occurred in England, and only two on the Continent. Death may follow the external use of zinc chloride. Some years ago, a quack at Barnstaple, Devon, applied zinc chloride to a cancerous breast; the woman died with all the general symptoms of poisoning by zinc, and that metal was found in the liver and other organs.

The symptoms observed in fatal cases of chloride of zinc poisoning are—immediate pain in the throat, and burning of the lips, tongue, &c. There is difficulty in swallowing, an increase in the secretion of saliva, vomiting of bloody matters, diarrhœa, collapse, coma, and death. In some cases life has been prolonged for days; but, on the other hand, death has been known to occur in a few hours. In those cases in which either recovery has taken place, or in which death is delayed, nervous symptoms rarely fail to make their appearance. In a case recorded by Dr. R. Hassall, 3 ounces of Burnett's fluid were swallowed. The usual symptoms of intense gastro-intestinal irritation ensued, but there was no purging until the third day; after the lapse of a fortnight, a train of nervous symptoms set in, indicated by a complete perversion of taste and smell. In other cases, aphonia, tetanic affections of groups of muscles, with great muscular weakness and impairment of sight, have been noticed. Very large doses of zinc chloride have been recovered from, *e.g.*, a man had taken a solution equivalent to about 13 grms. (200 grains) of the solid chloride. Vomiting came on immediately, and there was collapse, but he recovered in sixteen days. On the other hand, .38 grm. (6 grains) has destroyed life after several weeks' illness.

§ 866. **Post-mortem Appearances.**—In poisoning by sulphate of zinc, the appearances usually seen are inflammation, more or less intense, of the mucous membrane of the stomach and bowels. In the museums of the London hospitals, I could only find (1882) a single specimen preserved illustrating the effects of this poison. This preparation is in St. George's Hospital Museum, and shows (ser. ix. 43 and 198) the stomach of a man who died from zinc sulphate, and whose case is reported in the *Lancet*, 1859. The mucous membrane is wrinkled all over like a piece of tripe; when recent it was vascular and indurated, but uniformly of a dirty grey colour; the lining membrane of the small intestine is very vascular, and in the duodenum and upper part of the jejunum the colour is similar to that of the stomach, but in a less marked degree; the stomach and intestines are contracted.

The pathological appearances after chloride of zinc vary according to the period at which death takes place. When it has occurred within a few hours, the lining membrane of the mouth and gullet shows a marked change in texture, being white and opaque, the stomach hard and leathery, or much corrugated or ulcerated. In cases in which life has been prolonged, contractions of the gullet and stomach may occur very similar to those caused by the mineral acids, and with a similar train of symptoms. In a case which occurred under Dr. Markham's[955] observation, a person died ten weeks after taking the fatal dose, the first symptoms subsiding in a few days, and the secondary set of

[953] Taylor notices this case, but adds that she died in three days. This is a mistake, as the soup was taken on the 12th of June, probably at mid-day, and the woman died on the 13th, at 8 P.M.

[954] "Observations toxicologiques sur le zinc," *Annales d'Hygiène Publique*, July 1878, p. 153.

[955] *Med. Times and Gazette*, June 11, 1859, p. 595.

symptoms not commencing for three weeks. They then consisted mainly of vomiting, until the patient sank from exhaustion. The stomach was constricted at the pyloric end, so that it would scarcely admit a quill.

In Guy's Hospital there is a good preparation, 1799^{35}, from the case of S. R., aged 22; she took a tablespoonful of Burnett's fluid, and died in about fourteen weeks. There were at first violent vomiting and purging, but she suffered little pain, and in a day or two recovered sufficiently to move about the house; but the vomiting after food continued, everything being ejected about five minutes after swallowing. Before death she suffered from pneumonia. The stomach is seen to be much contracted—5 inches in length; it is ulcerated both near the pylorus and near the gullet; at the latter part there is a pouch-like portion of the mucous membrane of the stomach adherent to the spleen, which communicates by a perforation with an abscess formed and bounded by the stomach, diaphragm, and spleen; it contained 3 ozs. of dirty-looking pus. At the pylorus, in the centre, there is a second perforation, but extravasation of the contents is prevented by the adherent omentum and transverse colon. The muscular coats are thickened.

§ 867. **Detection of Zinc in Organic Liquids or Solids.**—In cases where the poison has been expelled from the stomach by vomiting, the muscles and bones would appear to be the best tissues to examine chemically; for Matzkewitsch investigated very carefully a dog poisoned by 100 parts of zinc, subcutaneously injected in the form of acetate, and found it distributed over the several organs of the body in the following ratios:—Muscles 60.5, bones 24.41, stomach and intestines 4.63, skin 3.70, place of injection 2.19, liver 1.75, lungs and heart 1.68, kidneys, bladder, and urine 1.14.

The only certain method of detection is to produce the sulphide of zinc, best effected by saturating a neutral or feebly acid liquid with hydric sulphide. If an organic liquid, which can be easily filtered, is operated upon, it may be strongly acidulated with acetic acid, and at once treated with hydric sulphide. If, however, zinc is sought for as a part of a systematic examination (as will most likely be the case), the solution will have been treated with hydrochloric acid, and already tested for arsenic, antimony, lead, &c., and filtered from any precipitate. In such a case the hydrochloric acid must first be replaced by acetic, which is effected by adding a slight excess of sodic acetate; the right quantity of the latter is easily known, if the hydrochloric acid originally added was carefully measured, and its specific gravity ascertained; 3.72 of crystallised sodic acetate saturating one of HCl. Lastly, should the distillation process, given before, have been adopted, the contents of the retort will only require to be treated with water, filtered, and saturated with sulphuretted hydrogen. In any of the above cases, should a white, dirty white or lightish-coloured precipitate (which is not sulphur) be thrown down, zinc may be suspected; it will, however, be absolutely necessary to identify the sulphide, for there are many sources of error. The most satisfactory of all identifications is the production of Rinman's green. The supposed sulphide is dissolved off the filter with hot nitric acid, a drop or more (according to the quantity of the original precipitate) of solution of cobalt nitrate added, the solution precipitated with carbonate of soda and boiled, to expel all carbonic anhydride; the precipitate is then collected on a filter, washed, dried, and ignited in a platinum dish. If zinc be present in so small a proportion as 1.100,000 part, the mass will be permanently green.

§ 868. Other methods of procedure are as follows:—The supposed zinc sulphide (after being well washed) is collected in a porcelain dish, and dissolved in a few drops of sulphuric acid, filtered, nitric acid added, evaporated to dryness, and heated to destroy all organic matter. When cool, the mass is treated with water acidulated by sulphuric acid, and again filtered. The solution may contain iron as well as zinc, and if the former (on testing a drop with ferrocyanide of potash) appears in any quantity, it must be separated by the addition of ammonia in excess to the ammoniacal filtrate; sodic carbonate is added in excess, the liquid well boiled, and the precipitate collected on a filter and washed. The carbonate of zinc thus obtained is converted into zinc oxide by ignition, and weighed. If oxide of zinc, it will be yellow when hot, white when cold: it will dissolve in acetic acid; give a white precipitate with sulphuretted hydrogen; and, finally, if heated on charcoal in the oxidising flame, and moistened with cobalt nitrate solution, a green colour will result. Zinc may also be separated from liquids by electrolysis. The simplest way is to place the fluid under examination in a platinum dish of sufficient size, acidify, and insert a piece of magnesium tape. The metallic film so obtained may be dissolved by hydrochloric acid, and the usual tests applied.

2. NICKEL—COBALT.

§ 869. The salts of nickel and cobalt have at present no toxicological importance, although, from the experiments of Anderson Stuart,[956] both may be classed as poisonous. The experiments of Gmelin had, prior to

[956] "Nickel and Cobalt; their Physiological Action on the Animal Organism," by T. P. Anderson Stuart, M.D., *Journ. of Anat. and Physiol.*, vol. xvii., Oct. 1882.

Stuart's researches, shown that nickel sulphate introduced into the stomach acted as an irritant poison, and, if introduced into the blood, caused death by cardiac paralysis. Anderson Stuart, desiring to avoid all local irritant action, dissolved nickel carbonate in acid citrate of soda by the aid of a gentle heat; he then evaporated the solution, and obtained a glass which, if too alkaline, was neutralised by citric acid, until its reaction approximated to the feeble alkalinity of the blood; the cobalt salt was produced in the same way. The animals experimented on were frogs, fish, pigeons, rats, guinea-pigs, rabbits, cats, and dogs—in all 200. The lethal dose of nickelous oxide, when subcutaneously injected in the soluble compound described, was found to be as follows:—frogs, .08 grm. per kilogram; pigeons, .06; guinea-pigs, .030; rats, .025; cats, .01; rabbits, .009; and dogs, .007. The cobaltous oxide was found to be much less active, requiring the above doses to be increased about two-thirds. In other respects, its physiological action seems to be very similar to that of nickelous oxide.

§ 870. **Symptoms—Frogs.**—A large dose injected into the dorsal lymph sac of the frog causes the following symptoms:—The colour of the skin all over the body becomes darker and more uniform, and not infrequently a white froth is abundantly poured over the integument. In an interval of about twenty minutes the frog sits quietly, the eyes retracted and shut; if molested, it moves clumsily. When quiet, the fore limbs are weak, and the hind legs drawn up very peculiarly, the thighs being jammed up so against the body, that they come to lie on the dorsal aspect of the sides of the frog, and the legs are so much flexed that the feet lie on the animal's back, quite internal to the plane of the thighs. Soon fibrillary twitchings are observed in the muscles of the abdominal wall, then feeble twitchings of the fingers, and muscles of the fore limbs generally; lastly, the toes are seen to twitch, and then the muscles of the hind limbs—this order is nearly always observed; now spasmodic gaping and incoördinate movements are seen, and the general aspect is not unlike the symptoms caused by picrotoxin. After this, tetanus sets in, and the symptoms then resemble those of strychnine; the next stage is stupefaction and voluntary motor paresis; the respiratory movements become feeble, and the paresis passes into paralysis. The heart beats more and more slowly and feebly, and death gradually and imperceptibly supervenes. The *post-mortem* appearances are well marked, *i.e.*, rigor mortis, slight congestion of the alimentary tract, the heart with the auricle much dilated and filled with dark blood, the ventricle mostly small, pale, and semi-contracted. For some time after death, the nerve trunks and muscles react to the induction current.

Pigeons.—In experiments on pigeons the symptoms were those of dulness and stupor, jerkings of different sets of muscles, and then death quietly.

Guinea-pigs.—In guinea-pigs there were dulness and stupefaction, with some weakness of the hind limbs.

Rats.—The symptoms in rats were almost entirely nervous; they became drowsy and apathetic, and there was paralysis of the hind legs.

Rabbits.—In rabbits, also, the symptoms were mainly those caused by an affection of the nervous system. There was paralysis, which affected either the hind legs only, or all four limbs. The cervical muscles became so weak that the animal was unable to hold its head up. Diarrhœa occurred and persisted until death. If the dose is not large enough to kill rapidly, the reflex irritability is decidedly increased, so that the slightest excitation may cause the animal to cower and tremble all over. Now appear twitchings and contractions of single groups of muscles, and this excitement becomes general. The respirations also become slower and more difficult, and sometimes there is well-marked dilatation of the vessels of the ears and *fundi oculi.* Convulsions close the scene.

§ 871. **Circulation.**—The effect of the salt on the frog's heart was also studied in detail. It seems that, under the influence of a soluble salt of nickel, the heart beats more and more slowly, it becomes smaller and paler, and does not contract evenly throughout the whole extent of the ventricle; but the rhythm of the ventricular and auricular contractions is never lost.

It is probable that there is a vaso-motor paralysis of the abdominal vessels; the blood-pressure falls, and the heart is not stimulated by the blood itself as in its normal state. In support of this view, it is found that, by either pressing on the abdomen or simply inverting the frog, the heart swells up, fills with blood, and for a time beats well.

Nervous System.—The toxic action is referable to the central nervous system, and not to that of peripheral motor nerve-endings or motor nerve-fibres. It is probable that both nickel and cobalt paralyse to some extent the cerebrum. The action on the nerve-centres is similar to that of platinum or barium, and quite different from that of iron.

§ 872. **Action on Striped Muscle.**—Neither nickel nor cobalt has any effect on striped muscle. In this they both differ from arsenic, antimony, mercury, lead, and iron—all of which, in large doses, diminish the work which healthy muscle is capable of performing.

§ 873. **Separation of Nickel or Cobalt from the Organic Matters or Tissues.**—It is very necessary, if any case of poisoning should occur by either or both of these metals, to destroy completely the organic matters by the process already detailed above. Both nickel and cobalt are thrown down, if in the form of acetate, from a neutral solution by sulphuretted hydrogen; but the precipitation does not take place in the presence of free mineral acid; hence, in the routine process of analysis, sulphuretted hydrogen is passed into the acid liquid, and any precipitate filtered off. The liquid is now made almost neutral by potassic carbonate, and then potassic acetate added, and a current of sulphuretted hydrogen passed through it. The sulphides of cobalt and nickel, if both are present, will be thrown down; under the same circumstances zinc, if present, would also be precipitated. Cobalt is separated from zinc by dissolving the mixed sulphides in nitric acid, precipitating the carbonates of zinc and cobalt by potassic carbonate, collecting the carbonates, and, after washing, igniting them gently in a bulb tube, in a current of dry hydrochloric acid; volatile zinc chloride is formed and distils over, leaving cobalt chloride.

§ 874. To estimate cobalt, sulphide of cobalt may be dissolved in nitric acid, and then precipitated by pure potash; the precipitate washed, dried, ignited, and weighed; 100 parts of cobaltous oxide (Co_3O_4) equals 73.44 of metallic cobalt. Cobalt is separated from nickel by a method essentially founded on one proposed by Liebig. The nitric acid solution of nickel and cobalt (which must be free from all other metals, save potassium or sodium) is nearly neutralised by potassic carbonate, and mixed with an excess of hydrocyanic acid, and then with pure caustic potash. The mixture is left exposed to the air in a shallow dish for some hours, a tripotassic cobalticyanide (K_3CoCy_6) and a nickelo-potassic cyanide (2KCy, $NiCy_4$) are in this way produced. If this solution is now boiled with a slight excess of mercuric nitrate, hydrated nickelous oxide is precipitated, but potassic cobalticyanide remains in solution, and may be filtered off. On carefully neutralising the alkaline filtrate with nitric acid, and adding a solution of mercurous nitrate, the cobalt may then be precipitated as a mercurous cobalticyanide, which may be collected, washed, dried, decomposed by ignition, and weighed as cobaltous oxide. After obtaining both nickel and cobalt oxides, or either of them, they may be easily identified by the blowpipe. The oxide of nickel gives, in the oxidising flame with borax, a yellowish-red glass, becoming paler as it cools; the addition of a potassium salt colours the bead blue. In the reducing flame the metal is reduced, and can be seen as little greyish particles disseminated through the bead. Cobalt gives an intense blue colour to a bead of borax in the oxidising flame.

IV.—PRECIPITATED BY AMMONIUM SULPHIDE.
Iron—Chromium—Thallium—Aluminium—Uranium.

1. IRON.

§ 875. It was Orfila's opinion that all the salts of iron were poisonous, if given in sufficient doses; but such salts as the carbonate, the phosphate, and a few others, possessing no local action, may be given in such very large doses, without causing disturbance to the health, that the statement must only be taken as applying to the more soluble iron compounds. The two preparations of iron which have any forensic importance are the perchloride and the sulphate.

§ 876. **Ferric Chloride** ($Fe_2Cl_6 = 325$).—Anhydrous ferric chloride will only be met with in the laboratory. As a product of passing dry chlorine over red-hot iron, it sublimes in brown scales, is very deliquescent, and hisses when thrown into water. There are two very definite hydrates—one with 6 atoms of water, forming large, red, deliquescent crystals; and another with 12 of water, less deliquescent, and crystallising in orange stellate groups.

The pharmaceutical preparations in common use are:—

Stronger Solution of Perchloride of Iron (Liquor Ferri Perchloridi Fortior).—An orange-brown liquid of specific gravity 1.42, and containing about 58 per cent. of ferric chloride.

Tincture of Perchloride of Iron (Tinctura Ferri Perchloridi), made by diluting 1 part of the strong solution with 1 volume of rectified spirit, and adding distilled water to measure 4.

Solution of Perchloride of Iron (Liquor Ferri Perchloridi).—Simply 5 volumes of the strong solution made up to 20 by the addition of water; hence, of the same strength as the tincture.

§ 877. **Effects of Ferric Chloride on Animals.**—A very elaborate series of researches on rabbits, dogs, and cats was undertaken a few years ago by MM. Bérenger-Féraud and Porte[957] to elucidate the general symptoms and effects produced by ferric chloride under varying conditions. First, a series of experiments showed that, when ferric chloride solution was enclosed in gelatine capsules and given with the food of the animal, it produced either no

[957] "Étude sur l'empoisonnement par le perchlorure de fer," par MM. Bérenger-Féraud et Porte, *Annales d'Hygiène Publique*, 1879.

symptoms or but trifling inconvenience, even when the dose exceeded 1 grm. per kilogrm.; anhydrous ferric chloride and the ferric chloride solution were directly injected into the stomach, yet, when food was present, death did not occur, and the effects soon subsided. In animals which were fasting, quantities of the solution equal to .5 grm. per kilogrm. and above caused death in from one hour to sixteen hours, the action being much accelerated by the addition of alcohol—as, for example, in the case of the tincture: the symptoms were mainly vomiting and diarrhœa, sometimes the vomiting was absent. In a few cases the posterior extremities were paralysed, and the pupils dilated: the urine was scanty or quite suppressed; death was preceded by convulsions.

§ 878. **Effects on Man.**—Perchloride of iron in the form of tincture has been popularly used in England, from its supposed abortive property, and is sold under the name of "steel drops." It has been frequently taken by mistake for other dark liquids; and there is at least one case on record in which it was proved to have been used for the purpose of murder. The latter case[958] is peculiarly interesting from its great rarity; it occurred in Martinique in 1874-1876, no less than four persons being poisoned at different dates. All four were presumed to have had immoral relations with a certain widow X——, and to have been poisoned by her son. In three of the four cases, viz., Char——, Duf——, and Lab——, the cause of death seems pretty clear; but the fourth, Ab——, a case of strong suspicion, was not sufficiently investigated. All three took the fatal dose in the evening, between eight and nine o'clock—Lab—— the 27th of December 1874, Duf—— the 22nd of February 1876, and Char—— on the 14th of May 1876. They had all passed the day in tippling, and they all had eaten nothing from mid-day, so that the stomach would, in none of the three, contain any solid matters. The chloride was given to them in a glass of "punch," and there was strong evidence to show that the son of the widow X—— administered it. Char—— died after about thirteen hours' illness, Duf—— and Lab—— after sixty-five hours' illness; Ab—— lived from three to four days. With Char—— the symptoms were very pronounced in an hour, and consisted essentially of violent colicky pain in the abdomen and diarrhœa, but there was no vomiting; Duf—— had also great pain in the abdomen and suppression of the urine. Lab—— had most violent abdominal pains; he was constipated, and the urinary secretion was arrested; there was besides painful tenesmus. According to the experiments of Bérenger-Féraud and Porte,[959] the perchloride in the above cases was taken under conditions peculiarly favourable for the development of its toxic action, viz., on an empty stomach and mixed with alcohol.

There have been several cases of recovery from large doses of the tincture, *e.g.*, that of an old man, aged 72, who had swallowed 85 c.c. (3 ozs.) of the tincture; the tongue swelled, there were croupy respiration and feeble pulse, but he made a good recovery. In other cases,[960] 28.3 c.c. (an ounce) and more have caused vomiting and irritation of the urinary organs. The perchloride is not unfrequently used to arrest hæmorrhage as a topical application to the uterine cavity—a practice not free from danger, for it has before now induced violent inflammation and death from peritonitis.

§ 879. **Elimination of Iron Chloride.**—Most of the iron is excreted in the form of sulphide by the fæces, and colours them of a black hue; a smaller portion is excreted by the urine.

§ 880. **Post-mortem Appearances.**—In the experiments on animals already referred to, the general changes noted were dryness, pallor, and parchment-like appearance of the cavity of the mouth, the mucous membrane being blackened by the contact of the liquid. The gullet was pale and dry, not unfrequently covered with a blackish layer. The mucous membrane of the stomach was generally healthy throughout; but, if the dose was large and very concentrated, there might be one or more hyperæmic spots; otherwise, this did not occur. The internal surface of the intestines, similarly, showed no inflammation, but was covered with brownish coating which darkened on exposure to the air. The liver, in all the experiments, was large and gorged with black and fluid blood; there were ecchymoses in the lungs and venous congestion. The kidneys were usually hyperæmic, and contained little hæmorrhages. There was also general encephalic engorgement, and in one experiment intense congestion of the meninges was observed. Few opportunities have presented themselves for pathological observations relative to the effects produced by ferric chloride on man. In a case related by Christison, in which a man swallowed 42.4 c.c. (1½ oz.) of the tincture, and died in five weeks, there was found thickening and inflammation of the pyloric end of the stomach.

The case of Char——, already alluded to, is that in which the most complete details of the autopsy are recorded, and they coincide very fairly with those observed in animals; the tongue was covered with a greenish fur, bordered

[958] Fully reported in Bérenger-Féraud's paper, *loc. cit.*

[959] *Dub. Med. Press*, February 21, 1849.

[960] *Provincial Journal*, April 7 and 21, 1847, p. 180; see also Taylor's *Principles and Practice of Medical Jurisprudence*, vol. i. p. 320, 2nd Edition.

at the edges with a black substance, described as being like "mud"; the lining membrane of the gullet was pale, but also covered with this dark "mud." The stomach contained a greenish-black liquid; the liver was large and congested; the kidneys were swollen, congested, and ecchymosed; the cerebral membranes were gorged with blood, and the whole brain hyperæmic.

§ 881. **Ferrous Sulphate, Copperas, or Green Vitriol**, $FeSO_47H_2O$ = 152 + 126; specific gravity, anhydrous, 3.138; crystals, 1.857; composition in 100 parts, FeO, 25.92; SO_3, 28.77; H_2O, 45.32.—This salt is in beautiful, transparent, bluish-green, rhomboidal prisms. The crystals have an astringent, styptic taste, are insoluble in alcohol, but dissolve in about 1.5 times their weight of water; the commercial article nearly always responds to the tests, both for ferrous and ferric salts, containing a little persalt. The medicinal dose of this salt is usually given as from .0648 to .324 grm. (1 to 5 grains), but it has been prescribed in cases requiring it in gramme (15.4 grains) doses without injury. Sulphate of iron has many technical applications; is employed by all shoemakers, and is in common use as a disinfectant. The salt has been employed for criminal purposes in France, and in this country it is a popular abortive. In recorded cases, the symptoms, as well as the pathological appearances, have a striking resemblance to those produced by the chloride. There are usually colic, vomiting, and purging; but in one case (reported by Chevallier), in which a man gave a large dose of sulphate of iron to his wife, there was neither vomiting nor colic; the woman lost her appetite, but slowly recovered. Probably the action of ferrous sulphate, like that of the chloride, is profoundly modified by the presence or absence of food in the stomach. Anything like 28.3 grms. (an ounce) of sulphate of iron must be considered a dangerous dose, for, though recovery has taken place from this quantity, the symptoms have been of a violent kind.

§ 882. **Search for Iron Salts in the Contents of the Stomach, &c.**—Iron, being a natural component of the body, care must be taken not to confound the iron of the blood or tissues with the "iron" of a soluble salt. Orfila attempted to distinguish between the two kinds of iron by treating the contents of the stomach, the intestines, and even the tissues, with cold acetic acid, and allowing them to digest in it for many hours before filtering and testing for iron in the filtrate, and this is generally the process which has been adopted. The acid filtrate is first treated with sulphuretted hydrogen, which gives no precipitate with iron, and then with sulphide of ammonium, which precipitates iron black. The iron sulphide may be dissolved by a little hydrochloric acid and a drop of nitric acid, and farther identified by its forming Prussian blue when tested by ferrocyanide of potash, or by the bulky precipitate of oxide, when the acid liquid is alkalised by ammonia. In the case of Duf——, the experts attempted to prove the existence of foreign iron in the liver by taking 100 grms. of Duf——'s liver and 100 grms. of the liver of a non-poisoned person, and destroying each by nitro-muriatic acid, and estimating in each acid solution the ferric oxide. Duf——'s liver yielded in 100 parts .08 mgrm. of ferric oxide, the normal liver .022—nearly three times less than Duf——'s.

To obtain iron from the urine, the fluid must be evaporated down to a syrup in a platinum dish, a little nitric acid added, heated, and finally completely carbonised. The residue is dissolved in hydrochloric acid. Normal urine always contains an unweighable trace of iron; and, therefore, any quantity, such as a mgrm. of ferric oxide, obtained by careful precipitation of the hydrochloric acid solution out of 200 to 300 c.c. of urine, would be good evidence that a soluble salt of iron had been taken. The hydrochloric acid solution is first precipitated by ammonia and ammonic sulphide. The precipitate thus obtained will not be pure iron sulphide, but mixed with the earth phosphates. It should be redissolved in HCl, precipitated by sodic carbonate, then acidified by acetic acid and sodic acetate added, and the solution well boiled; the iron will then be precipitated for the most part as oxide mixed with a little phosphate of iron.

Since, as before mentioned, a great portion of the iron swallowed as a soluble salt is converted into insoluble compounds and excreted by the fæces, it is, in any case where poisoning by iron is suspected, of more importance to examine chemically the fæces and the whole length of the alimentary canal, than even the contents of the stomach. In particular, any black material lying on the mucous membrane may be sulphide of iron mixed with mucus, &c., and should be detached, dissolved in a little hydrochloric acid, and the usual tests applied.

In the criminal cases alluded to, there were iron stains on certain linen garments which acquired an importance, for, on dissolving by the aid of nitric acid, they gave the reactions of chlorine and iron. Any stains found should be cut out, steeped in water, and boiled. If no iron is dissolved the stain should then be treated with dilute nitric acid, and the liquid tested with ferrocyanide of potash, &c. It need scarcely be observed that iron-mould is so common on shirts and any fabric capable of being washed, that great care must be exercised in drawing conclusions from insoluble deposits of the oxide.

2. CHROMIUM.

§ 883. The only salts of chromium of toxicological importance are the neutral chromate of potash, the bichromate of potash, and the chromate of lead.

Neutral Chromate of Potash, CrO_3K_2O = 194.7, containing 56.7 per cent. of its weight of chromic anhydride, CrO_3.—This salt is in the form of citron-yellow rhombic crystals, easily soluble in water, but insoluble in alcohol. Its aqueous solution is precipitated yellow by lead acetate or basic acetate; the precipitate being insoluble in acetic acid. If chromate of potash in solution is tested with silver nitrate, the red chromate of silver is thrown down; the precipitate is with difficulty soluble in dilute nitric acid.

§ 884. **Potassic Bichromate**, CrO_3K_2O = 295.2, containing 68.07 per cent. of its weight of chromic anhydride, CrO_3.—This salt is in beautiful large, red, transparent, four-sided tables; it is anhydrous and fuses below redness. At a high temperature it is decomposed into green oxide of chromium and yellow chromate of potash. It is insoluble in alcohol, but readily soluble in water. The solution gives the same precipitates with silver, lead, and barium as the neutral chromate. On digesting a solution of the bichromate with sulphuric acid and alcohol, the solution becomes green from the formation of chromic oxide.

§ 885. **Neutral Lead Chromate**, $PbCrO_4$ = 323.5, composition in 100 parts, PbO, 68.94, CrO_3, 31.06.—This is technically known as "*Chrome Yellow*," and is obtained as a yellow precipitate whenever a solution of plumbic acetate is added, either to the solutions of potassic chromate or bichromate; by adding chrome yellow to fused potassic nitrate, "chrome red" is formed; it has the composition CrO_32PbO. Neutral lead chromate is insoluble in acids, but may be dissolved by potassic or sodic hydrates.

§ 886. **Use in the Arts.**—Potassic bichromate is extensively used in the arts—in dyeing, calico-printing, the manufacture of porcelain, and in photography; the neutral chromate has been employed to a small extent as a medicine, and is a common laboratory reagent; lead chromate is a valuable pigment.

§ 887. **Effects of some of the Chromium Compounds on Animal Life.**—In the chromates of potash there is a combination of two poisonous metals, so that it is not surprising that Gmelin found the chloride of chromium, $CrCl_3$, less active than the neutral chromate of potash; 1.9 grm. of the last, administered to a rabbit by the stomach, caused death within two hours, while 3 grms. of chromous chloride had no action. Subcutaneous doses of .2 to .4 grm. of neutral chromate (according to the experiments of E. Gergens[961] and Carl Posner[962]) act with great intensity on rabbits. Immediately after the injection the animals are restless, and show marked dyspnœa; death often takes place within a few hours.

Diarrhœa does not seem, as a rule, to follow when the salt is administered by subcutaneous injection to animals; but Gmelin's rabbits had considerable diarrhœa when 1.9 grm. was introduced into the stomach. The same quantity, injected beneath the skin of a dog, caused loss of appetite, and, after six days, there was a dry exanthem on the back, and the hair fell off in patches; there was, however, neither diarrhœa nor vomiting. Bichromate of potash causes (according to the researches of Pelikan)[963] symptoms similar to those produced by arsenic or corrosive sublimate; it acts as a powerful irritant of the stomach and intestinal canal, and may even cause inflammation; on its absorption a series of symptoms are produced, of which the most prominent are albuminuria, bloody urine, and emaciation. From .06 to .36 grm. (1-5½ grains) is fatal to rabbits and dogs.

§ 888. **Effects of some of the Chromium Salts on Man—Bichromate Disease.**—In manufacturing potassic bichromate, the workmen exposed to the dust have suffered from a very peculiar train of symptoms, known under the name of "bichromate disease." It was first described in England by Sir B. W. Richardson.[964] It appears that if the workmen inspire the particles chiefly through the mouth, a bitter and disagreeable taste is experienced, with an increase of saliva. This increase of the buccal secretion gets rid of most of the poison, and in that case but little ill effect is experienced; but those who keep the mouth closed and inspire by the nose, suffer from an inflammation of the septum, which gradually gets thin, and ultimately ulcerated; finally the whole of the septum is in this way destroyed. It is stated that when a workman has lost his nasal septum, he no longer suffers from nasal irritation, and has a remarkable immunity from catarrh. The Chemical Works Committee of Inquiry report (1893) that the manufacture of bichromate of potash or soda is practically in the hands of three firms at Glasgow, Rutherglen, and

[961] *Arch. f. experiment. Pathol. u. Pharmakol.*, Bd. 6, Hft. 1 and 2, § 148, 1875.

[962] Virchow's *Archiv f. path. Anat.*, Bd. 79, Hft. 2, § 333, 1880.

[963] *Beiträge zur gerichtl. Medicin, Toxikol. u. Pharmakodynamik*, Würzburg, 1858.

[964] *Brit. and For. Med. Chirurg. Review*, Oct. 1863. See also a paper by the same writer, read before the Medical Society, reported in the *Lancet*, March 11, 1882.

Falkirk, and that they visited all of them, and found "that almost all the men working where dust was prevalent, more especially between the furnaces and the dissolving tanks, had either perforation of the septum of the nose, or had lost the septum altogether." The bichromate also causes painful skin affections—eruptions akin to eczema or psoriasis; also very deep and intractable ulcerations. These the workers call "chrome holes." These cutaneous maladies start from an excoriation; so long as the skin is not broken, there seems to be little local effect, if any. The effects of the bichromate are also seen in horses employed at the factories; the salt getting into a wound or crack in the leg, produces ulceration: horses may even lose their hoofs.

§ 889. Acute poisoning by the chromates is rare. In the ten years ending 1892, in England and Wales, 4 accidental deaths are ascribed to potassic bichromate and 1 to chromic acid. Falck has, however, been able to find in medical literature 17 cases, 6 of which were suicidal, 10 accidental, and in 1 the bichromate was used as an abortive. In a case of poisoning by the chromate of potash (related by Maschka),[965] in which a woman, aged 25, took for a suicidal purpose a piece of potassic chromate, which she described as the size of a hazel-nut (it would probably be at least 6 grms. in weight), the chief symptoms were vomiting, diarrhœa, pain in the stomach, and rapid collapse; death took place fourteen hours after swallowing the poison.

In poisoning by potassic bichromate, there may be much variety in the symptoms, the more usual being those common to all irritant poisons, *i.e.*, vomiting, diarrhœa, and collapse, with cramps in the limbs and excessive thirst; and the rarer affecting more especially the nervous system, such as narcosis, paralysis of the lower limbs, and dilatation of the pupils; occasionally there is slight jaundice.

In a case recorded by Dr. Macniven,[966] a man took a lump of bichromate of potash, estimated to be over 2 drachms (7.7 grms.). The symptoms commenced in fifteen minutes, and consisted of lightness in the head, and a sensation of great heat in the body, which was followed by a cold sweat; in twenty minutes he vomited; he then suffered from great pain in the stomach, giddiness, specks before the eyes, a devouring thirst, and there was loss of power over the legs. These symptoms, again, were followed by severe rigors and great coldness of the extremities. On the patient's admission to hospital, two hours after taking the poison, it was noted that the pupils were dilated, the face pale and cold, and the pulse feeble. He complained of intense epigastric pain, and a feeling of depression; there was some stupor; the stomach was emptied by emetics and by the stomach-pump, and the patient treated with tepid emollient drinks, whilst subcutaneous doses of sulphuric ether were administered. He made a good recovery.

In a case recorded by Mr. Wilson,[967] a man, aged 64, was found dead in his bed twelve hours after he had gone to rest. During the night he was heard to snore loudly; there were no signs of vomiting or purging, and bichromate of potash was found in the stomach.[968]

§ 890. Chromate of lead has also caused death. In one case[969] the breathing of chromate of lead dust seems to have been fatal; and there is also a double poisoning recorded by Dr. Linstow,[970] of two children, aged three and a half and one and three-quarter years respectively, who ate some yellow ornaments,[971] which were used to adorn a cake, and which contained chrome yellow (chromate of lead). The younger died in two and the elder in five days. The symptoms were redness of the face, dulness, and an inclination to sleep; neither complained of pain; the younger one had a little diarrhœa, but the elder neither sickness nor purging.

§ 891. **Post-mortem Appearances.**—We possess some very exact researches[972] upon the pathological changes induced by subcutaneous injections of solutions of potassic bichromate on animals, and especially on the changes which the kidneys undergo. If the animal is killed, or dies a few hours after the injection, there are apparently no striking appearances, but a closer microscopical examination shows considerable changes. The epithelium of the tubuli contorti exhibits a yellow cloudiness, and the outline of the cells is irregular and jagged. The glomeruli are

---

965 *Prager Vierteljahrsschr. f. d. prakt. Heilk.*, Bd. 131, § 37, 1877; Schmidt's *Jahrb.* 1878, Bd. 178, § 237. See also Schuchardt in Maschka's *Handbuch*, Bd. ii. p. 3.

966 "On a Case of Poisoning with Bichromate of Potash," by Ed. O. Macniven, M.B., *Lancet*, Sept. 22, 1883.

967 *Med. Gazette*, vol. 33, 734.

968 See also cases recorded by Dr. M'Lachlan, *Glasgow Med. Journ.*, July 1881; Dr. M'Crorie, *ibid.*, May 1881; Dr. R. A. Warwick, *Lancet*, Jan. 31, 1880; and Dr. Dunbar Walker, *ibid.*, Sept. 27, 1879—a summary of all of which may be found in Dr. Macniven's paper, *loc. cit.*

969 *Ueber tödtliche Vergiftung durch Einathmen des Staubes von mit Chromsäuren Blei-Oxyde gefärbten Garne.—Vierteljahrsschr. f. ger. Med.*, 1877, Bd. xxvii. Hft. i. p. 29.

970 *Ibid.*, Bd. xx. s. 60, 1874.

971 The ornaments were imitations of bees; each contained .27 grm. gum tragacanth, .0042 grm. neutral lead chromate.

972 C. Posner, *op. cit.*

moderately injected, and their capsules contain an albuminous exudation; the canaliculi are filled with round cells imbedded in a fluid which, on heating, coagulates, and is therefore albuminous or fibrinous; probably this is the first stage of the formation of fibrinous casts.

In the case quoted of the woman who poisoned herself with potassic chromate, very striking changes were found in the stomach and intestines. The stomach contained above a litre of dark chocolate fluid of alkaline reaction; the mucous membrane, in the neighbourhood of the cardiac and pyloric extremities, was swollen and red in sharply defined patches; portions of the epithelial layer were detached, the rest of the mucous membrane was of a yellow-brown colour, and the whole intestine, from the duodenum to the sigmoid flexure, was filled with a partly bloody, partly treacly-looking fluid; the mucous membrane, throughout its entire extent, was swollen, with numerous extravasations, and in places there were losses of substance. Similar appearances to these have been found in other instances; the anomalous case recorded by Mr. Wilson (*ante*) is an exception. In this instance a pint of inky, turbid liquid, which yielded to analysis potassic bichromate, was found in the stomach; but there were no marked changes anywhere, save a slight redness of the cardiac end of the gullet. In Linstow's two cases of poisoning by lead chromate, there were found in both fatty degeneration of the liver cells, and red points or patches of redness in the stomach and intestines. In the elder boy the changes in the duodenum were very intense, the mucous membrane was swollen and easily detached, in the upper part strongly injected with blood; in one place there was a perforation, and in several places the membrane was extremely thin. In the younger boy the kidneys seem to have been normal, in the elder congested and containing pus. Although it was clear that the two children died from lead chromate, a chemical analysis gave no result.

§ 892. **Detection of the Chromates and Separation of the Salts of Chromium from the Contents of the Stomach, &c.**—If in the methodical examination of an acid liquid, which has been already filtered from any precipitate that may have been obtained by sulphuretted hydrogen, this liquid is made alkaline (the alkali only being added in slight excess), and hydrated chromic oxide is thrown down mixed, it may be with other metals of the second class, the precipitate may then be fused with nitre and potassic carbonate, and will yield potassic chromate, soluble in water, and recognised by the red precipitate which it gives with silver nitrate, the yellow with lead acetate, and the green colour produced by boiling with dilute sulphuric acid and a little alcohol or sugar. If by treating a complex liquid with ammonium hydrosulphide, sulphides of zinc, manganese, and iron are thrown down mixed with chromic oxide, the same principles apply. If a chromate is present in the contents of the stomach, and the organic fluid is treated with hydrochloric acid and potassic chlorate, chromic chloride is formed, and dissolving imparts a green colour to the liquid—this in itself will be strong evidence of the presence of a chromate, but it should be supplemented by throwing down the oxide, and transforming it in the way detailed into potassic chromate.

A general method of detecting and estimating both chromium and barium in organic matters has been worked out by L. de Koningh.[973] The substances are burnt to an ash in a platinum dish. The ash is weighed; to the ash is added four times its weight of potassium sodium carbonate and the same amount of potassium nitrate; and the whole is fused for fifteen minutes. The fused mass is boiled with water and filtered; if chromium is present, the filtrate is of a more or less pronounced yellow colour, but manganese may produce a green colour and mask the yellow; this colour is removed by boiling with a little alcohol. The liquid is concentrated down to 20 c.c., filtered into a test-tube, and a colorimetric estimation made of the chromium present by imitating the colour by a solution of potassium chromate of known strength. To prove that the colour is really due to chromium, acetic acid and lead acetate are added, when the yellow chromate of lead is at once thrown down. (If lead was in the ash, a yellow precipitate may appear on the addition of acetic acid.) To the portion of ash insoluble in water strong hydrochloric acid is added, and to the acid solution a large excess of calcium sulphate is added; this precipitates barium as sulphate free from lead sulphate, for, if the latter should be present, it does not, under the circumstances, come down, being soluble in strong hydrochloric acid.

3. THALLIUM.

§ 893. Thallium was discovered by Crookes in 1861. Its atomic weight is 204; specific gravity, 11.81 to 11.91; melting-point, 290°. It is a heavy diamagnetic metal, very similar to lead in its physical properties. The nitrate and sulphate of thallium are both soluble in water, the carbonate less so, requiring about 25 parts of water for solution, while the chloride is sparingly soluble, especially in hydrochloric acid.

§ 894. **Effects.**—All the salts of thallium are poisonous. One of the earlier experimenters on the physiological action, Paulet, found 1 grm. (15.4 grains) of thallium carbonate sufficient to kill a rabbit in a few hours; there were

[973] *Arch. Pharm.* (3), xxvii. 944.

loss of muscular power, trembling of the limbs, and death apparently from asphyxia. Lamy[974] used thallium sulphate, and found that dogs were salivated, and suffered from trembling of the limbs, followed by paralysis. The most definite results were obtained by Marmé,[975] who found that .04 to .06 grm. of a soluble thallium salt, injected subcutaneously or directly into the veins, and .5 grm. administered through the stomach of rabbits, caused death. The action is cumulative, and something like that of mercury: there are redness and swelling of the mucous membrane of the stomach, with mucous bloody discharges; hæmorrhage may also occur from the lungs. Thallium is eliminated through the urine, and is also found in the fæces; it passes into the urine from three to five minutes after injection: the elimination is slow, often taking as long as three weeks. It has been found in the milk, in the tears, in the mucous membrane of the mouth, of the trachea, in the secretion of the gastric mucous membrane, and in the pericardial fluid; and in these places, whether the poison has been introduced by subcutaneous injection, or by any other channel. It seems probable that the reason of its being detected so readily in all the secretions is the minute quantity which can be discovered by spectroscopic analysis.

§ 895. **Separation of Thallium from Organic Fluids or Tissues.**—The salts of thallium, if absorbed, would only be extracted in traces from the tissues by hydrochloric acid, so that, in any special search, the tissues are best destroyed by either sulphuric or nitric acid, or both. In the ordinary method of analysis, when an acid liquid is first treated with sulphuretted hydrogen, and then made alkaline by ammonia and ammonic sulphide, thallium would be thrown down with the manganese and iron of the blood. From the mixed sulphides, thallium may be separated by oxidising and dissolving the sulphides with nitric acid, evaporating off the excess of acid, dissolving in a very little hot water, and precipitating thallous chloride by solution of common salt. The ease, however, with which thallium may be separated from solutions of its salts by galvanism is so great as to render all other processes unnecessary: the best way, therefore, is to obtain a deposit of the metal on platinum by a current from one or more cells, and then to examine the deposit spectroscopically. Thallium gives, when heated in a Bunsen flame, a magnificent green line, the centre of which corresponds with wave length 534.9; a second green line, the centre of which coincides with W.L. 568, may also be distinguished.

4. ALUMINIUM.

§ 896. **Aluminium and its Salts.**—A strong solution of acetate of alumina has irritant properties, and has given rise to accidents. The term alum, in a chemical sense, is given to a class of bodies of the type of $AlKSO_4$. Common alum is at the present time ammonia alum, $NH_4Al(SO_4)_2 + 12H_2O$; when made anhydrous by heat it is known by the name of burnt alum, and possesses caustic properties.

§ 897. **Action of Alum Salts.**—Death or illness has hitherto only taken place from the ingestion of large doses of alum or the acetate, and the symptoms in these cases have been those of an irritant poison; we are, however, indebted to Paul Siem[976] for a research on the absorbed substance, in which the local effects as far as possible have been reduced.

Siem's research was made on frogs, cats, and dogs. For frogs he employed a double salt, consisting of sodic and aluminic lactate, to which he ascribed the formula $Al_2(C_3H_5O_3)_3(C_3H_4NaO_3)_3$, equal to 15.2 per cent. of Al_2O_3. Twenty to thirty mgrms., administered by subcutaneous injection to frogs, caused death in from ten to twenty-four hours. After the injection there was restlessness, and, ultimately, general paralysis of the central nervous system. The circulation was not affected; the heart was the last to die.

For warm-blooded animals he used the double tartrate of sodium and aluminium. Beginning with a small dose subcutaneously administered, he gradually increased it, and found, under these circumstances, that the lethal dose for rabbits was 0.3 grm. per kilo. of body weight; for dogs 0.25 grm., and for cats 0.25 to 0.28 grm.; if, however, a single dose was administered, then cats could be killed by 0.15 grm. per kilo. The symptoms commenced ten to twelve hours after the injection of a large dose, but with a medium dose the symptoms might be delayed for from three to four days, then there was loss of appetite, constipation, emaciation, languor, and a disinclination to move. Vomiting and loss of sensation to pain followed, the power of swallowing even saliva was lost, and a condition supervened similar to bulbar paralysis. However true this picture may be when large doses are given subcutaneously, it does not follow that hydrate of alumina in small doses, given by the mouth, mixed with food, produces any symptoms whatever.

Alum baking-powders, containing from 30 to 40 per cent. of alum mixed with carbonate of soda, are in

[974] *Chem. News*, 1863.

[975] *Göttinger Gelehrt. Nachrichten*, Aug. 14, No. 20.

[976] *Ueber die Wirkungen des Aluminiums u. Berylliums, Inaug. Diss.*, Dorpat, 1886; Schmidt's *Jahrbuch*, vol. ccxi. 128.

commerce, and have been for a long time, many tons being sold yearly. When water is added to such powders decomposition takes place, the result being sodic sulphate and aluminic hydrate, carbonic acid being given off. Were the hydrate, in small doses, capable of producing indigestion or disease of the central nervous system, it seems astonishing that, considering the enormous number of persons who use alum baking-powders, there should not be some definite evidence of its effect. The author and his family for months together have used alum baking-powders without any apparent injury, and there is little doubt that alumina hydrate passes out of the system mainly by the bowel, without being absorbed to any great extent. In a trial with regard to an alum baking-powder at Pontypridd (1893), the prosecution advanced the theory, and supported it by eminent scientific opinion, that aluminium hydrate was dissolved by the hydrochloric acid of the gastric juice, forming chloride of aluminium, some of which might be absorbed and enter the circulation; that which was not absorbed in the stomach passed on, and, meeting the alkaline fluids of the intestines, was again separated as aluminium hydrate, and as such absorbed.

If this does occur, still there is no direct evidence of its toxic influence in the small quantities used in baking-powder. It may be pointed out, also, that with regard to the possible lethal effect of a non-corrosive salt of alum, presuming that the lethal dose for man is the same as that for a cat, the amount of alumina to kill a 68-kilogramme man would have to be equal to 17 grms., or about 3 ozs. of ammonia alum. This important question can only be settled by careful feeding of animals carried on for a long period of time.

§ 898. **Post-mortem Appearances.**—In the few cases in which persons have been killed by large doses of alum or its salts there have been found corrosion of the mouth, throat, and stomach, and hyperæmia of the kidneys and intestine. In the animals experimented upon by Paul Siem, hyperæmia of the intestine, fatty degeneration of the liver and hyaline degeneration of the kidneys were the chief changes noted.

§ 899. **Detection of Alumina.**—In all operations for the detection of alumina, glass and porcelain vessels are to be avoided. The substances should be burned to an ash in a platinum dish, the ash treated with hydrochloric acid, the acid driven off by heat, and a few drops of nitric acid added, and dissolved in hydrochloric acid, and the solution boiled and filtered. If organs of the body are operated upon, iron and phosphoric acid will be present in the ash; this will, indeed, be the case with most organic substances. The filtered solution is boiled, and, while boiling, poured into a strong solution of sodic hydrate contained in a silver or platinum dish; the iron will now separate as oxide, and can be filtered off. To the filtrate is added a little sodic phosphate; it is then feebly acidified with hydrochloric acid, and ammonia added just sufficient to render it alkaline; a light whitish cloud of alumina phosphate, should alumina be present, is thrown down, and can be collected, thoroughly washed, dried, ignited, and weighed as alumina phosphate.[977] The alumina phosphate is then fused with sodic sulphate in a platinum dish or crucible, and the fused mass treated with hot water; the sodic phosphate dissolves, and the alumina oxide may be filtered off and dissolved in a little hydrochloric acid or sulphuric acid.

A solution thus prepared has the following properties:—

Ammonium sulphide; white precipitate of hydroxide.

Potash or soda; white precipitate, soluble in excess.

Ammonia; white precipitate, only slightly soluble in excess.

There is also a blowpipe-test: if a little of the hydroxide be collected, moistened with cobalt nitrate, and heated on charcoal by the oxidising flame, alumina, under these circumstances, becomes of a blue colour.

5. URANIUM.

§ 900. **Uranium.**—The salts of uranium are intensely poisonous. The nitrate of uranium is used in photography and the arts, and is a common reagent in chemical laboratories.

According to Kowalewsky,[978] the acetate of uranium possesses an unusual power of uniting with albumin; the other soluble uranium salts act also in a similar way. Hence concentrated solutions of uranium salts corrode the mucous membranes, transforming, for example, the walls of the stomach into a dead uranic albuminate. If a non-corrosive salt of uranium is injected subcutaneously, glycosuria is produced, with fatty degeneration of the walls of the blood-vessels, and fatty changes in the kidneys, liver, &c. The animal wastes and ultimately dies; 0.5 to 2.0 mgrms. of UO_3 per kilogrm. will kill a cat, dog, or rabbit, if injected subcutaneously. The nitrate or acetate, when given by the mouth, produces gastro-enteritis and nephritis, with hæmorrhages in the substance of the kidney. Uranium is not used in medicine.

§ 901. **Detection and Estimation of Uranium.**—Uranium forms uranous and uranic salts. Both classes of salts

[977] One part of al. phosphate is equal to 0.42 Al_2O_3, 3.733 ammonia alum, and 4.481 potash alum.

[978] *Ztschr. f. Anal. Chemie*, xxiv., 1885, p. 551.

are not precipitated by SH_2, but are precipitable by ammonium sulphide, and, therefore, in toxicological analyses are likely to be met with in conjunction with iron.

The sulphides of iron and uranium may be dissolved in strong hydrochloric acid, boiled to expel SH_2, and the solution then oxidised with a little nitric acid; the solution is now alkalised with ammonium carbonate, which precipitates the iron as oxide and leaves the uranium in solution. On now acidifying with nitric acid in slight excess, a solution of sodic phosphate will precipitate uranium phosphate as a white precipitate, alkalies will give a yellow precipitate, alkaline carbonates a yellow precipitate soluble in excess. Barium carbonate also gives a precipitate, and is useful in separations. Uranium oxide gives a green glass in the oxidising flame with borax or with sodic metaphosphate.

V.—ALKALINE EARTHS.

Barium.

§ 902. The soluble salts of barium are undoubtedly poisonous, and are of frequent occurrence in the arts. The chloride of barium is used in the staining of wool, the nitrate and the chlorate in the green fires of the pyrotechnist, the oxide and the carbonate in the manufacture of glass. The chromate is used by artists under the name of "yellow ultramarine," while the sulphate, technically known as "permanent white," is, on account of its weight and cheapness, occasionally used as an adulterant of white powders and other substances. Barium sulphide, under various names, such as Bottcher's depilatory, Thompson's hair destroyer, *Poudre épilatoire*, and other names, is in commerce, and has caused poisonous symptoms.[979]

§ 903. **Chloride of Barium**, $BaCl_22H_2O$ 208 + 36; anhydrous, Ba, 65.86 per cent., Cl, 34.14; specific gravity, 3.75, is in commerce in the form of white, four-sided, tabular crystals; water dissolves about half its weight at ordinary temperatures, three-fourths at 100°. Its solution gives a white precipitate with sulphuric acid, quite insoluble in water and nitric acid.

The salt imparts a green hue to an otherwise colourless flame; viewed by the spectroscope, green bands will be visible. We may note that chloride of barium gives two different spectra—the one at the moment of the introduction of the salt, the other when the substance has been exposed for some time to a high temperature. This is caused by a rapid loss of chlorine, so that the first spectrum is due to $BaCl_2$, with a variable mixture of BaCl, the second to BaCl alone.

§ 904. **Baric Carbonate**, $BaCO_3$ = 197; specific gravity, 4.3; BaO, 77.69 per cent., CO_2, 22.31, in its native form termed *Witherite*, is a dense, heavy powder, insoluble in pure water, but dissolving in acetic, nitric, and hydrochloric acids, the solution giving the reactions of barium.

A rat-poison may be met with composed of baric carbonate, sugar, and oatmeal, flavoured with a little oil of aniseed and caraway.

§ 905. **Sulphate of Barium**, $BaSO_4$; specific gravity, 4.59; BaO, 65.66 per cent., SO_3, 34.34 per cent., is a pure white powder when recently precipitated, absolutely insoluble in water, and practically insoluble in cold dilute acids. It is quite unalterable in the air at a red heat; on ignition with charcoal, it may be converted almost entirely into sulphide of barium; and by ignition with $CaCl_2$ into chloride.

§ 906. **Effects of the Soluble Salts of Barium on Animals.**—One of the early notices of the poisonous characters of barium compounds was by James Watt,[980] who found that *witherite*, given to dogs, produced vomiting, diarrhœa, and death in a few hours. Sir Benj. Brodie[981] administered barium chloride, and noticed its paralysing effect on the heart. Orfila[982] made several experiments, and observed that 4 grms. of the carbonate produced death in dogs in periods varying from one to five hours; but in these experiments the gullet was tied. The later investigators have been Gmelin, Onsum, Cyon, and Böhm.[983] Gmelin found barium carbonate and barium chloride act in a very

[979] Barium carbonate and sulphate are usually enumerated as occasional adulterants of bread, but there is no modern authentic instance of this.

[980] *Memoirs of the Literary and Philosophical Society of Manchester*, 1790, vol. iii. p. 609.

[981] *Phil. Trans.*, 1812.

[982] *Traité des Poisons*, 3rd ed., t. i., Paris, 1826.

[983] Gmelin, C. G., *Versuche über die Wirkungen des Baryts, Strontians, Chroms, Molybdäns, Wolframs, Tellurs, u. s. w. auf den thierischen Organismus*, Tübingen, 1824; Onsum, J., Virchow's *Archiv*, Bd. 2, 1863; Cyon, M., *Archiv f. Anatomie, Physiologie, &c.*, 1866; Böhm, *Archiv f. experiment. Pathol.*, Bd. 3, 1874.

similar manner; and, indeed, it is improbable that barium carbonate, *as* carbonate, has any action, but, when swallowed, the hydrochloric and other acids of the stomach form with it soluble compounds. J. Onsum made eight experiments with both barium carbonate and chloride on animals. The respiration was quickened and, at the same time, made weak and shallow; the heart's action was accelerated; the animals became restless: and there was great muscular prostration, with paralytic symptoms; convulsions did not occur in any one of the eight animals. He found, on *post-mortem* examination, the right side of the heart full of blood from backward engorgement; he describes a plugging of the small arteries with little fibrinous coagula, having an inorganic nucleus, with constant hæmorrhagic extravasations. Onsum seems to have held the theory that the baryta salts circulated in the blood, and then formed insoluble compounds, which were arrested in the lungs, causing minute emboli, just in the same way as if a finely-divided solid were introduced directly into the circulation by the jugular vein.

Onsum stands alone in this view. Cyon found no emboli in the lungs, and refers the toxic effect to a paralysing influence on the heart and voluntary muscles, and also on the spinal cord. Cyon, to settle the embolic theory, injected into the one jugular vein of a rabbit barium chloride, and into the other sodic sulphate, but the small arteries and capillaries of the lungs remained clear. Böhm, operating on frogs, found a great similarity between the action of small doses of barium salts and that of certain organic poisons; as, for example, cicutoxin, .012 to .02 grm. subcutaneously injected into frogs, acted as a heart-poison. So also Blake[984] found the heart slowed, and concluded that barium chloride had a direct action on the cardiac muscle, and also a toxic influence on the nervous system. F. A. Falck, in experiments on rabbits, found a great reduction of temperature after poisoning with barium chloride (3° to 12.6°).

§ 907. **Effects of the Salts of Barium on Man.**—There were about fifteen cases of poisoning by barium salts on record by the end of 1883—three of which were suicidal, but most of them were due to accident or mistake. In three cases, barium chloride was taken instead of Glauber's salts; in one, instead of Carlsbad salts; in another, a mixture of barium nitrate and sulphur, instead of pure sulphur; in a sixth case, a mixture of barium acetate and raspberry syrup, instead of sodic ethylsulphate; in a seventh, a chemist put a larger dose than was ordered by the prescription; and in four cases barium carbonate had been mixed with flour, and this flour used in the making of pastry. Of the fifteen cases, nine, or 60 per cent., proved fatal; the fifteen cases have now (1894) been increased to twenty-six.

Fatal Dose.—The recorded cases of poisoning have not satisfactorily settled the question as to the least fatal dose of the barium salts. 6.5 grms. (about 100 grains) of the chloride have destroyed the life of an adult woman in fifteen hours; 14 grms. (½ oz.) of the nitrate of baryta have killed a man in six and a half hours; and the carbonate of baryta has destroyed a person in the relatively small dose of 3.8 grms. (60 grains). On the other hand, certain Continental physicians have prescribed barium chloride in large medicinal doses; for example, Pirondi[985] and Lisfranc[986] have gradually raised the dose of barium chloride from 4 decigrams up to 3 grms. (48 grains) daily, given, of course, in divided doses. Pirondi himself took in a day 7.7 grms. (119 grains) without bad effect.

§ 908. **Symptoms.**—The local action of barium salts must be sharply distinguished from the action of the absorbed salts. Kobert divides the symptoms into seven groups:—

(1) Local, consisting in *malaise*, nausea, salivation, vomiting, and pain in the stomach. This group merges so much into the next as hardly to admit of precise separation.

(2) Excitation of the alimentary canal, both of the nervous and muscular apparatus. Hence vomiting, painful colic, and acute diarrhœa. All these phenomena may be produced in animals by subcutaneous injection, and, therefore, do not depend alone upon local action.

(3) Excitation of the brain motor centres, which leads to convulsions, or may result in paralysis. About half the recorded cases of barium poisoning in the human subject have been convulsed; the other half paralysed. In one case mania resulted.

(4) Weakness or destruction of the power of muscular contraction; this produces in frogs, when the muscular test movements are recorded graphically, a veratrin-like convulsion curve. In the human subject the effect is that of great muscular weakness.

(5) Digitalin-like influence on the heart and blood-vessels, showing itself in great slowing of the pulse, præcordial anxiety, and strong beating of the heart (not only sensible to the patient, but which can be heard and felt

[984] *Journ. of Anat. and Physiol.* 2nd series, 1874.

[985] *De la Tumeur Blanche de Genou*, éd. 2, Paris, 1836.

[986] *Gaz. Med. de Paris*, 1835, No. 14.

by the bystanders). The arteries are incompressible and rigid, the blood-pressure strikingly raised. The blood-vessels of old people do not stand the pressure, hence hæmorrhages in the lungs, stomach, and other organs. Frogs die with the heart in systole.

(6) Catarrhal affection of the conjunctiva, the mucous membrane of the respiratory tract, and the nose.

(7) Formation of insoluble baryta salts in the blood-vessels, according to Onsum. This has not been observed in man, and the fact is disputed (see *ante*).

In Dr. Tidy's case,[987] in which a man, suffering from rheumatism, but otherwise healthy, took a mixture of barium nitrate, flowers of sulphur, and potassic chlorate, instead of sulphur, the symptoms were blisters on the tongue, a burning pain in the gullet and stomach, with vomiting, diarrhœa, convulsions, aphonia, and coldness of the extremities. A case, copiously detailed by Seidel,[988] in which a pregnant woman, twenty-eight years old, took carbonate of baryta for the purpose of self-destruction, is interesting. She probably took the poison some little time before six in the evening; she vomited and had great pain in the stomach, but slept during the night without further sickness. The next morning, after drinking some coffee, the sickness was renewed; nevertheless, at 7 A.M., she repaired to her employment, which was distant an hour's walk; she probably suffered much on the way, for she did not arrive until 9 A.M. The vomiting, accompanied by diarrhœa, continuing, she was sent to bed at 2 P.M. She was very cold, and complained of great weakness; the vomiting now ceased. At 8 P.M. she shivered violently, could scarcely swallow, and the respiration was oppressed. At 11 she seemed a little improved; but at 3 A.M. she was found much worse, breathing rapidly, but fully conscious; at 4 A.M. she was again seen, but found dead; she thus lived about thirty-four hours after taking the fatal dose.

§ 909. **Distribution of Barium in the Body.**—Neumann has shown that, after repeated injection of insoluble barium sulphate into the veins of rabbits, barium is to be found in the liver, kidneys, spleen, and spinal cord, but not in the muscles, thymus, or brain. G. Linossier[989] has made a similar series of experiments, but with the more soluble carbonate, and this salt was injected into animals for a period of thirty days. All the organs contained some barium; lungs, muscles, and the heart only contained traces, the liver rather more, the kidneys, brain, and spinal cord still more, and, lastly, the bones a considerable quantity, as much as 0.056 per cent.

§ 910. **Post-mortem Appearances.**—The *post-mortem* appearances are usually changes in the stomach and intestinal tract, but there are only rarely traces of great inflammation. It is true, that in a case recorded by Wach,[990] perforation of the stomach was found; but, since there was old-standing disease of both liver and stomach, it is not clear that this is to be attributed entirely to poison. In the case of suicide just detailed, the mucous membrane of the stomach was much ecchymosed; over the whole were strewn little white grains, sticking to the mucous membrane, and there were also ecchymoses in the duodenum.

§ 911. **The Separation of Barium Salts from Organic Solids or Fluids, and their Identification.**—In the usual course of examination of an unknown substance, the matter will already have been extracted by hydrochloric acid, and the solution successively treated with hydric and ammonic sulphides. The filtrate from any precipitate, after being boiled, would in such a case give a precipitate if treated with sulphuric acid, should a salt of barium soluble in hydrochloric acid be present.

If there, however, should be *special* grounds to search for baryta in particular, it is best to extract the substances with pure boiling water, to concentrate the solution, and then add sulphuric acid, collecting any precipitate which may form. If the latter is found to be sulphate of baryta, it must be derived from some soluble salt, such as the nitrate or the chloride. The substances which have been exhausted with water are now treated with hydrochloric acid, and to the acid filtrate sulphuric acid is added. If sulphate of baryta is thrown down, the baryta present must have been a salt, insoluble in water, soluble in acids—probably the carbonate. Lastly, the organic substances may be burnt to an ash, the ash fused with carbonate of soda, the mass, when cool, dissolved in HCl, and the solution precipitated with sulphuric acid. Any baryta now obtained was present, probably in the form of sulphate; nevertheless, if obtained from the tissues, it would prove that a soluble salt had been administered, for (so far as is known) sulphate of barium is not taken up by the animal fluids, and is innocuous.

The sulphate of barium is identified as follows:—

(1) A part of the well-washed precipitate is boiled with distilled water, filtered, and to the filtrate a solution of

[987] *Pharm. Journ.*, June 1868.

[988] Eulenberg's *Vierteljahrsschrift f. ger. Med.*, Bd. 27, § 213.

[989] *Compt. rend. Soc. Biol.* (8), iv. 122-123.

[990] Henke's *Zeitschrift f. Staatsarzneik.*, 1835, Bd. 30, Hft. 1, § 1.

chloride of barium added. If there is no precipitate, the sulphate can be none other than baric sulphate, for all the rest, without exception, are soluble enough to give a slight cloud with baric chloride.

(2) The sulphate may be changed into sulphide by ignition on charcoal, the sulphide treated with HCl, the solution evaporated to dryness, and the resulting chloride examined spectroscopically; or, the sulphide may be mixed with chloride of calcium, taken up on a loop of platinum wire, heated strongly in the flame of a Bunsen burner, and the flame examined by the spectroscope.

(3) A solution of the chloride of barium obtained from (2) gives a yellow precipitate with neutral chromate of potash, insoluble in water, but soluble in nitric acid.

APPENDIX.

Treatment by Antidotes or otherwise of Cases of Poisoning.

§ 912. All medical men in practice are liable to be summoned hastily to cases of poisoning. In such emergencies not a moment is to be lost, for valuable lives have ere this been sacrificed simply from the delay caused by searching for medicines and instruments, and visiting the patient unprovided with suitable remedies. Hence it is far the safest plan for every medical man to provide himself with an "*antidote bag*," which, to be complete, should be furnished with the following requisites:—

I. Instruments:—

(1.) A **stomach-pump** or **tube**,[991] with proper mouth gags.

(2.) A **hypodermic syringe**.

(3.) An ordinary bleeding **lancet**.

(4.) A **glass-syringe** with suitable canula, which may, in case of necessity, be used for transfusion.

(5.) **Bistoury**, **forceps** and **tubes** suitable for performing **tracheotomy**.

A small **battery** (interrupted current).

II. Emetics:—

(1.) *Sulphate of zinc.*

(2.) *Apomorphine.*

(3.) *Mustard.*

(4.) *Ipecacuanha.*

The *sulphate of zinc* may either be carried in 30-grain powders or in the ordinary solid crystalline state, together with a little measure made out of a small pill-box which, when exactly full, is found to contain from 25 to 30 grains.

A still more convenient form is that of the compressed tablets, sold as a speciality by one or more firms. The same remarks apply to *ipecacuanha.*

The *apomorphine hydrochlorate* should be in solution, a suitable strength is 2 per cent.; a few drops of this substance, injected hypodermically, will cause vomiting in a few minutes.

Besides the above list, the bag should be furnished with a selection of the so-called antidotes.

III. Antidotes:—

(*a.*) *Chemicals neutralising the poison.*

Acetic acid and **calcined magnesia**.

(*b.*) *Precipitants of alkaloids.*

---

[991] The stomach-tube is simply a tube of india-rubber, from 6 to 8 feet in length, one end of which should be a little stiff, and have a solid rounded extremity pierced with two lateral oval holes—catheter-like; but, on an emergency, any india-rubber tube of a suitable length will do. It is used by passing the proper end gently down the throat into the stomach; if the patient is insensible, or, as in some determined suicides, obstinate, the jaws must be forcibly opened by the handle of a spoon, and some solid substance placed between the teeth so as to give sufficient room for the entry of the tube. If the tube is now passed in the median line well into the grasp of the pharynx, it is actually drawn down into the stomach by the pharyngeal muscles, so that the operator has, as it were, only to "pay out" a sufficient quantity of the tubing. Holding the tube in a perpendicular position, it may then be filled with water by means of a small funnel. When full, the end must be pinched and brought down to the ground to deliver in a basin; it will then act as a syphon and the contents of the stomach will be syphoned off. The tube is elevated again above the body, and the stomach filled with water; this syphoned off, and the process repeated. Coffee, also, or antidotes may be conveniently introduced. If the recumbent position is necessary, the patient must, of course, be placed on a bed or table, in order that there should be sufficient fall for the syphon.

Tannin—A solution of **iodine in potassic iodide.**

(*c.*) *Narcotics, or anæsthetics,* for the treatment of the tetanic class.

Chloral—chloroform.

(*d.*) *Substances which act physiologically.*

French oil of turpentine.—A solution of **atropine sulphate** for hypodermic use (strength .8 per cent.); hypodermic dose from 5 to 6 drops.

Solution of **nitrate of pilocarpine** (strength 5 per cent.); dose, 10 drops or more.

Muscarine—a solution in water (strength 5 per cent.); dose, 10 drops.

Morphine meconate in solution (strength 10 per cent.); dose, from 5 drops.

A solution of **nitrate of strychnine** (strength 2 per cent.); hypodermic dose, from 2 to 3 drops.

Potassium Permanganate in crystals.

To these may be added a bottle of **Wyeth's dialysed iron** for use in arsenic poisoning, a flask of **brandy**, some **chloric ether**, **aromatic spirits of ammonia**, and some really good **extract of coffee.**

TREATMENT.

§ 913. Acid Carbolic.

Use the **stomach-tube** or **pump**, unless there is great destruction of the mucous membrane. In the latter case, excite vomiting by injecting subcutaneously from 5 to 6 drops of the **apomorphine** solution; or give an emetic of **zinc sulphate**, **ipecacuanha**, or **mustard**.

The stomach may, by the aid of the tube, be washed out with a weak alkaline solution of **soda**; **albumen** may also be given, and such stimulants as **brandy** and **water**, **chloric ether**, and **aromatic spirits of ammonia**.

It is important to apply warmth to the extremities.

Inject subcutaneously from 2 to 3 drops of the **atropine hypodermic** solution.

Nitrite of amyl by inhalation is said to have been useful.

In desperate cases **bleeding**, followed by **transfusion**, is to be considered.

Acids—Mineral, including Sulphuric, Nitric, Hydrochloric, Glacial Acetic Acids.

Stomach-tube or **pump**, inadmissible.

Neutralise by calcined **magnesia**, **lime**, **chalk**, or **soda,** but not with potash, if there is choice.

If no neutralising agent can be immediately procured, then dilute with plenty of water.

Other remedies are—**oil**, **milk**, **white of eggs**, **gruel**.

It is often recommended in such cases to administer hypodermically a little **morphine**.

Aconite—Aconitine.

Use at once the **stomach-tube** or **pump**, or give emetics of **sulphate of zinc**, or hypodermic solution of **apomorphine**.

Keep the patient in the recumbent posture.

After the stomach has been emptied, give **atropine**, either by hypodermic injection or by the mouth, say 4 drops of the P.B. solution; failing atropine, 20 drops of the tincture of **belladonna**. The dose may be repeated more or less frequently according to the condition of the patient.

If there is great tendency to heart-syncope, tincture of **digitalis** in ½-drachm doses by the mouth, or in hypodermic doses of from 10 drops upwards.

Apply a mustard poultice to the pericardium; aid vomiting and elimination of the poison by plenty of water, to which may be added brandy or any form of alcohol.

Inhalations of **nitrite of amyl** are said to have been useful. If the breathing stops, try **artificial respiration**.

Alcohol.

Empty the stomach by the **tube** or **pump**, and then wash it out with warm coffee; if the stomach-tube is not at hand, then empty the stomach by hypodermic injection of 5 drops of **apomorphine**, or by a **mustard** emetic, or **sulphate of zinc**. Keep the body very warm, but the cold **douche** may be applied to the head.

Endeavours should be made to rouse the patient, if insensible, by shaking, shouting at him, &c.

Inhalations of **amyl nitrite** are said to be useful.

Alkalies—Ammonia—Potash—Soda.—**Stomach-pump** or **tube** not to be used.

Vomiting nearly always present, or may be produced by administering plenty of lukewarm water; after which give **dilute vinegar**, or the juice of **lemons** or **oranges**; **olive oil**, the **white of eggs**, **barley water**, **arrowroot**, and always plenty of **water** may be administered.

There may be œdema of the glottis, especially if ammonia has been taken. In such a case, and death threatening from suffocation, perform **tracheotomy**. In poisoning by ammonia, with croupous respiration, keep the room warm, and fill it with steam by means of a bronchitis kettle.

Relieve pain by small doses of **morphine** injected subcutaneously.

Ammonia.—See Alkalies.

Antiarin.—See Digitalis.

Antimony—Tartar-Emetic—Antimonial Wine, &c.

The stomach will generally have been emptied by vomiting. In those rare cases in which this does not take place, use the **stomach-pump** or **tube**, or give hypodermic injection of **apomorphine**.

Follow this with doses of **strong tea**, or give half-a-drachm of **tannin** or **gallic acid** in warm water.

Give also demulcent drinks, and stimulants in small doses, frequently repeated.

Keep the patient very warm by hot blankets and wraps.

The interrupted galvanic current to the heart may be useful.

Apocynin.—See Digitalis.

Arsenic.

Use the **stomach-pump** or **tube**, or empty stomach by emetics, such as hypodermic solution of **apomorphine**, or give **mustard** or **sulphate of zinc**. The stomach should then be washed out by large quantities of water, most conveniently administered by the pump or tube.

If the tube or pump is not at hand, then administer at once either **dialysed iron**, or the freshly-precipitated **hydrated oxide of iron**, obtained by precipitating the ordinary perchloride by means of carbonate of soda or ammonia, avoiding excess of the latter. If the operator has sufficient chemical knowledge to precipitate the iron with fair exactness, so that there is no great excess of ammonia, or of sodic carbonate, then filtration is unnecessary. In other cases, filter through a handkerchief.

Oil, **mucilaginous drinks**, the **white of eggs**, and, if faintness exists, small doses of **stimulants** may all be given.

If the skin is cold, warmth must be applied to the body by means of hot blankets, &c.

Pain may be relieved by **morphine**.

Atropine—Belladonna—Tincture of Belladonna.

Empty the stomach by means of the **stomach-pump** or **tube**.

Give an enema of **coffee**.

Administer half a grain of **pilocarpine nitrate**; or, if that is not at hand, **morphine** or **opium** in suitable doses will act to a certain extent antagonistic to the poison.

A subcutaneous dose of **muscarine** may be administered instead of pilocarpine, but is not quite so good.

Hot water to the feet, alternate **douches** of cold and hot water are found useful.

If the respiration seems likely to stop, **artificial respiration** must be practised.

Belladonna.—See Atropine.

Benzene.

If swallowed, then empty the stomach by **pump** or **tube**, or by the hypodermic injection of **apomorphine**; or give emetics, such as **zinc sulphate**, **mustard**, or **ipecacuanha**.

If the vapour has been *inhaled*, this is unnecessary.

Plenty of **fresh air**.

A subcutaneous dose of **atropine**, say 1-60th of a grain, or from 30 to 40 drops of **belladonna** tincture.

Alternate **douches** of hot and cold water to the chest, **artificial respiration**, if necessary. The heart to be maintained by mild interrupted shocks of the **battery** over the region of the heart.

Bichromate of Potash.—See Chromium.

Brucine.—See Strychnine.

Calabar Bean—Physostigmine.

Use **stomach-pump** or **tube**, or emetics, such as **sulphate of zinc**, **mustard**, or **ipecacuanha**; or, better still, hypodermic solution of **apomorphine**.

Give hypodermic doses of 1-60th grain **atropine** until the pupils dilate. This treatment seeming to fail, **chloral** in 10-grain doses, every quarter of an hour, has been recommended.

In certain cases **strychnine** has been used in hypodermic doses of 1-12th of a grain.

Stimulants and **artificial respiration** will probably be necessary in some cases.

Camphor.

Use **stomach-pump** or **tube**, or empty the stomach by emetics.

Hypodermic injections of **brandy**, inhalations of **ether**, the alternate hot and cold **douche**, warmth to the extremities by hot blankets, &c., seem to be the best methods of treatment.

Cantharides—Cantharidine.

Use **stomach-pump** or **tube**, if the mucous membrane of the throat is not inflamed; or, administer hypodermic dose of **apomorphine**, or give emetics—**sulphate of zinc, mustard,** or **ipecacuanha**.

Allay pain with **morphine**. Give plenty of water and **demulcent drinks**.

Chloral.

Use **stomach-pump** or **tube**, and, when the stomach is emptied, introduce by the same means **warm coffee**, or give a hypodermic injection of **apomorphine**, or administer emetics of **sulphate of zinc**, or **mustard**, or **ipecacuanha.**

An **enema of coffee** will be useful.

Keep the limbs warm.

Administer hypodermically 2 or 3 drops of the solution of **strychnine** at intervals of from fifteen to twenty minutes.

Rouse the patient by various means, such as shouting, shaking, flapping the skin with a wet towel, &c.

Inhalations of **amyl nitrite** are recommended.

Artificial respiration may be necessary.

Chlorate of Potash.

Use the same treatment as for **nitrate of potash**.

Chloride of Zinc.—See Zinc.

Chloroform—(*Inhaled*).

Give plenty of **fresh air**, pull the tongue forward, and commence at once **artificial respiration**. If the heart has stopped, strike the chest two or three times very hard, over the region of the heart; this has been found occasionally to restore its beat. Apply the **battery**, but with a weak current only; one pole may be placed on the larynx, the other at the pit of the stomach.

Inhalations of **nitrite of amyl** are useful. The hot and cold **douche** may also be used.

Chloroform—(*Swallowed*).

Empty the stomach by **pump** or **tube**, or by emetics, such as 5 drops of the hypodermic solution of **apomorphine**, or **sulphate of zinc**, or **mustard**.

Give an enema of **hot coffee**.

Administer large draughts of **water**, which may advantageously contain a little **sodic carbonate** in solution.

Attempt to rouse the patient. **Nitrite of amyl** inhalations, and, if necessary, **artificial respiration** may be used.

Chromate of Potash.—See Chromium.

Chromic Acid.—See Chromium.

Chromium—Bichromate of Potash—Chromate of Potash—Chromic Acid.

Empty the stomach by **pump** or **tube**; administer a subcutaneous injection of **apomorphine**, or give **sulphate of zinc**, **mustard**, or **ipecacuanha** as emetics. Follow up by administering, suspended in water, calcined magnesia, or carbonate of magnesia, or chalk.

Demulcent drinks, such as **barley-water**, &c.

Cocculus Indicus.—See Picrotoxin.

Colchicum—Meadow Saffron—Colchicum Wine, Tincture, &c.

Use **stomach-pump** or **tube**, or empty the stomach by emetics, such as **sulphate of zinc**, or **mustard**, or **ipecacuanha**; or, better than all, give a hypodermic injection of 4 or 5 drops of the solution of **apomorphine**.

Give **tannin** or **gallic acid** in ½-drachm doses, or strong tea or coffee.

Allay the pain in the bowels and purging by small doses of **opium** or **morphine**.

Keep the extremities warm, apply hot fomentations to the abdomen; **stimulants** may be used, give plenty of **water** and **demulcent drinks**.

Colocynth.

Treatment on the same lines as that for Colchicum.

Conium—Hemlock.

Empty the **stomach** by the **pump** or **tube**, or give a hypodermic injection of 4 or 5 drops of the solution of

apomorphine, or emetics of **sulphate of zinc**, or **mustard**.
Keep up the temperature of the body by hot wraps.
Administer, as a drink, strong **tea**, **tannin**, **gallic acids**, or any harmless vegetable decoction containing tannin.
Stimulants may be administered.
If necessary, use **artificial respiration**.
Copper—Salts of.
Empty stomach by **pump** or **tube**, and either inject by the same means or administer **white of egg** in solution in water; if no white of eggs can be had, substitute milk; give plenty of **water** and **emollient drinks**.
Pain may be allayed by **opium** or **morphine**.
Corrosive Sublimate—Perchloride of Mercury—Nitrate of Mercury.
Empty the stomach by the **tube** or **pump**, and wash the organ out with plenty of white of egg, dissolved in water or milk. If the stomach-pump is not at hand, then give emetics, such as the solution of **apomorphine**, hypodermically, in from 4 to 5-drop doses, or a **zinc sulphate** emetic, or **mustard**, or **ipecacuanha**. Probably violent vomiting is already present, then stomach-tube or emetics are unnecessary: but, in any case, give plenty of albuminous fluids, such as **white of egg** in water or **milk**. If neither of these is at hand, chop any **fresh meat** up as finely as can be done in a short space of time, diffuse in water, and administer. Follow up with **demulcent drinks**, such as **barley-water**, **flour** and **water**, &c.
Pain may be allayed with a little **opium** or **morphine**.
Stimulants are admissible, if necessary.
Croton Oil.
Empty stomach by means of **tube** or **pump**, or give emetics of **mustard** or **sulphate of zinc**, or administer hypodermic injection of apomorphine.
Give 10 drops of **laudanum** every twenty minutes or half hour, until the pain and purging are somewhat abated, or else inject subcutaneously small doses of **morphine** at intervals.
Give plenty of **demulcent drinks**.
Two or three drops of **essence of camphor** in milk are useful.
Stimulants, such as **brandy**, **ammonia**, or **chloric ether**, are admissible.
Cytisine.—See Laburnum.
Curarine—Woorari—Urari.
The poison is of course introduced by a wound; if any is likely to be still in the wound apply a **ligature**, **suck the wound**, and then wash it with a slightly alkaline solution of **potassic permanganate**.
Keep up the **respiration artificially**, give plenty of **water** and a dose of spirits of nitre, apply warmth to the loins. By these means the poison will be rapidly separated by the urine; and, if the patient can only be kept alive by artificial respiration for a little time, he may recover, for elimination is very rapid.
Cyanide of Potassium.—See Prussic Acid.
Digitalis Group of Heart Poisons, *including*, besides the Digitalins, Antiarin, Apocynin, Neriin, Oleandrin, Evonymin, Thevetin, Scillain, Strophantin, and Erythrophlein.
Empty the stomach by the **tube** or **pump**, or administer a subcutaneous dose (4 drops) of **apomorphine**, or give a tablespoonful of **mustard** in water, or **sulphate of zinc**.
Follow up with strong **tea**, or half a drachm of **tannin**, or **gallic acid** in aqueous solution.
A very small dose of **aconitine nitrate** in solution (say 1-200th of a grain) may be injected subcutaneously and the effect watched; if in a little time it seems to do good, repeat the dose. On no account let the patient rise from the recumbent posture, or he may faint to death.
Stimulants in small doses may be given frequently by the mouth, or, if there is vomiting, by the bowel.
Ergot.
Use **stomach-pump** or **tube**, or empty the stomach by a **mustard** or **sulphate of zinc emetic**, or give a subcutaneous injection of **apomorphine**.
Give a purgative, such as a drop of **croton oil**, and assist its action by plenty of warm drinks.
Tannin and **gallic acid** have also been recommended, but are probably of but little use.
After the bowels have well acted, and the stomach has been emptied, give small doses of **opium** at intervals.
Dr. Murrell recommends 1-50th of a grain of **nitro-glycerin** every fifteen minutes.
The recumbent position is necessary, and the circulation should be maintained by warmth, and, if necessary, by friction.

Erythrophlein.—See Digitalis.
Ether.—The same treatment as with Chloroform.
Evonymin.—See Digitalis.
Fungi.—See Mushrooms.
Gelseminine.
If seen soon after taking the dose, use the **stomach-pump** or **tube**, or give a tablespoonful of **mustard**.
Administer a small dose of **atropine** subcutaneously, or give by the mouth tincture of belladonna in 20-drop doses.
Stimulants are admissible.
If necessary, use **artificial respiration**.
Rouse the patient by hot and cold **douches**.
Hemlock.—See Coniine—Conium.
Henbane—Hyoscyamine.—The same treatment as for Atropine.
Hydrochloric Acid.—See Acids, Mineral.
Hydrocyanic Acid.—See Prussic Acid.
Hyoscyamine.—The same treatment as for Atropine.
Iodine.
Empty the stomach by **pump** or **tube**, or administer emetics, such as the hypodermic solution of **apomorphine**, or give by the mouth **mustard** or **sulphate of zinc**.
Give plenty of **starch** diffused in warm water, or in the form of a dilute paste; or give any **farinaceous substance** whatever, such as **arrowroot**, **boiled rice**, or **flour**, or thin **gruel**.
Inhalations of **amyl nitrite** have been recommended.
Pain may be relieved by **morphine** or **opium**.
Jaborandi.—Treatment the same as Pilocarpine.
Laburnum Seeds—Cytisine.
Empty stomach by **tube** or **pump**, and wash it out with **tea** or **coffee**, or give (as an emetic) a hypodermic dose of **apomorphine**, or (by the mouth) **mustard** or **zinc sulphate**; follow up this treatment by an enema, or a brisk **purgative**.
Stimulants may be administered, the patient may be roused by the hot or cold **douche**.
Laudanum.—See Morphine.
Laurel Water.—See Prussic Acid.
Lead—Salts of.
Empty stomach by **pump** or **tube**, or administer subcutaneously a dose of **apomorphine**, 4 to 5 drops; or give by the mouth a **sulphate of zinc** or **mustard** emetic. Follow up with half a drachm of **dilute sulphuric acid**, or half an ounce of **magnesic** or **sodic sulphate**.
Milk and **albuminous fluids** may be given.
Allay pain with **opium** or **morphine**. Treat colic with hot fomentations.
Meadow Saffron.—See Colchicum.
Mercury, Salts of.—See Corrosive Sublimate.
Monkshood.--See Aconite.
Morphine—Opium—*Laudanum and preparations in which the Opium Alkaloids predominate.*
If taken by the mouth, give at once a solution of potassium permanganate and then empty the stomach, but, if taken by hypodermic injection, both these would be useless. The stomach in opium-poisoning is best relieved by the **pump** or **tube,** and should then be well washed out with hot **coffee**, leaving in the organ a pint or more. If the stomach-pump or tube is not at hand, a large subcutaneous dose of **apomorphine** (say 10 minims) may be given, or **mustard** or **zinc sulphate**, but there may be difficulty in obtaining vomiting from any emetic.
Attempt to rouse the patient by the **battery**, if at hand; by flips with a towel, and by shaking. In all books will be found the usual direction that you are to keep walking the patient about; but this treatment is questionable, and likely to favour the toxic action of morphine on the heart.
Ammonia may be applied to the nostrils.
Hot **coffee** may also be introduced into the bowels by an **enema** apparatus, or by a simple tube.
The alternate **cold and hot douche** to the head is good, but the body should be kept warm with hot wraps.

Small subcutaneous doses of **atropine** (say 1-20th of a grain) may be administered, repeating the close every twenty minutes, and watching the effect.

If necessary, apply **artificial respiration**.

Inhalations of **nitrite of amyl** have been used.

Muscarine.—See Mushrooms.

Mushrooms—Muscarine—Poisonous Fungi Generally.

Empty stomach by **stomach-pump** or **tube**, or give a subcutaneous dose of **apomorphine**, or administer by the mouth either **mustard** or **zinc sulphate**.

Inject as soon as possible a subcutaneous dose of 2 to 4 drops of the solution of atropine; or, after the stomach has been emptied, give **tincture of belladonna** every half hour, in from 20 to 30-min. doses.

It is equally important to remove the remains of the fungi from the intestines, and for this purpose it is well to give a dose of **castor oil**, and to use an enema.

Stimulants may be given. The body should be kept warm.

Neriin.—See Digitalis.

Nicotine—Tobacco.

Unless the stomach has been already emptied by vomiting, use **stomach-pump** or **tube**, or give an emetic of **mustard** and plenty of water.

Inject subcutaneously a small dose of **strychnine** (say 1-25th of a grain of the nitrate), or give half a drachm of tincture of **nux vomica**.

Stimulants, such as **brandy**, **chloric ether**, &c., may be given.

Keep the body warm, but the **cold douche** may be applied to the head.

Tannin and vegetable infusions containing **tannin** may also be given, but it is questionable if they are of much use, unless any remnants remain in the stomach.

Keep the patient lying down for fear of fatal syncope.

Nitre—Nitrate of Potash.

Empty the stomach immediately by the **pump** or **tube**, or give a subcutaneous dose of **apomorphine** (from 2 to 3 drops), or administer by the mouth a tablespoonful of **mustard**, or a scruple of **sulphate of zinc**.

Dilute the poison, and attempt to wash it out of the system by giving plenty of **water** or **mucilaginous drinks**.

Apply hot fomentations to the loins, and keep the patient as warm as possible.

Stimulants that are likely to increase the kidney congestion are to be avoided.

Inhalations of **nitrite of amyl** have been recommended.

Nitric Acid.—See Acids, Mineral.

Nitro-Benzene.

Empty the stomach at once by the **stomach-pump** or **tube**, and wash the organ out with plenty of warm water, to which advantageously a little spirit may be added; or give emetics, such as **zinc sulphate** or **mustard**.

Administer stimulants, either by the stomach-tube, as an enema, or by subcutaneous injection.

Keep up the respiration artificially, if necessary, and maintain the heart's action by application of weak, interrupted shocks to the chest-wall, by means of the **battery**.

Rouse the patient by the **douche**.

Atropine subcutaneously has been recommended.

Nitrous Oxide Gas.

The treatment is the same essentially as for chloroform (*which see*).

Inhalations of **oxygen** may do good, but oxygen is very rarely at hand.

Nux Vomica.—See Strychnine.

Oleandrin.—See Digitalis.

Opium.—See Morphine.

Oxalic Acid—Binoxalate of Potash—Sodic Oxalate.

Unless the patient has already vomited freely, empty the stomach at once by emetics of **zinc sulphate** or **mustard**; or the **stomach-pump** or **tube** may, in most cases, be used. If the acid has been taken, neutralise by **chalk**, **lime water**, or, better, by **saccharated lime water**; but on **no** account neutralise by carbonate of soda or any alkali, for the alkaline oxalates are extremely poisonous.

Assist elimination by the kidneys by giving plenty of water; apply hot fomentations to the loins.

An enema may be given, if necessary, to empty the bowels well.

Phosphorus.

Empty the stomach by **tube** or **pump**, and, at the same time, wash the organ out with water to which has been added a drachm of **French turpentine**, or give emetics. The best emetic for phosphorus is said to be **sulphate of copper**, 4 or 5 grains dissolved in water, and given every ten minutes until vomiting is produced.

In default of sulphate of copper, then **sulphate of zinc** or **mustard**.

Give ½-drachm doses of **turpentine**, floating on water or on mucilage, every half hour. Inhalations of turpentine vapour, much diluted, are also of service. The American and German turpentines are said to be of no avail. Probably the turpentine will freely purge the patient; but, if not, the bowels should be opened by a suitable purgative, such, for instance, as **magnesic sulphate**.

Physostigmine.—See Calabar Bean.

Picrotoxin—Cocculus Indicus.

Use **stomach-pump** or **tube**, or empty stomach by usual emetics, *e.g.*, **mustard**, **zinc sulphate**, or **apomorphine**, subcutaneously.

Chloral, in doses of from 10 to 20 grains, may be given every half hour to allay or prevent tetanus, the effects being, of course, watched. For the same purpose **bromide of potassium** has been recommended. In severe cases, it may be combined with choral, 1 drachm of the bromide with 20 grains of chloral.

Pilocarpine.

The best treatment is a subcutaneous dose of **atropine** (say 1-60th of a grain) or tincture of **belladonna** by the mouth in 20-minim doses, to be repeated every twenty minutes until the pupils dilate.

Potash.—See Alkalies

Prussic Acid.[992]

Use **stomach-pump** or **tube**, or, if not at hand, an emetic of **mustard** or **sulphate of zinc**.

If the breathing has stopped, try **artificial respiration** and weak shocks to the heart.

1-60th of a grain of **atropine** subcutaneously is recommended to assist the heart's action.

A **brandy enema** may be given, or brandy injected under the skin.

The body must be kept warm, but the cold **douche** may be advantageously applied to the head.

Salts of Sorrel.—See Oxalic Acid.

Savin.

If the patient has not already emptied the stomach by repeated vomiting, and the throat is not inflamed, use the **stomach-pump** or **tube**, and wash the organ out with water, or give any one of the usual emetics—such as **mustard**, **sulphate of zinc**, or **ipecacuanha**.

If the bowels have not acted well, give a dose of **castor oil**; allay pain with small doses of morphine.

Scillain.—See Digitalis.

Snakes, Bite of.

Suck the wound, and apply an alkaline solution of **permanganate of potash**.

In severe cases of cobra poisoning and other extremely venomous snakes, death threatening, the only likely means of saving life would be bleeding at one arm and **transfusing** blood by the other.

Ammonia may be given by the mouth, and also smelt.

In cobra poisoning and venoms which kill mainly through the respiration, the breathing must be kept up artificially; and, should there be signs of the heart failing, weak, interrupted **galvanic** shocks may be applied to the walls of the chest.

Lacerda's plan of injecting permanganate of potash under the skin is not alone useless but mischievous, for it takes up time which might be more valuably employed.

---

[992] J. Kossa, considering that potassium permanganate ought, theoretically, to act as a chemical antidote to potassium cyanide, by checking the paralysis of the respiratory centres, has performed some experiments. Rabbits were shown to be fatally affected in a few minutes by 0.01 grm. of the poison, but if, at the time of administration, 0.5 grm. of permanganate dissolved in 50 c.c. of water was also introduced into the stomach, doses of cyanide up to 0.1 grm. failed to cause death. Larger quantities (0.2 grm.) proved fatal under similar conditions, but the action of the poison was much delayed. Successful experiments were also performed with aqueous solutions of hydrocyanic acid containing 0.1 per cent. It is suggested, therefore, that, in cases of cyanide poisoning, ½ to ⅓ litre of a 3 to 5 per cent. solution of permanganate should be administered immediately (*Vratch*, through *Nouv. rem.*, ix. 567).

Soda Caustic.—See Alkalies.

Solanine—Solanum Dulcamara—Bitter Sweet—Woody Nightshade.—The same treatment as for Atropine (*which see*).

Stramonium.—The same treatment as for Atropine.

Strophantin.—See Digitalis.

Strychnine—Brucine—Nux Vomica.

Empty the stomach as quickly as possible by an emetic of **mustard**, or **zinc sulphate**, or by a hypodermic solution of **apomorphine** (4 drops).

The **stomach-pump** or **tube** inadmissible; for, if tetanus is present, it cannot be applied; or, if absent, it is likely to excite a spasm.

Place patient at once under **chloroform** or **ether**, and keep up a gentle narcosis for several hours, if necessary.

Darken the room, stifle all noise; if in a town, and opportunity permit, have straw or peat placed at once before the house to deaden noise.

If the spasms threaten the respiration, **artificial respiration** is absolutely necessary; and, to facilitate this, it would be justifiable, in a dangerous case, to perform **tracheotomy**, of course under chloroform.

Chloral may be given in place of chloroform, but the latter is best; the dose of **chloral** should be, at least, half a drachm, and if no effect is produced in half an hour, then doses of 20 grains should be given at intervals of a quarter of an hour.

If neither chloroform nor chloral is at hand, the juice from a recently-smoked pipe may be diffused in a little water and a few drops injected subcutaneously, and the effect watched. If there is a marked improvement the treatment may be persevered in.

Bromide of potassium in combination with chloral has been recommended.

Nitrite of amyl inhalations are said to be of use.

Curarine in a subcutaneous dose of one-third of a grain is antagonistic so far that it paralyses the voluntary muscles.

Sulphuric Acid.—See Acids, Mineral.

Tartar Emetic.—See Antimony.

Tartaric Acid.—The same treatment as for Oxalic Acid (*which see*).

Thevetin.—See Digitalis.

Tobacco.—See Nicotine.

Turpentine.

Empty stomach by **tube** or **pump**, or administer the usual emetics, such as **mustard**, or **sulphate of zinc**, or **ipecacuanha**, or give hypodermically 3 or 4 drops of the solution of apomorphine.

If purging is not already present, empty the bowel by enema; give plenty of water and demulcent drinks to aid elimination by kidneys.

Apply hot fomentations to the loins.

Allay pain with **opium** or **morphine.**

Veratrine.

Empty the stomach by the **tube** or **pump**, or give any one of the usual emetics—such as **mustard**, or **zinc sulphate**, or **ipecacuanha**.

Keep the patient lying down.

Stimulants may be administered.

An enema of **hot coffee** has been recommended.

Keep the body warm with wraps, hot blankets, &c.

White Precipitate.—The same treatment as for Corrosive Sublimate.

Wasps, Bees, Hornets—Sting of.

An **onion** immediately applied to the part stung is a favourite popular remedy; but **ammonia** is better.

Extract the sting, if it remains in the wound.

Give **stimulants**, if necessary.

Zinc.

The only salt likely to cause poisonous symptoms is the chloride, which is used in the arts, and is the active principle of Burnett's disinfecting fluid.

Stomach-pump or **tube** inadmissible. Give plenty of **water**, in which **carbonate of soda** is dissolved; or, if that is not at hand, **carbonate of potash**.

Eggs and **milk** should also be given.

Solutions of **tannin**, strong **tea**, and the like, also, to some extent, neutralise the poison.

The pain in the abdomen is to be allayed in the usual way—by hot fomentations and small frequent doses of **morphine** or **opium**.

DOMESTIC READY REMEDIES FOR POISONING.

§ 914. Large households, more especially those in which no one possesses any special medical knowledge, would do well to furnish an ANTIDOTE CUPBOARD, for use in cases of emergency. This cupboard may contain:—

(1.) *The Multiple Antidote*, which consists of saturated solution of sulphate of iron 100 parts, water 800, magnesia 88, animal charcoal 44 parts. It is best to have the animal charcoal and magnesia mixed together in the dry state and kept in a well-corked bottle; when required for use, the saturated solution of sulphate of iron is mixed with eight times its bulk of water, and the mixture of charcoal and magnesia added with constant stirring. The multiple antidote may be given in wine-glassful doses, frequently repeated, in poisoning by arsenic, zinc, opium, digitalis, mercury, or strychnine; it is of no use in phosphorus poisoning, or in poisoning by the caustic alkalies or antimony.

(2.) *Calcined Magnesia*, for use in poisoning by acids.

(3.) *French Turpentine*, for poisoning by phosphorus.

(4.) Powdered ipecacuanha in a well-corked bottle; the bottle containing a small pill-box which is cut down, so that when full it contains 30 grains—the proper dose as an emetic. A similar small supply of sulphate of zinc may also be provided.

(5.) A tin of mustard.

(6.) A bottle of vinegar.

If, then, provided with such a supply, any member is known to have taken poison, and yet the precise poison is not known, give a **sulphate of zinc** or **ipecacuanha emetic**, and follow it up by the **multiple antidote**, which is in itself not poisonous.

If Phosphorus has been taken, then give the **French turpentine** as directed under Phosphorus.

If Acids, neutralise by the **calcined magnesia** (see Acids, mineral).

If Alkalies, neutralise with **vinegar** (see Alkalies).

INDEX.

A

B

D

E

U

V

W

X

Y

www.ingramcontent.com/pod-product-compliance
Lightning Source LLC
LaVergne TN
LVHW060018210926
848481LV00013B/3733